COMPLEMENTARY and ALTERNATIVE MEDICINE

An evidence-based approach

JOHN W. SPENCER, PHD
University of Maryland University College,
School of Undergraduate Studies,
Adelphi, Maryland

JOSEPH J. JACOBS, MD, MBA
Medical Director,
Office of Vermont Health Access,
Waterbury, Vermont;
Former Director,
Office of Alternative Medicine,
National Institutes of Health,
Bethesda, Maryland

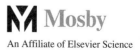

Mosby
An Affiliate of Elsevier Science

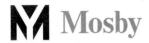 Mosby

An Affiliate of Elsevier Science

11830 Westline Industrial Drive
St. Louis, Missouri 63146

NOTICE

Complementary and alternative medicine is an ever-changing field. Standard safety precautions must be followed, but as new research and clinical experience broaden our knowledge, changes in treatment and drug therapy may become necessary or appropriate. Readers are advised to check the most current product information provided by the manufacturer of each drug to be administered to verify the recommended dose, the method and duration of administration, and contraindications. It is the responsibility of the licensed prescriber, relying on experience and knowledge of the patient, to determine dosages and the best treatment for each individual patient. Neither the publisher nor the author assumes any liability for any injury and/or damage to persons or property arising from this publication.

Previous edition copyrighted 1999

International Standard Book Number 0-323-02028-3

Publishing Director: Linda Duncan
Publishing Manager: Inta Ozols
Publishing Services Manager: Pat Joiner
Associate Developmental Editor: Melissa Kuster Deutsch
Project Manager: Gena Magouirk
Designer: Mark A. Oberkrom
Cover Art: Harry Sieplinga

Printed in U.S.A.

Last digit is the print number: 9   8   7   6   5   4   3   2   1

Contributors

Andrew Baron
Student,
Temple University,
Philadelphia, Pennsylvania

David A. Baron, MSEd, DO
Professor and Chair,
Department of Psychiatry and
    Behavioral Science,
Temple University School of
    Medicine,
Philadelphia, Pennsylvania

Iris R. Bell, MD, PhD
Director of Research,
Complementary Medicine Program,
University of Arizona School of
    Medicine,
Tucson, Arizona

Kathleen M. Boozang, JD, LLM
Associate Dean and Professor of Law,
School of Law,
Seton Hall University,
Newark, New Jersey

Tacey Ann Boucher, PhD
Project Coordinator,
Center for Addiction and Alternative
    Medicine Research,
Minneapolis Medical Research
    Foundation,
Minneapolis, Minnesota

Cheryl Bourguignon, RN, PhD
Assistant Professor and Postdoctoral
    Fellow,
Center for the Study of Complementary
    and Alternative Therapies,
University of Virginia,
Charlottesville, Virginia

Milton L. Bullock, MD
Director,
Division of Addiction and Alternative
    Medicine,
Department of Medicine,
Hennepin County Medical Center,
Minneapolis, Minnesota

Opher Caspi, MD
Faculty,
Complementary Medicine Program,
University of Arizona School of
    Medicine,
Tucson, Arizona

Chung-Kwang Chou, PhD
Chief EME Scientist and Director,
Corporate EME Research Laboratory,
Motorola Florida Research Laboratories,
Plantation, Florida

Ann C. Cotter, MD
Medical Consultant,
Center for Research in Complementary
    and Alternative Medicine,

Kessler Medical Rehabilitation Research
    and Education Corporation,
West Orange, New Jersey

Patricia D. Culliton, MA, Dipl Ac
Director,
Alternative Medicine Clinic,
Department of Medicine,
Hennepin County Medical Center,
Minneapolis, Minnesota

Karen D'Huyvetter, ND
Postdoctoral Fellow,
Center for the Study of Complementary
    and Alternative Therapies,
University of Virginia,
Charlottesville, Virginia

Ellen M. DiNucci, MA
Project Coordinator,
Complementary and Alternative
    Medicine Program,
School of Medicine,
Stanford University,
Palo Alto, California

Daniel I. Galper, PhD
Postdoctoral Fellow,
Center for the Study of Complementary
    and Alternative Therapies,
University of Virginia,
Charlottesville, Virginia

William L. Haskell, PhD
Director,
Complementary and Alternative
    Medicine Program;
Deputy Director,
Center for Research in Disease Prevention;
Professor,
School of Medicine,
Stanford University,
Palo Alto, California

Micah Hill
Research Assistant,

Complementary and Alternative
    Medicine Program,
Center for Research in Disease Prevention,
Stanford University,
Palo Alto, California

James F. Kleshinski, MD
Assistant Professor of Medicine,
Medical College of Ohio,
Toledo, Ohio

Fredi Kronenberg, PhD
Director,
Center for Complementary and Alternative
    Medicine in Women's Health,
College of Physicians and Surgeons,
Columbia University,
New York, New York

May Loo, MD
Assistant Clinical Professor,
Stanford University;
Director,
Neurodevelopmental Program,
Santa Clara County Valley Medical
    Center,
San Jose, California

Frederic M. Luskin, PhD
Research Associate,
Center for Research in Disease
    Prevention,
School of Medicine,
Stanford University,
Palo Alto, California

Debra E. Lyons, RN, PhD, FNF
Assistant Professor and Postdoctoral
    Fellow,
Center for the Study of Complementary
    and Alternative Therapies,
University of Virginia,
Charlottesville, Virginia

Victoria Maizes, MD
Faculty,

Complementary Medicine Program,
University of Arizona School of
 Medicine,
Tucson, Arizona

Farshad F. Marvasti
Research Assistant,
Complementary and Alternative
 Medicine Program,
Center for Research in Disease Prevention,
Stanford University,
Palo Alto, California

Angele V. McGrady, PhD
Professor and Administrative Director,
Complementary Medicine Center,
Department of Psychiatry,
Medical College of Ohio,
Toledo, Ohio

Patricia Aikins Murphy, CNM, PhD
Consulting Epidemiologist,
Center for Complementary and Alternative
 Medicine in Women's Health,
College of Physicians and Surgeons,
Columbia University,
New York, New York

Kathryn A. Newell, MA
Research Coordinator,
Complementary and Alternative
 Medicine Program,
School of Medicine,
Stanford University,
Palo Alto, California

Phuong Thi Kim Pham, PhD
Program Director,
National Cancer Institute,
National Institutes of Health,
Bethesda, Maryland

Aron Primack, MD
Health Scientist Administrator,
Fogarty International Center,

National Institutes of Health,
Bethesda, Maryland

Ru-Long Ren, MD
Department of Pathology,
Ball Memorial Hospital,
Muncie, Indiana

Samuel C. Shiflett, PhD
Principal Investigator and Director,
Center for Health and Healing,
Beth Israel Hospital,
New York, New York

Ann Gill Taylor, RN, EdD, FAAN
Professor and Director,
Center for the Study of Complementary
 and Alternative Therapies,
University of Virginia,
Charlottesville, Virginia

Christine Wade
Research Manager,
Center for Complementary and Alternative
 Medicine in Women's Health,
College of Physicians and Surgeons,
Columbia University,
New York, New York

Thanks to those who contributed to the
 first edition:

Bruce J. Diamond
M. Eric Gershwin
Robert M. Hackman
Thomas L. Hardie
James M. Horner
Sangeetha Nayak
James A. Peightel
Cherie Reeves
Nancy E. Schoenberger
Leanna J. Standish
Judith S. Stern
Roberta C.M. Wines
Diane Zeitlin

Preface

The initial reason for writing *Complementary and Alternative Medicine: An Evidence-Based Approach* was the need to examine research evidence and claims purported by advocates, clinicians, and researchers of complementary and alternative medicine (CAM) regarding its effectiveness. Both of us had previous experience with certain of these therapies since we had worked with American Indians who used alternative spiritual-indigenous medical approaches to health-related problems. Joseph Jacobs, a Mohawk, grew up using many of these healing practices. Later, we were involved at a national level establishing the first Office of Alternative Medicine (OAM) at the National Institutes of Health (NIH). The office was set up as a mandate from Congress to scientifically evaluate the claims made by the CAM community regarding treatment efficacy and safety.

We have attempted to be sensitive to and aware of the continuing debate over the need to study CAM. An early concern voiced by conventionally trained physicians, health providers, and scientists that its evaluation was a waste of time, partially because CAM had no scientific basis and partially because it simply was not useful, and in some cases, safety concerns could be raised, is still heard today. Our first edition evaluated many CAM therapies used for a variety of medical conditions. While there was no definitive or consensual finding regarding treatment efficacy, this should not be surprising given the paucity of research effort and financial expenditure for CAM evaluation. Therapies such as acupuncture, massage, and "psychological" (biofeedback, meditation-relaxation) have been increasingly used by consumers and also studied and evaluated, and a pattern of valid and reliable outcomes, under certain conditions, appears to be evolving.

Our second edition provides updated information on CAM since the late 1990s, as well as several new areas that are both important and relevant to the practice of CAM. Our goals for this second edition remain unchanged from our earlier work.

We want the book to contain the most recent and updated material concerning CAM and to be able to serve as a reference for physicians, health care providers, and scientists. We recognize that this is a formidable task because of the huge and not very well-defined areas of CAM. It is not possible to cover every study or therapy, but we tried to establish some general guidelines within which therapies and medical conditions were evaluated based on reported usage, recent demographic evaluations, and study quality. We hope by providing an evidence base for CAM that we continue to contribute to a database that allows the consumer, clinical scientist, and practicing healthcare provider to make knowledgeable decisions about CAM usage. That knowledge about healthcare practices regarding their integration with conventional medicine, where appropriate, will benefit patients and make available the safest and highest quality of medicine.

ORGANIZATION OF THE BOOK

We, as editors, have sought to allow the various chapter contributors the freedom to review and discuss those therapies that in their opinion merit the most focus. We have encouraged the use of as many databases as possible pursuant to establishing a firm evidence base. Besides using the federal *Medline NIH Database,* each author has supplemented their chapters differently. One major addition is our attempt to allow for more discussion(s) regarding the *quality* of the studies with less emphasis on simple quantity. We have also attempted in Appendices B and C to provide readers with more information about where clinical and research data regarding CAM exist. With such a quickly and continuously growing field, however, today's information about CAM is almost outdated by tomorrow.

    Complementary and Alternative Medicine: An Evidenced-Based Approach is organized around three major themes. The first part, *Basic Foundations* (Chapters 1 and 2), evaluates what is known about CAM focusing on definitional, usage, and research (clinical and preclinical) strategies; positioning of evidence-based medicine; and education/training. During the late 1990s, the movement by the Cochrane group to provide more systematic reviews for CAM therapies is an encouraging sign to place more emphasis on stronger research methodology. Although there are clear and major differences of opinion regarding the usefulness of certain research methodologies, by allowing for closer scrutiny of many different types of designs we suggest that a more relevant clinical and scientific outcome may evolve. The debate concerning the "placebo response" is a noteworthy example of the many research and clinical questions reviewed in this text. Its place in the healing process as well as its "control" attributes cannot and should not be ignored. A greater knowledge base concerning the potentially strong influence of the mind\brain in many healthcare issues may be an outgrowth of the "placebo" study and debate.

    The second and largest part, *Clinical Research Outcomes: Use of Complementary and Alternative Therapies in General Medicine,* evaluates and reviews clinical research. In Chapter 3, CAM's role in treating asthma and allergies is presented carefully, reviewing the evidence and allowing readers to form their own conclusions regarding CAM contributions. Chapter 4 reviews and updates what has been done in the area of cancer. Although there is no major change in the reported efficacy of CAM in the treatment of cancer, potentially useful approaches may be on the horizon. Noteworthy is the American Cancer Society's recent contribution of common herbal use with cancer. Chapter 5 reviews atherosclerotic vascular disease, focusing on the importance of both prevention and the integration of CAM to maximize benefit. Chapter 6 has more information on the use of herbs with diabetes mellitus. Quality of life remains an important issue. Chapter 7 reviews CAM therapies in the treatment of neurological conditions with an appropriate focus on rehabilitation issues. Chapter 8 evaluates CAM in the field of psychiatry. Importantly, the continued tracking and review of the use of St. John's wort for the treatment of mild to moderate depression and the issue of safety with kava-kava for anxiety management is featured. Chapter 9 discusses the use of CAM in the treatment of alcohol and chemical dependency. While many therapies have at times produced "positive findings," there still remains a challenge in producing consistency and replicable results. The complexity of many factors that are associated with substance abuse and its treatment needs much more evaluation and clarification in all treatment protocols. Chapter 10 directs attention to the ubiquitous area of pain control by the use of CAM methods. Recent studies that have evaluated manipulation procedures or the use of massage points to some useful findings. Also encouraging is the work of acupuncture in the treatment of fibromyalgia. Chapters 11 to 13 feature populations that increasingly constitute significant numbers of CAM consumers: children, women, and the elderly. The uniqueness of these populations and their importance in more accurately framing research questions around specific targeted areas needs strong emphasis. Of special concern are attention-deficit disorder as a possible medically overtreated health problem, the nausea and vomiting associated with pregnancy, and Alzheimer's and osteoarthritis and the important realm of quality-of-life issues.

In the final part, *Future Directions and Goals for Complementary and Alternative Medicine,* a new chapter, Legal and Ethical Issues (Chapter 14), directs attention to the impact and interaction(s) that must occur between CAM and the legal field, as well as updating and reviewing the important issues of accreditation and licensing of CAM providers. This is extremely relevant to the validation of CAM as being clinically trustworthy and safe. A second new chapter, Integration of Clinical Practice and Medical Training with Complementary and Alternative and Evidence-Based Medicine (Chapter 15), features the place for CAM in the context of integrative medicine and its part for healthcare and society. While one aspect of an evidence-based medicine may arguably be the inclusion of science and experimentally driven procedures such as statistics, the individual patient should not be "left out of the equation." Importantly, this concept and evidence-based medicine as one part of CAM should be directed at medical students at various levels or stages of training. Chapter 16 provides a review of the importance and needs of the consumer in a driven business market. At the federal level, regulation of CAM for both consumer protection and validation of usefulness and safety is necessary. A final summary (Chapter 17) puts forward potential emerging CAM therapies that should be tracked and watched for future outcomes. A list of goals that are attainable and relevant to the development of CAM and evidence-based medicine is provided.

Note: John Spencer and Joseph Jacobs are writing as individuals, and as such anything contained within does not reflect any present or past policy of the NIH or any other organization/association they have been or are currently affiliated with.

Acknowledgments

Many people have provided varying degrees of assistance in the writing of this second edition. In addition to those we listed in the first edition, many of whom were helpful in this edition, we would like to acknowledge Karen Keating and Fern Ingber for their help with Chapters 1 and 16 respectively. We are especially grateful to Jennifer Watrous, Melissa Kuster Deutsch, Gena Magouirk, Kellie White, and Inta Ozols at Elsevier Science.

We, as editors, would like to especially thank the following individuals for reviewing chapters from the first and second editions of *Complementary and Alternative Medicine: An Evidenced Based Approach:*

Marjorie Bowman   Sadja Greenwood   Neil Sonenklar
Laurel Archer Copp   Robert Michael   William Stuart
Richard Cumberlin   David Scheim   Jackie Wootton

John W. Spencer, PhD
Joseph J. Jacobs, MD, MBA
Fall, 2002

Contents

PART ONE

Basic Foundations

CHAPTER 1

Essential Issues in Complementary and Alternative Medicine

JOHN W. SPENCER

The debate between proponents and critics of complementary and alternative medicine (CAM) continues to renew both old and new arguments and biases at the start of the twenty-first century. The opinions of health providers, consumers, and researchers remain divided on whether this "unproven form of medicine" can be or ever will be demonstrated as being cost-effective, accessible, and most importantly, medically useful and safe. Even writing about CAM, especially when using terminology not familiar to the general public, can be fraught with difficulties and complexities. New sensitivities in medical language need to evolve as CAM becomes better understood through its study, evaluation, and ultimate acceptance or rejection. That is, definitions and descriptions of CAM should remain flexible as more information about this evolving field becomes available.

This chapter discusses six areas that are important in shaping the best "descriptors" of CAM: definitional, historical antecedents, usage-demographic factors, clinical/research methodologies, evidence-based issues, and training/education. These areas are not mutually exclusive but rather interact and are mutually influential. Chapter 16 focuses on tangential but important areas of consumer involvement, the CAM market, and federal/state regulations.

Definitional Considerations

Complementary or alternative medicine can be defined as a single or group of potentially classifiable procedures that are proposed to either substitute for or add to more conventional medical practices in the diagnosis/treatment or prevention areas of health. A single definition of CAM cannot exist, however, without considering many cofactors, and even these can be problematic. For example, consider the following:

COMPLEXITY OF FIELD

The field of CAM is multifaceted and multilayered in terms of its components. Many disparate therapies help delineate CAM's scope, including acupuncture, homeopathy, herbal therapies, hypnosis, and systems such as naturopathy. The focus, theoretic basis, and history of many therapies allow them to be grouped by a taxonomy or classification that becomes *one part* of their defining dimension.[54] For example, CAM can be part of a larger category of procedures, such as chiropractic, that is nested within a licensed, regulated, and professionally independent system, whereas CAM therapies of guided imagery and botanicals are placed in "mind-body" and "popular-health reform" categories, respectively. (See Appendix A and Suggested Readings, especially Novey, 2000.)

The assumption, however, that all of CAM is some type of a vague or "weird" form of health practice that is generally excluded from more conventional medicine is simply not true. Physical therapy, massage, biofeedback, hypnosis, and chiropractic procedures form the basis of many common health therapies that are ancillary to medicine as practiced by the vast majority of physicians who generally emphasize the use of pharmaceuticals as first line treatment. It is true, however, that CAM therapies are not at present partially or fully adopted as "standard treatments" by conventional medicine.

SCIENTIFIC CREDIBILITY

Any description of CAM should acknowledge that CAM has not been proven to be either *completely safe* or *useful* for many health-related areas. Attempts to show convincing treatment efficacy through clinical research have failed in part because of poor scientific quality and insufficient evidence (see later sections in this chapter and the described evidence base in subsequent chapters including strategies for integration of CAM with conventional medicine described in Chapter 14).

MEANINGFUL TERMINOLOGY

The actual terms *alternative* and *complementary* need to be closely evaluated because their use in the clinical setting relative to conventional treatments can become an important distinction. Words such as "alternative," "untested," "unproven," "unconventional," and "unorthodox" generally include medical or health therapies that become *replacement* or *substitute* (alternative) therapies for orthodox treatments. An example is shark cartilage used in place of more conventional therapy for cancer treatments (radiation or chemotherapy).

Complementary therapies include those treatments that are used with and in addition to conventional treatments, such as treatment of hypertension or diabetes by the use of conventional medication and complementary biofeedback or relaxation procedures. Thus biofeedback complements the biologic effects of blood pressure medication, possibly allowing for lower doses and minimizing drug side effects while optimizing treatment effects.

Use of chiropractic manipulation illustrates well the difficulty in attempting to form an all-encompassing definition for CAM. Manipulation is typically used for the treatment of low back pain. Good scientific evidence exists that chiropractic procedures can significantly reduce associated pain.[4,9] A measurable physical response can be defined and directly linked with muscle-nerve interactions with known mechanisms of action that can be used to describe how manipulation produces its effect. The question might be asked, "Just how alternative is this practice?" In terms of general medicine, however, manipulation may still be considered an "alternative" to surgery.

When chiropractic manipulation is used to treat medical conditions for which minimal scientific data exist to support its use and for which no rationale exists that would explain its physiologic action, the definition and use become more controversial. For example, is there acceptable scientific evidence for the use of chiropractic manipulation to treat psychiatric depression or otitis media? The second part of a more complete definition must include *how* CAM use is framed or applied for a specific treatment.

INSURANCE AND SOCIETAL INVOLVEMENT

Health insurance plans for CAM continue to evolve and partly depend on the need to document that particular therapies are useful and safe. Currently, medical reimbursement for CAM service delivery overall is significantly less than for conventional medicine. Societal considerations, including educational and management characteristics about CAM, form a further part of the definition. CAM is proposed to be part of a social process. Part of CAM's definition includes practices that are ongoing, evolving processes in which a procedure such as acupuncture moves through and into classifications or categories based on use and subsequent integration.[115] Therefore CAM could be referred to as *ancillary, limited, marginal,* "quasi," or *preliminary.* As consumer demands change and more information becomes available about treatment efficacy and safety, a particular therapy or practice could move from one and through other classifications.

DEFINITIONAL DESCRIPTION BY FEDERAL CONSENSUS

In the mid 1990s the then Office of Alternative Medicine at the National Institutes of Health (NIH) convened a panel to provide a definition and description of CAM activities.[75] CAM was described as "seeking, promoting, and treating health," but it was noted that the boundaries between CAM and other more dominant or conventional systems were not always clearly defined. The panel concluded that CAM's definition must remain flexible.

The definitions of CAM described in this text and in clinical or research settings are incomplete. Changes to any definition of CAM will continue as more information becomes available about the entire CAM process,[14] including study and evaluation.

◪ Historical Considerations

ANCIENT TIMES TO TWENTIETH CENTURY

In ancient China a system of medical care developed as part of philosophical teaching. Principles were recorded in and subsequently translated from *The Yellow Emperor's Classic of Internal Medicine* as follows[110]:

> It is said that in former times the ancient sages discoursed on the human body and that they enumerated separately each of the viscera and each of the bowels. They talked about the origin of blood vessels and about the vascular system, and said that where the blood vessels and the arteries (veins) met there are six junctions. Following the course of each of the arteries there are the 365 vital points for acupuncture. Those who are experts in using the needle for acupuncture follow Yin, the female principle, in order to draw out Yang. And they follow Yang, the male principle, in order to draw out Yin. They used the right hand in order to treat the illness of the left side, and they used the left hand in order to treat the illness of the right side.

Normal activities of the human body resulted from the balance between *yin* and *yang*. A breakdown of yin and yang balance was thought to be the general pathogenesis of all diseases. A patient with depression would be in a state of excessive yin, whereas a patient with mania would have excessive yang. Restoration of yin and yang balance led to recovery from illness.

Diagnosis involved close observation, listening, questioning, and recording various physiologic activities (Figure 1–1). Much of *traditional Chinese medicine* (TCM) as practiced today contains many of these same assumptions, including the respect for the unique aspect of the individual patient.

Chinese *materia medica*, an important part of TCM, is composed of materials derived from plants, animals, and minerals. The classic Chinese textbook on materia medica is *Bencao Gangmu*, written by Li Shi-Zhen during the Ming Dynasty (1552–1578). It listed 1892 medical substances and contained more than 1000 illustrations and 10,000 detailed descriptions. Through trial and error, worthless and less effective agents were eliminated from further consideration. The Chinese have accumulated a vast experience on disease prevention and treatment by using the Chinese materia. The 1990 edition of *The Pharmacopoeia of the People's Republic of China* collected 506 single drugs and 275 forms of complex preparations. One hundred preparations or drugs are being studied in pharmacology, chemical analysis, and clinical evaluation.[66] Ethnobotany, as currently practiced, owes much to the early accumulation of this information.

A similar but distinct system, *Ayurveda*, was developed on the Indian subcontinent more than 5000 years ago, emphasizing an integrated approach to both prevention and treatment of illness. Again, "imbalance" was a major part of the explanation of disease. A focus of awareness or level of consciousness was proposed to exist within each individual. This "inner" force was a major part of the practice of good health. Mental stress was involved in producing poor health, and techniques such as meditation were developed to aid in healing. Other ayurvedic components included lifestyle interventions of diet, herbs, exercise, and yoga.

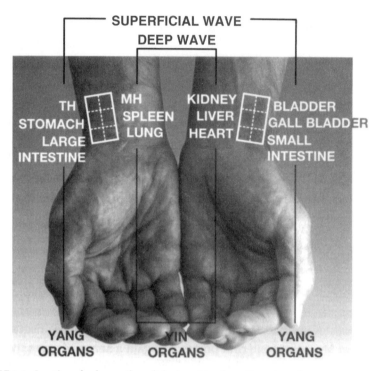

FIGURE 1–1. Location of pulses on the radial artery. At each position, yin and yang organs are coupled. The kidney pulse on the right is the kidney *yang,* or "vital gate." At least 28 qualities of the pulse, such as "superficial," "deep," and "short," relate to certain medical diseases or syndromes (internal, cold, excess). The seasons influenced the pulse, as did age, gender, and constitution. (*From Helms JM:* Acupuncture energetics: a clinical approach for physicians, *Berkeley, Calif, 1995, Medical Acupuncture Publishers.*)

In the second century AD, the ideas of the Greek physician Galen shaped what would eventually become modern scientific medicine. In his influential guide, *Anatomical Procedures,* Galen noted the following reasons to study the human body[90]:

> Anatomic study has one use for the man of science who loves knowledge for its own sake, another for him who values it only to demonstrate that nature does naught in vain, a third for one who provides himself from anatomy with data for investigating a function physical or mental, and yet another for the practitioner who has to remove splinters and missiles efficiently, to exercise parts properly, or to treat ulcers, fistulae and abscesses.

Galen's ideas eventually became the groundwork for evaluating and treating patients by focusing on the use of visual and physical objectivity. This was subsequently emphasized in medical education during the twelfth century. Greek philosophy and medicine were eventually incorporated into parts of Arabic and Latin cultures in the western Mediterranean region.

During the Newtonian era of the eighteenth century, the emphasis was on an objective approach to observations of any phenomenon. The replacement of the "rational philosophy" of the ancient tradition with the implementation of a stronger "experimental documentation" was continuing. Anomalous events that could not be explained by a theory were questioned or ignored.[40] The following three examples reflect this paradigm shift and illustrate foundational arguments that still exist between proponents and critics of CAM:

1. French scientist Anton Mesmer observed that after electrical stimulation of nerves and muscles, "forces" such as twitching could be recorded. He concluded that a magnetic fluid flowed throughout the body and that disease was the result of too much or too little fluid in one part of the body. His peers discredited Mesmer for being unable to reproduce any result that would verify his suggestions. His clinical results were said to result from "mental suggestion."

2. Methodist minister John Wesley collected many "written ideas" for maintaining health and healing based on what people told him was useful or produced healing. No theory or observation could support any of his claims.

3. German physician Samuel Hahnemann tested many common herbal and medicinal substances to establish what medical symptoms they might produce in humans. He experimented by diluting a solution and then subjecting it to vigorous shaking, called *succussion.* The dilution limit (i.e., that point when volume of solvent did not contain a single molecule of solute) was often exceeded. He treated sick patients by prescribing the medicine that most closely matched the symptoms of their illness, but in doses so small that their therapeutic value was questioned. Most of Hahnemann's results were not reproducible, and the subjectivity of his "therapies" was questioned.

By the mid-1800s, medicine in the United States was a mix of many different contributions and philosophies from various countries. The practice of medicine changed greatly with the advent and use of vaccines and antibiotics.[43] A second, equally important change occurred at the beginning of the twentieth century. Abraham Flexner, a U.S. educator, was charged with evaluating medical education. His 1910 report, *Medical Education in the United States and Canada,* was partly responsible for the diminution of CAM practice in the United States.[56] Although the study was intended to upgrade medical education in general, medical schools with a biomedical focus were favored and positioned to receive most of the money from large philanthropic organizations and foundations. By 1914 the number of U.S. medical schools had, partly because of economic considerations, decreased by approximately 40%. Remaining institutions generally favored a biomedical approach. Other important changes included the enactment of state licensing laws through the efforts of the American Medical Association (AMA) and the passage of the Pure Food and Drug Act of 1906.[103]

An important trend in early-twentieth-century medicine that influenced CAM was the evolution of "manual manipulation" as a major ancillary health therapy to general medicine,[40] initially promoted by Andrew Still and David Palmer. Still was an "osteopath" who advocated bone setting and manipulation of painful joints. Disease was thought to be the result of misplaced bones within the spinal cord. Palmer helped start the system called "chiropractic," which held that all diseases were caused by impingement of nerves passing through the spine. Most osteopaths were trained with some emphasis on basic science and surgery. Osteopaths used findings from biomedical research, including microscopic analysis of bacteria, antibiotics, analgesics, and antiinflammatory drugs. Chiropractors were slower to expand into scientific inquiry, although more recently this has changed with scientific evaluation of their procedures.[4]

ETHNOLOGIC CONTRIBUTIONS

The *cross-cultural*, as distinct from the historical, record of systems of healing is voluminous. Anthropologists have studied a wide variety of "folk medical systems" (e.g., shamanism, magic) and native cultural theories of illness and curing. Even with wide variations, however, it is possible to identify features common to other, non-modern medical systems, especially those recorded in cultures of the developing world. These theories are typically embedded in overarching native religious systems.[25] The causes of disease that are frequently described include the following:

- Loss of one's soul(s) in whole or in part
- Spirit possession
- Intrusion of human-filled object, where *mana* is an impersonal, supernatural force
- Intrusion of illness-causing spirit
- Violation of taboos, especially those involving correct relations to deities, including one's ancestors
- Spirit attack, including capricious "jokester" spirits
- Homeopathic and contagious magic
- Disturbances or violation of social rules and relationships

At present the alternative medical practitioner in many cultures is likely to be as much guru, shaman, and charismatic figure as physician in the mainstream Western secular sense.

Illness and healing can take on a cultural meaning that is relative to specific treatments,[58] diagnostic issues,[99] or both. For example, the healer/clinician in any society offers treatment to patients who bring stories of their own illnesses and special mental, emotional, and ethical concerns. The structure of the illness is really the manner in which it is meaningful to patient, family, and healer. Illness is a form of suffering that involves both mind and body. Self-awareness of pain or discomfort can be bound by various cultural and religious beliefs and can involve a host of properties, many of them psychologic. Symptoms of illness or enduring illness in one society may not be as relevant in another.

A continual dichotomy, or differing emphasis, exists between conventional medicine (and its treatment of the patient using modern scientific technology) and the more culture-bound approach emphasized in many CAM therapies, in which illness is often tied to personal beliefs and complaints or patients' judgment of illness.

NATIONAL INSTITUTES OF HEALTH

In 1991, Congress appropriated funds to start the Office of Alternative Medicine (OAM) at the NIH. The establishment of the OAM was seen as demonstrating congressional and public intent to expand the range of available health treatment modalities, especially for conditions treated unsuccessfully by conventional medicine, such as cancer. Many scientists viewed the appropriation as a waste of taxpayers' money, especially because of the negative stigma associated with alternative medicine and "quackery." Within this same time frame, however, the Office of Technology Assessment (OTA) published a lengthy report expressing the need for more clinical research evaluating alternative treatments for cancer.[109]

As a first step to "investigate and validate" alternative treatments as mandated by the U.S. Congress, the OAM released its first Request for Applications (RFA) in 1993 for a one-time, 1-year, exploratory grant that could not exceed $30,000. The purpose of this grant was to develop a foundation of scientific data that could lead to more extensive studies, possibly through funding by specific institutes at the NIH.[96] More than 450 applications were received and reviewed. Subsequently, 42 pilot projects were funded, and a broad range of therapies and health conditions were evaluated (Table 1-1).

Subsequently, about 25% of these studies were published in peer-reviewed journals. One lesson learned from this first program was the difficulty in completing any research project with limited financial resources made available through individual grants. This was most obvious in the costly areas of subject recruitment and data analysis.

Later, a group of CAM centers were funded to conduct research on a variety of health problems, including pain, asthma/allergies, human immunodeficiency virus/acquired immunodeficiency syndrome (HIV/AIDS), cancer, women's health, drug abuse/alcoholism, stroke/neurologic conditions, aging, cardiovascular issues, psychiatry, and pediatrics. More specialized centers evaluated chiropractic procedures as well as the role of botanicals in health (see Appendix B). The World Health Organization (WHO) designated the OAM itself as a collaborating center in traditional medicine. This involvement with WHO was seen as providing for the study of more traditional healing practices and allowing relevant findings to be made available to both the public and U.S. scientists.

In 1998 the OAM was elevated to "center" status and is now called the National Center for Complementary and Alternative Medicine (NCCAM), with a budget exceeding $70 million. Opportunities now exist for more funding of individual grants (research, education/training) and centers, creating multiple opportunities for co-funding with other institutes as well as establishing an intramural research component for the evaluation of CAM on the NIH campus.

The involvement of the NIH has renewed interests, debates, and controversies about CAM. Journals relevant to CAM include *Alternative Therapies, Alternative Therapies in Clinical Practice, Alternative Therapies in Health and Medicine, Journal of Alternative and Complementary Therapies, Mind-Body Medicine, Acupuncture and Electro-therapeutics Research,* and *Chinese Medical Journal.* Many self-help books devoted to health and healing and emphasizing CAM procedures are increasingly available in bookstores. The Internet contains hundreds of websites on CAM. The quality of this information is mixed, and little scientific evidence is presented for claims made.

TABLE 1–1. **COMPLEMENTARY AND ALTERNATIVE MEDICINE (CAM) THERAPIES AND MEDICAL/HEALTH CONDITIONS TREATED**

CAM Therapy	Medical/Health Condition
Acumoxa	Breech birth
Acupuncture	Unipolar depression
	Osteoarthritis
	Dental pain
	Attention deficit
Acupuncture/herbs	HIV (sinusitis)
	HIV survey
Antioxidant vitamins	Cancer cell function
Ayurvedic herbals	Brain chemistry
Ayurvedic medicine	Health status survey
Biofeedback	Diabetes mellitus type 2
	Pain survey
Dance therapy	Cystic fibrosis
Electrochemical DC	Cancer (preclinical)
EEG normalization	Mild head trauma
Energetic therapy	Basal cell carcinoma
Ethnomedicine	Hepatitis survey
Herbal	Hot flashes
	Skin warts
	Premenstrual syndrome
Homeopathy	Health status survey
	Mild brain injury
Hypnosis	Bone fracture healing
	Low back pain
Macrobiotic diet	Cancer
Manual palpation	Device evaluation
Massage	Bone marrow transplant
	Infant growth
	HIV
	Postoperative pain
Music therapy	Head injury
Prayer	Substance abuse
Qi Gong	Pain
T'ai chi	Balance disorder
Therapeutic touch	Stress
	Immune function
Transcranial electrostimulation	Chronic pain
Visual imagery	Asthma
	Breast cancer
	Immune function
	Drug use
Yoga (hatha)	Obsessive-compulsive disorder

From Exploratory Grant Program, Office of Alternative Medicine, U.S. National Institutes of Health, 1993, Bethesda, Md.
HIV, Human immunodeficiency virus; *DC,* direct current; *EEG,* electroencephalogram.

◼ Clinical-Demographic Considerations

USE OF CAM THERAPIES IN THE 1990s

In the early and mid-1990s, numerous demographic surveys were published to better understand CAM. The data obtained generally included numbers of patients using a particular CAM therapy and demographic information. Often missing were use and ways the particular therapy could be integrated with conventional medicine, follow-up data on longer-term benefits, cost issues, and evaluation of population distributions using multivariate statistics. Still, the reported information was useful and helped shape future research questions leading to efficacy studies.

Although surveys can produce important information about use of CAM therapies, they can also be misleading if done improperly or incompletely. Great care must to be taken to ensure that neither interviewer bias nor subject bias exists. Questions that are vague, not validated, or not clinically relevant should be avoided. Subjects with preconceived or negative views about CAM are not good candidates. Incorrect survey information may be collected and results skewed when variables such as sample size, age, gender, ethnicity, education, and income are not carefully profiled and analyzed. Depending on the question or hypothesis explored, either stratified or randomized subject selection is useful. "Usage" does not imply that the therapy is always efficacious for specific groups or sample populations. Surveys simply measure impressions of individuals and are limited to what information they provide or remember to provide. Surveys, however, can be the first step toward uncovering a general degree of documentation about CAM usage.

Europe

The use of complementary therapies throughout Europe and Asia has been well researched. Fisher and Ward[37] reported that 20% to 50% of European populations used complementary therapies. Consumer surveys indicate that in the Netherlands and Belgium, use of CAM is as high as 60%, and in Great Britain, 74% are willing to pay additional insurance premiums to cover complementary therapies. One CAM therapy, *homeopathy*, has grown in popularity, especially in France, and remains extremely popular in Great Britain. Reilly[79] provided one of the early surveys of physicians and medical students in Europe concerning their knowledge and use of CAM. He reported that physicians had positive attitudes toward their patients' use of CAM.

The most frequently used therapies included *hypnosis, manipulation, homeopathy*, and *acupuncture*. Interestingly, physicians' personal use of CAM therapies was linked to greater interest in training. In Germany, 95% of physicians themselves reportedly used herbal therapy or homeopathy.[50] Of 89 physicians surveyed in Israel, 54% reported that certain complementary therapies might be clinically useful, and 42% had referred patients for specific treatments.[84] German medical students indicated a significant interest in learning about acupuncture (42%) and homeopathy (55%) and thought that these therapies had the potential to be effective.[7] Further, in Canada, a cross section of 200 general practitioners revealed that 73% thought they should have some knowledge about certain alternative treatments.[111] Chiropractic procedures were popular, and efficacious treatments were reported for musculoskeletal and chronic pain.

Ernst et al.[35] combined and evaluated 12 separate surveys of perceived effectiveness of complementary therapies among physicians. The individual surveys were conducted throughout Europe and the Middle East and included the United Kingdom, New Zealand, Germany, the Netherlands, Sweden, and Israel. On a scale of 1 (low) to 100 (high), the average score was 46, indicating that the therapies were considered to be "moderately effective." Younger physicians viewed complementary medicine as promising. The most popular therapies were manipulation, acupuncture, and homeopathy. Respondents' views regarding whether the use of complementary therapies would be more effective than a placebo were not evaluated.

An extensive description of the practice or research of CAM in Europe and other countries such as China and India is beyond the scope of this chapter and text, but this does not lessen the importance of these areas. In many ways CAM has fared much better in terms of its acceptance and integration with conventional medicine in Europe, partly because of different, less restrictive regulations. Recently, recommendations have been made for the reexamination of health care and service delivery in the United Kingdom, because a reported 750,000 consultations may occur annually, and 40% of medical practices may provide access to CAM.[104] Vincent and Furnham[113] provide additional information on CAM practice outside the United States.

United States

The trend of CAM usage in the United States continues to be on the increase, although certain CAM practice areas may have reached a numeric plateau. Cassileth[22,23] was among the first to report on the use of certain unorthodox therapies for the treatment of cancer (see Chapter 4). In the early 1990s, Eisenberg et al.[34] evaluated the use of unconventional treatments for general medical conditions. They interviewed 1539 adults and recorded that 34% had used at least one alternative therapy in the previous year; 72% of the respondents did not inform their physician that they were using unconventional approaches. The greatest usage was by middle-aged individuals (25 to 49 years of age). The major complaints most often cited included back problems, anxiety, depression, and headaches. Therapies most often used included chiropractic, relaxation, imagery, and self-help groups. Expenditures associated with the use of these therapies were estimated at $14 billion, of which $10 billion was paid by the patient. In a later survey conducted through 1997, CAM usage continued to increase by more than 8% from 1993.[33]

Survey and clinical use of CAM therapies in the United States during the 1990s has been reported for such divergent conditions as chronic arthritis treated by acupuncture,[73] epilepsy treated by prayer,[28] and voice disorders treated by laryngeal massage.[29] In a focused regional 1995 survey of U.S. family physicians' knowledge of, use of, training in, and particularly important, evidence expected of complementary medicine for acceptance as a legitimate practice, Berman et al.[15] reported a wide range of attitudes and revealed notable trends. Diet/exercise, biofeedback, and counseling/psychotherapy were most often used in medical practice. Additionally, most physicians sampled thought that standards of acceptance for conventional medicine using scientific rules of evidence should be equally applied to complementary medicine. In a 1998 study, Berman et al.[16] reported that psychologic therapies such as biofeedback, relaxation, counseling/psychotherapy, and diet/exercise were seen as more "legitimate" by physicians. TCM, electromagnetic therapies, and American Indian medicine were less accepted, whereas chiropractic therapies and acupuncture were increasing in acceptance. Age was an important variable; the longer the physician was in practice, the more a less favorable attitude existed toward the practice of CAM.

WHY PATIENTS USE CAM

The reasons that patients choose to use CAM are multifaceted, complex, personal, and biased. CAM patients may have strong negative opinions about conventional medicine.[50,59] Some mistrust institutions and new technologies; others view conventional medicine as an impersonal and profit-motivated system. When conventional treatments are not helpful, patients often blame the physician. When a communication problem exists with their health care provider, patients may start "doctor shopping" and request additional tests to reassure themselves that earlier opinions were in error. At this point, patients are more likely to try CAM therapies.

Predictive parameters of useful communication between physician and patient include (1) the type of disease being treated, (2) the difficulty or complexity of the treatment, (3) the patient's "interpretation" (i.e., attitude) of the treatment, and (4) the patient's involvement in the treatment decision-making process.[85] Furnham and Forey[39] evaluated two separate and matched groups of patients seen by either a general practitioner (GP) or an alternative practitioner (AP) to determine influence of attitudes. The AP group was more skeptical about whether conventional medicine worked, and they believed that CAM would be more useful in improving health.

Both physician and patient must work to achieve better communication with each other. Education is useful because referrals for alternative therapies can be substantial. In community settings in Washington state, New Mexico, and southern Israel, for example, 60% of all physicians made referrals at least once in the preceding year and 38% in the previous month. Patients requested these referrals because of a closer alliance with their cultural beliefs, the lack of success of conventional treatments, and the physician's belief that patients had a "nonorganic" profile. No correlation existed between the rate of referral and the physician's level of knowledge, beliefs about effectiveness, or understanding of alternative therapies.[18] Useful information concerning additional patient and physician communication issues is presented in Chapter 14.

Since 1998, relevant information has continued to be published on the use of CAM (Table 1-2). More emphasis is being placed on obtaining larger samples and examining diversity issues such as age, gender, and ethnicity. Additional studies are needed, however, especially evaluating longer-term follow-up and replication.

It is important to recognize the continued difficulty with sampling, return rates on surveys, and the validity of the self-reporting issue. Clearly, however, CAM usage is on the increase; a majority of CAM therapies that still appear to be "borderline conventional" are those used by psychologists, psychiatrists, massage therapists, and chiropractors. Acupuncture appears to be one therapy increasing in use and is more

TABLE 1-2. DEMOGRAPHIC STUDIES IN COMPLEMENTARY AND ALTERNATIVE MEDICINE

Study/Reference	Demographic Studied (Number of Subjects)	Results	Comments
Eisenberg et al,[33] 1998	Prevalence of CAM use (2055), U.S. sample, 1990–1997; 67% response rate	Use up 8% (33.8%–42.1%): Out-of-pocket expenses, disclosure to physicians least change from previous survey; popular CAM therapies were herbal medicine, massage, megavitamins used for chronic back pain, headache, anxiety, depression	Selected sample, telephone survey; nonminority focus
Berman et al,[16] 1998	Physician survey of CAM training, attitudes, practice (783)	Most popular/usable in practice: psychologic therapies, diet, exercise Best predictor of use: attitude training Older physicians less positive toward CAM	Limited sample by specialty
Druss et al,[31] 1999	Prevalence of CAM use (16,068), 77% response rate, Medical Expenditure Panel Survey	6.5% used CAM and conventional therapies 1.8% used only CAM Most popular: chiropractic therapies	Wide-based sampling, more representative
Furnham,[38] 2000	Classification of CAM use (600); rate on familiarity with, use, knowledge, and efficacy of CAM	Highest rated: acupuncture, herbal medicine, massage, yoga Lowest rated: ayurvedic chelation, ozone	Separated most important factors of familiarity, efficacy with public perception
Harris and Ress,[47] 2000	Prevalence of CAM use in general population; systematic review analysis; 12 studies from 638 met criteria	Increased use of CAM in 1990s Most prevalent therapy: chiropractic and massage Great variation in methods, sample size, representation	Age/gender demographics missing Importance of consistent, valid survey methodologies
Sturm,[106] 2000	Prevalence of CAM use as risk-taking behavior (9585), 64% response rate from community surveys, "chiropractic" not included	CAM patients perceive selves more as risk takers than general public Female gender important predictor for CAM use	Separate analysis for chiropractic therapies would have been useful. What is "risk behavior"?
Brolinson et al,[19] 2001	Nurses' perceptions of CAM use (1000), 57% response rate, wide U.S. survey	50% judged hypnotherapy, chiropractic, acupressure, acupuncture, and healing touch as safe. 30%–40% used multivitamins, meditation, relaxation, and massage. Most regarded CAM training as poor.	Low response rate; more in-depth information needed in survey questionnaire

Study	Description	Findings	Comments
Cappuccio et al,[21] 2001	Prevalence of CAM use in multiethnic populations (1577), 64% response rate; men and women; age range: 40–59	10.4% use overall Women and blacks in higher socioeconomic groups more likely to use CAM than whites and Asians Popular therapies: vitamin supplements, oil, garlic	Stratified sample; broader coverage of CAM therapies needed
Eisenberg,[32] 2001	Patients' perceptions of CAM therapies (831), 60% response rate, U.S. telephone survey	79% said both conventional and CAM superior together rather than separate Confidence in CAM provider same as for conventional provider Up to 72% did not tell physician of CAM use because "not important." CAM therapies best for pain, less for "hypertension"	Sampling bias; question "accurate memory" of CAM usage by participants; Reasons for CAM use multifaceted, but is not related to fear of conventional provider disapproval Important finding
Greger,[44] 2001	Consumers' dietary supplement use; review of multiple studies	Increase in supplement use by 40% (92%–96%) Predictive factors: female, higher income, white, older, lifestyle (exercise) Toxicity issues unknown Most users receive information from nonphysicians.	Urgent need for more information specific to vitamins and supplements Incomplete data on long-term effects
Kessler,[55] 2001	Prevalence of CAM use by long-term trends in U.S. (2049), 60% response rate; stratified by age, gender, ethnicity, education, and U.S. region	67% used one CAM therapy that increased in use over lifetime 30% use: under age 54 50% use: ages 33–53 70% use: ages 18–33 Most often used therapies: psychologic, acupuncture, diet/vitamins	Important descriptor for "residual health" Sample bias; self-reporting accuracy issues Does suggest increasing interest in and need for CAM
Long et al,[68] 2001	Benefits of CAM therapies by sampling CAM professional organizations (66)	Top treatable conditions using CAM: stress/anxiety, headaches, back pain, respiratory problems, insomnia, cardiovascular problems Most popular therapies: aromatherapy, massage, nutrition reiki, yoga	Question bias/nonbias of CAM organizations in the referral process
Standish et al,[102] 2001	Prevalence of CAM use by HIV-positive men and women (1675)	63% used vitamin C 53% used vitamin E 53% used garlic Most consulted therapists: massage (49%); acupuncturists (45%) CAM activities: aerobic exercise (63%); prayer (58%); massage (53%); meditation (46%)	Important for understanding CAM use with chronic disease Outcome information continues to be important

(Continued)

TABLE 1–2. **DEMOGRAPHIC STUDIES IN COMPLEMENTARY AND ALTERNATIVE MEDICINE—cont'd**

Study/Reference	Demographic Studied (Number of Subjects)	Results	Comments
Chandrashekara et al,[24] 2002	Prevalence of CAM use for arthritis (114)	43% used CAM Most common therapies: ayurveda, homeopathy Family income or community does not influence use	Important finding was majority of patients lost faith in usefulness of conventional medicine; Common belief was fewer adverse effects with CAM
Langmead et al,[60] 2002	Prevalence of CAM use for inflammatory bowel disease (239)	26% of patients use herbal remedies Profiles included younger, single adults Gender or ethnicity was not a predictive factor	Small sample size Issues of poor quality of life and/or social and emotional factors being related to CAM use is relevant finding.

HIV, Human immunodeficiency virus.

"alternative/complementary" in the true sense of the word. Research papers by Harris and Ress[47] and Wootton and Spaber[120] illustrate how the field of CAM usage and demographics continues to expand through more focused regional and national studies that can be combined for systematic review analysis.

◼ Clinical Research Methodology Considerations

INCONSISTENCY OF MODELS FOR CAM

Although strong research methodology can lead to outcome results that are both accurate and reproducible, a debate exists between advocates of CAM and conventional scientists and physicians concerning which forms of research designs are appropriate or even needed to determine efficacy.[65]

One reason for the disparity between CAM and conventional medical research is completely opposite theoretic models. The *biomedical approach* focuses on a disease orientation, which suggests that a specific agent is responsible for a specific illness or disorder. Hypothesis testing and linear reasoning with logic and causation are the main components. CAM therapies are based more on a philosophy that uses a *comprehensive approach* concerned with multidimensional factors that may or may not be studied independently. Causation and mechanisms of therapeutic action, or how something "works," are not always seen as important. One central goal of CAM is to improve the "wellness" of the patient. Rather than just removing a disease-producing agent, "quality of life" is emphasized by treating functional or somatic problems with ancillary and important psychologic, social, emotional, and spiritual aspects.

Many CAM research studies are not focused, do not use hypothesis testing or large number of subjects, and tend to rely more on verbal reports from the patients.[53] The quality of most CAM studies, as judged by Western-trained scientists, is not always considered acceptable.[77] Relevant examples include acupuncture and homeopathy.[57,112]

IMPORTANCE OF CAM VALIDATION

Strengths and weaknesses of clinical research in a particular area should be evaluated using a scientific consensus development approach. In the mid-1990s the then OAM and NIH sponsored a conference evaluating the quality of research on acupuncture.[1] An independent, nonfederal panel reviewed the scientific evidence and concluded that few well-performed research studies assessed the efficacy of acupuncture with either placebo or "sham" controls. Future research was encouraged to include and evaluate enrollment procedures, eligibility criteria, clinical characteristics of the subjects, methods for diagnosis, and accurate description of protocols, including types and number of treatments, outcomes used, and statistical analysis.

Significantly, needle acupuncture was reported to be most efficacious for postoperative and chemotherapy-associated nausea and vomiting and for nausea associated with pregnancy. Acupuncture was somewhat efficacious for postoperative dental pain. For the remaining health areas, however, the panel found that most of the scientific literature was mixed regarding positive treatment outcomes; determination could not be made in many cases because of poor study design. The panel also reported that the incidence of reported adverse effects with the use of acupuncture was lower than with many drugs. Future proposed study areas included: (1) the demographics of acupuncture use; (2) efficacy of acupuncture, with evaluation of whether different theories of acupuncture produce different treatment outcomes; and (3) ways to integrate research and acupuncture findings into the health care system.

These conference findings highlight the important factors to be considered when evaluating differences between conventional medicine and CAM approaches.[8] Because of varied treatment reactions, a patient receiving acupuncture may have the contact points changed throughout the procedure, making it difficult to describe a specific effect of procedures, points used, therapist-patient interaction, or a combination of these factors. Because CAM therapists are an integral part of the therapeutic procedure, however, their communication with patients is crucial. The relative or absolute importance of isolating some or all of the many cofactors involved in treatment outcome continues to be a central debate between various research methodologists. That is, by eliminating certain nonspecific effects or "nuisance variables" (patient belief, experimenter attitude or role), the therapy situation can change, as might the treatment outcome.

Table 1–3 presents types of evidence required for the validation of research. Each of the items listed, when appropriate and realistic, should be part of any practice or research protocol, regardless of CAM or conventional clinical orientation. The use of this type of evidence is important to the consumers who use CAM therapies and to the federal and state agencies that attempt to regulate practices and that need to integrate research findings, which should be collected under valid and objective conditions.

TABLE 1–3. **TYPES OF EVIDENCE IN EVALUATION OF COMPLEMENTARY AND ALTERNATIVE MEDICINE**

Evidence	Validation Question
Experimental	Is the practice efficacious when examined experimentally?
Clinical (practice)	Is the practice effective when applied clinically?
Safety	Is the practice safe?
Comparative	Is the practice the best therapy for the problem?
Summary	Is the practice known and evaluated?
Rational	Is the practice rational, progressing, and contributing to medical and scientific understanding?
Demand	Do consumers and practitioners want the practice?
Satisfaction	Is the practice meeting patients' and practitioners' expectations?
Cost	Is the practice inexpensive to operate and cost-effective? Is the practice provided by insurance?
Meaning	Is the practice the appropriate therapy for the individual?

SUBJECT SELECTION

Most methodologists insist that adequate numbers of subjects by gender, age, education, and similarity of medical condition should be minimal conditions for inclusion in any clinical protocol. Each subject should have an equal chance of either receiving or not receiving treatment (*randomization*). This application ensures that the study will have more equated samples with which to evaluate, leading to less variance in the analyzed outcome. Further, a no-treatment or placebo control group should be ensured; the patient and examiner should be unaware of group placement (*blinding*); and the medical condition to be treated should be clearly diagnosed with specified criteria for each subject/group. Certain medical journals now require that parameters explicitly related to randomization be described to facilitate validation and future replication.[41] Also, the registering of all clinical protocols to create a complete national database should be an ongoing goal that is a primary focus for all researchers.

Ethically, conceptually, and practically, however, randomized trials may present problems in research design, especially for CAM.[42,113] For example, if a therapy is new and safe, a good chance exists that it may also be effective. Patients may not want to participate in or may resent being in a study in which they could be randomized into a control group. A subject's belief that he or she might be in a "no-treatment" group could impact personal attitude and influence the subject's response to the therapy or to the experimenters. Further, the clinical trial may seem artificial and pose no relevance to the clinical practice itself. Randomized controlled trials are not designed to evaluate individual differences. Some patients may respond to a treatment only in part, and others may not respond at all. Treatment nonresponders need to be more completely described and understood (e.g., beliefs, motivations, demographics). The same analysis is necessary for "no-treatment" responders.

Many CAM practitioners also argue that randomization actually "biases out" any positive finding. That is, by controlling all or many of the nonspecific random or nuisance factors that are of concern to conventional research, variables such as group/family support, strength of the therapeutic relationship, or knowledge of group placement may reduce any treatment effect.

A recent analysis of randomized trials revealed that many CAM studies need to craft controlled groups more carefully to evaluate all treatment effects, both specific and nonspecific.[48] This would include and impact the development and formulation of accurate hypotheses and more complete rationales for the type of design used. Also, clear details were lacking in many CAM studies about what and when subjects were informed regarding an explanation of the study, including its rationale, risks, and certain procedures. Appropriate information about human consent in research, has been provided at workshops for the CAM community describing its importance and how to obtain consent.[95]

Suggestions for improvement of CAM studies include the following:

1. To ensure homogeneity of groups, patients might be evaluated first using a standard physician interview with conventional diagnostic techniques. Then patients might be evaluated again using a CAM practitioner, with eventual subcategorizing of each patient based on findings important to the *specific therapy* under

evaluation.[118] For example, in evaluating acupuncture, pulse and tongue character-istics would be documented, and in homeopathy, a collection of symptoms with specific remedies. The treatment protocol is balanced because both conventional and individual symptom pattern diagnoses are incorporated. One difficulty is the large number of patients required, along with associated expense and time required to complete the protocol.

2. In a simpler design, each patient serves as his or her own control. Variables such as gender, genetic factors, social strata, and personality are matched, and each subject is evaluated over time, generally before, during, and after treatment. The important variable of *washout* of effects, allowing adequate time for residual treatment effects to dissipate, should be an integral part of the design. In certain designs a *crossover* to the treatment group can be studied. The use of a crossover prevents subjects from developing attitudes or beliefs that they will never be treated, thus complicat-ing or negating treatment outcomes.

3. In an "n-of-1" design, each patient is studied individually by one physician/ researcher, and results are instantaneously recorded. Individual clinical trial packages can be developed, including standardized questionnaires and measurement devices. If similarities in patient profiles and other variables occur, data may be pooled together, although care should be taken when equating. Using this design, Guyatt et al.[46] reported that 81% of trials were completed, and the results increased physicians' confidence in their practice management. The n-of-1 design could be used to begin early studies of certain CAM therapies by first individually profiling patients' respon-siveness in clinical practice settings and then entering results into a registered data-base. Subsequently, larger scale clinical trials would then be developed.

4. Ensure that adequate informed consent procedures are used in all studies and that these studies are registered into a national database to aid replication.

A relevant issue in the selection of subjects for research is the *actual number* used in either treatment or no-treatment groups. Most studies evaluating treatment efficacy in CAM use too few subjects per group. The mythical number of 50 per group is either inappropriate or not always feasible. The best way to ensure that the results are accurate and reproducible is to use a "power analysis" to determine actual sample size needed, done before or after the study.[26,27]

SUBJECT EXPECTATION AND ROLE OF PLACEBO

When patients are treated for any illness or health condition, explanations for improvement include the following[108]:

1. The treatment itself may be responsible for change.
2. Most illnesses including pain simply remit on their own over time and heal (*natu-ral history*), or extreme symptoms simply return to a closer approximation of the original health state (*regression to the mean*).
3. Patients improve on their own simply because they "think" someone is doing something for them (*Hawthorne effect*), or they mistakenly think the symptoms and complaints are related to a disease or illness, but in actuality, these symptoms are related more to psychosocial stress.

4. The patients were originally misdiagnosed by physician or caregiver and in fact did not have a particular illness.
5. Some unexplained, nonspecific effect operates, such as a positive or negative attitude toward ancillary caregivers, or the patient has or develops a positive attitude or belief that the treatment will be either beneficial (*placebo*) or negative, that is, not beneficial (*nocebo*).

The term *placebo* refers to a sham treatment that physicians may use to "please" (its Latin meaning) either anxious patients or those who are difficult to treat. It contains no active pharmaceutical substance(s). In clinical trials the placebo is considered a "non-treatment" and given with the assumption that because of its inactivity, patients will not respond as they would to active treatments.[36]

Beecher[11] postulated that placebos can change patient functioning structurally and physiologically. For example, Levine et al.[63] have demonstrated that the "placebo" response might be partially endorphin mediated because naloxone, which blocks endorphin release, could reverse "placebo treatment effects" for reducing postoperative dental pain in some patients. A specific transmitter-mediated "placebo central nervous system (CNS) pathway," while an intriguing possibility, has not been established. The brain's involvement (CNS) with placebo administration has been recently demonstrated.[69] Subjects receiving a placebo were reported to show increased brain glucose metabolism (positron emission tomography [PET] scan activities) in prefrontal areas of the cortex, as well as "anterior cingulate, premotor, parietal, posterior insula and posterior cingulate." Decreases were observed in the "subgenual cingulate, parahippocampus and thalamus." Interestingly fluoxetine antidepressant responders had similar response profiles and additionally showed changes in "brainstem, striatum, anterior insula and hippocampus." Also, placebos have unique pharmacokinetics, including dose response,[78] side effects,[17] and residual long-term effects.[70] All of these studies suggest that placebos are more than simply "inert."

One of the more interesting aspects of placebo responses is describing the varied conditions under which they might work.[117] In any clinical study a certain number of patients will respond positively to placebos. Generally the number varies across studies but may range from 30% to 70%. Oh[76] has suggested that placebos appear to work in patients with pain and disorders of autonomic sensation, such as nausea, psychoneuroses, phobias, and depression, and in disorders of blood pressure and bronchial airflow. Attempts to define and predict which subjects might be "placebo responders" based on gender, personality, and attitudes about drugs, physicians, nurses, and hospitals have not yielded consistent results. Variables that require closer evaluation include: a) positive patient expectation of treatment outcome; b) favorable response to a specific practitioner; and c) high degree of patient compliance.[108] Placebos may operate by decreasing patient anxiety[36] or by helping highly anxious patients maximize their responsiveness to placebos.[88] Placebos could simply work as a classically conditioned response.[114] However, none of these explanations has been consistently verified, and although they may play a role in "placebo responding," these hypotheses remain incomplete and speculative.

A recent systematic review evaluated more than 4000 patients randomized to receive either placebos (pharmacologic or nonpharmacologic studies) or no treatment. No significant effect was reported for placebos compared with a "no-treatment condition," thus questioning the continued use of placebos in certain research protocols.[51] Clearly, interwoven in the debate to use placebos is the ethical issue of their action or lack of action in patients who may have chronic or life-threatening diseases. It also becomes more problematic for describing and understanding the broad range of nonspecific effects superimposed on and influencing individual differences in patients. In drug clinical trials, placebos may have some indications; it is equally important to understand, however, that patients respond favorably to a treatment procedure for many reasons, and that it becomes impossible to always describe reasons for improvement accurately. This type of analysis should be an important goal though for future research regardless of what type of medicine—CAM or conventional—is evaluated. The NCCAM has recently held a conference on placebos and a report will be published through British Medical Journal (BMJ) Books subsidiary in 2002.

Another way to evaluate recovery and healing responses after therapy is by "remembered wellness."[12] As an alternative to the term "placebo responding," Benson describes that after an active or passive therapeutic intervention, a memory of past events occurs and helps to trigger a physical response. The patient remembers a time when peace, strength, and confidence were an active part of consciousness and good health. This process involves the individual's own "belief" system and includes prior learning, previous experiences (environment), and genetic interactions (biologic factors).

According to Benson,[12] a good way to access "remembered wellness" is through relaxation. The quieting of both the mind and the body assists in healing. Relaxation has been demonstrated in clinical research studies to reduce physiologic responses, such as sweat, muscle/nerve (electroencephalographic), temperature, and heart rate, and thus subsequently treat anxiety,[93] as well as high blood pressure, pain, headaches, and a variety of other illnesses.[13,49,107]

Benson is describing the continually evolving interaction(s) between mind/brain and body (Figure 1–2) as a suitable area for clinical research; (also see Spencer and Shanor,[98] who describe mind-body approaches for "usage" in health).

Clinical and preclinical basic studies have revealed intriguing relationships between the CNS and the immune system. The seminal work of Ader and Cohen[2] on ways to modify the immune system through conditioning of the immunosuppression response helped to shape the field of psychoneuroimmunology. Other work has emphasized the important role of stress management and its positive effects on cardiovascular and stroke-related illnesses in disease prevention.[3]

"Belief in some type of a treatment outcome," either positive or negative, can become an integral part of a multi-interactive process that has specific relationships with CAM. *Spiritual belief* and its impact on healing in mental health areas have been reviewed and found to be of importance.[61] Patients who are committed to a more religious orientation report a better overall satisfaction with life and lower levels of depression and stress. Also, clinical psychologists report that many of their patients use religious language such as prayer when discussing the many emotional issues around treatment of mental health problems.[87] The potential of spiritual healing using a patient's belief system and including counseling[94] may have huge, untapped ramifi-

ZIPPY BILL GRIFFITH

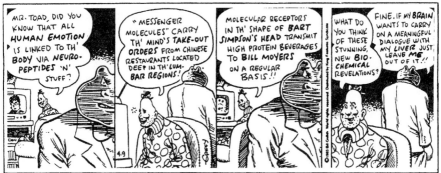

FIGURE 1–2. *Zippy* cartoon: "My Kidney, My Self." *(Courtesy Bill Griffith; reprinted with special permission of King Features Syndicate.)*

cations helped to many health-related areas. For example, one of my previous graduate students recently reported that prayer (self and group) helped to reduce anxiety and depression and helped to increase the seeking of social support and positive self-talk in Christian women diagnosed with stage II breast cancer when compared with a smaller, nonpraying group of similarly diagnosed women.[86] A manualized group treatment protocol was used to ensure consistent week-by-week agendas and to aid in study replication. Because of the small sample size, inference is limited. Extension of sample size and replication will be needed.

SUBJECT ASSESSMENT MEASURES

One of the major weaknesses in research evaluating CAM therapies has been the use of incomplete, biased, or often invalidated treatment outcome measurements. This variable severely limits statements about degree of efficacy and the ability to make clinical generalizations.

A common outcome measurement used in CAM studies is the "self-report," which can produce helpful information under certain guidelines.[92] Generally, direct questions with yes-or-no answers are asked, boxes are checked, or a ranking scale (e.g., 1 to 10) is used. The truthfulness of the respondent is major concern in this type of analysis. Factors that can influence accuracy include motivation, deception, willingness to please, medical condition, and psychometric properties, such as reliability and validity of the particular items used.

Rather than using a single outcome measure, most CAM therapies should consider using multidimensional assessments to maximize external validity. Meaningful clinical effects can be described by monitoring the cases in which a treatment is both beneficial and safe and by determining longevity. In addition to evaluating major medical parameters such as basic laboratory studies or physiologic functioning,[100] ancillary functions including quality of life, hospital visits, and abilities to work (e.g., functional capacities such as job-related duties of lifting weight), are all useful and relevant. Further, WHO has developed a system to evaluate CAM therapies by describing their impact on psychologic and physical level of independence, social relationships, and spiritual domains.[121] More recent work has suggested that broad and subjective health scales and self-reports should be included at various stages of treatment to evaluate progress.[67] Examples of these scales include the Karnofsky Performance Status Scale, quality of life index,[101] and symptom distress scale.[71]

Other measurements should include individual patient concerns and predictions about illness and treatment outcome. Through this analysis, influences of belief and attitude and their potential interaction with study results can be more fully developed. The more appropriate term, *subjective health status*, is of greater use than "quality of life," which is difficult to define, understand, and accurately measure.[62]

Multivariate analysis is a tool that can be used to understand CAM methodology. Importantly, more studies are including greater and more complete statistical sophistication. For example, the predictive value of CAM therapeutic approaches can be evaluated using structural equations.[5] Patients who had previously undergone coronary artery bypass grafting improved their psychologic adjustment after surgery; 85% practiced CAM. Patients who used prayer, exercise, or diet modification in their lifestyle had less depression and less psychologic distress (Figure 1–3). This important finding demonstrates how multiple variables can be appropriately evaluated in CAM research and produce meaningful outcome statements. This finding is also clinically significant for individual patients who want to improve their health after surgery because it demonstrates the importance of belief as a cofactor in health recovery.

An approach to patient measurement and evaluation in CAM that may be less costly than conducting large-scale, controlled randomized trials is the use of systematic *clinical auditing*. Certain patient characteristics are documented, including diagnosis, type of therapy used, and outcome results from large samples of individuals. This observational information describes the clinical practice through questionnaires sent during set periods after hospital admission. In one report, 1597 patients were evaluated over 1 year at a hospital for TCM in Germany.[72] Each patient was initially seen by both a German and a Chinese physician, and general data and documentation were collected. Approximately 66% of the patients had chronic pain, and common diagnoses included nervous system diseases and musculoskeletal conditions. Most patients were treated with either acupuncture or Chinese herbal remedies. At discharge, 38% revealed a greater than 50% symptom resolution, and 32% had less than 50% improvement; 24% had no change in their condition; 6% reported an increase in symptoms. Interestingly, the authors reported that 97.1% of the patients gave valid and reproducible health information.

Retrospective studies of cancer CAM treatments have also revealed that individual documentation of demographic, clinical, and treatment outcomes is possible if strong record-keeping procedures are in place.[81] This is important information for describing mortality issues as well as noting changes in health status through close monitoring. When using the clinical audit, researchers should be aware that collected data may be subject to bias through the use of self-reports, thus limiting accuracy of information. Criteria for inclusion and exclusion of all patients must be explicitly stated, and any coding of diagnoses should reflect precise, accurate parameters. The

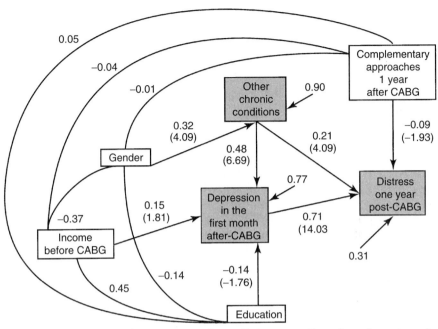

FIGURE 1–3. Model of complementary approaches predicting current distress in cardiac patients after surgery. Arrows between boxes represent a direct effect, with appropriate correlation coefficients and statistical t-test values in parentheses. Curved lines between boxes show bivariate associations with correlations. Stand-alone arrows (0.90, 0.77, 0.31) directed at darker boxes (endogenous variables) represent random error within the study. *CABG* = Coronary artery bypass grafting (surgery). *(From Amy AI: Personal communication, 1997.)*

clinical audit should be one way of collecting useful information about CAM in large-sample populations.

SYSTEMATIC REVIEW AND META-ANALYSIS

Data from one clinical research trial generally are not sufficient to provide adequate information regarding treatment efficacy, safety, or cost benefit. Rather, a focused evaluation of a specific topic (e.g., acupuncture, herbal therapies) must be done, with data pooled from several clinical trials and then analyzed and interpreted together. The two main objectives are to quantify any potential finding and evaluate the consistency of findings across several samples of patients. To be included in a meta-analysis, a study should meet these specified criteria: (1) adequate number of subjects in the study; (2) appropriate type of statistic to be used; (3) clearly stated hypothesis; (4) full description of all valid outcome measures used; (5) complete analysis of all data, and (6) listing of potential nuisance variables and limitations.[74] The relevance of meta-analysis to CAM is that it can become an acceptable format for including and determining which particular research studies accurately focus on specific parameters.

When evaluating groups of research articles, it is also important to determine how far back the evaluation should be made (generally 5 years), who and what will determine how treatment efficacy is described and established, and how publication bias will be handled. For example, does a bias exist against the publication of negative findings? Also, and especially relevant for CAM, in the absence of any negative findings, do collated, positive findings report a positive effect that may be falsely truncated? Sixteen studies reporting the significant effects of an herbal preparation or type of massage for the treatment of migraine headache may not be meaningful if 75 studies found no effect. Generally, however, the criteria used for inclusionary acceptance into a meta-analysis will serve to reduce a large number of reviewed studies to a very small number actually evaluated in the analysis. Further, many meta-analyses and systematic reviews do not consider commentary from other researchers published separately from the individual study results.

Recently, several articles have reviewed publication bias.[80,105] Small sample or poor methodology reduces the quality of studies found in a meta-analysis, as does exaggeration of treatment effects. Some "within subject variance" might be a useful parameter for deciding inclusion and/or combination with other clinical trials. Also, during review for journal publication, reviewers may reflect a bias toward nonacceptance of CAM studies even though the research may be technically strong.

Meta-analysis and systematic review can lead to better generalizations about treatment outcome. They do not provide the total answer, however, and care must be taken to avoid placing too much emphasis on any one type of methodology.

DATABASES

One of the early difficulties in evaluating CAM was finding adequate published research, which was often nonexistent, poorly done, or reported in foreign journals. Also, much of CAM continues to be published in a group of CAM clinical research journals that physicians either are unaware of or do not read. In the last several years, however, more conventional medical journals are publishing methodology and other issues regarding CAM. For example, Ai and Spencer[6] used a focused statistical procedure for evaluating CAM treatment in back and musculoskeletal rehabilitation; and the *Annals of Internal Medicine* has published a section devoted to CAM. The largest U.S. medical database is *Medline*, which is located through the National Library of Medicine at NIH. A subset of this database developed by CCAM features articles specifically describing and evaluating CAM. Additional information that can be indexed using Medline includes previous consensus and technology conferences. Some CAM articles are not included on Medline; other relevant and searchable databases include Psych Info, CHID, and Ovid Technologies (see Appendix B). CISCOM, the database for the Research Council for Complementary Medicine in England, uses part of the British Library and covers papers published since the mid-1960s. Other data sources distinct from bibliographic (text-based) resources are important because they can be used for standard case-level statistical analysis, subgrouping of investigations, and modification of data from original analyses.

The major internationally focused database is the Cochrane Library, which has formed a comprehensive registry of randomized control trials and systematic reviews.[82] The goal of the Cochrane Library is to facilitate decision making about potential treatments and their efficacy and safety using an evidence-based approach. This database includes a complementary therapy research evaluation section. Medline periodically accesses Cochrane reviews, and the clinical query feature of PubMed (Medline) can help search for systematic reviews using Cochrane abstracts from a Database of Abstracts of Reviews of Effectiveness (DARE). The Cochrane abstracts can be found at *www.update-software.com/cochrane/*. Full text articles require a paid subscription. In January 2002, 50 articles listed Cochrane reviews focused on CAM.

Transferring Clinical Research Information from Databases

For the clinician evaluating medical research, it becomes imperative that quick, current, and reliable information can support accurate decision making. Textbooks and journals may not be adequate because they do not always reflect the relevance of daily practice, and clinicians may have little time to form a plan for integration into patient care. For example, a survey of physicians revealed that when questioned regarding their perceived needs, most physicians cited the need to learn more about certain treatments, guidance on use, and personal psychologic support, including affirmation, commiseration, and feedback.[91]

As more patients ask questions about CAM, deficiencies in current information become apparent. The best tool for communicating research information should be electronic, portable, fast, and easy to use. A summary of clinical outcome studies in specific health categories cross-referenced by CAM therapy could be indexed. Databases can be set up so that when an individual patient is seen, information can be recorded in a clinical protocol with subjective comments and the records then electronically collated. The approach used should lead to better management of clinical information. Optimal treatment and effective patient-provider interaction should improve relationships among health care providers, patients, and the general public.

▨ Evidence-Based Medicine Considerations

One of several ways that CAM has a potential to be more fully accepted and integrated into conventional medicine is through the use of an *evidence-based analysis*,[64] which is a major feature of the clinical chapters in this book, and especially Chapter 14, where its interface with clinical practice is more fully described. Interest and information about evidence-based medicine (EBM) have been reported primarily for conventional medicine since the early 1990s. Currently, more than 7000 citations on Medline list EBM's applicability and results in medical and health articles. EBM involves critical appraisal of various types of research articles and information, including individual expert opinion, through searching the medical literature and then reporting and using the results with the strongest scientific base. The "best" type of clinical-research evidence remains somewhat debatable partly because of various types of designs currently in use and partly because of the types of questions asked and expectation(s) and usage of the results. (Again, refer to Chapter 14 to examine the posited types of designs that may have relevance.) The use of EBM will, however, have an influence on patient referral profiles and likely clinical benefits.

REPORTING CLINICAL VERSUS RESEARCH SIGNIFICANCE AS EVIDENCED BASED

Statistically based research as described previously is important for determining certain relationships, but the more important question is the extent to which the findings have clinical significance. That is, does a finding from a group of carefully selected research patients, with all nuisance variables controlled, mirror the individual patient in the clinician's office? How can interpretation be made of treatment effects that are simply numbers that describe group differences? Were the differences meaningful (real), or were they more relative to a particular diagnosis, population, age, or gender? Can treatment effects be extended to factors such as quality of life? For example, a patient with cancer may have debilitating effects such as hiccups from the chemotherapy, or an AIDS patient may have diarrhea from the multiple medications. In both cases the use of CAM needs to be considered for conditions beyond the disease process itself.

In attempting to evaluate CAM through EBM, the clinician must understand that information needs to be developed and reviewed concerning the extent to which CAM can move patients from *outside* the range of a dysfunctional healthy population to *inside* (or toward) the range of a more functional population.[52] The term *clinical significance* must be understood in the context of a change associated with the return of certain parameters of a normative group, including individual well-being. As they are weighing and deciding on treatments using EBM, clinicians must understand that their own beliefs as well as their patients' beliefs are shaped, are communicated, and may become an integral part of the evaluation quotient.[20]

Useful parameters that should be considered when making a determination of the clinical research that is to form an evidence base include: (1) whether the journal uses peer reviewers; (2) whether any consensual evidence has been reached through judges reviewing evidence; and (3) whether clinical guidelines have been written that would guide practice. Because CAM is still in its nascent state of thorough and systematic research evaluation, few consensus or technology assessments have been done. A panel convened in the mid-90s reported that a clinical research evidence base was insufficient to allow for any practice guidelines to be written at that time.[119]

CRITIQUING EBM

Although EBM can be useful in informing the clinician as well as the public, it is equally important to be aware of its shortcomings. Science produces empiric evidence, but clinical experience must be factored into any decision making, and areas of disagreement will always arise regarding interpretation of the scientific literature. This is especially true when studies do not report on comparisons between therapies but rather simply use placebo groups; the former is really of more interest to the clinician. Reviewing articles is time consuming, and the evaluation of all studies must have a "bottom line" prominently featured. Other intervening or additional variables, such as culture, safety, cost-effectiveness analysis, and involvement of family or significant others, must be factored into any clinical outcome analysis.

In the current decade, EBM is poised to be one of several prominent factors producing quality information that will be useful to the clinician. As CAM grows in terms of defining its own scope of practice and limitations, EBM will play a role in increasing CAM's credibility as well as improving the understanding of the practice of medicine at several levels. EBM must be a part of CAM's reference data, along with all aspects of training and education.

⚑ Training and Education Considerations

In this section, CAM's involvement with education and training is discussed. The focus is primarily within the undergraduate medical school programs. A more detailed description of the evolution of CAM at the graduate residency level of training, including subsequent integration with conventional medicine, can be found in Chapter 14.

The movement to provide CAM instruction within the medical school curriculum has gained momentum in the past few years. Box 1–1 lists medical schools (as of 2001) that offer either elective (68% stand alone) or required (31% part of another course) courses in CAM; Box 1–2 presents the medical schools that provide continuing medical education (CME) in CAM; and Box 1–3 lists postgraduate education opportunities. A 1998 survey reported that many CAM courses were devoted to such topics as acupuncture, chiropractic techniques, herbal therapies, homeopathy, and mind-body approaches.[116] Most courses were taught at an introductory level of expertise. The subject content of courses appears to vary greatly, indicating a possible need to standardize at least introductory CAM curricula. Certainly, students who desire additional "hands-on training" in CAM should be accommodated.

Almost a century ago, Dock[30] noted that, "There is a large number of reformers going about the country longing to give medical students more work. Some think that what a young doctor needs is a course of lectures on ethics, others, lectures on medical history, and so on." There has never been adequate time in the curriculum for all the things a medical student needs to know. One of the most common complaints made by external curriculum review committees is that the curriculum is too "dense," that too many hours of lecture are devoted to too much detail. The goal of curriculum reform is to allow time for more self-directed activities rather than adding more courses.

Course offerings in CAM within medical schools will meet resistance. One part of the difficulty is scheduled instruction time, but another is the lack of clear, clinical, and scientific evidence that the therapies are useful. However, a good justification for courses that introduce CAM to medical students is that patients will refer themselves to CAM practitioners while undergoing treatment by physicians. If the physician understands something about the CAM practitioner's therapeutic interventions, the activities can be potentially complementary, integrative, and more useful. At the very

BOX 1–1. U.S. Medical Schools Currently Offering Course(s) in Complementary and Alternative Medicine

Albany Medical College
Albert Einstein College of Medicine
Allegheny University School of Medicine
Boston University School of Medicine
Brown University School of Medicine
Case Western Reserve University School of Medicine
Chicago Medical School
City University of New York School of Medicine
Columbia University College of Physicians and Surgeons
Cornell Medical College
Dartmouth Medical School
Duke University School of Medicine
East Tennessee State University James H. Quillen College of Medicine
Eastern Virginia Medical School
Emory University School of Medicine
George Washington University School of Medicine
Georgetown University School of Medicine
Harvard Medical School
Howard University College of Medicine
Indiana University School of Medicine
Jefferson Medical College, Thomas Jefferson University
Johns Hopkins School of Medicine
Loyola University of Chicago School of Medicine
Mayo Medical School
Medical University of South Carolina
Michigan State University of Medicine
Morehouse School of Medicine
Mount Sinai School of Medicine
New York Medical College
Northeastern Ohio Universities College of Medicine
Northwestern University School of Medicine
Ohio State University College of Medicine
Oregon University School of Medicine
Pennsylvania State University College of Medicine
Rush Medical College
Southern Illinois University School of Medicine
St. Louis University School of Medicine
State University of New York at Brooklyn School of Medicine
State University of New York at Buffalo School of Medicine
State University of New York at Syracuse School of Medicine
Stanford University School of Medicine
Temple University School of Medicine
Tulane University School of Medicine
Tufts University School of Medicine

BOX 1–1. U.S. Medical Schools Currently Offering Course(s) in Complementary and Alternative Medicine

Uniformed Services University of the Health Sciences
Universidad Central del Caribe School of Medicine, Puerto Rico
University of Arizona School of Medicine
University of California, Los Angeles School of Medicine
University of California, San Diego School of Medicine
University of California, San Francisco School of Medicine
University of Chicago Pritzker School of Medicine
University of Cincinnati School of Medicine
University of Colorado School of Medicine
University of Connecticut School of Medicine College of Medicine
University of Illinois at Chicago School of Medicine
University of Illinois at Rockford College of Medicine
University of Iowa College of Medicine
University of Kansas School of Medicine
University of Louisville School of Medicine
University of Maryland School of Medicine
University of Medicine and Dentistry of New Jersey Medical School
University of Miami School of Medicine
University of Michigan School of Medicine
University of Minnesota School of Medicine
University of Nebraska School of Medicine
University of Nevada School of Medicine
University of New Mexico School of Medicine
University of North Carolina, Chapel Hill School of Medicine
University of Pennsylvania School of Medicine
University of Pittsburgh School of Medicine
University of Southern California School of Medicine
University of Texas, Dallas Southwestern Medical School
University of Texas Medical Branch at Galveston
University of Vermont College of Medicine
University of Virginia School of Medicine
University of Utah School of Medicine
University of Washington School of Medicine
University of Wisconsin Medical School
Vanderbilt University School of Medicine
Virginia Commonwealth University School of Medicine
Wake Forest University School of Medicine
Washington University School of Medicine
Wayne State University School of Medicine
West Virginia School of Medicine, Robert C. Byrd Health Sciences Center
Wright State University School of Medicine
Yale University School of Medicine

BOX 1–2. U.S. Medical Schools Offering Continuing Medical Education (CME) Courses in Complementary and Alternative Medicine

Columbia University College of Physicians and Surgeons
Botanical Medicine in Modern Clinical Practice

Harvard Medical School
Alternative Medicine: Implications for Clinical Practice
Clinical Training in Mind/Body Medicine

University of Arizona School of Medicine
Program in Integrative Medicine

University of California at Los Angeles School of Medicine
Medical Acupuncture for Physicians
Integrative East-West Medicine

University of Colorado Health Sciences Center
The Scientific Basis for Using Holistic Medicine to Treat Chronic Disease

University of Massachusetts Medical School
Evidence-Based Botanical Medicine

University of Minnesota School of Medicine
Complementary Care: From Principles to Practice
The Scientific Basis for the Holistic Treatment of Chronic Disease

University of New Mexico School of Medicine
Alternative Medicine

University of Vermont College of Medicine
The Scientific Basis for Using Holistic Medicine to Treat Chronic Disease

Wayne State University School of Medicine
A Course in Clinical Hypnosis: Basic Level

---

least, harmful interactions can be avoided. A recent survey revealed that many physicians are not familiar with herbal medicines or their potential toxicity with or without additional allopathic medicines, and the physicians are not versed in how to find such information.[89] Also, although integration with conventional medicine might be a goal to help maximize treatment benefit, health care providers still need to learn the vocabulary and nomenclature necessary for understanding CAM.

Required courses in CAM will not soon be part of the first 2 years of the medical student's training. Opportunities exist during clinical rotation, however, when it is appropriate to have students learn about the application of various CAM techniques and their potential integration with conventional treatment strategies. As CAM gains acceptance and questions are included on the national licensing examinations, CAM emphasis may be included in the predoctoral curriculum. OAM in the mid-1990s sponsored a conference on CAM in medical and nursing education, with participants sharing their experiences of teaching CAM in a variety of formats. The different approaches for teaching CAM included the following:

BOX 1–3. U.S. Medical Schools Offering Postgraduate Opportunities in Complementary and Alternative Medicine

Beth Israel Medical Center
Residency in Urban Family Practice
New York, NY

Montefiore Medical Center
Residency Program in Social Medicine
Bronx, NY

University of Arizona School of Medicine
Fellowship Program in Integrative Medicine
Department of Medicine
Tucson, Ariz

University of Maryland School of Medicine
Fellowship in Pain/Complementary Medicine
Division of Complementary Medicine
Baltimore, Md

University of Washington
Residency Program in Family Medicine
Ambulatory Pediatric Medicine
Seattle, Wash

- Present a series of visiting lectures for weekly discussions.
- Offer seminars on particular health maintenance approaches (e.g., t'ai chi) in which students could learn through participation.
- Offer CME credit and formal lectures describing CAM and specific methodology skills necessary to evaluate CAM so that physicians can more completely discuss its value with their patients.
- Develop the ability to evaluate the CAM research literature critically.

Critical evelution of the research is important because the future providers of health care in the United States will need to have some basis for making judgments about claims of CAM. Personal experiences and testimonies can be informative, but it is extremely important to have objective evidence for claims made. A recent paper discusses the need for organizing at least an introductory course in CAM around critical thinking and evaluation.[83] Accumulating evidence indicates the following[10,45]:

1. Medical students view CAM as a useful supplement to orthodox medicine and a helpful learning tool for practitioners of conventional medicine.
2. Practitioners should have some understanding of how CAM works.
3. Therapies not tested scientifically should not be encouraged.
4. Acupuncture, chiropractic, and massage therapy are believed to be more useful than faith healing, naturopathy, and homeopathy.
5. Although the students were not optimistic that they would receive adequate training in CAM, the most preferred teaching model would be by direct observation.

Agreement seems to be widespread on the general value of CAM instruction in medical schools, but there is less agreement on the practical problems of time and funding. CAM will be conceded as important but will most likely remain as an elective and limited in most curricula. Areas within the medical schools where CAM may become integrated are *behavioral* and *family* medicine because these areas include the patients most likely to use certain CAM therapies. Importantly, however, the integration of any type of unproven medical practice in the absence of strong evidence that it is useful and safe would be a waste of time. It may be necessary to provide content information about CAM so that physicians can discuss and understand their patients' questions. This form of integration will occur before medical students are taught a more hands-on approach to CAM.

SUMMARY

The major issues that impact the practice of CAM have evolved from many other areas, with many commonalities. Historical antecedents reveal that CAM is partially rooted in ancient cultures and beliefs, as well as in more modern, eclectic groups of practices. Some therapies have been "incorporated" into conventional medicine, including the use of certain plant products (e.g., foxglove in digitalis, *Rauwolfia* plants for antihypertensive drugs), diet, exercise, and vitamins for prevention and treatment of heart disease and joint manipulation for pain.[40] Definitions of CAM should attempt to be simple and flexible for change.[75]

Most of medical science, including physicians, has been slow to accept CAM, primarily because little information exists to demonstrate that these therapies are helpful and safe. All practicing health providers need to become more knowledgeable about CAM therapies as more consumers increasingly use these procedures. Practice guidelines will help make the profession more credible.

To date, the quality of CAM research has generally been poor. A science-based evaluation is required to develop more focused and creative ways to evaluate targeted areas in CAM.[97] Relevant outcome research should include an evidenced-based approach. Researchers should continue to standardize information about certain therapies such as herbal medicine using a broad range of activities, including active substances used throughout the world, and listing the most successful plants and therapies. Closer evaluation, replication, extension, and further development of other research strategies, as discussed in later chapters, are needed. This is true for the evaluation of treatments, diagnostic methods, and techniques.

The argument is made that the acceptance of CAM will depend on how well it is able to demonstrate both clinically and scientifically that its therapies are both safe and useful.

REFERENCES

1. Acupuncture, National Institutes of Health Consensus Development Conference Statement, 1997, Bethesda, Md.
2. Ader R, Cohen N: Behaviorally conditioned immunosuppression, *Psychosom Med* 37:333, 1975.

3. Adler N, Matthews K: Health psychology: why do some people get sick and some stay well? *Annu Rev Psychol* l45:229, 1994.

4. Agency for Health Care Policy and Research: Acute pain management: operative or medical procedures and trauma, Pub No AHCPR 92-0032, Rockville, Md, 1992.

5. Ai A, Peterson C, Bolling SF: Psychological recovery following coronary artery bypass graft surgery: the use of complementary therapies, *J Altern Complement Med Res Paradigm Pract Policy* 3(4):343, 1997.

6. Ai A, Spencer J: The use of structural equation models for analyzing the multi factors associated with neuromuscular rehabilitation, *J Back Musculoskel Rehabil* 10(2):97, 1998.

7. Andritzky W: Medical students and alternative medicine: a survey, *Gesundheitswesn* 6:345, 1995.

8. Anthony HM: Some methodological problems in the assessment of complementary therapy. In Lewith GT, Aldridge D, editors: *Clinical research methodology for complementary therapies*, London, 1993, Hodder and Stoughton.

9. Assendelft WJ et al: The relationship between methodological quality and conclusions in reviews of spinal manipulation, *JAMA* 274(24):1942, 1995.

10. Baugniet J, Boon H, Ostbye T: Complementary/alternative medicine: comparing the views of medical students with students in other health care professions, *Fam Med* 32:3178, 2000.

11. Beecher HK: The powerful placebo, *JAMA* 159:1602, 1955.

12. Benson H: *Timeless healing: the power of biology and belief,* New York, 1996, Scribner.

13. Benson H, Crassweller SE: Relaxation response: bridge between psychiatry and medicine, *Med Clin North Am* 61:929, 1977.

14. Berman BM, Larsen D, editors: *Alternative medicine: expanding medical horizons—a report to the National Institutes of Health on alternative medical systems and practices in the United States,* Pub No 94-066, Bethesda, Md, 1994.

15. Berman BM et al: Physicians' attitudes toward complementary or alternative medicine: a regional survey, *J Am Board Fam Pract* 8:36l, 1995.

16. Berman BM et al: Primary care physicians and complementary-alternative medicine: training, attitudes and practice patterns, *J Am Board Fam Pract* 11:272, 1998.

17. Blackwell B, Bloomfield SS, Buncher CR: Demonstration to medical students of placebo responses and non-drug factors, *Lancet* 1:1279, 1972.

18. Borkan J et al: Referrals for alternative therapies, *J Fam Pract* 39(6): 545, 1994.

19. Brolinson PG et al: Nurses' perceptions of the effectiveness of alternative and complementary therapies, *J Community Health* 26, no 3 Jun, 175, 2001.

20. Brophy JM, Lawrence J: Placing trials in context using Bayesian analysis, *JAMA* 273(11):871, 1995.

21. Cappuccio FP et al: Use of alternative medicines in a multi-ethnic population, *Ethn Dis* 11(1):11, 2001.

22. Cassileth BR: Contemporary unorthodox treatments in cancer medicine: a study of patients, *Ann Intern Med* 101:105, 1984.

23. Cassileth BR et al: Survival and quality of life among patients receiving unproven as compared with conventional cancer therapy, *N Engl J Med* 324:1180, 1991.

24. Chandrashekara S et al: Complementary and alternative drug therapy in arthritis, *J Assoc Physicians India* 50: 225, 2002.

25. Child A: Illness and healing. In *Religion and magic in the life of traditional peoples,* Englewood Cliffs, NJ, 1993, Prentice-Hall.

26. Cohen J: The differences between proportions. In *Statistical power analysis for the behavioral sciences,* New York, 1977, Academic Press.

27. Cohen J: A power primer, *Psychol Bull* 112(1):155, 1992.

28. Danesi MA, Adetunji JB: Use of alternative medicine by patients with epilepsy: a survey of 265 epileptic patients in a developing country, *Epilepsia* 35(2):344, 1994.

29. D'Antoni ML, Harvey PL, Fried MP: Alternative medicine: does it play a role in the management of voice disorders? *J Voice* 9(3):308, 1995.

30. Dock G: Medical ethics and etiquette, *Physician Surgeon* 28:481, 1906.

31. Druss BG, Rosenheck RA: Association between use of unconventional therapies and conventional medical services, *JAMA* 282(7):651. 1999.

32. Eisenberg DM: Perceptions about complementary therapies relative to conventional therapies among adults who use both: results from a national survey, *Ann Intern Med* 135: 344, 2001.

33. Eisenberg DM et al.: Trends in alternative medicine use in the United States, 1990–1997, *JAMA* 280(18):1569, 1998.
34. Eisenberg DM et al: Unconventional medicine in the United States: prevalence, costs and patterns of use, *N Engl J Med* 328:246, 1993.
35. Ernst E, Resch KL, White AR: Complementary medicine: what physicians think of it—a meta-analysis, *Arch Intern Med* 155:2405, 1995.
36. Evans FJ: The placebo response in pain reduction, *Adv Neurol* 4:289, 1974.
37. Fisher P, Ward A: Complementary medicine in Europe, *Br Med J* 309(6947):107, 1994.
38. Furnham A: How the public classify complementary medicine: a factor analytic study, *Complement Ther Med* 8:82, 2000.
39. Furnham A, Forey J: The attitudes, behaviors and beliefs of conventional vs. complementary (alternative) medicine, *J Clin Psychol* 50(3):458, 1994.
40. Gevitz N: Unorthodox medical theories. In Bynum WF, Porter R, editors: *Companion encyclopedia of the history of medicine*, London, 1993, Routledge.
41. Glass RM, Flanagin A: New requirements for authors submitting manuscripts to JAMA, *JAMA* 277:74, 1997.
42. Gordon G: Is there a need to devise clinical trials that do not depend on randomized controlled testing? *Adv J Mind Health* 9(2), 1993.
43. Gordon JS: The paradigm of holistic medicine. In *Health for the whole person*, Boulder, Colo, 1980, Westview.
44. Gregor JL. Dietary supplement use: consumer characteristics and interests, *J Nutr* 131:1339S, 2001.
45. Greiner KA, Murray JL, Kallail KJ: Medical student interest in alternative medicine, *J Altern Complement Med* 6(3):231, 2000.
46. Guyatt GH et al: The n-of-1 randomized controlled trial: clinical usefulness, *Ann Intern Med* 112:293, 1990.
47. Harris P, Rees R: The prevalence of complementary and alternative medicine use among the general population: a systematic review of the literature, *Complement Ther Med* 8:88, 2000.
48. Hart A: Randomized controlled trials: the control group dilemma revisited, *Complement Ther Med* 9:40, 2001.
49. Hatch JP, Fisher JG, Rugh JD: *Biofeedback studies in clinical efficacy*, New York, 1987, Plenum.
50. Himmel W, Schulte M, Kochen MM: Complementary medicine: are patients' expectations being met by their general practitioners? *Br J Gen Pract* 43(371):232, 1993.
51. Hrobjartsson A, Gotzsche PC: Is the placebo powerless? An analysis of clinical trials comparing placebo with no treatment, *N Engl J Med* 344(21):1594, 2001.
52. Jacobson NS, Truax P: Clinical significance: a statistical approach to defining meaningful change in psychotherapy research, *J Consult Clin Psychol* 59(1):12, 1991.
53. Jonas W: Evaluating unconventional medical practices, *J NIH Res* 5:64, 1993.
54. Kaptchuk TJ, Eisenberg DM: Varieties of healing. 2. A taxonomy of unconventional healing practices, *Ann Intern Med* 135:196, 2001.
55. Kessler RC et al: Long-term trends in the use of complementary and alternative medical therapies in the United States, *Ann Intern Med* 135:262, 2001.
56. King LS: The Flexner Report of 1910, *JAMA* 251(8):1079, 1984.
57. Kleijnen J, Knipschild P, Rietter G: Clinical trials of homeopathy, *Br Med J* 302(316):23, 1991.
58. Kleinman A: *The illness narrative: suffering, healing and the human condition*, New York, 1988, Basic Books.
59. Konner M: *Medicine at the crossroads*, New York, 1994, Vintage Books.
60. Langmead L et al: Use of complementary therapies by patients with IBD may indicate psychosocial stress, *Inflamm Bowel Dis* 8(3):174, 2002.
61. Larson D, Milano M: Religion and mental health: should they work together? *J Altern Complement Ther* 2(2):91, 1996.
62. Leplege A, Hunt S: The problem of quality of life in medicine, *JAMA* 278(1):47, 1997.
63. Levine JD, Gordon NC, Fields HL: The mechanism of placebo analgesia, *Lancet* 2:654, 1978.
64. Lewith GT: The use and abuse of evidence-based medicine: an example from general medicine. In Ernst E, editor: *Complementary medicine: an objective appraisal*, Oxford, 1996, Butterworth-Heinemann.

65. Lewith GT, Aldridge D, editors: *Clinical research methodology for complementary therapies*, London, 1993, Hodder and Stoughton.
66. Liu CA, Xiao PG: *An introduction to Chinese materia medicine*, Beijing, 1993, Peking Union Medical College, Beijing Medical University.
67. Liverani A, Minelli E, Ricciuti A: Subjective scales for the evaluation of therapeutic effects and their use in complementary medicine, *J Altern Complement Med* 6(3):257, 2000.
68. Long L et al: Which complementary and alternative therapies benefit which conditions? A survey of the opinions of 223 professional organizations, *Complement Ther Med* 9(3):178, 2001.
69. Mayberg H et al: The functional neuroanatomy of the placebo effect, *Am J Psychiatry* 159(5):728, 2002.
70. Max MB et al: Amitriptyline relieves diabetic neuropathy pain in patients with normal or depressed mood, *Neurology* 37:89, 1987.
71. McKorkle R, Young K: Development of a symptom distress scale, *Cancer Nurs* 1(5):373, 1978.
72. Melchart D et al: Systematic clinical auditing in complementary medicine: rationale, concept and pilot study, *Altern Ther Health Med* 3(1):33, 1997.
73. Michle W: Chronic polyarthritis treatment with alternative medicine: how frequent is self therapy with alternative methods? *Fortschr Med* 113(7):81, 1995.
74. Nony P et al: Critical reading of the meta-analysis of clinical trials, *Therapie* 50:339, 1995.
75. O'Connor B et al: Defining and describing complementary and alternative medicine, *Altern Ther Health Med* 3(2):49, 1997.
76. Oh VM: The placebo effect: how can we use it better? *Br Med J* 309:69, 1994.
77. Patel M: Problems in the evaluation of alternative medicine, *Soc Sci Med* 25(6):669, 1987.
78. Pogge RC: The toxic placebo. I. Side and toxic effects reported during the administration of placebo medicine, *Med Times* 91:1, 1963.
79. Reilly DT: Young doctors' views on alternative medicine, *Br Med J* 287:337, 1983.
80. Resch KI, Ernst E, Garrow J: A randomized controlled study of reviewer bias against an unconventional therapy, *J R Soc Med* 93:164, 2000.
81. Richardson MA et al: Assessment of outcomes at alternative medicine cancer clinics: a feasibility study, *J Altern Complement Med* 7(1):19, 2001.
82. Robinson A: Research practice and the Cochrane Collaboration, *Can Med Assoc J* 152(6):883, 1995.
83. Sampson W: The need for educational reform in teaching about alternative therapies, *Acad Med* 76(3):248, 2001.
84. Schachter L, Weingartern MA, Kahan EE: Attitudes of family physicians to non-conventional therapies: a challenge to science as the basis of therapeutics, *Arch Fam Med* 2(12):1268, 1993.
85. Schar A, Messerli-Rohrbach V, Schubarth P: Conventional or complementary medicine: what criteria for choosing do patients use? *Schweiz Med Wochenschr Suppl* 62:18, 1994.
86. Scott S, Spencer J: Faith supportive group therapy and symptom reduction for Christian breast cancer patients. Paper presented at National Conference of Christian Association for Psychological Studies, Richmond, Va, 2001.
87. Shafranske EP, Malony HN: Clinical psychologists' religious and spiritual orientations and their practice of psychotherapy, *Psychotherapy* 27(1):72, 1990.
88. Shapiro AK, Shapiro E: Patient-provider relationships and the placebo effect. In Matarazzo JD et al, editors: *Behavioral health: a handbook of health enhancement and disease prevention*, New York, 1984, Wiley-Interscience.
89. Silverstein DD, Spiegel AD: Are physicians aware of the risks of alternative medicine? *J Community Health* 26(3):59, 2001.
90. Singer C: *Galen on anatomical procedures*, New York, 1956, Oxford University.
91. Smith R: What clinical information do doctors need? *Br Med J* 313:1062, 1996.
92. Sobell LC, Sobell MD, Nirneberg TD: Assessment and treatment planning with substance abusers, *Clin Psychol Rev* 8:19, 1988.
93. Spencer J: Maximization of biofeedback following cognitive stress pre-selection in generalized anxiety, *Percept Mot Skills* 63:239, 1986.
94. Spencer J: So, is counseling useful? Lessons from research, *Christian Counseling Today* 7(4):78, 1999.

95. Spencer J: The use of human subjects in clinical research. In Primack A, Spencer J, editors: *The collection and evaluation of clinical data relevant to alternative medicine and cancer,* Conference report, Bethesda, Md, 1996, National Institutes of Health.

96. Spencer J, Beckner W, Jacobs J: *Demographics of the first exploratory grant program in alternative medicine at the NIH.* Paper presented at 29th Proceedings of U.S. Public Health Commissioned Officers Meeting, Baltimore, 1994.

97. Spencer J, Jonas W: And now alternative medicine, *Arch Fam Med* 6:155, 1997.

98. Spencer J, Shanor K: Mind-body medicine. In Shanor K, editor: *The emerging mind,* Los Angeles, 1999, Renaissance Books.

99. Spencer J, Thomas J: Psychiatric diagnostic profiles in hospitalized adolescent and adult Navajo Indians, *Soc Psychiatry Psychiatr Epidemiol* 27:226, 1992.

100. Spencer J et al: Microtremors during a sustained concentration task from boys previously exposed to opiates in utero, *J Child Adolesc Subst Abuse* 7(2)53: 1997.

101. Spitzer WO et al: Measuring quality of life of cancer patients: a concise QL index for use by physicians, *J Chron Dis* 34:585, 1981.

102. Standish LJ et al: Alternative medicine use in HIV-positive men and women: demographics, utilization patterns and health status, *AIDS Care* 13(2):197, 2001.

103. Starr P: *The social transformation of American medicine,* New York, 1982, Basic Books.

104. Steering Committee for Prince of Wales Initiative on Integrated Health Care: A way forward, *J Altern Complement Med* 4(2):209, 1998.

105. Sterne JA, Egger M, Smith GD: Investigating and dealing with publication and other biases in meta-analysis, *BMJ* 323:101, 2001.

106. Sturm R: Patient risk-taking attitude and the use of complementary and alternative medical services, *J Altern Complement Med* 6(5):445, 2000.

107. Surwit D: Diabetes: mind over metabolism. In *Mind-body medicine: how to use your mind for better health,* Yonkers, NY, 1993, Consumer Reports Books.

108. Turner J et al: The importance of placebo effects in pain treatment and research, *JAMA* 271(20):1609, 1994.

109. United States Congress, Office of Technology Assessment: *Unconventional cancer treatments,* Pub No OTA-H-405, Washington, DC, 1990, US Government Printing Office.

110. Veith I: *The Yellow Emperor's classic of internal medicine,* ed 2, Birmingham, Ala, 1988, Gryphon.

111. Verhoef MJ, Sutherland LR: General practitioners' assessment of and interest in alternative medicine in Canada, *Soc Sci Med* 41(4):511, 1995.

112. Vincent CA: Acupuncture as a treatment for chronic pain. In Lewith GT, Aldridge D, editors: *Clinical research methodology for complementary therapies,* London, 1993, Hodder and Stoughton.

113. Vincent C, Furnham A: *Complementary medicine: a research perspective,* Chichester, NY, 1997, Wiley & Sons.

114. Voudouris NJ, Peck CL, Coleman G: The role of conditioning and verbal expectancy in the placebo response, *Pain* 43:121, 1990.

115. Wardwell WI: Alternative medicine in the United States, *Soc Sci Med* 38(8):1061, 1994.

116. Wetzel MS, Eisenberg DM, Kaptchuk TJ: Courses involving complementary and alternative medicine at U.S. medical schools, *JAMA* 280(9):784, 1998.

117. White L, Tursky B, Schwarz GE: *Placebo theory research and mechanism,* New York, 1985, Guilford.

118. Wiegant FAC, Kramers CW, van Wijk R: The importance of patient selection. In Lewith GT, Aldridge D, editors: *Clinical research methodology for complementary therapies,* London, 1993, Hodder and Stoughton.

119. Woolf SH: Clinical practice guidelines in complementary and alternative medicine: an analysis of opportunities and obstacles, *Arch Fam Med* 6:149, 1997.

120. Wootton JC, Sparber A: Surveys of complementary and alternative medicine. Part 1. General trends and demographic groups, *J Altern Complement Med* 7(2):195, 2001.

121. World Health Organization Quality of Life Assessment (WHOQOL) Group: Position paper from the World Health Organization, *Soc Sci Med* 41:1403, 1995.

SUGGESTED READINGS

Ader R, Felton D, Cohen N: *Psychoneuroimmunology,* ed 3, San Diego, 2001, Academic Press.

Benson H: *Beyond the relaxation response,* New York, 1984, Berkeley Books.

Berman B, Larson DB, editors: *Alternative medicine: expanding medical horizons,* Washington, DC, 1995, US Government Printing Office.

Blumenthal M, Goldberg A, Brinchmann J: *Herbal medicine,* Expanded Commission E monographs, Newton, Mass, 2000, Integrative Medicine Communications.

Castleman M: *The healing herbs,* Emmaus, Pa, 1991, Rodale.

Charman RA: *Complementary therapies for physical therapists,* Boston, 2000, Oxford, Butterworth-Heinemann.

The complementary and alternative medicine (CAM) coding manual, V200R5, ed 2, Las Cruces, NM, 2000, Alternative Link.

Egger M, Smith D, Altman D, editors: *Systematic reviews in health care: meta-analysis in context,* ed 2, London, 2001, BMJ Books.

Engel L et al, editors: *The science of the placebo: toward an interdisciplinary research agenda,* London, 2002, BMJ Books.

Friedland DJ et al: *Evidence-based medicine: a framework for clinical practice,* Stamford, Conn, 1998, Appleton & Lange/Simon & Schuster.

Fritz S: *Mosby's Fundamentals of therapeutic massage,* St Louis, 1995, Mosby.

Fromm E, Nash MR, editors: *Contemporary hypnosis research,* New York, 1992, Guilford.

Geyman JP, Deyo RA, Ramsey SD, editors: *Evidence-based clinical practice: concepts and approaches,* Boston, 2000, Butterworth-Heinemann.

Goldberg B: *Alternative medicine,* ed 2, Puyallup, Wash, 2002, Future Medicine.

Grim LG, Yarnold PR, editors: *Reading and understanding multivariate statistics,* Washington, DC, 1997, American Psychological Association.

Jonas W, Jacobs J: *Healing with homeopathy,* New York, 1996, Warner Books.

Novey D: *Clinician's complete reference to complementary and alternative medicine,* St Louis, 2000, Mosby.

Peters D: *Integrating complementary medicine in primary care: a practical guide for health professionals,* New York, 2002, Churchill Livingstone.

Peters D: *Understanding the placebo effect in complementary medicine: theory, practice, and research,* New York, 2001, Churchill Livingstone.

Shanor K, editor: *The emerging mind,* Los Angeles, 1999, Renaissance Press.

Shapiro A, Shapiro E: *The powerful placebo: from ancient priest to modern physician,* Baltimore, 1997, Johns Hopkins University Press.

Standish L, Calbreese C, Galatino ML: *AIDS and complementary & alternative medicine: current science and practice,* New York, 2002, Churchill Livingstone.

Stuk G, Hammerschlag R, editors: *Clinical acupuncture: scientific basis,* Berlin, 2001, Springer.

CHAPTER 2

Preclinical Research in Complementary and Alternative Medicine

RU-LONG REN, CHUNG-KWANG CHOU, and JOHN W. SPENCER

Preclinical research is important for complementary and alternative medicine (CAM) because an understanding of study findings helps to determine the safety and efficacy of CAM therapies and leads to better treatment methods for diseases such as cancer. CAM includes lifestyle practices, clinical tests, and therapeutic modalities that are promoted for the prevention, diagnosis, and treatment of diseases.[9,25] Therefore the determination of the safety and efficacy of these practices is a priority.

When in vitro, in vivo, and clinical trials prove efficacy and safety, CAM therapies can become a part of mainstream medicine. If the safety and effectiveness of such treatments remain unproved, the methods or agents should be abandoned to save money and avoid unnecessary harm to the public. For example, Laetrile (amygdalin) was thought to have anticancer effects and achieved great popularity in the United States in the 1970s, eventually being legalized for use in 27 states. Public interest resulted in a National Cancer Institute (NCI) study that showed no effect for Laetrile against cancer.[54]

Some CAM treatments have already been used in clinics as effective methods. Because systematic preclinical studies are lacking, however, the optimal therapeutic method may not be established, and the maximum effects may not be achieved. For example, electrochemical treatment (EChT) for cancer has been used in China and Europe in thousands of patients. Although shown to be an effective, safe alternative therapy for some cancers,[48,60,85,86] EChT is not a well-established method. We believe that if an optimal method is established and the mechanisms of EChT cell death are understood through a number of preclinical studies, EChT will provide a more effective and understandable alternative therapy for some localized cancers.

In describing the development of preclinical studies in CAM, this chapter uses the example of *cancer*, a major medical health problem in many cultures. Preclinical studies are defined as basic research and clinical trials (Phases I to III). It is important to recognize that basic research in CAM attempts to understand an *existing* therapy rather than developing a new one, which is the case for much of conventional research. Ernst[27] correctly points out that basic research for CAM can be positive if guidelines for quality and an understanding of needs are operative and can be tied to appropriate clinical practice. This effort is no easy task, however; as the chapters in this text clearly illustrate, the beginning of the twenty-first century is marked by conundrum and debate surrounding CAM research, evidence-based knowledge, and clinical practice.

⬥ Development of a New Drug in Conventional Medicine

In most countries, tests of drugs and medical devices are regulated by legislation and closely monitored by government agencies. In the United States, federal consumer protection laws require that drugs and devices used for the prevention, diagnosis, or treatment of disease be demonstrated as both safe and effective before being marketed.[52] To meet these requirements, preclinical and clinical evaluations of a new treatment must follow several steps in the evaluation of its potential effectiveness and safety. The regulatory agencies also require full disclosure of how products are manufactured, how devices are designed, and how they function. This section describes the process of the discovery, development, and regulation of a new drug.* The process involves substantial time, effort, and resources, as described by Berkowitz and Katzung[5] and Grever and Chabner.[32]

The first step in the development of a new drug is to discover or synthesize a potential *new drug molecule.* Most new drug candidates are identified (1) through empiric, random screening of biologic activity of many natural products resulting from rational chemical modification of a known molecule or (2) by designing a molecule based on an understanding of biologic mechanisms and chemical structure. A variety of biologic in vitro and in vivo assays (at the molecular, cell, organ, and whole-animal levels) are used to define a drug's activity and selectivity. Subsequently, more potent, less toxic derivatives often can be developed through these studies.

The second step in the development of a new drug is to conduct *pharmacologic studies* that include safety and toxicity tests. Candidate drugs that survive the initial screening and profiling procedures must be carefully evaluated for potential risks before beginning clinical testing.

Preclinical toxicology is frequently the third step in the progression of a new drug from discovery to initial Phase I clinical trials in humans. The major types of preclinical toxicologic studies are (1) acute toxicity, (2) subacute and chronic toxicity,

---

*References 2, 5, 13, 32, 49, 90

(3) effects on reproductive functions including teratogenicity, (4) carcinogenicity, and (5) mutagenicity.[5,32,33,74] The major objectives of the preclinical toxicologic studies include the definition of the qualitative and quantitative organ toxicities, the reversibility of these effects, and the initial safe starting dose proposed for humans. Important quantitative estimates include the *no-effect dose,* which is the smallest dose that is observed to kill any animal, and the *median lethal dose,* which is the dose that kills approximately 50% of the animals.

It is important to recognize the limitations of preclinical testing. There is no guarantee that the human subject will accommodate a new drug in the same way as an animal species. Extrapolation of toxicity data from animals to humans is not completely reliable. For any given compound, the total toxicity data from all species have a very high predictive value for its toxicity in humans; however, there are limitations on the amount of information that is practical to obtain. In addition, because large numbers of animals are needed to obtain preclinical data, toxicity testing is time-consuming and expensive. For statistical reasons, rare adverse effects are unlikely to be detected, as in clinical trials.

The fourth step in the development of a new drug is *human evaluation.* Testing in humans begins after sufficient acute and subacute animal toxicity studies have been completed. Chronic safety testing in animals is usually conducted concurrent with clinical trials. Evaluation in humans includes three formal phases of clinical trials. Only after showing positive Phase III results on efficacy and safety can the new drug be permitted to be marketed for further postmarketing surveillance.[2,5,72]

The objective of *Phase I* trials is to determine a dose that is appropriate for use in Phase II trials. There are several different types of Phase I trials.[72] These trials are non-blind, or "open." A small number of healthy volunteers or patients with advanced disease resistant to standard therapy are included in such trials. However, it is important that the patients have normal organ functions because important pharmacokinetic parameters, such as absorption of drugs, the half-life of maximum tolerated dose, and metabolism, are often determined in this phase of trials. Many predictable toxicities are detected. Phase I trials establish the drug's effects as a function of dosage. Because of the small sample size of Phase I trials, the pharmacokinetic parameters are generally determined imprecisely.

In *Phase II* trials the treatment is normally disease type specific, and the goal is to identify the disease types suitable for treatment. The drug is studied for the first time in patients with the target disease to determine the drug's efficacy. A broader range of toxicities may be detected in this phase. A small number of patients are studied in great detail. A single-blind design is often used.

Phase III is the controlled clinical trial in which the new treatment is compared with a conventional therapy. Based on the information gathered in Phases I and II, this trial will further establish drug safety and efficacy in a much larger number of patients. Certain toxic effects, especially those caused by sensitization, may become apparent for the first time during Phase III. Double-blind and crossover techniques are frequently employed. Phase III studies can be difficult to design and execute and are usually expensive because of the large numbers of patients involved and the massive amount of data that must be collected and analyzed.

▟ Electrochemical Treatment for Cancer

Electrochemical treatment (EChT) of cancer involves inserting platinum electrodes into tumors of conscious patients. A constant voltage of less than 10 V is applied to produce a 40-mA to 80-mA current between the anodes and cathodes for 30 minutes to several hours, delivering 100 coulombs (C) per cubic centimeter (cm^3). As a result of electrolysis, electrophoresis, and electroosmosis, cells near the electrodes are killed by the microenvironmental changes. From 1993 to 1998 this method was investigated at the City of Hope National Medical Center in Duarte, California.[18,69,88]

Nordenström[59-61] was the first in recent years to use *direct current* (DC) for the treatment of human tumors. He treated 26 lung metastases in 20 patients. Twelve of the 26 metastases regressed totally. Two patients with 5 of the 26 tumors were still alive 10 years later. In Japan, Nakayama[55] and Matsushima et al.[47] treated human cancer with EChT combined with chemotherapy and radiation. Matsushima et al.[48] summarized 26 patients treated with EChT, including two cases of breast cancer (the majority of the 26 cases were inoperable because of poor general condition of the patient or an advanced cancer stage). Symptoms improved (pain relief) in almost 50% of the patients. A decrease in tumor size to some degree was observed in 21 measurable lesions, two tumors disappeared completely, and no tumor cells remained in one patient who underwent a histopathologic examination. These results showed the usefulness of EChT alone to treat tumors, because the two tumors that completely disappeared had not responded to other, previous treatments. The main complication was pain during treatment; however, pain spontaneously disappeared and did not require specific treatment.

In 1987, Nordenström introduced EChT to China. Because of the large patient load and authority of physicians in China, physicians were able to use EChT on thousands of patients with various cancers.[85] Xin[86] summarized the results of 2516 cases on 23 types of tumors. The primary cases were cancer of the lung (593), liver (388), skin (366), and breast (228). The 5-year survival rates were 31.7%, 17%, 67%, and 62.7%, respectively. In addition, EChT produces minimal trauma compared with surgery. Also, unlike radiation therapy or chemotherapy, no serious side effects occur with EChT, and treatment can be repeated. Chinese physicians concluded that EChT is a simple, effective local therapy. The local control rates were considered satisfactory compared with those of conventional therapy. This method has been approved by the Chinese Ministry of Public Health and is used in approximately 1000 hospitals.[85]

PRECLINICAL ISSUES

Although EChT is already prevalent in clinical practice in China, and a number of clinical studies have shown that EChT has an antitumor effect, EChT has not been widely accepted in world clinics. The reason is that EChT is not a well-established method. The data lack essential preclinical studies, and reliable control of the clinical trials is missing. Review of literature pertaining to this topic shows that precise guidelines regarding electrode insertion and electrical parameters (i.e., voltage, current, treatment duration) are not available.

Therefore EChT can be a feasible treatment for some cancer patients, but we are not certain that the method presently used has achieved its optimal effectiveness. More basic research to address preclinical issues is necessary before EChT can be used for patients in the United States. Compared with the steps of preclinical evaluation of conventional medicine, the following research priorities must be given to EChT preclinical evaluation.

METHODOLOGY STUDIES

To make EChT a reliable, effective method for treating cancers, a standardized treatment must be determined. At this time, published clinical studies have shown various electrode insertion methods and distributions; different electrode placements have been used in Europe and China. Optimal electrode distribution has not been determined.

Electrode Insertion

Nordenström[60] of Sweden introduced the *biologically closed electric-circuit* (BCEC) concept. He named it the "third circuit" in the human body, after cardiovascular and lymphatic circuits. The BCEC circulates through the vascular interstitial closed circuit (VICC). Nordenström[62] believes that EChT is an artificial activation of the BCEC through the VICC. The flow of ionic current triggers interactions between the induced electromagnetic fields and the cancer tissue.

Therefore Nordenström has been treating his lung cancer patients with the anode inserted in the tumor center and the cathode in normal tissue several centimeters away from the tumor boundary. European researchers and physicians have followed this method. In China, Xin et al.[87] modified the technique, putting both anode and cathode into the tumor, with the anode in the center and cathodes in the periphery. Chinese physicians have found that placing both the anodes and cathodes in tumors not only protected the normal tissue but also had a greater effect on the tumor.

To resolve the discrepancies of whether both the anode and the cathode should be inserted within the tumor or whether the cathode should be in normal tissue, a detailed animal study should be conducted to test whether induced cell damage occurs around the anode and cathode during EChT. The morphologic responses of the EChT-treated cells near the anode and cathode should be studied to understand their pathologic mechanism. By comparing the cellular changes in tumors with those of normal muscles after EChT, this preclinical study would determine whether the placement of the cathode in normal tissue can cause problems.

Electrode Configuration

Another important preclinical issue in the study of EChT is electrode configuration. The studies described earlier would answer the questions of where the electrodes should be inserted and how many electrodes should be used. After several thousand patient treatments, Chinese physicians found that for superficial tumors, vertically inserting the electrodes into the tumor resulted in many cases of cancer cells recurring at the base of the tumor, because the electric field generated at the tip is too small to destroy cells at the base of the tumor. However, by horizontally inserting an adequate number of electrodes at the tumor base, much better results were produced.

We also observed this phenomenon in our animal studies.[18] Our preliminary mouse study,[18] using either two or five vertical electrodes or two horizontal electrodes through the central part of the tumor, did not produce a high cure rate (Figures 2–1 and 2–2). Later, in our rat study we adapted the tumor base method by inserting either six or seven electrodes at the tumor base perpendicular to the long axis of the tumor. Eighteen of 24 rats were cured for more than 6 months (Figures 2–3 and 2–4). From the Chinese clinical experience and our animal results, we believe that inserting electrodes at the base of the tumor is the best method of EChT treatment of superficial tumors.

Spacing of Electrodes

The number of electrodes to be used depends on the tumor size and nature. Because the effective volume of the treatment is limited to the vicinity of the electrodes, covering the tumor region with an adequate number of electrodes was thought to be essential. In China it was reported that the effective volume around each electrode is about 3 cm in diameter; therefore spacing between electrodes is usually kept at less than 2 cm. However, it is not known for what type of tumor this range is effective. Japanese practitioners have used 3-cm to 4-cm spacing. In Slovenia the cathode (not the anode) was

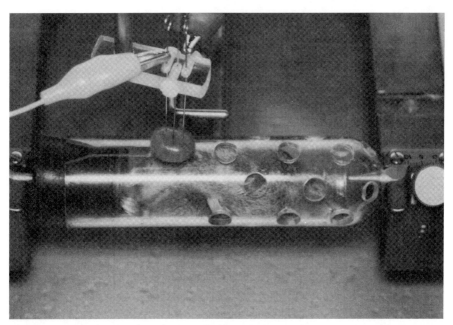

FIGURE 2–1. Two platinum electrodes vertically inserted into C3H/HeJ mice RIF-1 tumor at a spacing between 4 and 10 mm, depending on tumor size. A thermocouple for temperature measurement is in the central position.

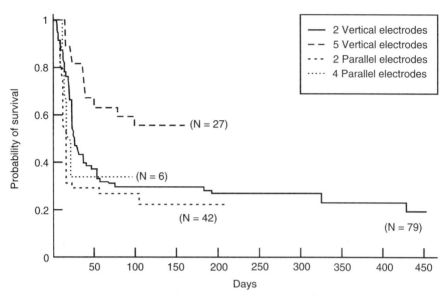

FIGURE 2–2. Electrochemical treatment survival curves showing results for four groups of C3H/HeJ mice. The best results were with four electrodes inserted parallel to the body. (*Modified from Chou CK et al: Bioelectromagnetics 18:14, 1997.*)

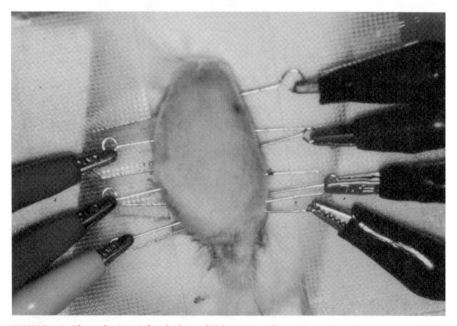

FIGURE 2–3. Electrodes inserted at the base of Fisher 344 rat fibrosarcoma. Insertion was perpendicular to the long axis of the tumor, and an arrangement of alternating cathodes and anodes was used.

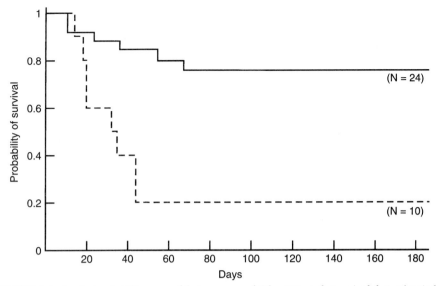

FIGURE 2–4. Survival probability curves of the two groups of Fisher 344 rats that received electrochemical treatment. Ten rats were treated with two arrays of electrodes, and 24 rats were treated with multiple electrodes at the tumor base. The difference in survival was significant (log-rank test; $p = .001$). *(Modified from Chou CK et al:* Bioelectromagnetics *18:14, 1997.)*

inserted in the skin tumor, and a plate electrode was pasted on the skin at 3 to 4 cm from the edge of the melanoma skin lesion.[66]

Because each cancer tumor has its own tissue conductivity, the effective volume differs for each different tumor; therefore the tissue conductivity must be determined. Rat tumor morphologic changes after EChT can be used to study the effect of spacing.

Dosage: Voltage and Electrical Dose

Although EChT is already clinically prevalent in China, and Chinese physicians have concluded that EChT is a simple, effective local therapy, the dosage guidelines have not been determined. Nordenström[60] stated that "because few indications existed to guide an optimal choice of voltage and amount of electric energy to be given, an arbitrary amount of current of 100 coulombs per centimeter of tumor diameter (at 10 V potential) was chosen to be the preliminary dose." Xin[86] treated his patients with 40-mA to 80-mA current, 8 to 10 V, at 100 C/cm³. The 100 C/cm³ value is more appropriate than the per-centimeter-diameter value because the dose should be related to the volume, not the diameter, of the tumor. Although 100 C has been used widely, the dosage guidelines used by Nordenström and Xin are arbitrary, and no scientific basis exists for these values.

Electrical dose (coulombs) is a product of current (A) and time (seconds). Higher current reduces treatment time but also causes pain. Lower current prolongs the treatment. Therefore a compromise with acceptable current density over a reasonable time is desirable. Notably, however, the arbitrary definition of dose is in coulombs per cubic centimeter. From the data published in China, apparently the charge is obtained by multiplying the DC passed between two electrodes by the time the current is applied, then dividing by the volume of the tumor. Clearly, the charge density is not uniform throughout the treated tumors and, the charge density, or *dose distribution*, is not appreciated. Many factors may affect the dose distribution. The charge density could be the source of the varying results when needles are implanted parallel or perpendicular to the body surface, or when changes in the numbers of needles and needle spacing are made. It would be advantageous to design dose experiments in which the researcher would be dealing with uniform charge density distribution rather than the highly non-uniform distributions obtained with needle electrodes. The lack of dosage guidelines has become a bottleneck in EChT development.

ANIMAL STUDIES

To provide fundamental knowledge about EChT electrode configuration, spacing, and dosage and to help formulate a standardized EChT method for breast cancer, we completed an animal research project supported by Army Breast Cancer Research Program.[69] Rat breast cancers were initiated by injecting 1×10^6 rat breast cancer cells (MTF-7, grown in logarithmic phase) to the right fat pad of the mammary gland of Fisher 344 female rats. A total of 259 rats were used for this study; 130 were used for a survival study and 129 for a pathology study. Rats were randomly divided into designated experimental groups when the tumors were grown to approximately 2 cm³.

In the survival study, 120 rats were randomly divided into three groups, and the electrode spacings were 3, 5, and 10 mm. In each group, 40 rats were divided into four subgroups of 10, and each group was treated with one of four levels of constant 8-V doses: 40, 60, 80, and 100 C. A four-channel BK29A ECT machine was used to administer the dosages. Platinum electrodes were horizontally inserted into the tumor base with predetermined spacing. Ten rats used as controls were anesthetized, and electrodes were inserted into each tumor bottom with 5-mm spacing, but no electricity was applied. Changes in tumor size, body weight, and local control rates were monitored for 3 months after EChT. The rats were euthanized by carbon dioxide if the tumors grew to 3.5 cm³. Local tumor control rate was less than 40% in the 40 C and 60 C groups and more than 70% in the 80 C and 100 C groups. Sixty-six rats died of primary tumors, including all 10 rats in the control group. Once a rat's primary tumor was controlled, no recurrence was found. The main reason for terminating the primary tumor–free rats (51 rats) was lymph node metastasis. Thirteen tumor-free rats survived for more than 6 months.

In the pathology study, 129 rats were randomly divided into three groups, and the electrode spacings were 5, 10, and 15 mm. In each group the 43 rats were divided into four experimental subgroups of 10 and one control subgroup of 3. Each experimental subgroup was treated with one of four levels of 8-V EChT: respectively, 10, 20, 40, and 80 C. The result indicated a significant dose effect on EChT-induced tumor necrosis. At 10, 20 40, and 80 C, the fractions showing necrosis were 39.7%, 52.3%, 62%, and 77.7% respectively ($p < .001$). Electrode spacing was not an important factor within a given range. At 5, 10, and 15 mm of spacing, the fractions showing the necrosis were 54.1%, 60.4%, and 59.2%, respectively ($p = .552$). The overlap rate of necroses was similar in the 5-mm and 10-mm groups (82.5% and 85%) and lower in the 15-mm group (65%).

Based on the survival and pathology studies, we concluded that the tumor response to EChT, local control, survival rates, and necrosis percentages were significantly increased with increasing dose. The changes in electrode spacing (3, 5, and 10 mm) did not significantly affect the tumor responses to EChT within the same dose. For a diameter of 2.0-cm to 2.5-cm rat breast cancer, EChT should be applied with 5 to 10 mm of spacing and a minimum dosage of 80 C. Again, animal study results cannot simply transfer to the clinical setting for patient therapy. For breast cancer patients, more studies need to be conducted to determine the dosage guideline.

PRECLINICAL SAFETY AND TOXICITY TEST

Electrochemical treatment must be carefully evaluated for potential risks before clinical use. Unlike therapies with chemical agents, EChT is a local therapy, and no foreign agent is injected into the body. Some toxicity tests can be ignored, such as effects on reproductive functions, including teratogenicity, carcinogenicity, and mutagenesis.

Based on published clinical data, EChT is used mainly in the treatment of patients who are not candidates for conventional therapy because of age, overall medical condition, or both. Compared with surgery, EChT is less traumatic, and therefore recovery is quicker. No serious side effects result from EChT compared with radiation therapy or chemotherapy. Because EChT destroys both normal and tumor tissue, however, there is a potential risk, depending on patient sensitivity, for certain parameters (e.g., voltage, current) to influence either quality or quantity of treatment. To bridge the gap between the animal studies and clinical evaluation, Phase I clinical trial is necessary. The following risks should be documented in preclinical tests:

1. Local pain is the main acute complication during electrode insertion and EChT procedure.
2. Tumor necrosis and ulceration are usually observed when superficial lesions are treated with EChT. The absorption of necrotic tissue may cause fever and leukocytosis after EChT.
3. If not well insulated, the skin can be burned by the chemical reaction. The healing time depends on the size and location of the lesion. Platinum electrode bases should be insulated to prevent skin injury at the entrance site.
4. During electrode insertion, blood vessels and nerves may be punctured. Therefore bleeding and pain may be observed during insertion.

MECHANISM OF ACTION

Besides methodology and dosage studies, more basic research, such as study of mechanisms, is necessary before EChT can be accepted for the treatment of patients in the United States. Mechanisms of EChT antitumor effects remain uncertain. Very probable and often mentioned mechanisms are biochemical reactions in the vicinity of the electrodes and DC effects on tumor cells. Biochemical reactions include changes in the pH and ion compositions of the extracellular matrix, both of which exert an influence on cell growth and survival.[50,51,82]

As noted earlier, EChT involves electrolysis, electrophoresis, and electroosmosis. *Electrolysis* results in the decomposition of electrolytes and pH alteration. During *electroosmosis*, water moves from the anode to the cathode, a process that dehydrates cells near the anode and hydrates cells near the cathode. Water volume change within the cell disturbs the cell structure and its function. In addition to the changes in pH and water volume, chloride (Cl_2), which is formed at the anode as a result of Cl^- electron loss, may play a role in cell growth inhibition by its oxidizing effect. In addition, the platinum ions, possibly formed by electrolysis of the platinum electrodes, may play a role in EChT killing effects. Although EChT-induced cell death may involve complicated processes, the pH alteration and ion movement are the most obvious and important factors in EChT.[44] Therefore basic research should focus first on pH and ion alteration in tumor cell killing.

Yen et al.[88] evaluated the effectiveness of EChT on human cancer cells (KB cells) and found that EChT delayed KB cell growth by using 0.3 C/ml (1.5 C in 5 ml of culture medium; 3 V, 400 μA for 62.5 minutes). From the results of a colony-forming assay, it was clearly demonstrated that increasing the EChT dose decreases tumor cell survival. The authors also measured the pH changes during EchT; pH at the anode decreased to 4.53 and at the cathode increased to 10.46. These results indicate that EChT is effective for killing human KB cells in vitro and that the toxicity effect is related to charge, current, and treatment time. The effect of pH alteration on cells is one of the mechanisms of EChT.

In EChT preclinical research, morphologic studies lead to better understanding of the mechanisms of action. Both light and electron microscopy were used to study the morphologic changes in human KB cells treated with DC. Figures 2–5 and 2–6 show scanning electron microscopic views of control and treated (0.05 C/ml) human KB cancer cells. Control cells are in a polygonal shape. Microvilli are abundant on cell surfaces. After EChT cells shrink, the number of microvilli decreases, and there are holes on cell surfaces. Transmission electron microscopy shows a normal tumor cell with rich mitochondria and polysomes in cytoplasm. After 0.2 C/ml EChT, there are decreased microvilli, mild mitochondrial swelling, polysome disaggregation, lysosome distention, and nuclear chromatism with focal aggregates in cells. At a higher EChT level (0.4 C/ml), the plasma membrane bursts, and the distended organelles escape. Microscopic studies reveal morphologic changes at EChT levels corresponding to inhibition of cell proliferation.

CLINICAL TRIALS

Although EChT has been used in some countries as an alternative method for cancer treatment, it is necessary to conduct clinical trials in the United States to verify its value. According to a U.S. Food and Drug Administration (FDA) exemption regulation for investigational devices, EChT was considered a "significant-risk" device. Therefore we submitted a clinical protocol to both the Institutional Review Board at the City of Hope and the FDA for Phase I clinical trial approval. A quality assurance of

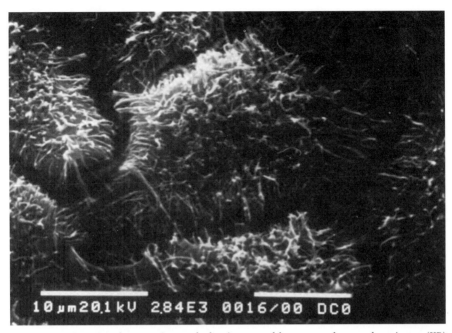

FIGURE 2–5. Scanning electron micrograph showing normal human oropharyngeal carcinoma (KB) cells. Microvilli are abundant on cell surfaces.

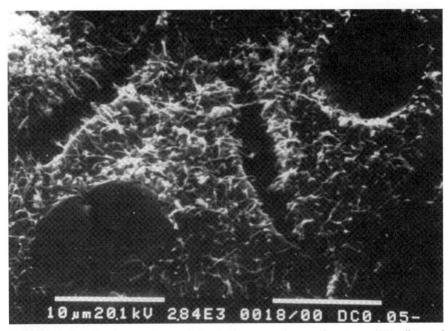

FIGURE 2–6. Scanning electron micrograph showing human oropharyngeal carcinoma (KB) cells treated with 0.05 C/ml of electrochemical treatment (EChT). After EChT, cells shrink, microvilli collapse, and holes appear on the cell membrane.

the equipment must be submitted to ensure the safety of its operation. The Phase I study asked for 25 recurrent, superficial, measurable malignant tumors for treatment. The purposes of these clinical trials were to evaluate the tumor response of EChT and to record the acute and late toxicities of EChT in the treatment of superficial tumors.

Our group (the authors and radiation oncologists) treated five patients at the City of Hope. The first patient had a diagnosis of $T_4N_0M_0$ carcinoma of the larynx. His treatment was laryngectomy and a full course of radiation therapy. EChT was used for multiple painful, subcutaneous metastases. He developed complete response in treated sites and tolerated EChT well. The second patient had lung cancer with subcutaneous multiple scalp and distant metastases. EChT was given to a scalp nodule to relieve pain. The patient had complete response with excellent pain relief that lasted for 3 months, then tumor regrowth occurred at the tumor margin. The third patient had a diagnosis of large, metastasized osteosarcoma of the left forearm. ECT achieved less than 50% response attributable to incomplete treatment. There was no complication from EChT. The fourth patient had a large, ulcerated T_4 breast cancer. Despite multiple-course chemotherapy, the patient developed multiple, extensive, painful, ulcerated local recurrences on the left-side chest wall. EChT was used to treat one of the nodules (6 cm) on the left upper arm. She developed an ulcer at the site of the tumor where the tumor was destroyed as a result of EChT. The fifth patient developed a painful left axial node metastasis (6×7 cm). She was given two courses of EChT. She had partial response and had excellent pain relief.

From these five preliminary patient results it appears that EChT is effective, safe, and well tolerated.

N Hyperthermia Treatment for Cancer

Numerous reports have shown a synergistic effect of heat and radiotherapy or of heat and chemotherapy.[15] The effective temperature range of hyperthermia treatments is very small: 41° to 45° C. At lower temperatures the effect is minimal. At temperatures higher than 45° C, normal cells are damaged. During hyperthermic treatment, temperatures in tumors are usually higher than in normal surrounding tissue because of the difference in blood flow. In addition, it is generally believed that tumors are more sensitive to heat. This is explained by the hypoxic, acidic, and poor nutritional state of tumor cells.[43] The synergism of radiation and hyperthermia is accomplished by thermal killing of hypoxic and S-phase cells (DNA synthesis) that are resistive to radiation. Hyperthermia has been used in combination with chemotherapy because heating increases membrane permeability and the potency of some drugs.

HISTORICAL CONSIDERATIONS

The interest in the use of heat in cancer treatment can probably be attributed to a clinical observation in 1866 made by M. Busch, a German physician. He described a patient with a neck sarcoma that disappeared after the patient had a high fever associated with erysipelas. Similar reports were made 20 years later. These findings led to studies using bacterial toxins extracted from the bacteria-causing erysipelas. In 1893, W. C. Coley, a surgeon in New York, administered to cancer patients bacterial toxins extracted from *Streptococcus* and *Serratia marcescens*. In 1898, Swedish gynecologist F. Westermark used a coil containing hot water as a controlled, localized source of heat in the treatment of uterine tumors. Such early studies and observations were followed by many reports of tumors responding to both whole-body and localized hyperthermic treatments that were induced by a variety of techniques.

Among the heating methods, *electromagnetic* (EM) heating earned an important role. After the German physicist Heinrich Hertz demonstrated the physical nature of EM waves and described their characteristic features, EM heating became a very popular but controversial treatment method for various diseases. As technology developed, higher-frequency EM fields were used. Short-wave *diathermy* became the standard approach, with frequencies of up to 100 MHz by 1920 and from 100 up to 3000 MHz by 1930. Meanwhile, many of the early reports describing the use of various forms of diathermy claimed frequency-specific effects for the EM energy involved. Mittleman et al.,[53] recognizing the need for careful dosimetry, measured the temperatures and related them to absorbed energy.

Although details of many experimental studies were published during the first half of the twentieth century, the biologic evidence was insufficient and interest in the clinical use of hyperthermia declined, principally because of lack of sufficient preclinical studies. In the 1960s, Cavaliere et al.[10] carried out a series of biochemical studies on the effects of elevated temperature on normal and malignant rodent cells. They observed that heat caused a greater inhibition of respiration in tumor tissues than in normal tissues and concluded that neoplastic cells were more sensitive to heat than their normal counterparts.

These preclinical studies did provide a stimulus to further research in the field. In the past 30 years there has been a systematic investigation of the possible anticancer effects of hyperthermia, with a variety of experimental studies being reported and critical analyses of a vast collection of clinical reports. The results confirm that temperature elevations of only a few degrees have profound effects on cells and tissues and that hyperthermia undoubtedly has an antitumor effect. Numerous biologic studies, mostly involving temperatures in the range of 41° to 46° C, have demonstrated a clear rationale for expecting hyperthermia to have a greater effect on tumors than on normal tissue. In addition, there has been significant progress in the application of heating systems and noninvasive thermometry techniques for clinical hyperthermia. The development and potential usefulness of hyperthermia as a technique to treat cancer have been demonstrated.[24,64,70,78,80] In the United States the FDA has approved five hyperthermia systems (BSD 1000, Cheung Laboratory HT 100A, Cook VH 8500, Clini-Therm Mark I and IV, and Labthermic Sonotherm 1000), which meet the FDA premarket evaluation standard for clinical use.

PRECLINICAL ISSUES

In vitro, in vivo, and clinical studies have all shown that in conjunction with radiation therapy and chemotherapy, hyperthermia is effective for treating cancer.[73] A summary of

25 nonrandomized studies from 1980 to 1988, including one study involving 1556 superficial tumors treated with radiotherapy and those treated with radiation therapy plus hyperthermia, shows that the average complete response rates for tumors were 34% and 64%, respectively. Clearly, hyperthermia is beneficial. However, a multiinstitutional randomized Phase III study conducted in the United States did not clearly demonstrate that hyperthermia in combination with radiation therapy improved tumor response compared with radiation therapy alone.[65] Inadequate heat delivery was considered to be the reason for failure. Some reports have shown that the effective temperature range of hyperthermia treatment is very small: 41° to 45° C; at lower temperatures the effect is minimal. At temperatures higher than 45° C, normal cells are damaged.[21,67]

The clinical use of hyperthermia has been hampered by a lack of adequate equipment to effectively deliver heat to deep-seated and even large superficial lesions and by a lack of thermometry techniques that provide reliable information on heat distribution in the target tissues. Therefore, besides the biologic considerations, the hyperthermia preclinical studies should mainly solve the problems of how to generate heat and how to control elevated temperatures in tumors. This section reviews the main methods of hyperthermia treatment and the steps necessary to evaluate the amount of heat delivered for each method. In addition, we use our intracavitary applicator as an example to discuss how much preclinical work should be performed before an applicator can be used in a clinic.

HEATING METHODS

The first step in preclinical studies evaluating hyperthermia is to develop an *effective heating method*. Techniques developed for heat induction over the past two decades include *whole-body heating* by hot wax, hot air, hot-water suit, or infrared irradiation and *partial-body heating* by either radiofrequency (RF) EM fields (including microwaves), ultrasound, heated blood, or fluid perfusion.[15]

Whole-Body Heating

For disseminated disease, many groups have studied whole-body hyperthermia (WBH) in conjunction with chemotherapy and radiation therapy.[3,7,71] Methods of WBH include hot wax, hot water, water blanket, water suit, extracorporeal heated blood, and radiant heat. The high morbidity and labor-intensive methods associated with WBH have caused concerns. Except for the extracorporeal blood-heating technique, which requires extensive surgical procedures, all other methods depend on conduction of heat from the body surface to the core. The preclinical studies have indicated that the core temperature should be kept below 41.8° C; above this temperature the brain and liver can be damaged.[26]

Local Heating

Local hyperthermia is produced by coupling energy to tissue through three accepted modalities: RF coupling at frequencies ranging from 100 kHz to 100 MHz, microwave coupling at higher frequencies (300 to 2450 MHz), and mechanical coupling by means of ultrasound (1 to 3 MHz).

EXTERNAL TECHNIQUES. Two RF methods have been used to provide subcutaneous heating. In the first method the tissues were placed between two capacitor plates and heated by displacement currents. This method is simple, but overheating of the fat, which is caused by the perpendicular electrical field, remains a major problem for obese patients. A water bolus is necessary to minimize fat heating.

The second RF method is inductive heating by magnetic fields that are generated by solenoidal loops or "pancake" magnetic coils to induce eddy currents in tissue. Because the induced electrical fields are parallel to the tissue interface, heating is maximized in muscle rather than in fat. However, the heating pattern is generally toroidal with a null at the center of the coil.

In the microwave frequency range, energy is coupled into tissues by waveguides, dipoles, microstrips, or other radiating devices. The shorter wavelengths of microwaves compared with longer wavelengths of RF provide the capability to direct and focus energy into tissues by direct radiation from a small applicator. Engineering developments have focused on the design of new microwave applicators. A number of applicators of various sizes operate over a frequency range of 300 to 1000 MHz.[38,42,58] Most are dielectrically loaded and have a water bolus for surface cooling.

INTRACAVITARY TECHNIQUES. Certain tumor sites in hollow cavities may be treated by intracavitary techniques. The advantages of intracavitary hyperthermia include (1) better energy deposition because of the proximity of an applicator to a tumor and (2) the reduction of normal tissue exposure as compared with externally induced hyperthermia. Clinical and research studies have examined hyperthermia in combination with either radiation therapy or chemotherapy in cancers of the esophagus, rectum, cervix, prostate, and bladder.

Microwaves and lower-frequency RF energy (13.65 to 2450 MHz) have been used for intracavitary hyperthermia. The main problem is that tumor temperature values are unknown. Most temperatures were measured on the surface of the applicators, which can be very different from those in the tumor. Furthermore, thermocouples or thermistors have been used to measure temperatures by many investigators who did not know the perturbation problem caused by the metallic sensors.[11] One solution to this problem is to measure tissue temperature in animals and then extrapolate the results to humans.[17]

INTERSTITIAL TECHNIQUES

RESISTIVE HEATING. Tissues can be heated by alternating RF currents conducted through needle electrodes. The operating frequency should be higher than 100 kHz to prevent excitation of nerve action potentials. Interstitial techniques for radiation implants, as primary or boost treatments, have been practiced successfully by radiation oncologists for many years. Other advantages of this technique include better control of temperature distributions within the tumor, compared with those of externally induced hyperthermia, and sparing of normal tissue, especially the overlying skin.[83]

MICROWAVE TECHNIQUE. Small microwave antennas inserted into hollow plastic tubing can produce satisfactory heating patterns at frequencies between 300 and 2450 MHz.[37]

A common frequency used in the United States is 915 MHz. A small coaxial antenna can irradiate a volume of approximately 60 cm³. With a multinodal coaxial antenna the extent of the heating pattern can be extended to approximately 10 cm in a three-node antenna.[41] For large tumors a single microwave antenna cannot heat the entire tumor to a therapeutic temperature, and an array of microwave antennas must be used. Because the antennas couple to each other, the spacing, phasing, and insertion depth affect the heating patterns of array applicators.[12,92]

FERROMAGNETIC SEED IMPLANTS. The technique of ferromagnetic seed implants is capable of delivering thermal energy to deep-seated tumors. When exposed to RF magnetic fields (about 100 kHz), the implants absorb energy and become heated. At the Curie point the implants become nonferromagnetic and no longer produce heat. The surrounding tissue is then heated by thermal conduction. Blood flow and tissue inhomogeneities in the tumor may affect the temperature distribution, which can be compensated for by the self-regulation of the implants. It is possible to maintain a temperature close to that of the Curie point.[46] Another method that exposes magnetic fluid in a tumor to an RF magnetic field (0.3 to 80 MHz) has been shown to be feasible for inducing selective heating.[40]

HEAT APPLICATOR DEVELOPMENT

The temperature elevation in tumors and tissues is determined by the energy deposited and the physiologic responses of the patient, as well as by blood flow and thermal conduction in the tissues. When EM methods are used, many factors affect the energy deposition, including frequency, intensity, and polarization of the applied fields, as well as the geometry and size of the applicator.[14] Along with these factors that affect heat delivery and coupling, the importance of designing an ideal applicator cannot be overemphasized. However, it is impossible to develop effective heat delivery and coupling applicators without sufficient preclinical tests. The following example describes the steps we employed before the applicator was used in patients.

Esophageal Applicator

The closed-end applicator, which was 76 cm long, consisted of a 6-mm-diameter polyurethane tube with a 2.67-mm, Teflon-lined center channel for an antenna and six 1.23-mm-diameter, Teflon-lined peripheral channels for nonperturbing temperature sensors or intraluminal radiation seeds. The microwave antenna was a 90-cm monopole made from flexible QMI-6000 cable (2.1 mm outer diameter [OD]) with a length of 10 cm from the tip to the center of a 1-mm gap. The center conductor was connected to the outer conductor at the tip, not at the gap, to give better heating results. The antenna can accommodate up to 130 W at 1 gigahertz (GHz).

Heating Pattern

Once an applicator was designed, heating patterns in human simulated (phantom) tissues had to be determined. A 28 × 28 × 8.5–cm Plexiglas box was filled with muscle phantom material[16] and covered with polyester silk screen. The surface temperature of the phantom interface was recorded by a thermographic camera. To simulate a clinical application, the applicator was placed on a thin plastic sheet on the phantom with the tip of the antenna at a depth of 13 to 18 cm. The applicator was then covered with a large mass of phantom muscle. After 30 to 45 seconds of 50-W, 915-MHz microwave exposure, the phantom was separated and a second thermogram obtained with the applicator removed. The thermograms of a 10-cm monopole before and after exposure were recorded (Figure 2–7). The point of *maximum heating rate* is 5 cm anterior to the junction. The *heating length* (greater than 50% heating rate) is longer than 15 cm; the voltage standing-wave ratio is 3:5.

ANIMAL STUDIES

After the heating tests in phantoms, we conducted heating tests on animals, using Yucatan and domestic pigs.[17] The chest region was exposed and Teflon tubes for inserting Luxtron fiberoptic probers were attached to the esophageal muscle at various locations relative to the microwave antenna junction; five sensors were near the aorta side and five on the opposite side. A Teflon tube was attached longitudinally along the outer surface of the esophagus for temperature mapping. Temperatures inside the

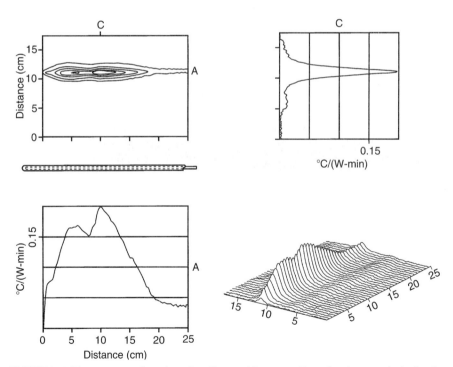

FIGURE 2–7. Thermograms of esophageal applicator with antenna No. 5 showing quantitative heating patterns. *(Modified from Chou CK et al. In Blank M, editor: Electricity and magnetism in biology and medicine, San Francisco, 1993, San Francisco Press.)*

applicator and the helical tubing were also mapped. Forty watts of 915-MHz power was applied. When a steady state was reached, temperatures were recorded. The esophagus was removed during autopsy to determine any obvious tissue effects. Histologic study was performed with light and electron microscopy.

Figure 2–8 shows the temperature of pig No. 5, which received treatment with 40 W of forward power (11 W reflected). Curve 1 shows temperatures in the esophageal wall near the aorta; curve 6 shows temperatures in the esophageal wall on the opposite side. The aorta side in general was similar to the other side. Curves 2 and 3 show the temperatures in the peripheral lumens inside the applicator; data of curve 4 were measured in the helical tube on the surface of the applicator. Curve 5 data were measured by a bare Luxtron 2000 sensor in the esophagus outside the applicator that measured the inner surface temperatures of the esophagus. Between 5.5 and 8.0 cm from the applicator, these temperatures ranged from 43.3° to 45.3° C. Curve 7 shows the temperatures outside the esophageal wall. The maximum temperature inside the esophageal muscle, which was measured 6 cm distal to the gap, was 44.4° C; this result was consistent with the thermogram. The temperatures in the peripheral lumens proximal to the gap were higher than the distal temperatures because of antenna self-heating attributable to current loss; this situation differs from the RF heating. Postmortem examination of the esophagus showed edema 5 to 6 cm distal to the antenna gap, which was consistent with the animal temperature measurement and the thermograms.

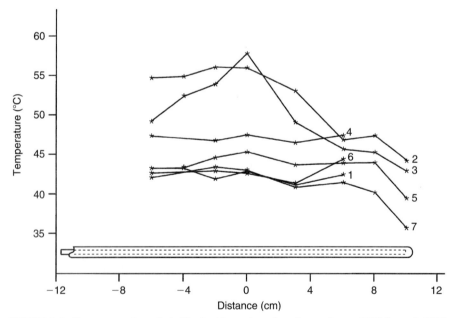

FIGURE 2–8. Temperature data of pig No. 5 with esophageal applicator. *Power:* 40 W forward, 11 W reflected. (*Modified from Chou CK et al. In Blank M, editor:* Electricity and magnetism in biology and medicine, *San Francisco, 1993, San Francisco Press.*)

Light microscopy showed vacuolization and swollen oval cellular nuclei in the heated area. Collagen in the lamina propria from the heated area seemed to be stretched, and the collagen bundles were parallel to the epithelial surface. Nuclei of fibroblasts in the collagen fabric were elongated along its fibers in the heated region of the esophagus; organization of this collagen in pig No. 5 was less complicated than in the control pig. Electron microscopy of epithelial cells in the heated area showed numerous vacuoles in the cytoplasm and cell boundaries.

CLINICAL TRIALS

Through comprehensive basic studies, we found that the designed applicator could provide good heat distribution and penetration for esophageal intracavitary hyperthermia. These results provided sufficient data to design protocols from which to evaluate the efficacy and safety of a clinical trial.

To evaluate the efficacy and tolerance of intracavitary hyperthermia combined with external radiation therapy and low-dose brachytherapy in the management of esophageal cancer, 25 patients with primary esophageal cancer received treatment following a clinical trial protocol.[68] Hyperthermia was applied with the previously described applicators. Temperature measurements were obtained while moving fiberoptic temperature sensors at 1.0-cm intervals in each of the applicator's six peripheral channels (Figure 2–9).

The 1-year and 2-year overall survival rates were 72% (18 of 25) and 32% (8 of 25), and the disease-free survival rates were 47% and 30%. The toxicity was mild. The acute toxic effect was pain in swallowing. The major late complication was mild esophageal fibrosis and difficulty in swallowing. No serious side effects such as fistulas or perforations were seen. These results indicate that hyperthermia is safe and feasible for treating esophageal carcinoma. Further Phase II and III studies should be implemented.

CURRENT STATUS AND FUTURE STUDIES

Although several thousand cancer patients have received treatment with hyperthermia, it has not become part of routine cancer treatment modalities. In most centers the use of hyperthermia is still part of a developing project. Through centuries of practice, however, hyperthermia has significant potential as an adjuvant therapy. To obtain good clinical results, researchers need not only better and more flexible heating systems, but also the ability to better plan and implement the individual patient treatments. The clinical use of heat has been hampered by a lack of adequate equipment for effective delivery of heat in deep-seated and even large superficial lesions and a lack of thermometry techniques that provide reliable information on heat distribution in the target tissue.

Despite the slow pace of investigation into thermal effects in U.S. clinics, several important studies are ongoing and strong interest persists in Europe and Asia.[22,63,78] Recently, Falk and Issels[28] provided an overview on the current clinical application of hyperthermia combined with conventional treatment modalities (e.g., ionizing

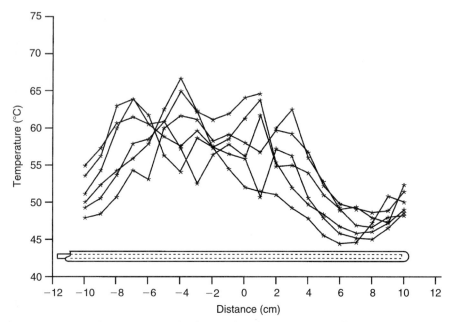

FIGURE 2–9. Typical temperature graph of an esophageal cancer patient undergoing treatment with intracavitary hyperthermia. Temperatures were obtained by moving fiberoptic temperature sensors at 1.0-mm intervals in the six peripheral channels of the applicator. *Power:* 42 W forward, 8.5 W reflected. (*Modified from Ren RL et al:* Int J Hyperthermia *14:245, 1998, www.tandf.co.uk/journals.*)

radiation and chemotherapy) in the treatment of malignant disease. The clinical application of hyperthermia with increase of tissue temperatures (range 40° to 44° C) has been integrated in multimodal anticancer strategies. This review described selected Phase I or II trials ($n = 17$) and Phase III trials ($n = 16$), investigating the effect of hyperthermia combined with radiotherapy (10 trials), chemotherapy (15 trials), or both (8 trials) in more than 2200 patients. The trials were performed for a variety of solid tumors (melanoma, head/neck cancer, breast cancer, cancer of gastrointestinal/urogenital tract, glioblastoma, sarcoma) in pediatric and adult patients.

Research has produced a scientific basis for the simultaneous application of hyperthermia with ionizing radiation and/or systemic chemotherapy. Hyperthermia is becoming more accepted clinically because of technical improvements in achieving a selected increase in temperature in superficial and deep-seated tumors. At present, the combination of hyperthermia and chemotherapy or radiochemotherapy is further being tested in clinical protocols (Phase II/III) to improve local tumor control and relapse-free survival in patients with high-risk or advanced tumors of different entities.

According to the literature, hyperthermia would provide a significant, worthwhile improvement in cancer control if researchers continue their preclinical scientific studies more carefully. Future preclinical studies should improve research methodology through the following:

1. Better biologic knowledge regarding the effects of thermal cytotoxicity in normal and tumor tissue (e.g., sequencing of modalities, impact of thermotolerance)
2. Better physics and engineering support regarding homogeneity of the power deposition (e.g., improved treatment planning methods, improved power deposition/tumor volume ratio, noninvasive thermometry control)

Recent Developments in CAM Preclinical Research

Preclinical research in CAM therapies should use both animal and human models at various levels of analysis. In the absence of strong and systematic preclinical studies, many CAM treatments may not achieve optimal and maximum benefits because the information is incomplete about all systems involved. This section discusses five common CAM therapies and related findings from preclinical research.

ACUPUNCTURE

As shown by its many references in this text, acupuncture continues to be used as a major CAM therapy. Acupuncture has been intensively studied, especially since the 1970s, when a debate arose about its potential for activating opiate receptors in the brain. Clearly, acupuncture has been shown in both animal and human studies to do more than simply superficially stimulate skin receptors.

One major thrust of research has been the description of physiologic and chemical change after acupuncture, especially activation of central nervous system structures. Yun et al.[91] used an animal model in which stress was first induced artificially, then electroacupuncture stimulation given, to demonstrate that a brain-derived neurotrophic factor messenger ribonucleic acid (mRNA) level of expression was restored within the hippocampus. RNA isolation and reverse transcription was used. In an intact rat model in which immobilization was used as a stressor, electroacupuncture stimulation reduced experimentally controlled alcohol drinking and increased dopamine levels in the striatum, thus providing a neurochemical correlate with the described behavior.[89] Importantly, these effects were specific to the acupuncture stimulation point ST 36 (Tsu-San-Li). In another study, a potential connection between cardiovascular reflex responses and brain stem activation was evaluated. The gallbladder pressor response, which is inhibited by electroacupuncture, can be reversed (attenuated) when mu- and delta-opioid antagonists are directly injected into the medulla of cats.[45] Possibly then, endogenous neurotransmitters, such as beta-endorphins and enkephalins that act on mu- and delta-opioid receptors, are involved in acupuncture effects, especially the described feeling of "relaxation."

Positron emission tomography (PET) scans in humans have shown that acupuncture activates major areas in the brain possibly related to pain control,[6] including the cerebellum bilaterally and cortical frontal areas. A second PET study describing subcortical areas and pathways showed that a prominently described point of analgesic efficacy (Li 4, Heku) not only activated cortical areas but also hypothalamic nuclei extending to the midbrain.[35] Electrophysiologic measurements have been used to describe brain activity, especially cortical changes during acupuncture insertion.[84] At Li 4, somatosensory-evoked potentials, (the first two waveform components) differed in terms of latency and amplitude when compared with a control point after electroacupuncture. Differences could also be described when median nerve electrical stimulation was used. Future investigations need to provide a complete mapping of activation in cortical and brain stem pathways during acupuncture, especially comparing specific and sham points with both single-unit and correlate waveform activity.

Acupuncture also influences the autonomic nervous system. Haker et al.[34] reported that acupuncture activates sympathetic activity (blood pressure, heart rate) but that the activity depends on the area of stimulation. Ear stimulation, for example, increases more parasympathetic activity. Other measures of autonomic activity and possible involvement of skin temperature and plethysmography need further evaluation to determine potential co-relationships.

HERBAL THERAPIES

The use of herbs, especially when they are given orally, presents a formidable task for the preclinical researcher. Determination of toxicologic issues, including dose response curves and standardization of extract analysis, is important but rarely done. Often the focus should be a better understanding of neurochemical mechanisms of action.

Calapai et al.[8] demonstrated that when *Hypericum perforatum* is orally administrated to mice, its major action may be through the cytokine interleukin-6 (IL-6), which is presumably produced by lymphocytes and other cells such as astrocytes. Although tryptophan level was not changed in the diencephalon, serotonin and 5-hydroxyindoleacetic acid (5-HIAA) levels were increased. Another type of analysis used is an "animal depression model," in which a form of experimental stress is induced, such as shock, isolation, or physical restriction. *H. perforatum* "protected" the animal from inhibiting or reducing response and instead allowed for an appetitive behavior task to be performed (the reverse of "anhedonia" as a human descriptor).[30] Interestingly, extraneuronal dopamine, assessed from the nucleus accumbens, did not decrease over 3 weeks of treatment, which is similar to findings describing conventional antidepressant medication action.

In another type of analysis, Fornal et al.[29] explored brain stem single-unit activity of serotonergic neurons during administration of St. John's wort in awake cats. Conventional antidepressants such as fluoxetine and sertraline decrease serotonergic neuronal activity, presumably by their action on inhibitory receptors. St. John's wort did not change neural activity, however, and thus its role in monoamine activity remains to be clarified.

Questions have recently been raised regarding the safety of the extract kava (*Piper methysicum*), for which closer evaluation is needed regarding long-term effects involving potential organ damage. One recent study has shown that human platelets MAO-B are reversibly inhibited and platelet homogenates (IC50, 1.2 fm) disrupted after administration of either kava extract or kava pyrones in vitro.[77]

HOMEOPATHY

The central issue in the evaluation of homeopathy is the determination whether biologic activity can be maintained after ultrahigh levels of dilution. Significant scientific skepticism remains because in many cases no molecules are present in the final dilution, and any debatable physiologic activity/energy must come from the water or dilution medium. Systematic reviews of preclinical research have reported little replication, negative results, or methodology that is questionable (preclinical research[81] and clinical human research[39]). The systems studied range from animals, plants, and isolated organ systems to cells in vitro.[79] Scattered reports indicate that ultradilutions can produce protection from experimentally induced catalepsis, as found, for example, in a whole-rat model.

Because most conventional journals will not publish assessments of homeopathy, especially preclinical studies, an objective debate seems limited. An important future direction is the need for integration from preclinical science describing "homeopathy clinical utility" in CAM. This integration could provide opportunities for conventional medicine to develop more sophisticated and working hypotheses that can be tested.

MANUAL THERAPIES

Various theories have been advanced regarding mechanisms involved in healing using therapies solely focused on utilization of somatic structures such as spinal manipulation. However, Nanesl and Szlazak[56] were unable to find clinical support for these therapies in treating internal diseases. Generally, the model used to test and evaluate manual therapies is to monitor nerve root and neuromuscular responses to either spinal manipulation or actual thrust movement. With different "loads" and force, different afferent nerve and motor pathways become sensitive at skin, muscle, and tissue points.

A recent comparison study of spinal manipulation and massage reported that spinal manipulation using the tibial nerve H-reflex response amplitude increased alpha motoneuron activity after therapy to a greater extent than did massage.[23] Paraspinal and limb massage did not inhibit motor neuron activity. Using intraoperative recordings, Colloca et al.[19] were able to show that amplitude and discharge frequencies of the evoked response were sensitive to the contact point and applied force vector created by the spinal manipulation thrust. Animal studies likewise have evaluated nerve root excitability, including mechanosensitive afferents.

These basic studies are designed to describe more completely and precisely the events occurring during manual manipulation. Such CAM research may have implications for future understanding of mechanisms of action, especially in regard to safety issues.

MIND-BODY THERAPIES AND MEDITATION

Generally, most preclinical studies evaluating mind-body techniques involve humans. Variables evaluated include environmental-situational or internal stress, attitudes, frustration, and tension as precursors to more serious health issues, such as cardiovascular disease or depression (see also Chapters 5 and 8). The major focus of the research is on the correlation of some type of "behavioral state," activated through meditation, Qi Gong, or yoga breathing, with a physiologic function.

Studies have shown that regional cerebral blood flow in areas such as the cingulate or orbital gyri and inferior frontal areas of the prefrontal cortex is increased during meditation and presumed focused concentration.[57] Likewise, Critchley et al.[20] reported, through PET scan analysis, an increase in neural activity in the left anterior cingulate and globus pallidus during biofeedback relaxation. Importantly, this same activation was not observed during biofeedback without relaxation or random feedback, indicating the importance of conscious control and motivation/learning. Other well-documented methods (e.g., electroencephalography) have shown changes after meditation, generally to higher alpha amplitudes, greater coherence, lower breath rates, and greater theta synchronization in anterior frontal regions.[1,76]

Barnes et al.[4] reported that the stressed-induced cardiovascular reactivity of subjects with diagnosed high blood pressure decreases (are reduced) at rest after meditation. Also heart rate and cardiac output likewise are reduced. Oxygen consumption and respiratory rate are reduced (decrease) during yoga.[75] Norepinephrine and epinephrine levels are lower after transcendental meditation, perhaps reflecting changes in the sympathetic nervous–adrenal medulla system.[36]

A second stage for much of this research is to determine how well biologic measures can be used to predict best-case responders to mind-body therapies. Correlation does not indicate causality, but understanding the mechanisms activated during a particular therapy and noting time course can be useful.

One of the major questions directed at preclinical research is the extent to which it makes some *contribution* to clinical practice. The time from basic "bench" type of research information being incorporated into clinical practice guidelines can be many years.[31] One way to "track" research information is to analyze the bibliographic listings of papers cited in clinical guidelines. In this way an evidence base can be reviewed. Using this procedure, Grant et al.[31] were able to determine the pattern of research citations. They report an 8-year lag time from publication of the research paper to publication of clinical guidelines. Also, many papers cited were more clinical than preclinical, and publication bias was evident in that international research data were often not quoted. Conventional practice guidelines at most cite only basic research 8% of the time. It is important to remember, however, that a paper's citation in a practice guideline does not indicate that a health issue was either addressed or changed. Also, citation does not suggest "importance," and a more precise type of "weight analysis" should be assigned.

Clearly, research itself should be researched. The following chapters show how an *evidence base* becomes a strong component of clinical practice. More work is needed to determine what constitutes minimal or maximal but adequate information that can bridge the gap from preclinical to clinical medicine, and how this information can be more rapidly downloaded and integrated into relevant practice guidelines for either conventional or CAM practice.

To date, funding in the area of preclinical research has been sparse. The intramural programs, though various institutes at the U.S. National Institutes of Health, are working toward forming collaborative research protocols with the National Center for Complementary and Alternative Medicine (NCCAM), and forthcoming efforts should be productive.

SUMMARY

As long as conventional medicine has its limitations, people will continue to seek help from CAM. Usually the origins of CAM are not scientific but rather are traditionally or culturally based. If a CAM therapy has initial proof that it is useful, scientists should conduct systematic preclinical studies to understand its mechanisms and variables for controlling its effectiveness. The examples of EChT and hyperthermia treatment with conventional medicine offer scientific details and present endeavors toward practicing these treatment methods in hospitals and clinics. Pyrites cannot stand the fire test, but gold can; preclinical study is the fire test of CAM.

REFERENCES

1. Aftanas LI, Golocheikine SA: Human anterior and frontal midline theta and lower alpha reflect emotionally positive state and internalized attention: high-resolution EEG investigation of meditation, *Neurosci Lett* 310(1):57, 2001.
2. American Medical Association: Prescription practices and regulatory agencies. In *Drug evaluations annual*, Chicago, 1992, The Association.
3. Anhalt D et al: The CDRH helix: an in vivo evaluation, *Int J Hyperthermia* 6:241, 1990.
4. Barnes VA, Treiber FA, Davis H: Impact of transcendental meditation on cardiovascular function at rest and during acute stress in adolescents with high normal blood pressure, *J Psychosom Res* 51(4):597, 2001.
5. Berkowitz BA, Katzung BG: Basic and clinical evaluation of new drugs. In Katzung BG, editor: *Basic and clinical pharmacology*, Norwich, Conn, 1995, Appleton & Lange.
6. Biella G et al: Acupuncture produces central activation in pain regions, *Neuroimage* 14(1, pt 1):60, 2001.
7. Bull JMC et al.: Chemotherapy resistant sarcoma treated with whole body hyperthermia (WBH) combined with 1–3-bis (2-chloroethyl)-1-nitrosourea (BUCN), *Int J Hyperthermia* 8:297, 1992.
8. Calapai G et al: Interleukin-6 involvement in antidepressant action of *Hypericum perforatum*, *Pharmacopsychiatry* 34(suppl 1):S8, 2001.
9. Cassileth BR, Chapman CC: Alternative cancer medicine: a ten-year update, *Cancer Invest* 14:396, 1996.
10. Cavaliere R et al: Selective heat sensitivity of cancer cells, *Cancer* 20:1351, 1967.
11. Cetas TC: Temperature. In Lehmann JF, editor: *Therapeutic heat and cold*, Baltimore, 1990, Williams & Wilkins.
12. Chan KW et al: Changes in heating patterns of interstitial microwave antenna arrays at different insertion depths, *Int J Hyperthermia* 5:499, 1989.
13. Chappell WR, Mordenti J: Extrapolation of toxicological and pharmacological data from animals to humans, *Adv Drug Res* 20:1, 1991.
14. Chou CK: Evaluation of microwave hyperthermia applicators, *Bioelectromagnetics* 13:581, 1992.
15. Chou CK: Electromagnetic heating for cancer treatment. In Blank M, editor: *Electromagnetic fields: biological interactions and mechanisms*, Washington, DC, 1995, American Chemical Society.
16. Chou CK et al: Formulas for preparing phantom muscle tissue at various radio frequencies, *Bioelectromagnetic*, 5:435, 1984.
17. Chou CK et al: Intracavitary hyperthermia and radiation of esophageal cancer. In Blank M, editor: *Electricity and magnetism in biology and medicine*, San Francisco, 1993, San Francisco Press.

18. Chou CK et al: Electrochemical treatment of mouse and rat fibrosarcomas with direct current, *Bioelectromagnetics* 18:14, 1997.
19. Colloca CJ et al: Neurophysiologic response to intraoperative lumbosacral spinal manipulation, *J Manipulative Physiol Ther* 23(7):447, 2000.
20. Critchley HD et al: Brain activity during biofeedback relaxation: a functional neuroimaging investigation, *Brain* 1124(pt 5):1003, 2001.
21. Dahl O, Mella O: Hyperthermia and chemotherapeutic agents. In Field SB, Hand JW, editors: *An introduction to the practical aspects of clinical hyperthermia*, London, 1990, Taylor & Francis.
22. Datta NR et al: Head and neck cancers: results of thermoradiotherapy versus radiotherapy, *Int J Hyperthermia* 6:479, 1990.
23. Disman JD, Bulbulian R: Comparison of effects of spinal manipulation and massage on motoneuron excitability, *Electromyogr Clin Neurophysiol* 41(2):97, 2001.
24. Dunlop PRC, Howard GCW: Has hyperthermia a place in cancer treatment? *Clin Radiol* 40:76, 1989.
25. Eisenberg DM et al: Unconventional medicine in the United States: prevalence, cost, and patterns of use, *N Engl J Med* 328:246, 1993.
26. Engelhardt R: Hyperthermia and drugs, *Recent Results Cancer Res* 104:136, 1987.
27. Ernst E: Back to basics? How important is basic research in CAM? *Altern Ther Health Med* 7(5):30, 2001.
28. Falk MH, Issels RD: Hyperthermia in oncology, *Int J Hyperthermia* 17:1, 2001.
29. Fornal CA et al: Effects of standardized extracts of St. John's Wort on the single unit activity of serotonergic dorsal raphe neurons in awake cats: comparisons with fluoxetine and sertraline, *Neuropsychopharmacology* 25(6):858, 2001.
30. Gambaerana C et al: *Pharmacopsychiatry* 34(suppl 1):S42, 2001.
31. Grant J et al: Evaluating "payback" on biomedical research from papers cited in clinical guidelines: applied bibliometric study, *BMJ* 320:1107, 2000.
32. Grever MR, Chabner BA: Cancer drug discovery and development. In DeVita VT Jr, Hellman S, Rosenberg SA, editors: *Cancer: principles and practice of oncology*, ed 5, Philadelphia, 1997, Lippincott-Raven.
33. Grever MR, Schepartz S, Chabner BA: The National Cancer Institute: cancer drug discovery and development program, *Semin Oncol* 19:622, 1992.
34. Haker E, Egekvist H, Bjerring PE: Effects of sensory stimulation (acupuncture) on sympathetic and parasympathetic activities in health subjects, *J Auton Nerv Syst* 79:52, 2000.
35. Hsieh JC et al: Activation of the hypothalamus characterizes the acupuncture stimulation at the analgesic point in human: a positron emission tomography study, *Neurosci Lett* 307(2):105, 2001.
36. Infante JR et al: Catecholamine levels in practitioners of the transcendental meditation technique, *Physiol Behav* 72(1–2):141, 2001.
37. Iskander MF, Tumeh AM: Design optimization of interstitial antennas, *IEEE Trans Biomed Eng* 36:238, 1989.
38. Johnson RH, Preece AW, Green JL: Theoretical and experimental comparison of three types of electromagnetic hyperthermia applicator, *Phys Med Biol* 35:761, 1990.
39. Jonas WB: A systematic review of the quality of homeopathic clinical trials, *BMC Complement Altern Med* 1(1):12, 2001.
40. Jordan A et al: Inductive heating of ferromagnetic particles and magnetic fluids: physical evaluation of their potential for hyperthermia, *Int J Hyperthermia* 9:51, 1993.
41. Lee DJ et al: A new design of microwave interstitial applicators for hyperthermia with improved treatment volume, *Int J Radiat Oncol Biol Phys* 12:2003, 1986.
42. Lee ER et al: Body-conformable, 915-MHz microstrip array applicators for large surface area hyperthermia, *IEEE Trans Biomed Eng* 39:470, 1992.
43. Lepock JR, Kruuv J: Mechanisms of thermal cytotoxicity. In Gerner EW, Cetas TC, editors: *Hyperthermic oncology*, vol 2, Tucson, Ariz, 1992, Arizona Board of Regents.
44. Li KH et al: Effects of direct current on dog liver: possible mechanisms for tumor electrochemical treatment, *Bioelectromagnetics* 18:2, 1997.
45. Li P, Tjeng-A-Looi S, Longhurst JC: Rostral ventrolateral medullary opioid receptor subtypes in the inhibitory effects of electroacupuncture on reflex autonomic response in cats, *Auton Neurosci* 89(1–2):38, 2001.

46. Mack CF et al: Interstitial thermoradiotherapy with ferromagnetic implants for locally advanced and recurrent neoplasms, *Int J Radiat Oncol Biol Phys* 27:109, 1993.
47. Matsushima Y, Amemiya R, Liu JS: Direct current therapy with chemotherapy for the local control of lung cancer, *Nippon Gan Chiryo Gakki Sh* 24:2341, 1989.
48. Matsushima Y et al: Clinical and experimental studies of anti-tumoral effects of electrochemical therapy (ECT) alone or in combination with chemotherapy, *Eur J Surg Suppl* 574:59, 1994.
49. Mattison N, Trimble AG, Lasagna L: New drug development in the United States: 1963 through 1984, *Clin Pharmacol* 43:290, 1988.
50. Miklavcic D, Sersa G, Kryzanowski M: Tumor treatment by direct electric current: tumor temperature and pH, electrode material and configuration, *Bioelectrochem Bioenerg* 30:209, 1993.
51. Miklavcic D, Sersa G, Novakovic S: Tumor bioelectric potential and its possible exploitation for tumor growth retardation, *J Bioelectricity* 9:133, 1990.
52. Miller HI, Young FE: Drug approval process at the Food and Drug Administration: new biotechnology as paradigm of science-based activist approach, *Arch Intern Med* 149:655, 1989.
53. Mittleman E, Osborne SL, Coulter JS: Short-wave diathermy power absorption and deep tissue temperature, *Arch Phys Ther* 22:133, 1941.
54. Moertel CG et al: A clinical trial of amygdalin (Laetrile) in the treatment of human cancer, *N Engl J Med* 306:201, 1982.
55. Nakayama T: Anti-tumor activities of direct current therapy combined with fractional radiation or chemotherapy, *J Jpn Soc Med Radio* 48:1269, 1988.
56. Nanesl D, Szlazak M: Somatic dysfunction and the phenomenon of visceral disease simulation: a probable explanation for the apparent effectiveness of somatic therapy in patients presumed to be suffering from true visceral disease, *J Manipulative Physiol Ther* 18(6):379, 1995.
57. Newberg A et al: The measurement of regional cerebral blood flow during the complex cognitive task of meditation: a preliminary SPECT study, *Psychiatry Res* 106(2):113, 2001.
58. Nikawa Y, Okada F: Dielectric loaded lens applicator for microwave hyperthermia, *IEEE Trans Microwave Theory Tech* 39:1173, 1991.
59. Nordenström BEW: Preliminary clinical trials of electrophoretic ionization in the treatment of malignant tumors, *IRCS Med Sc* 6:537, 1978.
60. Nordenström BEW: *Biologically closed electric circuits*, Stockholm, 1983, Nordic Medical.
61. Nordenström BEW: Electrochemical treatment of cancer. I. Variable response to anodic and cathodic fields, *Am J Clin Oncol* 12:530, 1989.
62. Nordenström BEW: The paradigm of biologically closed electric circuits (BCEC) and formation of an international association (IABC) for BCEC systems, *Eur J Surg Suppl* 574:7, 1994.
63. Overgaard J et al: Randomized trial of hyperthermia as adjuvant to radiotherapy for recurrent or metastatic malignant melanoma, *Lancet* 345:540, 1995.
64. Perez CA, Emami B: Clinical trials with local irradiation and hyperthermia: current and future perspectives, *Radiol Clin North Am* 27:525, 1989.
65. Perez CA et al.: Randomized phase III study comparing irradiation and hyperthermia with irradiation alone in superficial measurable tumors, *Am J Clin Oncol* 14:133, 1991.
66. Plesnicar A et al: Electric treatment of human melanoma skin lesions with low-level direct electric current: an assessment of clinical experience following a preliminary study in five patients, *Eur J Surg Suppl* 574:45, 1994.
67. Raaphrost GP: Fundamental aspects of hyperthermic biology. In Field, SB, Hand JW, editors: *An introduction to the practical aspects of clinical hyperthermia*, London, 1990, Taylor & Francis.
68. Ren RL et al: A pilot study of intracavitary hyperthermia combined with radiation in the treatment of esophageal carcinoma, *Int J Hyperthermia* 14:245, 1998.
69. Ren RL et al: Variations of dose and electrode spacing for rat breast cancer electrochemical treatment, *Bioelectromagnetics* 22:205, 2001.
70. Seegenschmiedt HM et al: Superficial chest wall recurrences of breast cancer: prognostic treatment factors for combined radiation therapy and hyperthermia, *Radiology* 173:551, 1989.
71. Shen RN et al: Whole body hyperthermia: a potent radioprotector in vivo, *Int J Radiat Oncol Biol Phys* 20:525, 1991.

72. Simon RM: Clinical trials in cancer. In DeVita VT Jr, Hellman S, Rosenberg SA, editors: *Cancer: principles and practice of oncology*, ed 5, Philadelphia, 1997, Lippincott-Raven.

73. Sneed P, Phillips TL: Combining hyperthermia and radiation: how beneficial? *Oncology* 5(3):99, 1991.

74. Suffiness M, Newman DJ, Snader K: Discovery and development of antineoplastic agents from natural sources, *Bioorg Marine Chem* 3:131, 1989.

75. Telles S, Reddy SK, Nagedra HR: Oxygen consumption and respiration following two yoga relaxation techniques, *Appl Psychophysiol Biofeedback* 25(4):221, 2000.

76. Travis F: Autonomic and EEG patterns distinguish transcending from other experiences during transcendental meditation practice, *Int J Psychophysiol* 42(1):1, 2001.

77. Uebelhack R, Franke L, Schewe HJ: Inhibition of platelet MAO-B by kava pyrone-enriched extract from *Piper methysticum* Forster (kava-kava), *Pharmacopsychiatry* 5:187, 1998.

78. Valdagni R, Amichetti M: Report of long-term follow-up in a randomized trial comparing radiation therapy and radiation therapy plus hyperthermia to metastatic lymph nodes in stage IV head and neck patients, *Int J Radiat Oncol Biol Phys* 28:163, 1994.

79. Vallance AK: Can biological activity be maintained at ultra-high dilution? An overview of homeopathy, evidence, and Bayesian philosophy, *J Altern Complement Med* 4(1):49, 1998.

80. Van der Zee J et al: Low-dose reirradiation with hyperthermia: a palliative treatment for patients with breast cancer recurring in previously irradiated areas, *Int J Radiat Oncol Biol Phys* 15:1407, 1988.

81. Vickers A: Independent replication of pre-clinical research in homeopathy: a systematic review, *Forsch Komplementarmed* 6(6):311, 1999.

82. Vodovnik L, Miklavcic D, Sersa G: Modified cell proliferation due to electrical currents, *Med Biol Eng Comput* 30:21, 1992.

83. Vora N et al: Primary radiation combined with hyperthermia for advanced (stage III-IV) and inflammatory carcinoma of breast, *Endocuriether Hyperthermia Oncol* 2:101, 1986.

84. Wei H et al: Early-latency somatosensory evoked potentials elicited by electrical acupuncture after needling acupoint LI-4, *Clin Electroencephalogr* 31(3):160, 2000.

85. Xin YL: Organization and spread of electrochemical therapy (ECT) in China, *Eur J Surg Suppl* 574:25, 1994.

86. Xin YL: Advances in the treatment of malignant tumors by electrochemical therapy (ECT), *Eur J Surg Suppl* 574:31, 1994.

87. Xin YL et al: Electrochemical treatment of lung cancer, *Bioelectromagnetics* 18:8, 1997.

88. Yen Y et al: Electrochemical treatment of human KB cells in vitro, *Bioelectromagnetics* 20:34, 1999.

89. Yoshiumoto K et al: Electroacupuncture stimulation suppresses the increase in alcohol-drinking behavior in restricted rats, *Alcohol Clin Exp Res* 25(6 suppl):63, 2001.

90. Young FE, Nightingale SL: FDA's newly designated treatment: INDs, *JAMA* 260:224, 1988.

91. Yun SJ et al: Effect of electroacupuncture on the stress-induced changes in brain-derived neurotrophic factor statement in rat hippocampus, *Neurosci Lett* 318(2):85, 2002.

92. Zhang Y, Joines WT, Oleson JR: Prediction of heating patterns of a microwave interstitial antenna array at various insertion depths, *Int J Hyperthermia* 7:197, 1991.

SUGGESTED READINGS

Bioelectromagnetics 18(1), 1997. This special issue includes the following reports: Li KH et al: Effects of direct current on dog liver: possible mechanisms for tumor electrochemical treatment; Chou CK et al: Electrochemical treatment of mouse and rat fibrosarcomas with direct current; and Xin YL et al: Electrochemical treatment of lung cancer.

Chou CK: Radiofrequency hyperthermia for cancer therapy. In Bronzino JD, editor: *CRC Biomedical engineering handbook*, Boca Raton, Fla, 1995, CRC Press.

Nordenström B et al, editors: Proceedings of the IABC International Association for Biologically Closed Electric Circuits (BCEC) in Medicine and Biology, *Eur J Surg* 160(suppl 574):7, 1994.

Seegenschmiedt HM, Fessenden P, Vernon CC: *Thermo-radiotherapy and thermo-chemotherapy*, London, 1995, Springer. This work was supported in part by the National Cancer Institute grant CA 33572 and the Army Breast Cancer Research Grant DAMD 17-96-1-6184.

PART TWO

Clinical Research Outcomes: Use of Complementary and Alternative Therapies in General Medicine

CHAPTER 3

Asthma and Allergies

ROBERT M. HACKMAN, JUDITH S. STERN, and
M. ERIC GERSHWIN
This chapter is published in its entirety from the first edition.

An estimated 14 million Americans suffer from asthma, and the incidence is rising at an alarming rate. Asthma is especially prevalent in children but affects people of all ages. Mortality from asthma is increasing as the number of hospital admissions for the treatment of asthma has increased; the number of deaths attributed to asthma has nearly doubled since 1976. Moreover, despite the thoughts of William Osler that "an asthmatic does not die of asthma, but rather pants one's way into old age," the number of older Americans with reactive airway disease is also increasing, even in the absence of direct tobacco exposure.[4,21,30,128]

Asthma is a common lung disease characterized by reversible airway obstruction and airway inflammation.[21,30] It is characterized by paroxysmal bronchospasm, inflammation, hypersecretion of mucus, airway wall edema, and bronchial hyperreactivity. The reasons for the unsettling increase in incidence and mortality are complex, and successful therapeutic approaches are elusive. However, throughout the world hundreds of unproved, yet potentially applicable treatment programs are used that rely on complementary/alternative medicine (CAM) for the management of asthma and sinusitis. These programs rely on a variety of protocols including nutrition, botanic medicine, homeopathy, and acupuncture. While conventional therapy is typically directed toward reducing airway inflammation and attenuating bronchial hyperreactivity, investigation of CAM approaches toward treatment and prevention of asthma may help yield new medical modalities to address an important personal and public health problem.[39,41,128]

◼ Epidemiology

Asthma is a chronic condition of varying severity, affecting approximately 3% to 5% of the population.[27,50] Over 15 million asthma-related visits are made to physicians,[77] and asthmatics experience well over 100 million patient days of restricted activity annually. Medical care costs related to asthma treatment exceed $4.6 billion a year.[77] Although the public primarily associates asthma with children, 40% of people with asthma first develop the disease after the age of 40 years.[28] In 1989, more than 479,000 hospitalizations were recorded in which asthma was the first listed diagnosis.[77]

Black children are 2.5 times more likely to have asthma than white children, and blacks of both sexes are about twice as likely as whites to die of asthma.[73,105] It is not clear why prevalence of asthma and its complications are more common among black cohorts compared with whites. Certain health-damaging behaviors, such as smoking or inhaling second-hand smoke, are more common in blacks than in whites. Blacks also have less access to health care. In addition, an underlying genetic predisposition to asthma may influence the higher incidence in blacks.[34]

According to the U.S. National Health Interview Survey on Child Health,[37] asthma is the leading cause of school absence in the United States. The data strongly suggest that childhood asthma is reaching epidemic proportions. Childhood asthma is a major reason for health care usage, totaling over 3.4 million patient visits from 1980 to 1981[84] and 149,000 hospitalizations in 1987.[78] With such an alarming rise in the incidence of childhood asthma, some investigators are calling for new perspectives on asthma care, including the use of complementary therapies to augment conventional care.[50,106]

The incidence of asthma in seniors (those 65 years of age and older) is 5.2%, and, as stated earlier, 40% of people with asthma first develop the disease after the age of 40 years. Greater disability among seniors has been linked to a history of asthma. A number of factors appear to influence the relatively high incidence of asthma among seniors. In 10% of asthmatics an acute inflammatory response to aspirin and related nonsteroidal antiinflammatory agents precipitates an attack.[110] Seniors are the most common users of aspirin and related nonsteroidal antiinflammatory agents, thus increasing their risk of aspirin-induced asthma. A second factor that may precipitate asthma, particularly among seniors, is sinusitis. Sinusitis is proposed to be a leading—and commonly undiagnosed—cause of asthma.[103]

◼ Risk Factors and Pathogenesis

Like most chronic diseases, asthma appears to have both genetic and environmental factors that precipitate the disease. We have shown that when appropriate quantitative genetic models are applied to data from large-scale twin studies, support exists for the notion that genetic factors are important in the etiology of asthma.[116] We have also reviewed the primary environmental factors that trigger genetically predisposed individuals to develop asthma.[116] The most significant environmental variables include allergen exposure, air pollution, cigarette smoke exposure, respiratory viral infections, and oxygen radical damage. Perhaps increased exposure of susceptible individuals to such triggers helps explain the increase in asthma incidence and mortality.

Substantial data suggest that in asthmatics' airways T lymphocytes are activated and encourage interaction with eosinophils, contributing to ongoing airway inflammation and bronchial hyperreactivity.[26,48] The major mechanism by which lymphocytes interact with other immune/inflammatory cells is through cytokine production. Cytokines act via specific receptors and form a network by which interleukins, interferons, lymphokines, monokines, and a variety of factors are related.[15]

Exposure to certain environmental hazards such as cigarette smoke and chemical fragrances can play a significant role in potentiating asthma because they act as triggers.[105] Common triggers include viral infections, cold air, sinusitis, dust, pollens, animal dander, and foods. Many of these aggressions may result in the release of reactive oxygen species (ROS)[109] by inflammatory cells. Oxygen free radicals generated by neutrophils,[72] eosinophils,[17] and other cells[20] are implicated in asthma by a variety of mechanisms, including bronchoconstriction, induction of mucus secretion, and microvascular leakage.[6,29] Reactive oxygen species can also cause an autonomic imbalance between muscarinic-receptor–mediated contraction and beta-adrenergic–mediated relaxation of pulmonary smooth muscle.[29,79] Neutrophils from asthmatics produce increased amounts of superoxide anion compared with those from normal subjects after stimulation by either N-formyl-methionyl leucyl-phenylalanine or phorbol-myristate acetate. Selenium levels in sera from asthmatics have been found to be lower than normal, although the extent to which the antioxidant capability of the circulating blood cells is compromised is not clear.[108]

For many years the upper and lower airways of humans have been regarded as anatomically and fundamentally separate with little or no relationship. Diseases of the upper and lower airways may coexist. For example, 80% of patients with asthma have rhinitis symptoms, and 5% to 15% of patients with perennial rhinitis have asthma. A number of relationships between the upper and lower airways can be identified. The nose serves as an important filter of inspired air. Relatively large particles are captured by the hairs within the nostrils, and other noxious substances are trapped in mucus. Therefore nasal obstruction or a failure in the filter function increases the allergen/irritant burden to the lower airway, thus potentiating lower airway hyperresponsiveness.

Heating and humidification of inspired air are important functions of the nose. Such functions are largely provided by a highly vascularized mucosa of the turbinates and septum. If inspired air bypasses warming and humidification provided by the nose, cooler, drier air is delivered to the lungs, which can potentiate a phenomenon referred to as exercise-induced asthma (EIA). Exercise is an important trigger for bronchial asthma and is thought to be initiated by loss of water and heat from the lower airway. Reduction in severity of EIA can be achieved by breathing through the nose rather than the mouth during exercise.[102]

In both children and adults with asthma, certain viral upper respiratory tract infections (URIs) provoke wheezing. Respiratory syncytial virus is most common in young children, with rhinovirus and influenza virus being more prevalent in older children and adults.[12] Obstructive changes in small airway function of the lung associated with viral illness may persist for up to 5 weeks, even after clinical illness has resolved. Viral URIs also cause airway hyperreactivity.

An estimated 75% of patients admitted with status asthmaticus had abnormal sinus x-rays.[38] Although more objective evidence that sinusitis triggers or exacerbates asthma would be helpful in further clarifying this issue, the data suggest that patients who come to medical attention with difficult-to-control asthma will improve when coexistent sinusitis is cleared by medical and/or surgical treatment. This can be considered as strong suggestive evidence for an etiologic role of sinusitis in lower airway disease.[104]

⚫ CAM Therapies in the Treatment of Asthma

Complementary and alternative medicine therapies for asthma and allergies appear to be widely used by a number of health care professionals in the United States. In a recent survey approach among health professionals subscribing to a leading CAM research journal, we found that dietary therapies were the most commonly used method of intervention for asthma[26a] (Table 3–1). This was closely followed by environmental medicine, which also includes dietary manipulation. Nutritional supplements ranked third in prevalence of use. Taken together, these data suggest that

TABLE 3–1. **TOP 12 RANKINGS* OF COMPLEMENTARY/ALTERNATIVE MEDICINE (CAM) TREATMENTS USED FOR ASTHMA AMONG HEALTH CARE PROFESSIONALS SUBSCRIBING TO A LEADING CAM RESEARCH JOURNAL**

Therapy	UTILITY/ USEFULNESS		USAGE (%)	
	Survey Ranking by MD	Survey Ranking by Non-MD	MD	Non-MD
Dietary	1	1	74	75
Environmental medicine	2	7	69	62
Nutritional supplements	3	2	57[†]	65
Homeopathy	4	3	39[†]	47
Botanicals	5	12	40[†]	57
Meditation/prayer	6	8	45[†]	58
Mind-body therapy	7	5	37[†]	47
Acupuncture	8	4	19[†]	33
Detoxification	9	9	32[†]	47
Massage	10	6	27[†]	48
Chiropractic	11	10	7[†]	23
Osteopathy	12	13	11	15

From Davis PA, Gold EB, Hackman RM, Stern JS, Gershwin ME: The use of complementary/alternative medicine for the treatment of asthma in the United States, *Invest Allergol Clin Immunol* 8:73, 1998.

*Ranking of 1 (most useful) to 20 (least useful) and usage (percentage of total respondents using a particular form of therapy).

MD, Doctor of Medicine.

[†]Different from non-MD, $p < 0.05$, chi-squared analysis.

nutritional therapies are the therapies most commonly used by CAM professionals in treating asthma. Other interventions commonly cited for asthma included homeopathy, botanicals, and prayer/meditation.

HISTORY

Most current conventional asthma treatments were first alternative therapies. That is to say, most of the pharmacologic treatments used by physicians to manage asthma were initially discovered as a result of the traditional use of plants and animal glands for the treatment of asthma. Many CAM remedies currently employed in the United States and Europe stem from folk remedies previously used in Europe. Most European practices originated in the Middle East and were derived over centuries from work of physicians in ancient Akkadia, Sumeria, Mesopotamia, and Egypt.[124,126] Originally rooted in the concept of magical energy in plants, systematic investigations by physicians in ancient Greece and Rome eventually developed a fairly rational pharmacopoeia by the first century A.D.

Nonbotanic Greco-Roman approaches were also used throughout Europe, including cupping, leeching, scarification, and venesection, supplemented by massage, exercises, baths, inhalations, fomentations, poultices, emetics, cathartics, and clusters.[124] Dietary prescriptions were routinely employed in the management of all diseases, and for asthma various herbs, spices, animal extracts, and food eliminations or additions were widely advocated by health experts of the time.

Moses Maimonides, the noted thirteenth-century physician, prescribed an integrated lifestyle for the asthmatic patient. His chief dietary remedy was a spicy herbal mixture of chicken broth that contained herbs such as fennel, parsley, oregano, mint, and onion.[24,31] It is now well known that hydration of the upper respiratory tract is helpful in alleviating some asthmatic symptoms, and robust consumption of broth is one way to accomplish such hydration. The role of vegetable and herbal extracts in soup broth remains to be examined, although onions and garlic have some protective effect against allergic reactions.

In eighteenth-century Europe, strong coffee was widely used for treatment of asthma.[127] The subsequent discovery that caffeine functions as an effective bronchodilator helped verify this practice. Although drinking tea was not particularly favored as an asthma treatment, tea leaves were the original source of theophylline, whose name means tea leaf. Another nineteenth-century European drug used to treat asthma was saltpeter, or potassium nitrate. Saltpeter was inhaled for the muscle-relaxing nitrate vapor. Potassium nitrate was also used in combination with *Datura stramonium* and other herbs in tobacco preparations.

Currently most conventional physicians are treating "alternative medicine" with caution when it comes to the treatment of asthma.[14,16,56] But out of the morass of alternative therapies, rigorous scientific exploration may reveal new, exciting approaches that may be viewed as "complementary." That is to say, therapies such as nutritional supplementation, botanic extracts, mind-body practices, and manipulation strategies may one day offer the physician and the asthma sufferer more options in their quest for a comprehensive approach to asthma[62] (Figure 3–1).

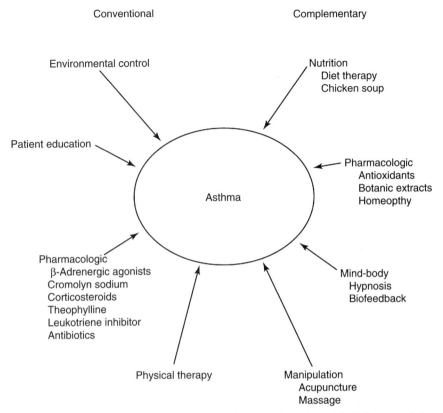

FIGURE 3–1. Conventional and complementary/alternative medicine (CAM) therapies currently in use for treatment of asthma.

NUTRITION

Dietary adjustments have been made throughout the ages to control asthma.[24] Unusual additions and rigorous elimination of articles of diet have had their advocates. Elimination and rotation diets are popular with some patients, who avoid items such as seafood (especially shellfish), chocolate, eggs, nuts, milk, cheeses, and certain liquors. In some cases a true food allergy can be avoided, but many patients subscribe to a limited diet without any clear evidence that the avoided foods are harmful. Undoubtedly, certain foods or additives can make asthma worse, but it is a challenge to construct a realistic elimination diet unless an obvious relationship between specific foods and an individual's asthma exists. For example, avoidance of restaurant salads or various packaged foods could be of importance in patients with sulfite sensitivity. Reports also exist of asthma-causing allergic reactions to vegetables[82] and fruits,[83] but such occurrences are rare. The concept of hypersensitivity to certain foods, most commonly staple foods in a person's diet (e.g., in the United States, milk, eggs, soy, wheat, corn, and rice), is embraced by physicians practicing "environmental medicine" (EM).

A recent report from India found that 83% of parents whose children have asthma believe that certain foods precipitate acute attacks.[55] This is in stark contrast to the estimated 8.5% of the population having true allergic reactions to food.[76] Reconciling the claim of widespread food hypersensitivity with the conventional physician's view of food allergies is impossible at the present time, since EM has not been documented in any systematic scientific manner.

The lung is particularly exposed to high levels of oxygen; thus oxygen-induced free radical damage is of concern. Antioxidants scavenge free radicals, and the role of antioxidants in pulmonary function and pathologies such as asthma has been investigated. Most of the research has focused on ascorbic acid (AA), since AA is the predominant antioxidant in the lung.

Low dietary AA intake has been associated with asthma, bronchitis, and wheezing in the National Health and Nutrition Examination Survey (NHANES II).[93] Recently, dietary analysis of patients suffering from seasonal allergic-type symptoms and asthma found that low AA intake was associated with more than a fivefold increased risk of bronchial reactivity.[104] Other epidemiologic studies have not found an association between AA intake and asthma.[114] Meta-analysis of existing human studies on dietary AA intake and asthma reports a majority of studies finding a positive association, while other studies find no relationship.[9]

In humans, acute AA supplementation (2 g) was found to improve forced expiratory volume in 1 second (FEV_1) pulmonary measures significantly better than a placebo.[11] AA supplementation has also been found to dramatically improve airway hyperresponsiveness in humans exposed to nitrogen dioxide.[74] This double-blind, placebo-controlled study found that 500 mg of AA taken four times per day for 3 days, followed by exposure to nitrogen dioxide, resulted in complete prevention of airway reactivity when assessed by a methacholine challenge test. Recently the effect of 2 g of AA on exercise-induced asthma (EIA) was assessed in those with EIA. Nine of the 10 individuals who received AA supplements 1 hour before exercise demonstrated significant improvement in pulmonary function as assessed by FEV_1. These benefits persisted for 2 weeks following the initial treatment, while the subjects consumed 0.5 g AA per day.[22] In other human studies, AA supplementation 1 hour before testing was able to reduce the duration and intensity of acute airway constriction induced by exercise,[91] histamine,[129] or methacholine.[75] Indomethacin was found to negate the beneficial effects of AA supplementation,[75,80] suggesting a mechanism involving prostaglandin and leukotriene metabolism. In contrast, other clinical studies have not found a role of AA in airway hyperreactivity.[52,112] The different findings in the various research studies on AA and asthma may be partly due to the wide range of vitamin C supplements used in the protocols, as well as the heterogeneous population that probably combines AA-sufficient and AA-deficient individuals. Most protocols to date use acute interventions, and the effect of longer-term treatment with dietary and supplemental AA remains an intriguing research area.

We have suggested other possible links between diet and asthma.[18] Potentially important dietary variables in regard to asthma are the amount and composition of polyunsaturated fatty acid (PUFA) intake. Much attention has been focused on the omega-3 class of fatty acids, such as eicosapentaenoic acid (EPA). EPA competitively inhibits formation of prostaglandins and leukotrienes derived from omega-6 PUFA, arachidonic acid, including LTC_4, LTD_4, and LTE_4, which activate ion transport,[61] mucus secretion,[67] and smooth muscle contraction, and LTB_4, which stimulates neutrophil chemotaxis.[8] In addition to being a competitive inhibitor of arachidonate, EPA is itself a substrate for the biosynthesis of leukotrienes as well as prostaglandins.[60,87]

Fish oils have been reported to aid in the relief of asthma symptoms among persons with mild asthma.[5] In a subsample of 2526 participants in the first National Health and Nutrition Examination Survey (NHANES I), a significant positive association between dietary fish oil intake and pulmonary function was reported.[94] Recently a placebo-controlled study found that addition of omega-3 polyunsaturated fatty acids in 27 patients with bronchial asthma resulted in less severe and less frequent attacks of asphyxia, and drug doses were reduced.[69] Provocation tests with allergen after 2 weeks of supplementation showed a significant decline in allergic response. In contrast, children with asthma given fish oil supplements for 12 weeks showed no significant differences in FEV1 compared with those receiving a placebo.[64]

Fish oils are rich in EPA and docosahexaenoic acid (DHA). These fish oils limit leukotriene synthesis and biologic activities by substituting substrate fatty acids as alternatives to arachidonic acid. Both EPA and DHA inhibit the conversion of arachidonic acid by the cyclooxygenase pathway to prostanoid metabolites and reduce the production of platelet-activating factor (PAF), which may be a possible mechanism of action to explain the apparent benefits of fish oil intake in those with asthma. However, obtaining sufficient fish oil from dietary sources may be problematic for many individuals,[105] since two to four servings weekly of cold-water fish such as salmon or mackerel are recommended. Supplements may be the best way to ensure adequate intake of essential fatty acids.

Zinc is a key nutrient with respect to modulation of immune function and has been implicated in asthma. Recently plasma zinc levels were found to be significantly lower among 22 asthma patients compared with 33 healthy controls (0.80 ± 0.01 mg/L among asthmatics vs. 0.89 ± 0.02 mg/L among controls [mean $\pm$ SE].[46] Plasma copper levels and the plasma zinc/copper ratio were also elevated in asthmatics compared with controls (1.28 ± 0.03 mg/L and 1.61 ± 0.04 vs. 1.06 ± 0.02 mg/L and 1.21 ± 0.02, respectively (mean $\pm$ SE). Both zinc and copper are involved in Zn/Cu-superoxide dismutase (SOD), a key antioxidant enzyme involved in free radical scavenging as well as in cytokine expression. Manganese-SOD has also been implicated in asthma. In a rat model of allergic asthma, Mn-SOD, but not Zn/Cu-SOD, showed significant induction when an asthmatic episode was evoked.[70] Pretreatment with recombinant human SOD resulted in a dramatic suppression of the asthmatic episode, with elimination of Mn-SOD induction.

Low dietary zinc intakes have been positively associated with bronchial hyperreactivity among persons with seasonal allergic symptoms and asthma.[105] Marginal dietary zinc intake may occur in many Americans,[115] and inadequate intake may modulate the severity of asthma, as we have proposed.[49] More specifically, we have suggested that physicians check zinc status of their patients as part of a comprehensive medical examination into the causes of asthma. Further, we suggest that dietary therapies and nutritional supplementation might be employed to replenish marginal or deficient zinc status. Excessive zinc intake due to occupational exposure has been reported to cause asthma[66]; although this level of exposure is unlikely in a normal population, it does illustrate the potential hazard of overconsumption of zinc if used to help treat asthma or other clinical conditions.

A potential link between nutrition and asthma involves magnesium.[117] An epidemiologic study of 2415 randomly selected persons in the United Kingdom found that airway hyperreactivity as measured by methacholine challenge was significantly lower among those consuming high-magnesium diets.[10] After adjusting for age, sex, and the effects of atopy and smoking, a 100-mg/day-higher intake of magnesium was related to a 28-ml-higher FEV_1, and an 18% reduction in relative odds of airway hyperreactivity. Low dietary intake of magnesium has been further associated with increased airway hyperreactivity among patients with asthma.[105] Intravenous magnesium is well known for its bronchodilating effect,[81,90] but evidence of the potential of dietary magnesium to impact asthma symptoms is still evolving. The bronchodilating effect of magnesium may be due to interference with calcium handling by bronchial smooth muscle cells.[33] An intriguing question for CAM research is whether dietary magnesium supplementation can attenuate severity of asthma symptoms.

Probiotics may also be a useful area of investigation in regard to nutritional influences on asthma. Consumption of microorganisms in yogurt and other beneficial bacteria is associated with a reduction in susceptibility to a variety of diseases. In recent studies we have found that daily consumption of 450 g of yogurt with live cultures (Dannon) is associated with a fivefold increase in gamma interferon by stimulated lymphocytes.[42] Since gamma interferon inhibits immunoglobulin E (IgE) synthesis, and since hyperproduction of IgE is implicated in asthma, probiotic supplementation may attenuate this sequence of events and reduce the severity of asthmatic symptoms. Further research is needed to confirm this hypothesis.

ASIAN HERBS

Chinese knowledge of botanic medicine dates back to the discovery of the herbal therapeutic Ma Huang around 3000 B.C. It was initially used as a stimulant but was also used for respiratory afflictions and other diseases.[125] The active ingredient in Ma Huang was subsequently found to be ephedrine, an effective bronchodilator. Ma Huang has been central to asthma treatment in traditional forms of Chinese medicine. Numerous composite preparations that are used in treatment of asthma rely on this botanic. For example, Ma Huang is combined with gecko lizard tails in Ge Jie Anti-Asthma Pill; other traditional mixtures are prescribed under such names as Minor Blue Dragon Combination.[124,125] Some preparations contain a compound with disodium cromoglycate–like activity, but many other favorite traditional Chinese remedies without Ma Huang have yet to show proven value. Traditional antiasthma agents such as Bupleurum, Pinellia, and Magnolia have not been found to be effective.[125]

Extracts of Ginkgo biloba have been shown to inhibit PAF, thus offering a scientific explanation for the use of this herb for treatment of asthmatic coughs.[7] Other traditional agents are known to antagonize PAF, including various fungal derivatives such as gliotoxin from a wood fungus and kadsurenone from haifentenga, a Chinese medication found in *Piper futokadsura*, and an extract of *Tussilago farfara*. This latter herb is known in the West as coltsfoot, and has long been used in both the West and in China as a mild antitussive. A comprehensive review of Chinese herbal medicines used to treat asthma has been published,[13] and the reader is directed to this exhaustive review for details beyond those provided in this chapter.

Traditional Chinese medicine may have introduced steroid therapy in a crude fashion through use of fetal and placental extracts and urine of pubescent children, practices sometimes used in the treatment of asthma. Although none of the Chinese herbal medications used to treat asthma have been found to have corticosteroid activity, it is quite possible that many components have antiinflammatory activity. For example, licorice has been extensively studied and does have such activity. *Ledebouriella seseloides*, *Rehmannia glutinosa*, and *Paeonia lactflora* also have antiinflammatory activity.[124]

In Japan a form of traditional practice, Kampo, has its origins in traditional Chinese medicine. Saiboku-To, a mixture of herbs that has been used for more than 200 years for treatment of asthma, is one such Kampo formula. Recent analytic studies suggested possible mechanisms for its effectiveness in treating asthma.[44,65] Another modern use of Saiboku-To in asthma aims at reducing the dose of steroids in steroid-dependent severe asthma.[113]

In Hawaii traditional use of *Sophora chrysophylla* has been reported for the treatment of asthma.[68] Locally termed "mamane," review of the historical use of this plant and the existing pharmacologic knowledge of other Sophora species suggests promising opportunities for future research.

AYURVEDIC HERBS

Ayurveda is a traditional form of medicine practiced throughout the Indian subcontinent. The practice is based on more than 7000 years of traditional use history. A multiple-intervention strategy is typically used in ayurvedic medicine, involving dietary adjustments, meditation and yogic practices, environmental alterations, and the use of herbal extracts.

Most ayurvedic medications used for asthma are still relatively unknown to Western scientists, but one plant, *Tylophora indica* asthmatica, has been a standard remedy in the treatment of respiratory disorders in which mucus accumulation is a symptom.[126] Chewing the leaves of *T. indica* was found to be an effective therapy in relieving asthmatic symptoms in an early double-blind, placebo-controlled crossover study.[100] Subsequent investigation found that an alcoholic extract of *T. indica* produced complete to moderate relief of asthma symptoms in 58% of patients after 1 week, compared with 31% of those taking a placebo.[101] The difference between the treatment and placebo groups became more marked during the following 12 weeks. In contrast, others have reported no effect of *T. indica* in FEV_1 measurements or symptom relief scores.[40]

The traditional drug vasaka, derived from *Adhatoda vasica* or the malabar nut tree, is smoked in cigarettes for asthma and tuberculosis. *A. vasica* is the source of bromhexine and ambroxol, two mucoregulating drugs used in Europe. Leaves of *Datura stramonium*, called "d'hatura" in India, contain a bronchodilator. Traditional use of this plant as a tobacco remedy for asthma originated in India, and *D. stramonium* cigarettes eventually became popular for treating asthma and bronchitis in Europe and North America.[128]

AFRICAN HERBS

Desmodium adscendens is a traditional botanic medicine used in Ghana as a treatment for asthma and other diseases associated with excessive smooth muscle contraction. Plant extracts inhibit contraction of guinea pig ileum caused by electrical field stimulation[1] and contractions of sensitized guinea pig airway smooth muscle induced by arachidonic acid or leukotriene D4.[2,3] This botanic contains several different elements that aid in relaxation of smooth muscle, acting to inhibit or reduce nicotinamide adenine dinucleotide phosphate (NADPH)–dependent monooxygenase pathway of arachidonic acid metabolism.[3] Recently *D. adscendens* has been shown to contain triterpenoid glycosides, which function as high-affinity activators of calcium-dependent potassium channels.[71] As such, this ethnomedicine contains the most potent known potassium channel opener yet discovered.

AMERICAN HERBS

North American plant derivatives were used in European respiratory therapeutics beginning in the sixteenth century. Important botanics included guaiac wood, ipecacuanha, tobacco, and chili peppers. As discussed previously, cigarettes containing *D. stramonium* were used and, often, also included horehound, mullein, coltsfoot, lobelia, cubebs, seaweed, and marijuana. Glyceryl guaiacolate (guaifenesin), which has mucus-loosening, expectorant properties, was eventually derived from guaiac wood. The mechanism of action of guaiac is the same as that produced by subemetic doses of ipecacuanha, which causes activation of the gastropulmonary mucokinetic reflex, thereby resulting in secretion of low-viscosity mucus.[123] Capsaicin, an active ingredient in cayenne and chili peppers, stimulates the mucokinetic reflex and releases and then depletes substance P stored in nonadrenergic noncholinergic nerves. The subsequent release of mucus, and possible bronchospasm, may help to decrease mucus production and prolong dilation of bronchial muscles.

In recent years isocyanates found in pungent vegetables such as onion have been shown to be protective against allergic reactions in the guinea pig.[31] Mandrake and related solaneous plants, a source of atropinic agents, offer benefits similar to those of *D. stramonium*. The related *Atropa belladonna* was long recognized in Europe to be a potent pharmacologic agent and appears to have been favored by observant lay healers as an antiasthma remedy hundreds of years before it became popular in the nineteenth-century medical community.

HOMEOPATHY

Homeopathy has a devoted group of users in western Europe and the United States. The treatment originated in Germany and was initially expanded to Europe and

America. The homeopathic physician believes that a constellation of physical, psychologic, and emotional domains must be considered to devise an individualized therapeutic program that uses very diluted extracts of botanics and other compounds. Each person is treated individually based on their "constitution," which creates a challenge in researching the effectiveness of specific homeopathic remedies that work in large, heterogeneous populations. Nonetheless, a number of studies in credentialed, peer-reviewed journals report the apparent effectiveness of homeopathy for certain asthmatic and allergic conditions.

Reilly and colleagues tested 28 patients with allergic asthma in a randomized, double-blind, placebo-controlled trial.[88] Before the intervention, patients were tested for allergic responses using skin pricks. The largest skin test wheal was used to determine the primary allergen. Also at this time, patients were tested for FEV_1, forced vital capacity (FVC), and pulmonary reactivity to inhaled histamine. A diary was begun to log drug use for asthma, and a visual analog–scaled questionnaire was administered to assess patients' symptom intensity. Four weeks later, patients were assigned to one of the two groups; those in the homeopathy group received extremely dilute preparations of their primary allergen, while those in the placebo group received inert material. Doses were taken orally, once daily for 4 weeks, at which time follow-up measurements were taken. Patients in the homeopathy group reported significant improvements in their symptom intensity within 1 week of starting the intervention compared with those receiving the placebo, and this difference persisted for the duration of the study. Measures of FEV_1 and FVC were significantly improved in the homeopathy group, and a median 53% reduction in bronchial reactivity to histamine was found in the homeopathy group, compared with a 7% increase in histamine reactivity in the placebo group. This study, published in *The Lancet* in 1994, has sparked vigorous discussion about the potential merits of homeopathy as a complementary treatment for asthma. Further research is needed to help focus such discussions.

Upon stepping back from the details of individual studies and assessing the broad field of CAM for asthma, one thing becomes clear. Despite mountains of traditional use history and current day testimonials, very little objective scientific research exists using the basic tenets of research design (Table 3–2). More research emphasis is urgently required for a number of reasons. First, a very real potential exists to make significant discoveries that help people who have asthma. Modern drugs have been successful at managing asthma symptoms but have limitations. Pharmaceuticals produce side effects, and many authorities believe that the drugs may not address the root causes of asthma. New approaches to help treat asthma at both the symptom and underlying disease levels are needed, and the areas of dietary therapies, nutritional supplements, and botanic extracts appear to offer the most promise for discoveries. A second reason for more research in CAM and asthma is that the consumer marketplace demands it. The sale of herbal remedies in the United States has been increasing at the rate of almost 20% per year since 1993. The sale of herbs is unregulated, and many false, misleading products exist. Research studies can help define which plants and plant fractions may be most useful as complementary therapies available to physicians and asthma sufferers. Quality standards in botanic extracts are desperately

TABLE 3–2. RESEARCH OVERVIEW OF SOME CAM THERAPIES USED FOR ASTHMA

Category	Practice	Research Strength	Key Citation (Reference No[s].)	Issues
Nutrition	Dietary: Avoid foods causing allergies	Excellent	76	Widely accepted by allopathic and CAM physicians
	AA (vitamin C) supplementation	Strong suggestive evidence	11, 22, 74	What is appropriate dosage? Do AA-depleted individuals respond differently than AA-replete persons?
	Essential fatty acids (fish oil) supplementation	Epidemiologic association; two small studies show promise in adults; one study in children showed no effect	5, 69, 94	Should doses be standardized to specific amounts of omega-3 and omega-6 fatty acids? What are appropriate dosage and duration? Do age differences exist?
	Zinc supplementation	Low zinc intake associated with seasonal asthma and allergies	104	No human clinical studies exist
	Magnesium supplementation	Strong epidemiologic evidence relating high magnesium intake to improved pulmonary function	10	No human clinical studies on magnesium supplementation exist
Botanics	Ma Huang (ephedra)	Excellent scientific studies	125	Side effects: Nervousness, cardiac arrhythmias, hypertension
	Other Chinese and Japanese single herbs and mixtures	Strong traditional use, but weak or mixed scientific results	13, 124	Studies fail to find benefits of some mixtures; traditionally used herb mixtures have not been studied using basic principles of research design
	Tylophora indica (from India)	One small study found benefit; one small study did not	40, 101	Repeat study using animal model; is this the very best herb from India to study?
	Other Indian herbs	Traditional use (ayurvedic) history but no scientific studies	126, 128	Systemic study of popular herbs required
Homeopathy	Native American plants	Traditional use history but no scientific studies	123	Systemic study required
	Ingestion of extremely diluted materials, typically botanic in origin	One significant, positive study	88	Repeat study with non-homeopaths conducting intervention; what are the active ingredients?

AA, Ascorbic acid.

needed by industry, government, and biomedical groups, and research laboratories are the place to start getting such standards established.

◤ CAM in the Treatment of Allergies

A variety of CAM treatments exist for allergies, eczema, summer hay fever, and rhinitis. These include therapies such as Chinese herbs, clinical ecology, acupuncture, hypnosis, applied kinesiology, nutritional and botanic supplementation, and homeopathy. Very little scientific evaluation of these therapies exists. Conventional physicians point to the lack of controlled studies and suggest that any benefit ascribed to the CAM treatment is most likely the result of suggestion or a placebo response. Some studies, however, suggest that further research into the area of CAM and allergies is warranted.

CHINESE HERBS

The best scientific evidence in the area of CAM and allergies comes from the study of a traditional Chinese herbal formulation used to treat atopic eczema. The formulation contained a blend of 10 herbs and had proved beneficial in open studies. Although traditional Chinese medicine considers every person as unique and botanic formulations are typically individualized for each patient, the same standard formula was used in six studies that have been published since 1992.

Initially, 40 adults with atopic eczema that was nonresponsive to conventional medical treatment were randomized into two groups for a double-blind, placebo-controlled, crossover study.[97] Herbal decoctions or placebos were consumed daily for 2 months, followed by a 1-month washout period, after which time the groups were crossed. Severity and extent of erythema and surface damage were significantly improved when subjects received the Chinese herbal formula compared with the placebo. No side effects were reported. A similarly designed study was also conducted with children who had nonexudative atopic eczema.[95] When the children received the herbal decoction, their eczema improved, compared with when they consumed the placebo. Ten of the 47 children who initially enrolled in the study withdrew, primarily because they found no relief. While such recidivism may have biased the study results, the similarity of results between the study with children and that with adults suggested that further research was warranted.

At the conclusion of the study with the children the opportunity to continue treatment was offered. All 37 children and parents chose to continue with the herbal treatments, and each child's progress was monitored for the following 12 months.[96] At the end of the year-long follow-up, 18 children showed at least 90% improvement in eczema symptoms, 5 showed moderate improvement, and 14 withdrew from the study (10 because of lack of response, 4 because of unpalatability of the decoction). Among those who completed the follow-up, 7 were able to discontinue treatment with the herbal formula and did not experience any relapse. The other 16 children were able to control their eczema with the herbs, with 12 of them able to reduce the frequency of intake from daily to once every 2 to 5 days. At recruitment into the initial blinded study, use of topical emollients averaged 60 g per day. At the end of the follow-up those who completed the study were using an average of 15 g per day. Only 4 children used 1% hydrocortisone ointment, and none applied it daily. Antihistamine use followed a similar pattern, with 17 of the 23 patients taking nightly antihistamines at the beginning of the controlled study and only 3 taking these drugs sporadically at the conclusion of the follow-up. Twenty-one of the 23 children who completed the study showed elevated IgE levels on admission to the blinded trial. By the end of the follow-up, 10 showed a decrease of greater than 10% in IgE and 3 showed more than a 10% increase. All showed a drop in peripheral blood eosinophil levels into the normal range during the 1-year follow-up. Serum aspartate aminotransferase (AST) levels exceeded 1.5 times the upper limit of normal in 2 children who enrolled in the follow-up. They were dropped from the study, and their AST levels returned to normal. The authors suggested that these 2 patients had idiosyncratic hepatotoxicity.

To investigate possible mechanisms of action of the traditional Chinese herbal formula cited above, the effect of an extract of these herbs or a placebo was tested on peripheral blood monocytes from nonatopic subjects.[57] Expression of CD23, a low-affinity IgE receptor thought to be involved in the pathology of atopic eczema, was assessed. The influence of interleukin 4 (IL-4), known to stimulate expression of CD23, was also monitored. The herbal formula was found to inhibit CD23 expression by as much as 60%, while the placebo had no effect on this parameter. Inhibition was dose dependent and was effective at a concentration as low as 250 µg/ml. When IL-4 was first added to the in vitro system, followed by the Chinese herbal extract or placebo, inhibition of CD23 was noted for the herbal extract for up to 12 hours, while no inhibition resulted from the placebo. The possibility of inhibition of CD23 expression by IL-4 due to cell death was assessed, but no effects were found for either the herbal or placebo preparation.

A more detailed study of immunologic changes among patients with atopic eczema who consumed the traditional Chinese herbal decoction has recently been published.[57] Eighteen patients consumed the formula for 8 weeks and showed an approximately 50% improvement in skin surface damage and erythema. Blood was collected from each patient at the beginning and end of the study period and measured for serum IgE complexes and total serum IgE. Peripheral blood mononuclear cells were derived and used to assess CD23 expression, IL-4 induction of CD23, and soluble interleukin 2 (IL-2) receptor. The treatment decreased serum IgE complexes but did not affect serum IgE or expression of CD23. A significant reduction in the ability of IL-4 to induce CD23 expression was found in monocytes isolated after the completion of the study, relative to pretest expression. At the start of the study soluble IL-2 levels were elevated in the serum of the patients compared with normal values. At the completion of the study soluble IL-2 values decreased significantly. Thus the benefits from the herbal remedy appear to correspond to a variety of changes in immunologic parameters. Antioxidant activity in aqueous decoctions of this Chinese herbal formula also have been reported recently.[51] Which herb(s) and which active compound(s) exert the immunologic effect await further identification, as does the role, if any, of antioxidants in modulating the immune response in this disease.

Other Asian herbs have been studied for their possible allergy treatment potential. The best study is of the dried rhizomes of *Alisma orientale*.[53] Methanol extracts were shown to significantly inhibit antibody-mediated allergic reactions in animal models of types I, II, III, and IV allergies. Four triterpenes and two sesquiterpenes isolated from the methanol fraction exhibited allergy-inhibiting effects, particularly for type III allergies.

The evidence on Chinese herbal medicine for skin disease is not entirely positive. Two cases of hepatitis have been reported in individuals consuming Chinese herbal formulas for skin conditions.[86] Both patients got better on discontinuing the use of the herbs, and recurrence of liver disease was noted on reintroduction of the formulas. Nine other cases of liver damage following the use of Chinese herbal medicines were also reported, although the authors did not provide case histories on these nine. Since the herbal formulas varied in composition and concentration of the different herbs, no clear indication of which ingredient(s) might be causing the liver toxicity was found. The effects did not appear to be dose dependent, and the authors suggested that the pathologic conditions were probably idiosyncratic. Two other cases of hepatitis[47] and one case of severe cardiomyopathy[35] induced by traditional Chinese herbs taken for skin conditions have been reported. The need for consumer caution and for physician inquiry into the use of herbal remedies in their patients is clearly warranted.

ACUPUNCTURE

The role of acupuncture in the treatment of allergic rhinitis has been reported, although these reports are case studies and clinical observations. An early study[59] described 22 patients with allergic rhinitis who received a series of six acupuncture treatments. Fifty percent of subjects were "virtually symptom-free" at the end of the regimen; an additional 36% had a moderate reduction in symptoms and 14% reported no relief. Measurement of serum IgE by radioimmunoassay, percentage of nasal eosinophils, and absolute blood eosinophil count were obtained before treatment, immediately following the final treatment, and 2 months later. Immunoglobulin E levels decreased in 64% of subjects at the end of the treatment regimen and in 76% of subjects at the 2-month follow-up. Those who reported subjective relief of symptoms also showed a drop in blood and nasal eosinophils.

The effect of acupuncture compared with antihistamine treatment was evaluated in 45 patients with allergic rhinitis.[19] Half of the subjects received 7 weeks of acupuncture treatment, and half consumed oral antihistamines. Data were collected before and immediately after the final treatment and at a 3-month follow-up. Symptom severity assessed by the patients and laboratory measures of serum and nasal secretion immunoglobulin (IgA) levels, blood eosinophil levels, and nasal clearance time were collected. X-rays of the paranasal sinus were also taken. Both groups recorded improvements in symptom relief, with the acupuncture group reporting significantly greater improvement than the antihistamine group. Symptom relief persisted at the 3-month follow-up. Similarly, both groups showed improved nasal clearance times, with the effect more lasting in the acupuncture group. Both groups showed significant declines in serum and nasal IgA levels, which still existed at the

3-month follow-up. No differences were found in blood eosinophil levels or in nasal sinus x-rays.

Desensitization treatment for allergic rhinitis was tested with 102 patients using positive allergens and acupuncture points on the head and face.[122] After two treatments allergen extracts were prepared and injected intradermally. The diameter of redness and degree of swelling were significantly less than when tested before acupuncture treatment. Cases were followed for up to 2 years, and the authors reported that 72% of cases had "significant curative effect" with another 24% showing improvement.

A recent study from China[111] reported the effects from a botanic extract (10% Cantharides), which was plastered and blistered on a key acupuncture point (Dazhui, Neiguan point) among 50 people with allergic rhinitis. The treatment was deemed "effective" for 88% of cases, with pretest to posttest measures of serum IgE and nasal eosinophil and basophil secretion levels, and an allergic mucosal provocation test showing statistically significant differences. No control group was used in this study.

Although numerous other acupuncture studies[*] also report positive effects, these are clinical observations and lack any control groups, making the reports difficult to evaluate scientifically. Research studies using the principles of contemporary science are clearly warranted in this area to help clinicians and patients make informed decisions regarding the potential of acupuncture as a complementary therapy for allergic rhinitis.

HOMEOPATHY

One of the first systematic studies on homeopathy assessed its effect on individuals with hay fever.[89] This double-blind, placebo-controlled study randomly assigned 144 patients with symptoms of grass pollenosis (hay fever) to either a treatment or a placebo group for 2 weeks, followed by 2 weeks of observation. The homeopathic remedy tested was an extremely diluted solution of a mixture of 12 grass pollens in the subject's geographic locale that were commonly associated with hay fever. Both patients and doctors kept logs of hay fever–related symptom intensity. Participants also recorded their use of antihistamine medication. The homeopathy treatment group showed a significant reduction in patient- and doctor-scored symptom intensity compared with the placebo group. When the data were adjusted for pollen count, the symptom score differences were even greater. Those in the treatment group also showed a reduction of approximately 50% in their use of antihistamines. The authors took great care to emphasize the statistical rigor of their study and concluded that the effects seen in the homeopathy group were beyond the effects of a placebo alone.

A survey of 102 patients treated in a homeopathic clinic of a large medical center in Israel reported that treatment of allergy-related conditions was the main reason for using this form of health care.[85] Most of the survey respondents were children and young adults (mean age, 22.7 years) in whom conventional Western medicine had been ineffective. Asthma, skin problems, and recurrent URIs were the three most frequently noted categories for which participants sought homeopathic care. More than

---

[*]References 23, 25, 32, 36, 43, 45, 54, 92, 98, 99, 118–121.

80% of participants were greatly satisfied with the homeopathic approach, and half of the respondents reported that their symptoms had improved. The survey bias of a self-selected population is obvious, and it is impossible to determine whether the benefits and satisfaction of patients are due to a placebo effect or are a result of the treatment. Since different patients received different homeopathic remedies, it is also impossible to assess which, if any, remedy was effective using scientifically accepted criteria. Nonetheless, such reports suggest a consumer demand for complementary therapies for allergy treatment, and rigorous study of homeopathy in the treatment of common allergic diseases is necessary to help patients and physicians more clearly identify treatments that may be beneficial.

A recent meta-analysis of 185 homeopathic trials[63] is the latest report pointing to the need for more rigorous research in this area. After applying the principles of scientific research design to the trials, 89 were found to have appropriate data for meta-analysis. The combined odds ratio was 2.45 in support of homeopathy. Four studies on the effect of a particular remedy used to treat seasonal allergies had a pooled odds ratio of 2.03 for relief of ocular symptoms after 4 weeks of treatment. The authors concluded that their results "are not compatible with the hypothesis that the clinical effects of homeopathy are completely due to placebo." Yet, they also note a lack of sufficient scientific study of homeopathy for any single medical condition and make a strong case for systematic scientific research in this area.

SUMMARY

A broad view of the research on CAM therapies for asthma or allergies may exist (Table 3–3); however more research and new research initiatives are required to make sense of an exciting yet confusing area of emerging biomedical importance. Between 1998 and 2002, the Cochrane Review group has evaluated several CAM therapies for treatment of asthma or allergy conditions. See www.update-software.com/cochrane/. (Editors.)

TABLE 3–3. **RESEARCH OVERVIEW OF SOME CAM THERAPIES USED FOR TREATMENT OF ALLERGIES**

Category	Practice	Research Strength	Key Citation (Reference No[s].)	Issues
Botanic	Specific Chinese herbal formula	Excellent results in children and adults	95, 96, 97	What are the active ingredients?
Acupuncture	Methods vary; needles only, herbal point stimulation; may or may not include herbal teas	Limited uncontrolled studies suggest some benefit	19, 59, 122	Standardize treatment; use basic principles of research design
Homeopathy	Ingestion of extremely diluted material, typically grass pollen, animal dander or other botanic	One study suggests benefits	89	Repeat study; what are the active ingredients?

REFERENCES

1. Addy ME: Some secondary plant metabolites in Desmodium adscendens and their effects on arachidonic and metabolism, *Prostagland Leukot Essent Fatty Acids* 47:85, 1992.
2. Addy ME, Burka JF: Effect of Desmodium adscendens fractions on antigen- and arachidonic acid-induced contractions of guinea pig airways, *Can J Physiol Pharmacol* 66:820, 1988.
3. Addy ME, Burka JF: Effect of Desmodium adscendens fraction 3 on contractions of respiratory smooth muscle, *J Ethnopharmacol* 29:325, 1990.
4. Alexander HL: A historical account of death from asthma, *J Allergy* 34:305, 1963.
5. Arm JP et al: Effect of dietary supplementation with fish oil lipids on mild asthma, *Thorax* 43:84, 1988.
6. Barnes PJ: Reactive oxygen species and airway inflammation, *Free Radic Biol Med* 9:235, 1990.
7. Barnes PJ, Chung KF, Page CP: Platelet-activating factor as a mediator of allergic disease, *J Allergy Clin Immunol* 82:751, 1988.
8. Barnes N, Piper PJ, Costello J: The effect of an oral leukotriene antagonist L-649, 923 on histamine and leukotriene D4-induced bronchoconstriction in the normal man, *J Allergy Clin Immunol* 79:816, 1987.
9. Bielory L, Gandhi R: Asthma and vitamin C, *Ann Allergy* 73:89, 1994.
10. Britton J et al: Dietary magnesium, lung function, wheezing, and airway hyperreactivity in a random adult population sample, *Lancet* 344:357, 1994.
11. Bucca C et al: Effect of vitamin C on histamine bronchial responsiveness of patients with allergic rhinitis, *Ann Allergy* 65:311, 1990.
12. Busse WE: The precipitation of asthma by upper respiratory infections, *Chest* 87(suppl):44, 1985.
13. But P, Chang C: Chinese herbal medicine in the treatment of asthma and allergies, *Clin Rev Allergy Immunol* 14:253, 1996.
14. Carlson CM, Sachs MI: Is alternative medicine an alternative for the treatment of asthma? *J Asthma* 31:149, 1994.
15. Casale TB, Smart SJ: Pathogenesis of asthma: mediators and mechanisms. In Gershwin ME, Halpern GM, editors: *Bronchial asthma: principles of diagnosis and treatment*, ed 3, Totowa, NJ, 1994, Humana.
16. Chanez P et al: Controversial forms of treatment for asthma, *Clin Rev Allergy Immunol* 14:247, 1996.
17. Chanez P et al: Generation of oxygen free radicals from blood eosinophils from asthma patients after stimulation with PAF or phorbol ester, *Eur Respir J* 3:1002, 1990.
18. Chang CC et al: Asthma mortality: another opinion—is it a matter of life and . . . bread? *J Asthma* 30:93, 1993.
19. Chari P et al: Acupuncture therapy in allergic rhinitis, *Am J Acupunct* 16:143, 1988.
20. Cluzel M et al: Enhanced alveolar cell luminol-dependent chemiluminescence in asthma, *J Allergy Clin Immunol* 80:195, 1987.
21. Cockcroft DW et al: Allergen-induced increase in non-allergic bronchial reactivity, *Clin Allergy* 7:503, 1977.
22. Cohen HA, Neuman I, Nahum H: Blocking effect of vitamin C in exercise-induced asthma, *Arch Pediatr Adolesc Med* 151:367, 1997.
23. Cortes JL: The practice of allergy in the People's Republic of China, *Ann Allergy* 46:92, 1981.
24. Cosman MP: A feast for Aesculapius: historical diets for asthma and sexual pleasure, *Ann Rev Nutr* 3:1, 1983.
25. Czubalski K et al: Acupuncture and phonostimulation in pollenosis and vasomotor rhinitis in the light of psychosomatic investigations, *Acta Otolaryngol* (Stockh) 84:446, 1977.
26. De Monchy JGR et al: Bronchoalveolar eosinophilia during allergen-induced late asthmatic reactions, *Am Rev Respir Dis* 131:373, 1985.
26a. Davis PA, Gold EB, Hackman RM, Stern JS, Gershwin ME: The use of complementary/alternative medicine for the treatment of asthma in the United States, *Invest Allergol Clin Immunol* 8:73, 1998.
27. Dodge R, Burrows B: The prevalence and incidence of asthma and asthma-like symptoms in a general population sample, *Am Rev Respir Dis* 122:567, 1980.

28. Dodge R, Cline MG, Burrows B: Comparisons of asthma, emphysema, and chronic bronchitis in a general population sample, *Am Rev Respir Dis* 133:981, 1986.

29. Doelman CJ, Bast A: Oxygen radicals in lung pathology, *Free Radic Biol Med* 9:381, 1990.

30. Dolovich J et al: Late-phase airway reaction and inflammation, *J Allergy Clin Immunol* 83:521, 1989.

31. Dorsch W et al: Antiasthmatic effects of onion extracts—detection of benzyl and other isothiocyanates (mustard oils) as antiasthmatic compounds of plant origin, *Eur J Pharm* 107:17, 1985.

32. Drasnar T, Palecek D: Classical acupuncture in the treatment of rhinitis vasomotorica and rhinitis pollinosa, *Cesk Otolaryngol* 30:104, 1981.

33. Durlach J: Commentary on recent clinical advances: magnesium depletion, magnesium deficiency and asthma, *Magnes Res* 8:403, 1995.

34. Evans R et al: National trends in the morbidity and mortality of asthma in the United States: prevalence, hospitalization and death from asthma over two decades—1965-1984, *Chest* 91(suppl):65S, 1987.

35. Ferguson JE, Chalmers RJ, Rowlands DJ: Reversible dilated cardiomyopathy following treatment of atopic eczema with Chinese herbal medicine, *Br J Dermatol* 136:592, 1997.

36. Fischer MV, Behr A, von Reumont J: Acupuncture: a therapeutic concept in the treatment of painful conditions and functional disorders—report on 971 cases, *Acupunct Electrother Res* 9:11, 1984.

37. Fowler MG, Davenport MG, Garg R: School functioning of U.S. children with asthma, *Pediatrics* 90:939, 1992.

38. Fuller C et al: Sinusitis in status asthmaticus, *J Allergy Clin Immunol* 85:222, 1990 (abstract).

39. Gershwin ME, Terr A: Alternative and complementary therapy for asthma, *Clin Rev Allergy Immunol* 14:241, 1996.

40. Gupta S et al: Tylophora indica in bronchial asthma: a double blind study, *Indian J Med Res* 69:981, 1979.

41. Hackman RM, Stern JS, Gershwin ME: Complementary and alternative medicine and asthma, *Clin Rev Allergy Immunol* 14:321, 1996.

42. Halpern GM et al: Influence of long-term yogurt consumption in young adults, *Int J Immunother* 7:205, 1991.

43. He S, Wang S, Peng Y: Treatment of allergic rhinitis with helium neon laser on acupoints, *J Tradit Chin Med* 10:116, 1990.

44. Homma M et al: A strategy for discovering biologically active compounds with high probability in traditional Chinese herbal remedies: an application of Saiboku-To in bronchial asthma, *Anal Biochem* 202:179, 1992.

45. Jia D: Current applications of acupuncture by otorhinolaryngologists, *J Tradit Chin Med* 13:59, 1993.

46. Kadrabova J et al: Plasma zinc, copper and copper/zinc ratio in intrinsic asthma, *J Trace Elem Med Biol* 10:50, 1996.

47. Kane JA, Kane SP, Jain S: Hepatitis induced by traditional Chinese herbs: possible toxic components, *Gut* 36:146, 1995.

48. Kay AB: Asthma and inflammation, *J Allergy Clin Immunol* 87:893, 1991.

49. Keen CL, Gershwin ME: Zinc deficiency and immune function, *Annu Rev Nutr* 10:413, 1990.

50. Kemper KJ: Chronic asthma: an update, *Pediatr Rev* 17:111, 1996.

51. Kirby AJ, Schmidt RJ: The antioxidant activity of Chinese herbs for eczema and of placebo herbs. I, *J Ethnopharmacol* 56:103, 1997.

52. Kreisman H, Mitchell C, Bouhuys A: Inhibition of histamin-induced airway constriction negative results with oxtriphylline and ascorbic acid, *Lung* 154:223, 1977.

53. Kubo M et al: Studies on Alismatis rhizoma. I. Anti-allergic effects of methanol extract and six terpene components from Alismatis rhizoma (dried rhizome of Alisma orientale), *Biol Pharm Bull* 20:511, 1997.

54. Lai X: Observation on the curative effect of acupuncture on type I allergic diseases, *J Tradit Chin Med* 13:243, 1993.

55. Lal A, Kumar L, Malhotra S: Knowledge of asthma among parents of asthmatic children, *Indian Pediatr* 32:649, 1995.

56. Lane DJ: What can alternative medicine offer for the treatment of asthma? *J Asthma* 31:153, 1994.

57. Latchman Y et al: Association of immunological changes with clinical efficacy in atopic eczema patients treated with traditional Chinese herbal therapy (Zemaphyte), *Int Arch Allergy Immunol* 109:243, 1996.

58. Latchman Y et al: Efficacy of traditional Chinese herbal therapy in vitro: a model system for atopic eczema–inhibition of CD23 expression on blood monocytes, *Br J Dermatol* 132:592, 1995.
59. Lau BH, Wong DS, Slater JM: Effect of acupuncture on allergic rhinitis: clinical and laboratory evaluations, *Am J Chin Med* 3:263, 1975.
60. Lee TH et al: Effect of dietary enrichment with eicosapentaenoic and dicosahexanoic acids on in vitro neutrophil and monocyte leukotriene generation and neutrophil function, *N Engl J Med* 312:1217, 1985.
61. Leikauf GD et al: Alteration of chloride secretion across canine tracheal epthelium by lipoxygenase products of arachidonic acid, *Am J Physiol* 250:F47, 1986.
62. Lewith GT, Watkins AD: Unconventional therapies in asthma: an overview, *Allergy* 51:761, 1996.
63. Linde K et al: Are the clinical effects of homeopathy placebo effects? A meta-analysis of placebo-controlled trials, *Lancet* 350:834, 1997.
64. Machura E et al: The effect of dietary fish oil supplementation on the clinical course of asthma in children, *Pediatr Pol* 71:97, 1996.
65. Makino S: Preventive therapy in Japan. In Morley J, editor: *Preventive therapy in asthma*, London, 1991, Academic.
66. Malo JL, Cartier A, Dolovich J: Occupational asthma due to zinc, *Eur Respir J* 6:447, 1993.
67. Marom Z et al: Slow reacting substance, leukotriene C4 and D4, increase the release of mucus from human airways in vitro, *Am Rev Respir Dis* 126:449, 1982.
68. Massey DG, Chien YK, Fournier-Massey G: Mamane: scientific therapy for asthma? *Hawaii Med J* 53:350, 1994.
69. Masuev KA: The effect of polyunsaturated fatty acids on the biochemical indices of bronchial asthma patients, *Ter Arkh* 69:33, 1997.
70. Matsuyama T et al: Superoxide dismutase suppressed asthmatic response with inhibition of manganese superoxide induction in rat lung, *Nippon Kyobu Shikkan Gakkai Zasshi* 31(suppl):139, 1993.
71. McManus OB et al: An activator of calcium-dependent potassium channels isolated from a medicinal herb, *Biochemistry* 32:6128, 1993.
72. Meltzer SM et al: Superoxide generation and its modulation by adenosine in the neutrophils of subjects with asthma, *J Allergy Clin Immunol* 83:960, 1989.
73. Mitchell EA: Racial inequalities in childhood asthma, *Soc Sci Med* 32:831, 1991.
74. Mohsenin V: Effect of vitamin C on NO2-induced airway hyperresponsiveness in normal subjects: a randomized double-blind experiment, *Am Rev Respir Dis* 136:1408, 1987.
75. Mohsenin V, Dubois AB, Douglas JS: Effect of ascorbic acid on response to methacholine challenge in asthmatic subjects, *Am Rev Respir Dis* 127:143, 1983.
76. Moneret-Vautrin DA, Kanny G, Thevenin F: Asthma caused by food allergy, *Rev Med Interne* 17:551, 1996.
77. National Heart, Lung and Blood Institute: Asthman statistics: data fact sheet, Bethesda, Md, May 1992, National Institutes of Health.
78. National Hospital Discharge Survey: Annual summary: 1987. Vital and Health Statistics, Pub PHS 89-1760, Series 13, No 99, National Center for Health Statistics, Hyattsville, Md, 1989, US Department of Health and Human Services.
79. Nijkamp FP, Henricks PA: Receptors in airway disease: beta-adrenoceptors in lung inflammation, *Am Rev Respir Dis* 141:S145, 1990.
80. Ogilvy CS, DuBois AB, Douglas JS: Effects of ascorbic acid and indomethacin on the airways of healthy male subjects with and without induced bronchoconstriction, *J Allergy Clin Immunol* 67:363, 1981.
81. Okayama H et al: Bronchodilating effects of intravenous magnesium sulphate in bronchial asthma, *JAMA* 257:1076, 1987.
82. Parra FM et al: Bronchial asthma caused by two unrelated vegetables, *Ann Allergy* 70:324, 1993.
83. Pastorello EA et al: Allergenic cross-reactivity among peach, apricot, plum, and cherry in patients with oral allergy syndrome: an in vivo and in vitro study, *J Allergy Clin Immunol* 94:699, 1994.
84. Patterns of ambulatory care in pediatrics: the National Ambulatory Medical Care Survey, United States, January 1980–December 1981 (data from the National Health Survey), Vital and Health Statistics, Pub PHS 84–1736, Series 13, No 75, National Center for Health Statistics, Hyattsville, Md, 1983, US Department of Health and Human Services.

85. Peer O, Bar Dayan Y, Shoenfeld Y: Satisfaction among patients of a homeopathic clinic, *Harefuah* 130:86, 1996.
86. Perharic L et al: Possible association of liver damage with the use of Chinese herbal medicine for skin disease, *Vet Hum Toxicol* 37:562, 1995.
87. Phinney SD et al: Reduced adipose 18:3w3 with weight loss by very low calorie dieting, *Lipids* 25:798, 1990.
88. Reilly DT et al: Is evidence for homeopathy reproducible? *Lancet* 344:1601, 1994.
89. Reilly DT et al: Is homoeopathy a placebo response? Controlled trial of homeopathic potency, with pollen in hay fever as model, *Lancet* 2:881, 1986.
90. Rolla G et al: Acute effects of intravenous magnesium sulfate for airway obstruction of asthmatic patients, *Ann Allergy* 61:388, 1988.
91. Schachter EN, Schlesinger A: The attenuation of exercise-induced bronchospasm by ascorbic acid, *Ann Allergy* 49:146, 1982.
92. Scheidhauer D, Gestewitz B: Acupuncture: a method in the treatment of vasomotor rhinitis, *Z Arztl Fortbild (Jena)* 83:37, 1989.
93. Schwartz J, Weiss ST: Dietary factors and their relation to respiratory symptoms: the Second National Health and Nutrition Examination Survey, *Am J Epidemiol* 132:67, 1990.
94. Schwartz J, Weiss ST: The relationship of dietary fish intake to level of pulmonary function in the first National Health and Nutrition Survey (NHANES I), *Eur Respir J* 7:1821, 1994.
95. Sheehan MP, Atherton DJ: A controlled trial of traditional Chinese medicinal plants in widespread non-exudative atopic eczema, *Br J Dermatol* 126:179, 1992.
96. Sheehan MP, Atherton DJ: One-year follow-up of children treated with Chinese medicinal herbs for atopic eczema, *Br J Dermatol* 130:488, 1994.
97. Sheehan MP et al: Efficacy of traditional Chinese herbal therapy in adult atopic dermatitis, *Lancet* 340:13, 1992.
98. Shevrygin BV, Karpova EP: Characteristics of acupuncture reflexotherapy in vasomotor and allergic rhinitis in children, *Vestn Otorinolaringol* 21, 1988.
99. Shevrygin BV et al: Status of the autonomic nervous system and reflexotherapy in children with vasomotor rhinitis, *Pediatriia* 46, 1989.
100. Shivpuri DN, Menon MPS, Parkash S: Cross-over double-blind study on Tylophora indica in the treatment of asthma and allergic rhinitis, *J Allergy* 43:145, 1969.
101. Shivpuri DN, Singhal SC, Parkash D: Treatment of asthma with an alcoholic extract of Tylophora indica: a cross-over, double-blind study, *Ann Allergy* 30:407, 1972.
102. Shturman-Ellstein R et al: The beneficial effect of nasal breathing on exercise induced bronchoconstriction, *Am Rev Respir Dis* 118:72, 1978.
103. Slavin RG: Chronic sinus disease and asthma. In: Gershwin ME, Halpern GM, editors: *Bronchial asthma: principles of diagnosis and treatment*, ed 3, Totowa, NJ, 1994, Humana.
104. Soutar A, Seaton A, Brown K: Bronchial reactivity and dietary antioxidants, *Thorax* 52:166, 1997.
105. Spector SL: Common triggers of asthma, *Postgrad Med* 90:50, 1991.
106. Spigelblatt LS: Alternative medicine: should it be used by children? *Curr Probl Pediatr* 25:180, 1995.
107. Stephen AM, Wald NJ: Trends in individual consumption of dietary fat in the United States: 1920–1984, *Am J Clin Nutr* 52:457, 1990
108. Stone J et al: Reduced selenium status of patients with asthma, *Clin Sci* 77:495, 1989.
109. Szczeklik A, Gryglewski RJ, Czerniawska-Mysik G: Clinical patterns of hypersensitivity to nonsteroidal anti-inflammatory drugs and their pathogenesis, *J Allergy Clin Immunol* 60:276, 1977.
110. Szczeklik A, Sladek K: Aspirin, related nonsteroidal anti-inflammatory agents, sulfites, and other food additives as precipitating factors in asthma. In Gershwin ME, Halpern GM, editors: *Bronchial asthma: principles of diagnosis and treatment*, ed 3, Totowa, NJ, 1994, Humana.
111. Tang ZM, Chen JX, Tan JS: Therapy of cantharides extract for perennial allergic rhinitis and its effect on total IgE in serum, *Chung Kuo Chung Hsi I Chieh Ho Tsa Chih* 15:334, 1995.
112. Ting S, Mansfield LE, Yarbrough J: Effects of ascorbic acid on pulmonary functions in mild asthma, *J Asthma* 20:39, 1983.

113. Toda S et al: Effects of the Chinese herbal medicine "Saiboku-To" on histamine release from and the degranulation of mouse peritoneal mast cells induced by compound 48/80, *J Ethnopharmacol* 24:303, 1988.

114. Troisi RJ et al: A prospective study of diet and adult-onset asthma, *Am J Respir Crit Care Med* 151:1401, 1995.

115. U.S. Department of Agriculture: 1986 Nationwide Food Consumption Survey: Continuing Survey of Food Intakes of Individuals–women 19 to 50 years and their children 1 to 5 years, 4 days, Report No 86-3, Hyattsville, Md, 1986, Nutrition Monitoring Division, Human Nutrition Information Service.

116. Waller NG, Teuber S, Gershwin ME: The genetics and epidemiology of asthma. In Gershwin ME, Halpern GM, editors: *Bronchial asthma: principles of diagnosis and treatment*, ed 3, Totowa, NJ, 1994, Humana.

117. Whang R: Magnesium deficiency: pathogenesis, prevalence, and clinical implications, *Am J Med* 82:24, 1987.

118. Xu J: Influence of acupuncture on human nasal mucociliary transport, *Chung Hua Erh Pi Yen Hou Ko Tsa Chih* 24:90, 1989.

119. Yang YQ: Progress on anti-allergy treatment with acupuncture, *Chung Kuo Chung Hsi I Chieh Ho Tsa Chih* 13:190, 1993.

120. Yu S, Cao J, Yu Z: Acupuncture treatment of chronic rhinitis in 75 cases, *J Tradit Chin Med* 13:103, 1993.

121. Zhao C, Yue F, Yao S: Treatment of allergic rhinitis by medicinal injection at fengmen acupoint, *J Tradit Chin Med* 10:264, 1990.

122. Zhou RL, Zhang JC: Desensitive treatment with positive allergens in acupoints of the head for allergic rhinitis and its mechanism, *Chung Hsi I Chieh Ho Tsa Chih* 11: 708, 721, 1991.

123. Ziment I: *Respiratory pharmacology and therapeutics*, Philadelphia, 1978, WB Saunders.

124. Ziment I: Five thousand years of attacking asthma: an overview, *Respir Care* 31:117, 1986.

125. Ziment I: The management of common respiratory diseases by traditional Chinese drugs, *Oriental Healing Art Int Bull* 13(2):133, 1988.

126. Ziment I: Historic overview of mucoactive drugs. In Braga PC, Allegra L, editors: *Drugs in bronchial mucology*, New York, 1989, Raven.

127. Ziment I: Unconventional therapy in asthma. In Gershwin ME, Halpern GM, editors: *Bronchial asthma: principles of diagnosis and treatment*, ed 3, Totowa, NJ, 1994, Humana.

128. Ziment I: Unconventional therapy in asthma, *Clin Rev Allergy Immunol* 14:289, 1996.

129. Zuskin E, Lewis AJ, Bouhuys A: Inhibition of histamine-induced airway constriction by ascorbic acid, *J Allergy Clin Immunol* 51:218, 1973.

SUGGESTED READINGS

Gershwin ME, Halpern GM, editors: *Bronchial asthma: principles of diagnosis and treatment*, ed 3, Totowa, NJ, 1994, Humana.

Robbers JE, Speedie, MK, Tyler VE: *Pharmacognosy and pharmacobiotechnology*, Baltimore, 1996, Williams & Wilkins.

Tyler VE: *The honest herbal: a sensible guide to the use of herbs and related remedies*, ed 3, New York, 1993, Pharmaceutical Products Press.

Tyler VF: *Herbs of choice: the therapeutic use of phytomedicinals*, New York, 1994, Pharmaceutical Products Press.

CHAPTER 4

Cancer

PHUONG THI KIM PHAM and ARON PRIMACK

Cancer is a major disease category in current health care for people of all ages. Even with beneficial programs, however, such as early detection of breast cancer with improved screening techniques, the overall incidence and mortality attributable to the major cancers (e.g., lung, breast, colon, prostate) have changed little over the past three decades, and conventional medical treatments are inadequate. Considerable progress has been made in genetic research explicating many reasons for susceptibility to cancer.

Radical surgical treatment for cancer has been replaced by more focused surgical approaches in combination with other methods, including radiation therapy, brachytherapy, chemotherapy,[303] and immunotherapy, with some improvement in results. Even with the burgeoning number of new chemotherapeutic agents, however, as well as the general acceptance of severe toxic effects and the many new products to ameliorate these potentially life-threatening toxicities, medical treatment of cancer has resulted in minimal statistical improvement over several decades. Although radiation therapy often can control local areas of disease, local recurrences, and specific complications, it falls short in overall cure rates and longevity.

This chapter delineates some of the cancer treatments in complementary and alternative medicine (CAM) and results of usage of these therapies. Rather than an all-inclusive listing of treatments attempted, used, or rejected, this discussion focuses on directions that have been taken and that need to be taken for CAM to be adjudicated, understood, and incorporated into medical treatment as CAM cancer therapies become scientifically validated.

⋏ Survey Results on Usage of CAM Therapies

Patients generally use CAM for chronic diseases such as back pain, headaches, arthritis, musculoskeletal pain, insomnia, depression, and anxiety.[49] However, patients with cancer are frequent users of CAM therapy as well, often for the accompanying chronic symptoms. Most patients who are using CAM therapy for their diabetes, cancer, and hypertension are also seen by conventional medical practitioners.[49] They have not circumvented the established medical system.

In a survey done in the 1980s and one of the first surveys on CAM usage, Cassileth et al.[55] reported that 54% of patients ($n = 304$) in a major cancer center were also using CAM, 40% of whom ultimately abandoned conventional therapy in favor of CAM. About 60% of the practitioners of CAM were physicians. Patients who used CAM were more likely to be white and well educated. The most common CAM therapies were metabolic treatments, diet treatments, megavitamins, imagery, spiritual treatments, and "immune" treatments. Patients chose CAM to assume personal responsibility for their care and because of an underlying belief that pollution and diet caused the cancer and therefore avoidance of pollution and modification of diet were the best approaches to its cure. Satisfaction with CAM treatment was reflected in the 43% of patients who believed vitamin therapy helped their cancer and 58% who believed vitamins helped their overall health.

Banner et al.[19] found that 28% of breast and cervical cancer patients in Hawaii used traditional Hawaiian remedies the year before the survey; 14% had sought help from a Hawaiian healer; and 6% said traditional therapy would be their first source of medical assistance. Further, Lerner and Kennedy[211] performed a statistically valid sampling study using telephone interviews of 5047 patients with cancer, almost all of whom were treated with conventional medicine, including surgery (69%), radiation therapy (33%), and chemotherapy (33%). Of these, 9% used at least one type of CAM. Women and men used CAM about equally, 9.2% and 8.7%. CAM usage rose proportionately with increased wealth, age less than 49 years, increasing education, and larger size of the household. Patients generally learned of these alternative methods of treatment from physicians, but the news media and television were also instrumental, along with word of mouth from family and friends. Some types of cancer were associated with CAM more often, including central nervous system (21%), lymphoma (14.5%), and ovarian (16%). The longer the patient had a malignancy, the more likely the patient was to seek alternative therapy. If the cancer was still in evidence at 5 years, 10% were using alternative therapy, and 6% with no evidence of disease used CAM. Diet therapies were more often used by women, mind-body therapies by men, and drug therapies equally.

More recently a survey of 453 outpatients at a comprehensive cancer center indicated that 69% of cancer patients used CAM treatment, excluding spiritual practices and psychotherapy.[306] Further, of 100 adult cancer patients in a private nonprofit south Florida hospital, 80% reported using some type of CAM.[31] The International Union Against Cancer (UICC) e-mail survey has also shown a large and heterogeneous group of CAM remedies used to treat cancer in both developed and developing countries worldwide.[57]

Lerner and Kennedy[211] reported that 44% of patients were using CAM after conventional therapy, presumably because of residual disease; 20% were using CAM simultaneously with conventional medicine; and 17% were using CAM before conventional therapy, possibly leading to delayed treatment and reduced chance of cure from the conventional approach.[28] The authors found that patients rarely discontinued their visits to their conventional therapist once they started CAM; 58% of these CAM users believed they were likely to be cured by the therapy, and 25% of CAM costs was covered through third-party health insurance.

Lerner and Kennedy[211] concluded that "it is evident that physicians must become familiar with questionable cancer therapies, must make it known to patients that they are available to discuss questionable methods, and must then, without criticism, direct patients to appropriate sources of care and additional information." They added the following:

> [Whereas] some questionable therapies are harmless or inexpensive, others have toxic effects and may be costly, and none [has] scientifically proven efficacy. Although the percentage of usage reported is relatively low, overall large numbers of patients are involved, especially in certain groups. The physician plays a key role in encouraging or preventing the use of questionable methods,[10,11] and substantial improvements in public and professional education are needed.

Cancer patients may use CAM more frequently than what standard history and physical examination might record. Because these therapies may interact with conventional treatments and cause significant side effects, it is crucial for medical oncologists to inquire with explicit questions about the use of CAM in order to guide patients using these therapies.[243]

The use of CAM in children[171,347,348] with cancer reveals that 10%, presumably through their parents, had previously consulted CAM practitioners, most often using chiropractic, homeopathy,[379] naturopathy, hypnotherapy with relaxation, and acupuncture. They were generally older children with better-educated mothers. Some children were given megavitamins, which could have serious negative consequences. The most common cancer-related medical conditions were respiratory illness, musculoskeletal problems, dermatologic conditions, gastrointestinal problems, and allergies. A recent study in Saskatchewan indicates that 36% of participating families reported using CAM for their child's cancer and that another 21% considered CAM.[38] CAM is used worldwide for cancer treatment (Table 4–1).

PHYSICIAN AND PATIENT ISSUES

The most common reasons that people with cancer seek CAM treatment are the (1) appeal of natural holistic remedies, (2) possibility of improving quality and quantity of life when the allopathic community says "nothing can be done," (3) need to have a sense of control over own life, (4) pressure from family and friends, and (5) mistrust of the conventional medical establishment and authority figures in general.[43] Further, allopathic medicine can be expensive. Scientific cancer medicine demands an appropriate, clear diagnosis, which requires a biopsy. Testing often includes costly radiographic imaging studies and laboratory evaluation. The therapy itself, including surgery, chemotherapy, and radiation therapy, can be very costly.

CAM, with its stress on natural products, teas, herbs, electric stimulation, massage, and so forth, often is much less expensive per treatment. Cancer patients often

TABLE 4–1.   STUDIES ON COMPLEMENTARY AND ALTERNATIVE MEDICINE (CAM) USAGE FOR TREATMENT OF CANCER

Study	Country	Patients	CAM Usage	Specific Findings	Most Common Therapies
Downer et al.[87]	Great Britain	415	16%	—	Healing relaxation, diet, homeopathy, vitamin
Lerner, Kennedy[211]	United States	5047	9%	—	Diet, mind/body, drug
Begbie et al.[26]	Australia	335	21.9%	Young adults, women, married/single, well educated, desire for "natural" therapies	Diet, psychologic, herbal remedies
Cassileth, Chapman[53]	United States	660	54%	—	Metabolic, diet, megavitamin, imagery, spiritual, "immune"
Fisher, Ward[107]	England	Not given	16% 16% 36% 24%	—	Acupuncture Homeopathy Manual Phytotreatment
Hauser[145]	Europe	Survey article	38% 33% 33%	Patients well educated; CAM recommended by friends/relatives	Diet Drug Electric
Risberg et al.[308,309]	Norway	642	20%	Younger/older adults, well educated, geographic differences	Healing by hands, herbal medicine, vitamin, diet, Iscador
Vd Zouwe et al.[388]	Holland	949	9.4%	—	—
Sawyer et al.[323]	Australia	48 children	46%	66% used at least one CAM modality, added rather than replaced conventional therapy	Positive imagery, hypnosis, relaxation, exercise, diet, vitamin, herbal
Morant et al.[255]	Switzerland	160	53%	Younger/older	Herbal teas, beetroot extracts, laying on hands, homeopathy, Iscador, magnetic, diet, acupuncture, psychologic
Pawlicki et al.[285]	Poland	70	25%	Caused delay in conventional medicine usage	—
Munstedt et al.[259]*	Germany	206	39%	—	Mistletoe, trace minerals, megavitamin, enzyme
Helary[151]	France	—	52%	—	—

Dady[80]	New Zealand	464	32%[†]	Ages 20–50 years	Diet, vitamin, Laetrile, magnetic resonance, faith healing
Richardson et al.[306]	United States	453	83.3%	Improve patient-provider communication and research to reduce potentially harmful drug-herb-vitamin interactions.	Spiritual, vitamin/herbal, movement/physical
Bernstein et al.[31]	United States	100	80%	Health care professionals must be educated about most common therapies as more patients use CAM remedies.	Vitamin, herbal, relaxation, massages, home remedies
Cassileth et al.[57]	33 countries	83		Large heterogeneous group of CAM remedies is used to treat cancer in both developed and developing countries.	Diet, shark products, vitamin, botanical
Metz et al.[243]	United States	196	40%	Of 79 patients using CAM, 84% were identified by directed questioning and 16% by standard history and physical examination.	Megavitamin, herbal, shark cartilage, hydrazine sulfate, mind-body

*Cancer in women.

†CAM advised generally along with conventional treatments.

seek an integrative approach to treatment, using both conventional medicine and CAM simultaneously. A huge amount of money is spent on CAM, but much less per treatment; exceptions include megavitamin therapy, chiropractic, antineoplastons, and dietary therapy in specialized spas, all of which may cost more than allopathic treatment. However, naturopathic treatment seems to be a small expense compared with allopathic medicine.[92–94]

Montbriand[252] found that 75% of her 300 informants did not tell their physician they were using some type of alternative therapy for treatment of cancer. With such a high prevalence of alternative treatments, it is important for conventional medical practitioners to know which therapies their patients are using. There is significant risk of product interactions,[79] such as interactions between herbal medicines and pre-scribed drugs,[169] and of clinical effects, which could confuse the patient's diagnosis. Some CAM treatments have potentially harmful effects[173] (Table 4–2).

TABLE 4–2. PLANTS AND PLANT PRODUCTS WITH POTENTIALLY ACTIVE INGREDIENTS AND POTENTIAL HERBAL TOXICITIES

Plant/Plant Product	Active Ingredient	Toxicity
Comfrey*	Pyrrolizidine alkaloids	Hepatic; primary pulmonary hypertension
Senecio/Crotalaria spp.	Pyrrolizidine alkaloids	Venooclusive disease
Heliostropium	Unknown	Hepatic failure
Ilex plants	Pyrrolizidine	Ascites, hepatic disease
Psoralea corylifolia (babchi)	Psoralen	Photosensitivity
Piper methysticum (kava,[97] kavakava)	Unknown	Stimulates then depresses central nervous system
Cantha edulis (khat)	Unknown	Psychosis, optic atrophy, pharyngeal cancer
Datura (thornapple, jimson weed)	Hyosciamine	Hallucinations
Valerian, skullcap†	Unknown	Liver damage
Taheebo	Unknown	Bleeding
Aloe vera	Unknown	Laxative: low vitamin K levels
Arnica	Unknown	Cardiac
Alfalfa	Canavanine	Splenomegaly, pancytopenia
Aristolochia (Virginia snakeroot)	Unknown	Nephrotoxicity; squamous cell carcinoma of stomach in rats
Coffee enemas	Unknown	Fluid/electrolyte imbalance
Ginseng	Sugars, steroids, saponins	Swollen tender breasts, vaginal bleeding, hypertension
Fungi (Psilocybe spp.)	Psliocybin, psilocin	Hallucinations
Lawsonia alba (henna dyes)	Unknown	Edema of face, lips, epiglottis, pharynx, neck, bronchi; anuria; acute renal failure
"Black powder" (phenylenediamine)	Unknown	Skin irritation, eczematoid dermatitis; vertigo; anemia; gastritis
Laetrile (vitamin B$_{17}$)	Hydrogen cyanide	Cyanide poisoning
Glycyrrhiza glabra (licorice)	Unknown	Hypokalemia, ventricular fibrillation
Margosa oil	Unknown	Fatty infiltration of liver, vomiting, drowsiness, metabolic acidosis

Modified from Tyler VE: *The new honest herbal: a sensible guide to herbs and related remedies,* Philadelphia, 1987, Stickley.
*Data also from Couet et al.,[74] Betz et al.,[32] and D'Arcy.[79]
† Data also from MacGregor et al.,[227] Chan et al.,[60] and Willey et al.[402]

Physicians also need to incorporate the beneficial effects of all types of treatments into their patients' treatment.[226] Lerner[210] has delineated the following guidelines for an effective physician role:

1. Avoid patient abandonment, which drives patients to the alternative medical practitioner completely.
2. Adopt a strategy of preemptive discussion, making it clear that this discussion is desired and valuable for the patient and the physician.
3. Clearly indicate that the physician is a valuable source of information about CAM practices.
4. Know the specific questionable methods that have been shown to be at best useless and at worst fraudulent.

Physicians should be clear in their goals of treatment and in the promise that conventional therapy offers, but brutal honesty and fearful predictions only tend to drive the patient to other sources of potential help, often promised without statistical validity.[49] Approximately 5% of cancer patients abandon conventional therapy and pursue alternative methods.[237] Knowing about CAM therapies,[251,380,381,414] discussing these alternative therapies early in the patient's treatment, and being honest about the patient's goals and the likelihood of help from conventional medicine and CAM enhance the physician-patient relationship. Seeking to help the whole patient, to look at patients in a humanistic way, is good medicine, whether practiced by the conventional therapist or the alternative practitioner.

Unfortunately, a recent survey indicates that although physicians may be aware of different forms of CAM treatments, they are still unaware of the existence of readily accessible reference materials on CAM remedies, such as *Physicians' Desk Reference for Herbal Medicines* and CAM journals[336] (see Appendix B). In addition, physicians' knowledge of the side effects and contraindications of 10 commonly used herbs was very limited. Recently the two journals *Scientific Review of Alternative Medicine* (http://www.hcrc.org) and *FACT: Focus on Alternative and Complementary Therapies* (http://www.ex.ac.uk/FACT/) were launched to cover scientific reports of CAM.

The goals of studies on CAM treatments are often complex and blurred. Standard chemotherapy, surgery, and radiation therapy studies hinged on measurements of disease-free survival and longevity. Although there were always questions about quality of life, these were often asked secondarily. In CAM studies, however, quality of life often becomes the key question, especially when treatments are given with only palliative intent. It will always be difficult to measure quality of life, and studies will need to be ever more carefully designed to use measurement and survey instruments that can accurately reflect differences across groups.[340]

CLINICAL RESEARCH ISSUES

Cancer therapy involves three types of specific multipatient studies. As discussed in Chapter 2 and previously, different phases of *preclinical studies* include techniques required to evaluate or synthesize a potential new drug molecule as well as conduct pharmacologic studies (safety and toxicity tests) and preclinical toxicologic studies (acute and chronic toxicity, teratogenicity, carcinogenicity, and mutagenicity).[68,69] *Phase I studies* are performed to determine the appropriate dose of a given material for study, not to seek anticancer effects of these therapies. *Phase II studies* are performed to seek potential clinical usefulness of a new drug or new drug combination. A number of patients, often with varying types of malignancies, are given a treatment at an acceptable dose level, as determined from Phase I studies. When greater than 20% potential response occurs, these drugs can then be entered into controlled *Phase III studies.* The newer agent or combination is compared with a control group using the best treatment to date, which might be another single agent, combination of treatments, or placebo.[25,175]

There are very few controlled *scientific studies* of CAM related to cancer treatment, and many CAM therapy practitioners are reluctant to conduct such research. However, some are actively engaged in careful *clinical studies*, which can be costly if controlled and well documented using high-level statistical analysis. Also, it is often difficult to control clinical studies in a double-blind format, although good records of quantifiable data should be kept, including tumor size and laboratory work. CAM practitioners often rely on the subjective views of the patient rather than objective evidence such as radiographs, laboratory work, and clinical measurement. Clear survey instruments can be developed to obtain subjective information in a reproducible way from patients about their lifestyle and quality of life, and future health care providers should obtain such data. (For a preliminary discussion of requirements of research design, see Chapter 1.) The following criteria should warn of questionable practices in the use of CAM, particularly for the treatment of cancer[15]:

- Lack of studies on effectiveness
- Practitioners who claim the medical community is keeping the cure from the public
- Treatment that primarily relies on diet and nutrition
- Claim that the "curative" treatment is harmless, painless, and without side effects
- Treatment with a "secret formula" that only a small group of practitioners can use
- Treatment by an untrained person[247]

Since 1991 the National Cancer Institute (NCI) has had a process for evaluation of data from CAM practitioners.[390] The Best Case Series Program provides an independent review of the medical records and primary source materials, including medical imaging (e.g., radiographs, ultrasound) and pathology (cytology, surgical), as well as an overall assessment of the evidence for a therapeutic effect.* To date, only one study provided sufficient data to carry forward to Phase III analysis. Unfortunately, only a few patients enrolled in the randomized trial.

In general, limited number of cases and limited data from medical records are the primary reasons preventing comparison of CAM to conventional treatment.[307] The NCI established the Office of Cancer Complementary and Alternative Medicine (OCCAM) in October 1998 to coordinate and enhance the activities of the NCI in the arena of CAM.

---

* See http://www.cancer.gov/occam/bestcase.html.

In 2001 the National Institutes of Health (NIH) funded more than $220 million in CAM research and training. The lead agency, the National Center for Complementary and Alternative Medicine (NCCAM), has an $89 million budget and funds more than 50 CAM projects on cancer treatment. Two research centers, Johns Hopkins University and the University of Pennsylvania, have been funded for $8 million over 5 years to study CAM cancer therapies. The NCI funded almost $50 million in CAM and CAM-related cancer research.

Although CAM cancer research has grown substantially over the last few years, more information concerning CAM is needed. Without formal standardization and regulation of CAM products and practitioners, while emphasis focuses on the individualized treatment, it will take more time and effort to carry out research in CAM modalities and incorporate them into standard care. Therefore the major obstacles to integrate CAM into medical science are still the burden of proof and standardization.

Efforts are increasing to integrate CAM into established research institutes. Tagliaferri et al.[366] reviewed potential methods to integrate certain CAM modalities into conventional adjuvant therapy for early-stage breast cancer. DiPaola et al.[84] describe research efforts in both conventional and CAM areas to improve the prevention and treatment of prostate cancer at the Cancer Institute of New Jersey. In collaboration with the NCCAM, the first OCCAM initiative provided supplemental funds to six NCI-designated cancer centers: Johns Hopkins Oncology Center, Wake Forest School of Medicine, University of Medicine and Dentistry of New Jersey, University of Colorado Cancer Center, University of California at San Francisco Cancer Center and Cancer Research Institute, and the University of Chicago Cancer Research Center. A total of $6 million has been funded over a 3-year period to stimulate CAM cancer research between CAM practitioners and researchers at the six cancer centers.

◼ CAM and Prevention of Cancer

Cancer prevention is a major subspecialty of conventional oncology.[230] The search for genetic predispositions and carcinogens is very active, but preventive activities are most useful in the area of *personal behavior modification*. Because these modifications, usually in the form of diet and specific chemical use, are being made in otherwise healthy individuals, such changes must be safe.[116]

A growing body of literature involves cancer prevention and CAM.[205] Although common lore indicates that civilization and pollution (i.e., the industrial world) are major causes, cancer is often found in less polluted areas. In fact, 56% of the world's 5 million cancer deaths in 1985 occurred in the developing world.[282,291] Three approaches for prevention of cancer are delineated by Reizenstein, Modan, and Kuller[302]: (1) control of environmental sources of carcinogens; (2) modification of personal habits, including cigarette smoking and diet; and (3) identification of specific genotypes. Of these, only personal habit modification is under the individual's direct control. It is also thought that this one approach would lead to the greatest potential decrease in cancer incidence.

A particularly novel approach to the prevention of cancer is by teaching personal habit modification through what might be called "cyberprevention." Shinke, Moncher, and Singer[335] described using interactive, culture-sensitive computer software to reduce risks of carcinogens, mainly cigarettes and poor diets, in a small study in one Native American population. Longer-term follow-up data were not available.

An ongoing study to determine the potential benefit of changing behavior is the Working Well Trial, which is being done at worksites across the United States under NCI auspices.[1] Because 80% of cancers may be attributable to lifestyle or environmental exposure, including smoking, diet, and occupational exposures, the focus is to change motivational factors and social norms in a more widespread way than would be possible in the clinical setting. Also, the American Cancer Society (ACS) has developed seven general recommendations to reduce cancer risk or diagnose the disease early, when it is most treatable[317]:

1. Choose most of the products from plant sources; that is, obtain vitamins, minerals, and other nutrients from food sources rather than from dietary supplements.
2. Choose foods low in fat, particularly from animal sources.
3. Reduce or eliminate sun exposure.
4. Be physically active, and stay within a recommended weight range for your age, height, and gender.
5. Reduce or eliminate consumption of alcoholic beverages.
6. Eliminate smoking and chewing tobacco.
7. Obtain a cancer-related checkup: every 3 years for people ages 20 to 40 and every year for people 40 and older.

◣ Diet

A potential link between cancer and diet has been suggested for more than 50 years. As early as 1933, a supposition was voiced that overweight people had a higher cancer risk than people of normal weight. The active study of this potential relationship began in the 1960s when the World Health Organization (WHO)[408] concluded that the majority of human cancers may be preventable largely through dietary modification. *The Surgeon General's Report on Nutrition and Health*[386] in 1988 showed a straight-line relationship between estimated daily dietary fat intake and breast cancer death rate. Colon cancer was correlated with dietary fiber intake and overall body weight. Several cancers were correlated with vitamin A or alcohol intake. Esophageal cancer was correlated with vitamin C intake, and both stomach and esophageal cancers were associated with poor nutritional status.

International surveys, migration studies, cohort studies, case control studies, and clinical trials data have all shown a relationship between diet and cancer, especially of the colon and rectum, breast, prostate, esophagus, lung, stomach, and liver.[133,134,136,362] A high-calorie, high-fat, low-fiber diet may increase the risk of cancer.[265,410] However, the fat intake by the general U.S. population is decreasing, potentially changing the comparison between control and treatment arms of studies.[111]

Colon cancer has been positively correlated with fat intake in a number of studies. Potentially premalignant adenomatous polyps are more common in countries of high animal fat consumption.[401] In an epidemiologic study of 24 European countries using mortality data, a direct correlation was shown between the consumption of animal (but not vegetable) fat and colon and breast cancer and an inverse relationship with fish oil consumption.[59] The authors surmised that fish oil is protective against these cancers and that animal fat is carcinogenic in colorectal and breast cancers.

Fish oils are potent modulators of eicosanoid production. *Eicosanoids* are derived from arachidonic acid[232] and include prostaglandins, thromboxanes, leukotrienes, and various hydroxy and hydroperoxy fatty acids. These substances have effects on inflammation, immune function, and tumor cell division. Recent epidemiologic and clinical studies indicate a potential role for treatment with eicosanoids in cancer prevention.[244] Some eicosanoids activate protein kinase C and may have potential action in animals, retarding tumor growth and inhibiting metastasis production.[236] Increased dietary fat leads to certain eicosanoids that result in increased levels of cytochrome-c oxidase II (COX-II), which may play an active role in the production of breast and prostate cancer.[314]

Controversy is ongoing over the role of dietary fat, cancer production, and cancer recurrence or spread.[72,111,313] There are marked differences in prevalence rates of breast cancer and prostate cancer in various parts of the world that correlate with increasing dietary fat intake, and these rates are changing with increasing dietary fat intake over time. In Japan, dietary fat intake and breast and prostate cancers have risen significantly.[411,412] Interestingly, Eskimos, with their high fatty intake—predominantly omega fatty acids—still have a very low incidence of breast cancer.

The blood levels of estrogenic compounds can be altered by diet. Fiber binds estrogen in the gastrointestinal tract, resulting in lower blood levels. The hypothesis that endogenously produced estrogen is related to the development of breast cancer is at least partly substantiated by the finding that *tamoxifen*, an estrogen blocker, reduces recurrence rates when used as adjuvant therapy after "curative" surgery and reduces occurrence of breast cancer in the contralateral breast when used in cases of carcinoma in situ.[90]

Estradiol and estrone blood levels were related to dietary fat intake in several studies and directly correlated with the prevalence of breast cancer.[187,334] Women who decreased the percentage of fat in their diet for 3 months lowered their circulating estrogen, estrone, and estradiol levels, whereas progesterone, luteinizing hormone, and follicle-stimulating hormone levels remained unchanged.[126,296,315,316] It remains to be determined, however, whether fat intake leads to lower cancer rates.[72]

Fat intake may influence breast cancer prevalence through mechanisms other than hormonal.[314] Fat-rich *linoleic acid*, an omega-6 fatty acid, enhances rat mammary carcinoma,[72] whereas olive oil, containing *oleic acid*, an omega-9 fatty acid, has no such effect. Epidemiologic studies in humans appear to be consistent with these findings in animals, and similar results are obtained with fish oil ingestion.[176,179] Eicosanoids produced by lipoxygenase activity have an enhancing role in growth, invasion, and metastases of cancers. Similar harmful effects were seen in prostate cancer cell growth.[313,316] A low-fat diet may decrease the production of these eicosanoids and thus inhibit growth, invasion, and metastases of breast or prostate cancer.

The nuclear grade of carcinoma in situ of the breast and of the prostate is also found to be proportional to the fat intake, being less aggressive in Japan with its low-fat diet than in the United States.[4,271,353] Akazaki and Stemmermann[4] reported that first-generation Japanese immigrants in Hawaii have a higher tendency for latent carcinoma to become invasive and aggressive compared with Japanese in Japan.

Total fat consumption from meat is directly related to risk of advanced prostate cancer.[120,398] In a population-based, case-control nutrition intake study in Utah of 358 patients with prostate cancer surveyed and matched with 679 controls, West et al.[398] found that dietary fat was the strongest risk factor to explain the aggressiveness of this cancer. Other factors that had no significant effect on the study population included the intake of protein, vitamin A, beta-carotene,[240] vitamin C, zinc, cadmium, and selenium. Fat intake from dairy products or fish was free from correlation. Heinonen et al.[150] reported the significant reduction in prostate cancer incidence and mortality in male smokers in a large, long-term study in Finland. Further studies are needed to corroborate this finding.

Recent clinical results indicate potential applications of *polyunsaturated fatty acids* (PUFAs) to cancer treatment. A double-blind study at the Harvard and Deaconess Medical Centers suggested a significant effect of postsurgical adjuvant supplementation with *eicosapentaenoic acid* (EPA) in limiting recurrence of colon cancer.[36] Twenty-seven patients with stage I or II colon carcinoma or potentially pre-malignant adenomatous polyps were randomly selected to consume 9 g daily of either fish oil with high EPA content or corn oil after excision of detectable lesions. S-phase labeling of tissue from proctoscopic mucosal biopsies, a predictor for incidence of new neoplasms, dropped from its baseline in the treated group but rose in the control group. The rate of metastases after curative breast cancer surgery also suggested a clinical benefit with the use of adjuvant supplementation with omega-3 PUFA.[39] Nanji et al.[263] offer a potential mechanism of action for these findings.

VITAMINS

Observational epidemiologic studies have suggested a possible decrease in the prevalence of cancer in people who consume higher amounts of fruits and vegetables, which are foods high in beta-carotene. This decreased prevalence may result from these foods' antioxidant[20] effect. Research literature is replete with anecdotal reports of antioxidant properties of many foods or food additives. For example, the spice turmeric has been found to exhibit such properties in vitro.[327]

Animal studies suggest the value of *vitamin A* and *retinoids* in regulating epithelial cell differentiation and maintenance. Animals receiving a vitamin A–deficient diet develop keratinization, squamous metaplasia, and gross tumors, with subsequent regression of this metaplasia on reintroduction of vitamin A into the diet.[254] Retinoids also inhibit tumor angiogenesis.[229,339] Chemoprevention of mammary carcinoma in some strains of rats and mice by vitamin A and retinoids has been shown, but hepatic toxicity may be significant, as well as dermatologic toxicity.[294] Metastases also decrease if retinoids are used as adjuvant treatment after removal of the primary tumor.

Further animal studies revealed that combining retinoids with oophorectomy, using dehydroepiandrosterone (DHEA), or with 2-bromo-alpha-ergocryptine (an inhibitor of pituitary prolactin secretion), had an additive effect. For example, in N-methyl-N-nitrosourea–induced rat mammary carcinoma, the combination of retinoids and selenium had an additive effect in cancer prevention. However, clinical studies in humans are needed to confirm these effects.

Although *vitamin K* is necessary for blood clotting, a possible link between the development of childhood cancers (leukemia) and injections of vitamin K supplements in newborns was suggested but not confirmed by subsequent studies.[317]

Matthew[235] reported that the blue-green microalgae of *Spirulina*, rich in carotenoids, reversed oral leukoplakia in tobacco chewers. Complete regression of lesions was observed in 45% of the 44 evaluable patients, with no toxicity, compared with only 7% of the placebo-treated patients. However, almost half the responders developed a recurrence within 1 year of discontinuance of *Spirulina* use.

Torun et al.[373] reported that compared with normal control subjects, patients with cancers from many different sites, including breast, head/neck, genitourinary, lung, and gastrointestinal, had a significantly decreased level of beta-carotene, vitamin E, and vitamin C. There was significantly increased level of *malondialdehyde*, a product of arachidonic acid metabolism and a potential mutagen and carcinogen whose increased level in serum may indicate increased lipid peroxidation in tissues.

The 1995 Western Electric Study, which evaluated 1556 employed middle-aged men over 37 years, is an example of how a large longitudinal analysis can produce useful information.[281] Men who ate a diet rich in vitamin C and beta-carotene fared better, with less heart disease and possibly less cancer. The correlation persisted after adjustment for age, cigarette smoking, blood pressure, serum cholesterol values, alcohol consumption, and other factors.

In 1996, Henneckens et al.[154] reported on 22,071 male physicians 40 to 84 years of age in the United States who were evaluated in a randomized, placebo-controlled, double-blind study to determine the potential effectiveness of alternate-day beta-carotene as a cancer preventive. Of the subjects, 11% were active smokers and 39% were former smokers when the study began in 1982. (A second part of this study, designed to determine the effectiveness of aspirin as a cardiac disease preventive, was discontinued before the study's predetermined end point because the aspirin had a statistically significant preventive effect.) The study was continued for more than 12 years. No differences were found in the overall incidence of early or late malignant neoplasms or in overall mortality, and no significant harmful effects were reported. In addition, no decrease in specific types of cancer was observed, including lung, colon/rectum, prostate, brain, and melanoma.

Omenn[279] followed 18,314 people at high risk for lung cancer because of their past or present smoking or exposure to asbestos. That study also showed no beneficial effect and, in fact, revealed an increase in lung cancer prevalence and death from lung cancer in the antioxidant-treated group. A randomized study of 755 former asbestos workers at high risk for cancer failed to find a decrease in sputum atypia between the beta-carotene or retinol arm and the placebo arm.[266]

In a double-blind controlled study, Albanes et al.[5] followed 29,133 eligible male cigarette smokers, randomly selected to receive beta-carotene, alpha-tocopherol, both, or placebo, for more than 5 years. The beta-carotene–treated group was observed to have no decrease in cancer but an increase in lung, prostate, and stomach cancer. Although the alpha-tocopherol–treated patients had a decrease in prostate and colorectal cancer and no change in lung cancer, they had an increase in stomach cancer and an increase in stroke, an unexpected finding, considering vitamin E's usual effect on platelets.

Greenberg and Sporn[131] followed 1805 patients who had had a recent non-melanomatous skin cancer and were randomly selected to receive 50 mg of beta-carotene daily or placebo. With yearly evaluations to detect new skin cancers, no reduction in the number of new nonmelanomatous skin cancers was detected.

In recent years, cruciferous vegetables, notably broccoli, have been touted as beneficial. Although rich in antioxidants of vitamin C and beta-carotene as well as folacin, cruciferous vegetables are also a source of hundreds of phytochemicals, which may stimulate the production of anticancer enzymes and chemicals that may block the effects of estrogen, among other, still-unidentified mechanisms.[221]

The craze to add antioxidants to treatment methods must be balanced by the need for scientifically valid studies. In two complex, nonrandomized, single-arm studies using beta-interferon, retinoids, and tamoxifen as maintenance therapy in patients with metastatic breast cancer, Recchia et al.[301] concluded that the combination as maintenance "is feasible and shows activity in metastatic breast cancer with an acceptable toxicity," but that further controlled studies would be needed to be able to confirm this statement.

In a randomized comparison of fluorouracil, epidoxorubicin, and methotrexate plus supportive care versus supportive care alone in patients with nonresectable gastric cancer, Pyrhonen et al.[300] showed that the chemotherapy-treated group had a better response rate and prolonged survival. Subjects in both arms of the study received vitamins A and E, however, so no conclusions can be drawn on the effectiveness of these antioxidants.

Studying chemoprevention by retinoids in the upper aerodigestive tract and lung carcinogenesis in a Phase II study, Lippman et al.[216] found a significant improvement in leukoplakia (67% in treated versus 10% in control group) with the use of high-dose *isotretinoin* in a short-term study. Because of the significant mucocutaneous toxic effects and short duration of remission of this isotretinoin treatment, the authors' subsequent study employed prolonged low-dose treatment. After a 3-month induction phase with high-dose isotretinoin, patients were randomly selected to receive either 9-month low-dose isotretinoin or beta-carotene. With follow-up to 5 years, the authors showed highly significant results, with progression of disease in only 8% of the isotretinoin-treated group versus 55% in the beta-carotene–treated group.

Pastorino et al.[283] reported a Phase III controlled study of *retinyl palmitate* compared with placebo used as adjuvant therapy in patients who had undergone curative surgery for stage I, non–small cell lung cancer. Although there was a decrease in second primary cancers in the retinyl palmitate–treated group and an increase in disease-free interval, no 5-year survival difference was found. The latter finding may be a result of the vigorous treatment received by the individuals who developed the second primary cancers.

Trace elements may have an antioxidant effect. *Copper* is required to maintain antioxidant defenses in vivo. Low copper states may produce prooxidant effects. Copper complexes have been shown to have anticancer, anticarcinogenic, and antimutagenic properties in vitro. *Zinc* has potential antioxidant effects as well, but its role in disease is unclear.[358] Zinc-deficient rats have an increase in single-strand deoxyribonucleic acid (DNA) breaks in the liver, and zinc leukocyte or plasma levels have been low in cancer patients, although little evidence suggests a zinc deficiency in these patients. The finding of decreased cancer rates in people who eat greater quantities of fruit may be related to their intake of these trace elements, which are found in these foods along with vitamins and beta-carotene.

Van Zandwijk[389] reported the use of *N*-acetylcysteine and glomerulus-stimulating hormone as antioxidants with potential antimutagenic and anticarcinogenic properties for prevention of lung cancer, as evidenced in a large European chemopreventive study. Ongoing European studies may determine the effectiveness of these agents and delineate possible toxicities.

SOYBEANS

Several review articles[185] have suggested that multiple soy products may suppress carcinogenesis, including a protease inhibitor called the *Bowman-Birk trypsin inhibitor* (BBI), also found in other beans and peas; inositol hexaphosphate (*phytic acid*); and the sterol *beta-sitosterol*.[109,146,184,242,250] Soybean isoflavones also appear to suppress carcinogenesis in animals. Other trypsin inhibitors with evidence of potential preventive effects on cancer include *saponins* and the phytoestrogen *genistein*, which may inhibit neovascularization and tumor cell proliferation.[22,109] BBI did not confer resistance on lung cancer cells in culture to irradiation or cisplatin-induced cytotoxicity but did confer such protection on mouse fibroblasts treated with both these methods.[186] Several NCI-sponsored human studies on individual soy components as potential chemopreventive agents in breast and prostate cancer are in progress.

The cancer-preventive effects of soybean products were reversed in animal studies by feeding the animals *methionine*. This finding may indicate that methionine deficiency in these animals is the cause of the decreased cancers.[146]

OTHER DIETARY PREVENTIVES

Recent studies indicate that high-fiber and high–folic acid intake is protective against colon cancer. Other cancers whose prevalence is inversely related to vegetable and fruit intake include those of the oral cavity, larynx, pancreas, bladder, and cervix. Whole-grain products seem to reduce the rate of colon cancer, possibly because of their increased fiber content.

Animal protein intake may increase urinary calcium loss, contributing to homocysteinemia, leading to an increase in the risk of various cancers, whereas low calcium intake has been associated with a risk of colon cancer.[401]

Folic Acid

A high dietary intake of folate appears to exert a protective action against adenomatous polyps in the colon.[172] A deficiency of folate appears to be correlated with cervical dysplasia (see earlier discussion).

Selenium

Garlic, which is high in selenium, has been found to inhibit colon cancer in mice,[396] possibly through its action as an antioxidant. Garlic inhibits skin tumor growth,[269] inhibiting carcinogenesis, and appears to have an immunostimulatory effect.[27] An epidemiologic study revealed that the prevalence of stomach cancer in the area of Georgia where there is the highest level of production of Vidalia onions, high in selenium, is significantly lower than in other parts of the state.[416] However, in one area of Japan where gastrointestinal tract carcinoma is common, high levels of selenium in the soil were not associated with a significantly high cancer mortality.[261]

Gupta et al.[139] studied plasma selenium levels in cancer patients and found that mean plasma selenium levels fell with increasing extent of disease and that patients with recurrent cancers had lower levels than those without recurrence. The authors believed that the low level is a causative factor in the cancer. One NCI study reported a 16% decrease in incidence of gastric cancer, a 4% reduction in esophageal cancer, and an overall 20% reduction in other cancers in a large group of Chinese adults taking vitamin E, beta-carotene, and selenium compared with a control group.[221] Because the study did not compare single variables, it is impossible to determine the role of each of the three additives. Clark, Combs, and Turnbull[71] reported a decrease in cancer incidence in patients with a history of basal cell or squamous cell carcinoma of the skin with supplementation with selenium. Goodwin, Lane, and Bradford[129] found that mean plasma selenium was elevated in 50 patients with untreated cancer of the oral cavity and oropharynx. On the other hand, mean erythrocyte selenium and glutathione peroxidase were depressed compared with age-matched controls. Additional research is needed to determine the role of selenium as a potential chemopreventive agent for head and neck cancer.

Molybdenum

Nakadaira et al.[261] found a correlation between molybdenum concentrations in soil sediment samples and death resulting from pancreatic cancer in women.

SUMMARY

Familiar drugs such as tamoxifen and aspirin have been found useful as chemopreventive agents for breast and colorectal cancer, respectively. Similarly, daily intake of folate supplement for 15 years may decrease the incidence of colorectal cancer. However, the pros and cons of each chemopreventive agent must be weighed against the risk of cancer for each individual.[332]

◣ Treatment of Cancer

The therapies described in this section have been reported in the literature as showing evidence of possible effectiveness. The listing is not meant to be all inclusive. Table 4–3 provides information on CAM in the treatment of specific malignancies.

ACUPUNCTURE

After being employed for thousands of years in China,[304] acupuncture is rapidly gaining popularity in the United States. Despite this long-term usage, there is no evidence of its effectiveness as treatment for cancer itself. Most claims for effectiveness are as a

TABLE 4–3. **TREATMENT RESULTS OF CAM THERAPIES FOR SPECIFIC MALIGNANCIES**

Malignancy	Treatment	Results	Study
Superficial bladder cancer	Keyhole limpet hemocyanin	Increased activity of natural killer cells	Kalble, Otto;[180] Lamm et al.[203]
Cervical dysplasia and cancer	NS	Low levels of beta-carotene, vitamins A and C	Romney et al.[311]
Cervical cancer	NS	Deficiency of folate, beta-carotene, vitamin C, riboflavin	Orr et al.[280]
Cervical smears abnormal	NS	Folic acid deficiency in Bantu women, corrected with folic acid treatment	Niekerk[267]
Cervical dysplasia	NS	Low levels of vitamin A, selenium	Dawson et al.[82]
Colorectal adenomas	NSAIDs or diet high in fresh fruits and vegetables	Lower incidence of adenomas	Janne et al.[172]
Esophageal cancer	Animal protein supplements in Chinese diet	Decreased rate of occurrence	Herbert[156,338]
Gastric cancer	Increased garlic and onion intake	Decreased rate of occurrence	You et al.[416]
Acute promyelocytic leukemia	Co-oxide in culture cells	Apoptosis, morphologic changes	Chen et al.,[62] Sun et al.[361]
Melanoma	Sesame/safflower oil in culture	Inhibited cell growth	Salerno, Smith[320]
Nonmelanoma skin cancer	Beta-carotene treatment	No change in number of new lesions over 5 years	Greenberg et al.[132]
Oral leukoplakia	*Spirulina fusiformis* vs. placebo	45% regression vs. 7% with placebo	Matthew[235]
Pancreatic cancer	Mistletoe extract	No improvement in tumor size or survival	Friess et al.[112]

NS, Nonspecific; *NSAIDs*, nonsteroidal antiinflammatory drugs.

treatment for the side effects of cancer, such as emesis associated with treatment or for control of pain. For the control of pain, acupuncture may activate "endogenous pain inhibitory systems" by the production of beta-endorphins and neuropeptides, which bind to opioid receptors, increase interleukin-2 (IL-2) levels, and increase natural killer (NK) cell activity.[12,34,35,48]

Measurements of CD3, CD4, and CD8 cells as well as soluble IL-2 receptor and beta-endorphin levels in the peripheral blood of patients with malignancies revealed an increase in CD3, CD4, and CD4/CD8 ratio and an increase in the beta-endorphin level after acupuncture, with a concomitant decrease in soluble IL-2 receptor levels.[34,35] Theoretically these findings might lead to clinical treatments for cancer patients, but further studies are needed. A preliminary review of *electroacupuncture with imagery* has revealed some potential usefulness.[382]

According to the 1997 NIH Consensus Development Conference on Acupuncture, acupuncture is an effective treatment for nausea and vomiting caused by chemotherapy drugs. A small clinical trial recently reported that acupuncture was also effective in reducing the number of hot flashes men experienced after hormonal therapy for prostate cancer.[142] Although generally considered safe, acupuncture performed improperly can cause fainting, local internal bleeding, convulsions, hepatitis B, dermatitis, nerve damage, and infection from contaminated needles at insertion sites. WHO publishes several guidelines on acupuncture, including research, training, safety, and nomenclature.*

ANTINEOPLASTONS

Antineoplastons are derived from glutamine, isoglutamine, and phenylacetate salts; antineoplaston AS5 is *phenylacetate* itself.[46] These chemicals inhibit incorporation of glutamine[292,344] into the proteins of tumor cells, which may cause G1-phase arrest. Antineoplaston A10 is thought to interfere with intercalation with DNA. Other antineoplastons inhibit methylation of nucleic acids; hypomethylation may activate tumor suppressor genes.[46] Antineoplaston A10 and AS2-1[44] have been shown to produce a deleterious effect on cell proliferation, cell morphology, cell cycle, and DNA in human hepatocellular carcinoma cell culture lines and in one patient with hepatocellular carcinoma.[377] Burzynski[46] stated that "it can be clearly observed that antineoplastons induce abnormal cells to undergo terminal differentiation and die."

Many Phase I trials on antineoplaston treatment have been performed in the United States and Japan. Tsuda et al.[376,377] reported responses in patients with ovarian cytoadenocarcinoma, anaplastic astrocytoma, recurrent renal cell carcinoma, brain metastases from prostatic carcinoma, brain metastases from breast cancer, lymphoma, and brain stem glioma. Their overall response rate was reported to be 32%. Sugita et al.[360] reported treatment success in a few patients with antineoplastons. Side effects included weakness, drowsiness, febrile reactions, nausea/vomiting, skin rash, and leukopenia/thrombocytopenia. Phase I studies of phenylacetate in patients with cancer have been performed,[371] and clinical Phase II studies would be needed to

---

*At http://www.who.int/medicines/library/trm/acupuncture/acupdocs.shtml.

determine the likelihood of clinical usefulness. Although an NCI study was begun to determine the usefulness of phenlyacetate treatment in patients with brain tumors, after a very slow accrual of patients, disagreements over study design prohibited the study from moving forward. (See Appendix B for websites presenting additional clinical trial data.)

AYURVEDA

Ayurveda (Sanskrit for "that which has been seen to be true about long life"[374]) treatment has been used in India for thousands of years. Smit et al.[341] found cytotoxicity in the flowers of *Calotropsis procera* and the nuts of *Semecarpus anacardium*. However, there are no randomized studies in humans to show the clinical effectiveness in cancer treatment.

Over the past 10 years, a form of Ayurveda medicine promoted vigorously through the Maharishi Mahesh Yogi has become quite popular,[145] with animal experiments showing cytotoxicity of Maharishi-4, a mixture of low-molecular-weight substances, including antioxidants such as alpha-tocopherol, ascorbate, beta-carotene, catechins, bioflavinoids, and flavoproteins in the treatment of 7,12-dimethylbenz [a]anthracene (DMBA)–induced mammary tumors in rats[331] and in the treatment of lung metastases in Lewis lung carcinoma in mice.[284] MAK-A, one such compound, induced biochemical and morphologic differentiation in murine neuroblastoma cells in culture.[295] MAK-4 and MAK-5 may have antioxidant properties.[89,101,270]

Ayurvedic healing techniques are based on the classification of people into one of three predominant body types, with specific remedies for disease and regimens for health promotion for each group. Ayurveda emphasizes regular detoxification and cleansing through all physiologic systems of elimination and all orifices. Toxicity has been reported with ayurvedic remedies. Hepatic venoocclusive disease was reported in patients taking *Heliostropium* species, causing rapidly progressive hepatic failure leading to death. A recent review of 166 species of plants used in the ayurvedic pharmacopoeia suggests that certain species may have some positive effects, at least in palliative care, and deserve further studies.[188]

CHIROPRACTIC

Chiropractic is generally reserved for the treatment of pain related to nonmalignant causes. Of concern is the possibility of negative outcomes resulting from manipulative treatments of patients with undiagnosed cancer. Few published studies are available on the complications of chiropractic manipulation. In one study, however, misdiagnosis of the patient's condition accounted for 26 of 135 complications after chiropractic treatment, 16 of which were in patients with neoplasms.[201] Because of the potential of paraplegia resulting from spinal manipulation in patients with cancer, malignancy is at the least a relative contraindication to chiropractic manipulation.[333] For example, a case of quadriplegia after chiropractic manipulation in a 4-month-old infant with congenital torticollis caused by a spinal astrocytoma has been reported.[329]

DIET AND NUTRITION

Diet is discussed earlier in relation to cancer prevention, but several diets are also used as treatment. So-called metabolic diets include anticancer diets with digestive enzymes; high-dose vitamin therapy, including vitamins A and C; pangamic acid (so-called vitamin B_{15}); amygdalin (Laetrile), or so-called vitamin B_{17}; an alleged vitamin preparation ("Plus 198"); and vitamin E and mineral supplements, with ancillary injections of intratumoral enzymes. Raw food consumption is increased, protein intake is decreased, and refined foods and additives are eliminated. Coffee enemas are used. Hair and blood analyses are also performed routinely. The ACS[9] has published its findings of serious risks to patients resulting from these "metabolic diets."

Macrobiotic diets were developed by Michio Kushi,[199] based on the yin-yang principle. These two elementary and complementary forms of energy are present within all people, according to ancient Asian spiritual traditions. For a person to achieve health and vitality, these two forces must be in equilibrium. A macrobiotic diet is considered a part of a whole-body regimen and philosophy, a more comprehensive way of life rather than just a diet. This diet obtains 50% to 60% of its calories from whole grains, 25% to 30% from vegetables, and the rest from beans, seaweed, and vegetarian soups. These strictly vegetarian diets have been touted as successful for the prevention of cancer, as well as its treatment. Although conventional medicine has recognized the potential benefit of increasing vegetables in the diet for prevention, there is no compelling evidence that this diet overall has a beneficial effect for prevention or treatment of cancer. No controlled trials of these diets have been made. The diets are potentially significantly deficient in vitamins D and B_{12}, as well as in protein, iron, and calories.[54,253]

Many anticancer diets have been described; they tend to be especially popular in Europe.[16,145] A partial listing follows:
- "Kousmine diet": raw vegetables and wheat that are "rich in vital energy"
- "Instinctotherapy": only raw products, including raw meat; no milk products
- "Moerman diet": lactovegetarianism plus "the eight essential substances: vitamins A, B, C, and E, iodine, sulfur, iron, and citric acid"
- "Breuss cancer cure": up to 1 L of vegetable juice daily and different teas for 42 days
- "Budwig's oil-protein diet": curd cheese/flaxseed oil mixture, with fruits/fruit juices
- "Anthroposophic diet": lactovegetarianism, unrefined carbohydrates, sour milk products
- "Bristol diet": raw and partly cooked vegetables, soybeans, peas, and beans
- "Gerson therapy": crushed fruits and vegetables, coffee enemas, nutritional supplements

Only the *Bristol diet* has been studied in a prospective, controlled trial.[17] Breast cancer patients attending a Bristol diet center showed no benefit compared with a control group. For cancer patients who were metastasis free at entry into the center, metastasis-free survival was, in fact, significantly worse than in the control group. Survival in patients with relapse was also poorer compared with controls. However, preenrollment differences in clinical staging, conventional treatment, and selective self-referral confuse and weaken the reported results.

Hoxsey herbal treatment includes an antimony-zinc-bloodroot paste, arsenic, sulfur, and talc as external treatments and a liquid mixture of licorice, red clover, burdock root, *Stillingina* root, barberry, *Cascara*, prickly ash bark, buckthorn bark, and potassium iodide for internal consumption. A mixture of procaine hydrochloride and vitamins, along with liver and cactus, is prescribed. The U.S. Congress Office of Technology Assessment (OTA) found that "taken together, the data indicate that many of the herbs used in the Hoxsey internal tonic or the isolated components of these herbs have antitumor activity or cytotoxic effects in animal test systems."[385] The OTA indicated that a paste made from these herbs had reliable beneficial effect on the treatment of basal cell carcinoma of the skin. Austin, Dale, and DeKadt[16] did find cures for patients placed on the Hoxsey regimen but did not find such responses for patients treated at the Gerson clinic. Review by the NCI of the "cures" from these treatments failed to reveal any evidence of effectiveness for these patients with cancer.

The *Gerson diet* is a no-sodium, high-potassium diet rich in carbohydrates and defatted liver capsules, with injections of liver extract and coffee enemas. The treatment has led to serious infections from the poorly administered liver extracts, as well as electrolyte imbalance resulting from the coffee enemas. No study published in the peer-reviewed literature has indicated any beneficial effect of this diet.

The *Kelley diet* employs enemas, diuretics, nasal irrigation, Sitz baths, deep-breathing exercises, and external body cleansing to rid the body of toxins; an expensive, restrictive diet generally follows. There have been no carefully performed studies to show any benefit. Gonzales in New York follows a similar system (although Kelley apparently disagrees) and has produced a best-case series for the NCI.[297,390] The hair analysis for nutritional assessment is believed to be of no value.[310]

Metabolic therapy, coffee enemas, laxatives, juices, "antineoplastic" enzymes, amygdalin, pangamic acid, and dozens of other products, including vitamins C and E, selenium, zinc, ribonucleic acid (RNA), DNA, and ground-up animal organs all have been used, and no studies have indicated effectiveness.[15,56]

Essiac ("Caisse" when spelled backwards; named after Rene Caisse, a Canadian nurse who popularized its use) is a combination of four herbs: burdock, Turkey rhubarb, sorrel, and slippery elm.[178] Researchers at the NCI and Memorial Sloan-Kettering Cancer Center have found that essiac has no anticancer effect.[54]

Cancell therapy is particularly popular in Florida and the Midwest. Through these medications, the practitioners claim to return the cancerous cell to a "primitive state," from which it can be rendered inert.[54,137] U.S. Food and Drug Administration (FDA) laboratory studies revealed that these are common chemicals, including nitric acid, sodium sulfite, potassium hydroxide, sulfuric acid, and catechol. The FDA found no basis for the claims of effectiveness of the Cancell treatment.[54] In 1989, the FDA was granted a permanent injunction against both principal manufacturers of Cancell/Entelev, prohibiting them or their agents from distributing the mixture across state lines and classifying the therapy as an unapproved new drug.

Table 4–4 summarizes a recent ACS publication and a review of additional diet and nutrition substances in cancer;[286] appropriate references are listed in the ACS book.[317]

TABLE 4–4 **AMERICAN CANCER SOCIETY AND OTHER REVIEWS OF DIET AND NUTRITION IN CAM CANCER RESEARCH**

Common Name	Scientific Name	Evidence	Conclusion	Complications
714-X[177, 286]	Trimethylbicyclo-nitramineo-heptane chloride	Laboratory/animal studies on camphor, a 714-X component; appears to promote immune response. No formal human clinical trial	More research needed to determine activity in cancer prevention/treatment	Potential side effects unknown, except local redness, tenderness, and swelling at injection site
Lactic acid bacteria	*Lactobacillus acidophilus*	Varied results in animal studies. No formal human study	More research needed to determine activity in cancer treatment/prevention	Possibly serious infections. Questionable product quality
Amino acids	Arginine, alanine, aspartic acid, etc.	One small human study needs further investigation. Conflicting results in laboratory/animal studies	More research needed to determine activity in cancer treatment/prevention	May interfere with effectiveness of chemotherapy drug asparaginase
Cassava, tapioca, manioc	*Manihot esculenta,* Crantz	No scientific evidence in cancer treatment/prevention	Gene therapy studies using linamarase gene from cassava plant require further investigation.	Cassava plant may produce cyanide, which can be deadly to humans.
Coenzyme Q10	Ubiquinone	Laboratory/animal studies show some antioxidant and anticancer activities. Human studies inconclusive because of design flaws or small number of patients	More studies needed with larger number of subjects to determine activity in cancer treatment	Headache, heartburn, fatigue involuntary muscle movements, diarrhea, skin reactions with high dose. Anticoagulant interactions
Ellagic acid: raspberries, strawberries, cranberries, etc.	Ellagic acid	Laboratory/animal studies show promising results. Human studies in progress	Human studies using berries containing ellagic acid needed to verify absorption and distribution into various human tissues	Raspberry leaf or its extraction may induce labor.
Fasting		No scientific evidence in cancer treatment/prevention	Risks outweigh benefit.	Immediate negative effects
Grapes	*Vitis vinifera, vitis coignetiae*	Laboratory/animal studies show some protective effects. One human trial shows some antioxidant activity in grape seed extract.	More research needed to determine if resveratrol, active ingredient in red grape skin, may benefit cancer treatment/prevention	Increased consumption of wine to increase resveratrol intake may increase risk of certain cancers.

Juicing		No scientific evidence in cancer treatment/prevention	Risks outweigh benefit.	Possibly severe diarrhea
Kombucha, Manchurian, Kargasok tea		No scientific evidence in cancer treatment/prevention	Risks outweigh benefit.	Death possible from acidosis and other complications.
Lycopene		Laboratory/animal studies show promising protective effects. Population studies and a human trial appear to show lower risk in certain types of cancer.	More research needed to determine if lycopene or other active ingredient in tomato and other fruits may benefit cancer treatment/prevention	No known side effects from lycopene in fruits and vegetables Supplement side effects unknown
Maitake mushroom	*Grifola frondosa*	Laboratory/animal studies show promising results. Human studies in progress	More research needed to determine if maitake D fraction (active ingredient) may benefit cancer treatment/prevention	No known side effects from mushroom itself Effects from maitake D fraction unknown
Modified citrus pectin (MCP), Pecta-sol		Laboratory/animal studies show potential inhibition of spread of prostate and melanoma cancer cells. No human study	More research needed to determine activity in cancer treatment/prevention	MCP may cause stomach discomfort.
Noni plant, Indian mulberry, Morinda, hog apple, etc.	*Morinda citrifolia*	Laboratory/animal studies show some positive effects in various compounds in noni juice. No human study	More research needed to determine activity of noni juice in cancer treatment/prevention.	Side effects unknown
Selected vegetable soup (SV), sun soup		Small human trial by soup developer found some positive effects in conjunction with conventional treatment.	More research needed to determine activity of SV with conventional cancer treatment	Insufficient data
Shiitake mushroom	*Lentinus edodes*	Animal studies show some positive effects of compounds. Human study of lentinan (one compound) showed positive effect on advanced/recurrent stomach/colorectal cancer.	More research needed to determine activity of mushroom and compounds in cancer treatment/prevention	Allergic reaction affecting skin, nose, throat, and lungs

Continued

TABLE 4-4 **AMERICAN CANCER SOCIETY AND OTHER REVIEWS OF DIET AND NUTRITION IN CAM CANCER RESEARCH —cont'd**

Common Name	Scientific Name	Evidence	Conclusion	Complications
Vitamin D		Laboratory/animal studies show reduced proliferation on certain tumor cell lines and inhibited metastasis in breast cancer models. Preliminary human studies show some promising effects.	More research needed to determine effectiveness and amount in cancer treatment/prevention	Overdose may lead to anorexia, nausea, vomiting, polyuria, polydipsia, weakness, pruritus, nervousness, and irreversible calcification of soft tissue in kidney and liver.
Wheatgrass	Agropyron	No scientific evidence in cancer treatment/prevention	Insufficient data	Insufficient data
Willard water		No scientific evidence in cancer treatment/prevention	Insufficient data	Insufficient data

Data from Rosenthal DS: *American Cancer Society's guide to complementary and alternative cancer methods*, Atlanta, 2000, American Cancer Society; National Cancer Institute database;[28b] and Lamson DW et al: Natural agents in the prevention of cancer. Part 2. Preclinical data and chemoprevention for common cancers, *Altern Med Rev* 6(2):167, 2001.[205]

HERBAL REMEDIES

Plant products have been used for centuries as medicines. At present, in most countries of the developing world, plant remedies are the most prevalent treatments, with recipes handed down from generation to generation. These remedies are readily available and are less costly than allopathic medicine, and practitioners are accessible and generally have a more culturally sensitive attitude.

Much of allopathic medicine is derived from plant product. An estimated 20% to 25% of U.S. prescriptions contain natural plant products.[305] Oncology drugs are no exception. Taxol and Taxotere are derived from the Western yew tree, epipodophyllotoxins from the mandrake plant, camptothecin[288] from the bark of a Chinese tree (bought at the rate of approximately $35,000/kg), and vinca alkaloids from periwinkle plants.

Approximately 114,000 plant extracts from 35,000 species were screened for anticancer activity between 1960 and 1981 in a mouse leukemia model. None proved effective in clinical trials during that time; therefore interest diminished.[305] Other countries, notably Japan, France, and China, continue to screen new plant materials. With the advent of newer models of evaluation, including cell culture lines, a screening program at the NCI has been renewed.[215,305] The NCI maintains a repository of 22,000 samples of natural products, primarily higher plants, adding about 6000 new samples yearly.

Any study of herbal products carries significant problems.[63,97] First, standardization of dosage and formulation is generally lacking. The plant contains many potentially effective compounds, with their inherent synergistic and competitive possibilities making it difficult to determine which products are beneficial and which are potentially harmful. Often, naturopaths employ several such plants simultaneously, making determination of effects of any one plant impossible. The studies are frequently poorly controlled, and scientific method is seldom employed. Biopsy proof of malignancy is often absent, as is direct clear measurement of end points. Careful, well-controlled statistical studies are needed.

Currently, hundreds of herbal remedies purported to have anticancer[75,317] benefits are available over the counter. Most of them have no such demonstrated benefit. Many are not reliably formulated in available products, and some are toxic (see later discussion). Nevertheless, a few remedies have demonstrated indications of potential anticancer activity, including polysaccharide krestin, which has demonstrated such activity in Phase III studies. Herbal agents[174] that merit closer study as potentially beneficial complementary treatments for cancer are described separately in the following sections.

POLYSACCHARIDE KRESTIN

Polysaccharide krestin (PSK) is a polysaccharide preparation isolated from the mushroom *Coriolus versicolor* (family Basidiomycetes), which consists predominantly of glucan and approximately 25% tightly bound protein.[378] PSK has been heavily reported in the medical literature and studied in vitro, in vivo in animal studies, and in controlled human clinical trials.[70,268] PSK is administered orally and has shown no toxicity. Murine colon cancer studies showed a suppression of growth of these cancers and augmentation of tumor-neutralizing lymph node activity of draining mesenteric nodes by PSK.[144]

PSK has shown significant effectiveness as clinical treatment as well as adjuvant therapy. In colon cancer as adjuvant therapy, PSK-treated patients had a 30% 8-year disease-free survival versus 10% for the control group. When added to radiation therapy as treatment for stage III non–small cell lung cancer, the 5-year survival was 22% versus control survival of 5%.[147] An 8-year disease-free survival for women with breast cancer with demonstrated vascular invasion was reported to be 75% with combination chemotherapy plus PSK, compared with 58% for those with only the chemotherapy.[165,166] As adjuvant therapy added to adjuvant chemotherapy of 5-fluorouracil plus mitomycin for gastric cancer, the 5-year disease-free survival was 71% versus 59% for the adjuvant chemotherapy alone.[262] Fukushima[113] reviewed the Japanese experience with gastric carcinoma treatment and concluded that PSK and other biologic response modifiers may have a role. In patients with colorectal cancer, PSK increased disease-free survival.[372]

In a randomized study of 158 patients with esophageal cancer treated with radiation therapy, a statistically significant improvement in survival was seen in those treated with PSK as well.[277] On the other hand, Suto et al.[364] found no survival benefit to PSK in hepatocellular carcinoma patients after treatment with various standard therapies. PSK greatly increased the motility and phagocytic activity of polymorphonuclear leukocytes, which may be significant based on other findings that the prognosis of cancer patients correlated positively with the degree of cellular infiltration around tumor sites.[372]

CHLORELLA

Chlorella pyrenoidosa is a one-celled green alga rich in proteins, vitamins, nucleic acids, and chlorophyll used extensively as a food supplement worldwide. *Chlorella* has not exhibited toxicity at any dose. The components with identified anticancer activity are water-soluble polysaccharides in the cell wall[352,383,391] and glyceroglycolipids.[256,257]

Chlorella has been shown to have antitumor activity in association with immune activation.[195,248,369] A study at the Medical College of Virginia of 15 patients with glioblastoma treated with *Chlorella* with or without other therapies, including radiation therapy or chemotherapy, resulted in a 2-year survival of almost 40%, with four of these six patients showing no tumor progression during that time.[241] Potential mechanisms of actions for *Chlorella* include (1) polysaccharide ingredients binding to tumor cell membranes, with subsequent effects on tumor cell growth, adhesion, invasion of normal tissues, metastasis, and vulnerability to immune attack; (2) increase in NK cell activity; (3) increase in helper/suppressor T cell ratio; and (4) stimulation of macrophage activity.[141,352]

WHO guidelines and standards on herbal/traditional medicine include research methodologies, uses, assessment, good manufacturing practices, safety, and efficacy.*

---

*At http://www.who.int/medicines/library/trm/guidelinesdocs.shtml.

CHINESE HERBS

Chinese herbal remedies form a subset of herbal medicine.[290] Several of these have been studied in vitro for cytotoxic activity (Table 4-5). Ko[193] has reviewed the clinical diagnosis and evaluation of Chinese herbal toxicity and has suggested methods to identify suspected herbs that cause adverse reactions. Although some studies[157,158] indicated benefits from traditional medicines, Ernst[96] emphasized the risk of heavy metal content (e.g., arsenic, cadmium, mercury, lead) in traditional Chinese medicines as well as in other traditional medicines. Therefore it is important that regulators, pharmacists, practitioners, and physicians as well as consumers are familiar with these risks and attempt to minimize them.

One specific Chinese herbal preparation deserves specific mention. *PC SPES* consists of reproducible extracts of seven different Chinese herbs and one American herb. The major component of PC-SPES, *baicalin*, inhibits the proliferation of human cancer cells by apoptosis and cell cycle arrest.[167] Specific studies in prostate cancer cell lines have revealed that exposure to PC SPES resulted in decreased secretion of prostate-specific antigen (PSA), as well as a less prominent decrease in intracellular PSA.[162] Preliminary study with SPES indicates a potential beneficial effect on metastatic growth and on pain resulting from cancer.[202]

Currently, clinical studies are under way to validate the anecdotal reports from patients taking PC SPES who have significantly decreased PSA and symptomatic improvement in patients with advanced prostate cancer. Side effects of high doses of the herbs must be evaluated in patients with advanced disease. Some evidence indicates an estrogenic effect. However, preliminary observations indicate some effectiveness in patients in whom diethylstilbestrol (DES) treatment failed previously. Because PC SPES contains concentrated phytoestrogenic components, precautions against thromboembolic phenomena may be appropriate.[21] Several NCCAM-sponsored trials are in progress. Nonetheless, as a result of an investigation and laboratory analysis, the California State Health Director warned consumers to stop using the dietary supplement/herbal products PC SPES and SPES capsules due to their contamination of warfarin and alprazolam, respectively. The manufacturer of the products, BotanicLab, has

TABLE 4–5 **CHINESE HERBAL REMEDIES**

Plant Source	Chemical Found	Cytotoxic Assay Cell Line	Study
Pteris multifida poir Pulsatilla chinensis	Deterpens Triterpenoids	Ehrlich ascites tumor cells P-388 murine leukemia, Lewis lung cancer, human large cell lung cancer	Woerenbag et al.[404] Ye et al.[413]
Guava leaf, mango steen peel, pomegranate leaf	Unknown	Human cell lines	Settheetham, Ishida[328]
Antrodia cinnamomea Trichosanthes	Zhankuic acid (steroid) Triterpenoids	P-388 murine leukemia B-16 melanoma	Chen et al.[61] Takada et al.[367]

voluntarily recalled PC SPES and SPES nationwide.[108] Subsequently, on June 1, 2002, BotanicLab officially closed.

CAPSAICIN

The use of hot peppers is common around the world. Often considered a food preservative or a sweating agent for people in hot climates, peppers are thought to be beneficial. Capsaicin (8-methyl-*N*-vanillyl-6-nonenamide), a major ingredient of these peppers, is used specifically for topical treatment of pain. It has also been shown to improve symptoms and reduce the size of the polyps associated with nasal hyperactivity.[102] However, the burning sensation caused by oral or topical use has caused some patients to stop using capsaicin, making it difficult to conduct placebo studies of the drug.

In mouse and human melanoma lines, capsaicin has been shown to inhibit plasma membrane–reduced nicotinamide adenine dinucleotide (NADH) oxidase and cell growth, leading to apoptosis.[258] Capasicin also has potential carcinogenic activity as a result of its covalent modification of protein and nucleic acids, and it may possess chemoprotective activity against some chemical carcinogens and mutagens.[363] On the other hand, in a case control study in Mexico, chili pepper consumers were at a significantly higher risk of developing gastric cancer than nonconsumers.[222]

Capsaicin is among a host of chemical compounds, including sulfides, indoles, and vitamins, that have significant influence on the cytochrome P-450 enzymes, which are responsible for the bulk of oxidation of xenobiotic chemicals.[138]

EVENING PRIMROSE OIL

In 1987, Van der Merwe and Booyens[387] reported *gamma-linolenic acid* (GLA) treatment of 21 patients with advanced malignancies. This therapy was based on the finding that GLA suppresses the proliferation of malignant cells in tissue culture and on the observation that evening primrose oil, containing a high level of GLA, reduces the rate of growth of transplanted mammary carcinoma in rats. Subjective improvement was observed in almost all 21 patients, and a survival benefit was reported in hepatocellular carcinoma patients, increasing from a mean of 40 days to 90 days, but using historical controls. Ongoing studies in Europe sponsored by Scotia Pharmaceuticals will help answer the question of clinical benefit. A single-course, 10-day infusion of lithium GLA for nonresectable pancreatic cancer is said to have significantly prolonged survival.[326] Intratumoral GLA is reported to shrink lesions significantly without toxicity.[81,260]

GARLIC

Garlic extract[182] has been reported to inhibit the first stage of tumor promotion in a two-stage mouse skin carcinogenesis model in vivo,[269] to inhibit dimethylhydrazine-induced colon cancer in mice,[396] and to inhibit growth of Morris hepatomas,[76] possibly as a result of diallyl sulfide, a thioether. Although no clinical study in humans has been reported, recent comparative epidemiologic studies with ecologic and case control approaches in high-epidemic and low-epidemic areas of China[368] suggest that frequent vegetable and garlic consumption contributes to low mortality rates for esophageal and stomach cancers in a low-epidemic area. Unfortunately, a recent study by Hoshino[160] suggests that some garlic preparations may cause undesirable effects, including gastrointestinal problems. Two recent reviews suggested that garlic might stimulate the immune response and therefore reduce the risk of cancer.[7,204] This inconsistency in the efficacy of garlic supplements may be a result of active compounds not being accurately identified and standardized. Song and Milners,[345] studies illustrate that the benefits of garlic may be lost because of the preparation or processing methods, such as heating.

GINSENG

Yun and Choi[418] found a lower overall rate of several cancers, including lung, hepatoma, and head/neck, in people who took extracts or powdered ginseng but not in those who used fresh ginseng or ginseng tea. Ginseng can cause swollen and tender breasts, headaches, tremors, manic episodes, insomnia, vaginal bleeding, and hypertension. In a more recent systematic review of 16 randomized clinical trials, Vogler et al.[392] concluded that ginseng root extract did not show effect on physical performance, psychomotor performance, cognitive function, the immune system, diabetes mellitus, or herpes simplex II infections. Efficacy of ginseng is either not known or unquestioned, and adverse reactions are not accurately described due to variation in production and potential ingredient contamination.[212]

MISTLETOE

Without empiric evidence of benefit, Steiner considered mistletoe a future cancer therapy but thought its spiritual quality would help integrate patients' "four different entities."[114] Mistletoe is commonly used in Europe, especially in Germany, where yearly expenditure is more than $750,000. It has been used as a sedative and for treatment of epilepsy, headache, paralysis, hypertension, lung ailments, and debility. Mistletoe is so popular that a stamp picturing the plant was issued in Guernsey, England, in 1978.

Animal studies in India have shown that *Iscador*, an extract from the semiparasitic plant *Viscum album*, was found to exhibit a dose-related inhibition of 20-methylcholanthrene–induced carcinogenesis in mice.[200] Yoon et al.[415] reported the inhibitory effect of Korean mistletoe (*Viscum album coloratum*) extract on tumor angiogenesis and metastasis of hematogenous and nonhematogenous tumor cells in mice, which he believed to be a result of the induction of tumor necrosis factor alpha[405] (TNF-α).

Further studies with mistletoe (*Viscum album*) lectins revealed that using the purified proteins from this plant induced apoptosis in lymphocytes in culture, as measured by the appearance of a hypodiploid DNA peak using flow cytometry.[47]

Mistletoe lectins have also been shown to have cytotoxic effects on breast cancer in cell culture.[325] In addition, it was postulated that cell killing may have been accomplished indirectly by damaging the cell membranes, with subsequent influx of Ca^{2+} and of DNA intercalating the dye propidium iodide and with cell shrinkage.

Although mistletoe has been regarded as a potentially dangerous plant, with the ability to cause seizures and even death, Spiller et al.[349] surveyed 92 people who had used this treatment and found that 11 were symptomatic from the mistletoe. The symptoms included gastrointestinal tract upset (six patients), mild drowsiness (two), eye irritation (one), ataxia (one child), and seizure (one child). Medical intervention was required in only one of these patients. Mistletoe preparations vary substantially depending on how they are prepared, which species they were obtained from, and the harvest season.

Numerous controlled clinical studies show no significant antitumor activity from mistletoe. Most treatment or prevention studies that have shown positive results are not considered scientifically dependable.[317] A recent European Phase III trial on the effect of an adjuvant mistletoe extract treatment in 477 patients with head and neck squamous cell carcinoma showed that 5-year survival of patients from the mistletoe group was no better than that in control patients.[354] In addition, no stimulation of the immune system or improvement in quality of life could be detected. A similar conclusion was drawn in an earlier Phase III trial of patients with high-risk melanoma.[91,191]

HERBAL REMEDY TOXICITY

As with synthesized drugs, plant products taken in excessive amounts may cause toxicity. Even prune juice, a natural laxative, may cause diarrhea if taken in excess. *Licorice* may cause hypertension as well as potassium loss. A recent review suggests that in high dosages for long periods, licorice can trigger pseudoaldosteronism, which may lead to hypokalemia, heart failure, and cardiac arrest.[192] However, Wang and Nixon[395] suggest that licorice might be a candidate in cancer chemoprevention studies when used with other botanicals such as green tea.

Many products can cause an allergic reaction, and many plants are carcinogenic in animals. Many herbal products are collected in their plant form, which may be contaminated with toxic insecticides, fertilizers, or infectious agents. Herbal remedies may contain lead, mercury, tin, zinc, or arsenic, which can be toxic in their own right.[96]

Herbal remedies are often believed to be harmless because of the "natural" characteristics. Although this is generally true, potential and demonstrated toxicities[60] occur. Because these herbs are often prescribed in otherwise healthy people and are presumed to be safe, it is of particular importance to delineate some of these side effects (Table 4–2).

Two herbal products deserve specific mention. First, *chaparral tea* can cause severe liver toxicity with cholestasis and hepatocellular injury, which resolved with discontinuation but recurred with challenge[6,23] in one reported case, leading to fulminant hepatic failure requiring a liver transplant.[130] Renal disease may also result from chronic chaparral tea ingestion.[342] The FDA has cautioned against the internal use of chaparral.

Second, short-term use of the Chinese herb *Jin bu huan* has been found to produce life-threatening neurologic and cardiovascular effects requiring intubation in children. Long-term treatment causes liver injury from a poorly defined hepatotoxic mechanism.[159,407] The chemical L-tetrahydropalmatine, a potent neuroactive substance, may play a role in this toxicity because it is 34% by weight, whereas in the natural plant it is only 1.5%. This product is sold without childproof packaging. Jin bu huan has been banned in the United States but apparently is still available. A recent study also shows hepatotoxic effects for additional Chinese herbal medicines (e.g., *Ma Huang, Sho-saiko-to*), pyrrolizidine alkaloid–containing plants, germander (*Teucrium chamaedrys*), *Atractylis gummifera*, and *Callilepsis laureola*.[357]

The recent ACS publication[317] and reviews* provide an updated list of unsafe and potentially safe herbal therapies (Table 4–6). The authors emphasize that an increase in public education, physician/pharmacist awareness, and patient-physician/pharmacist communication is needed to protect consumers from potential herbal remedy toxicity and herb-drug interactions. In addition, the lack of reliable research data, well-designed clinical trials, quality control, standardization of products, and postmarketing surveillance studies, as well as the increase in unregulated licensing, are key issues in the use of herbal therapies.

OTHER TOXICITIES

Supplementation in healthy individuals can be problematic because of the toxicities for these products, even if they are rare. Vitamin toxicities are uncommon but well defined, including *vitamin A*'s side effects of increased intracranial pressure and vomiting in children and its chronic use in adults potentially leading to hypercalcemia,[110] teratogenic abnormalities,[278] and rheumatologic complications.[51,110,189,266] Pennes et al.,[287] in a prospective study of patients receiving 13-*cis*-retinoic acid therapy, described the skeletal hyperostoses. The most common site of extraspinal hyperostoses is the knee.[403] Such arthropathies with arthralgias and myalgias may appear, often disappearing even with continued use.

Vitamin B complex overdose can lead to cardiovascular toxicities, including arrhythmias, edema, vasodilation, and allergic reactions. Megadoses of niacin can cause cardiac toxicity with arrhythmias and infarction, as well as liver toxicity and peptic ulceration. Long-term high-dose toxicities include gouty arthritis, hyperglycemia, hyperkeratosis, dry skin, and rashes.[253] Vitamin B_6 in megadose levels has caused peripheral neuropathies, with resulting numbness lasting up to 3 years.

Vitamin C toxicities include the development of renal stones and a risk of rebound scurvy when high-dose treatment is discontinued. Ascorbate has been found to inhibit mitoses and to induce chromosomal aberrations in cultured Chinese hamster ovary cells. The addition of copper and manganese enhanced both actions. Iron in both the ferrous and the ferric states also enhanced the chromosome-damaging capacity of ascorbate.[351,355,356]

---

*References 63, 97, 174, 182, 192, 193, 286, 290.

TABLE 4-6 **COMMON HERBS IN CANCER RESEARCH**

Common Name	Scientific Name	Evidence	Conclusion	Complications
Milk vetch, Huang qi/ch'i	Astragalus membranaceus	Laboratory/animal studies suggest enhancement of immune response. No human study.	More research needed to determine activity of Astragalus with conventional cancer treatment.	Abdominal bloating, low blood pressure, loose stools, dehydration.
Kilwart, milkbush, pencil tree	Euphorbia tirucalli, E. insulana	Laboratory/animal studies suggest promotion of tumor growth and suppression of immune system.	Risks outweigh benefit.	Burning of mouth and throat, skin inflammation, conjunctivitis, diarrhea, nausea, vomiting, stomach cramps.
Betulinic acid, Butalin, Bet A	—	Laboratory studies show antitumor activity in melanoma and nervous system tumors.	More research needed to determine if betulinic acid is potential antitumor drug.	Side effects are being studied.
Cat's claw, una de gato	Uncaria tomentosa	Laboratory/animal studies suggest alkaloids (active ingredients) may increase immune response. Human study in progress.	More research needed to determine activity in cancer treatment.	Contains tannins, which can cause gastrointestinal problems and kidney damage. Potentially serious drug-herb interactions.
Purple cone flower, Kansas snakeroot, black Sampson	Echinacea purpurea, E. angustifolia, E. pallida	Mixed results on enhancement of immune system. Human study: no reliable evidence of cancer resistance or alleviation of chemo/radiation therapy effects. Animal study: positive antitumor activity.[78,148]	More research needed to determine effectiveness, amount, and specific species of Echinacea in cancer treatment/prevention.	May cause liver damage and suppress immune system if used more than 8 weeks. Potentially serious drug-herb interactions.
Ginger root[182]	Zingiber officinale	Laboratory/animal studies suggest some antitumor promotional and antiproliferative effects. No human study; ability to reduce nausea/vomiting has mixed results.	More research needed to determine effectiveness, amount, and specific ingredients of ginger in cancer treatment/prevention and in treating nausea/vomiting.	Interference with blood clotting; prolongation of bleeding. Allergic reaction, upset stomach. Potentially serious drug-herb interactions.

Ginkgo biloba	Ginkgo biloba	Laboratory/animal studies show some positive antioxidant and chemopreventive effects.[3,122] No human study.	More research is needed to determine effectiveness of ginkgo in cancer treatment/prevention.	Potentially serious drug-herb interactions.[169] Headache, seizure (children), dizziness, upset stomach, bleeding.
Goldenseal, eye balm, eye root, goldsiegel, ground raspberry, Indian dye, Indian turmeric, jaundice root, yellow paint, yellow puccoon, yellow root	Hydrasis canadensis	No scientific evidence on effectiveness.	Testing needed for developmental problems and cancer of reproductive system.	High doses can lead to death from highly toxic effects.
Green, black, and Chinese tea	Camellia sinesis	Laboratory/animal studies show some positive antioxidant and chemopreventive effects. Human studies have mixed results.[293,359,375] NCI and NCCAM sponsoring studies.	Clinical trials needed to determine effectiveness of green tea in cancer prevention.	Allergic reactions. Nutritional and other problems with large amounts of tea due to its caffeine content and polyphenol activities.
Marijuana (pot, grass, cannabis, weed, hemp)	Cannabis sativa, delta-9-tetrahydro-cannabinol (THC)	Synthetic THC may be used to control chemotherapy-induced vomiting and nausea when other antiemetic drugs are useless. Additional studies sponsored by NCI are in progress.	More and better studies needed to evaluate use of marijuana as supportive care for cancer patients.	Smoking/eating raw marijuana may cause euphoria, low blood pressure, tachycardia, and heart palpitations. Marijuana also contains known carcinogens.
Milk thistle; Mary, Marian, and Holy Lady thistle; silymarin	Silybum marianum	Laboratory/animal studies show some positive antioxidant and chemopreventive effects of silymarin. No human study.	More research needed to determine effectiveness of silymarin in cancer treatment/prevention and in reducing chemotherapy side effects.	May act as mild laxative. Sweating, nausea, abdominal pain, diarrhea, vomiting, weakness.
Oleander, dogbane, Laurier rose, rose bay, anvirzel	Nerium oleander, Oleandri polium, Thevetia peruviana	No scientific evidence on effectiveness of oleander.	Should not be used.	May lead to fatal respiratory paralysis and cardiac effects.
Pau D'Arco; lapachol; lapacho morado, Colorado; ipe roxo, ipes, taheebo, tahuari; trumpet bush, trumpet tree	Tabebuia impetiginosa, T. avellanedae, T. heptaphylla, T. ipe	Laboratory/animal studies show some effects on certain tumor cells (sarcoma). Few studies of lapachol in humans show serious risk of side effects.	Should not be used.	Vomiting, diarrhea. High doses: liver and kidney damage. Low doses: interference with blood clotting.

Continued

TABLE 4-6 **COMMON HERBS IN CANCER RESEARCH**—*cont'd*

Common Name	Scientific Name	Evidence	Conclusion	Complications
Saw palmetto[194]	*Serenoa repens*	Scientific evidence shows relief of symptoms in benign prostatic hyperplasia (BPH). NCCAM co-sponsoring clinical trial for BPH.	More research needed to determine effectiveness of saw palmetto on BPH complications. May interfere with PSA measurement.	Headache, nausea, vomiting, upset stomach, dizziness, constipation, diarrhea, difficulty sleeping, fatigue, heart pain, hepatitis, and fibrosis.
St. John's wort,[214,239] goatweed, amber, Klamath weed, Tipton weed, Kira, Tension Tamer, Hypercalm	*Hypericum perforatum*	Scientific evidence shows effectiveness in treating mild to moderate depression. NIH sponsoring multicenter clinical trial using hypericin.[207]	More research needed to determine effectiveness of St. John's wort as effective antidepressant, especially in cancer patients.	Interactions[169] with alcohol, narcotics, amphetamines, anticoagulants, antibiotics, cold/flu medicine (pseudoephedrine), antidepressants, warfarin, indinavir, cyclosporine, digoxin, oral contraceptives, antiretrovirals. *

NCI, National Cancer Institute; *NCCAM*, National Center for Complementary and Alternative Medicine; *NIH*, National Institutes of Health; *PSA*, prostate-specific antigen.
*Interactions may result from induction of P-450 enzyme system. Serious adverse effects include photosensitization and induction of manic symptoms.

Vitamin D overdose becomes evident in elevated blood calcium levels and may cause symptoms of anorexia, nausea/vomiting, polyuria, polydipsia, weakness, pruritus, and nervousness, potentially with irreversible calcification of soft tissue in the kidney and liver. As newer, more highly active forms of vitamin D are developed, it becomes imperative to monitor even more carefully for this potential toxicity.

High-dose *vitamin E* therapy can interfere with blood coagulation by antagonizing vitamin K and inhibiting prothrombin production. As discussed earlier, in a recent study of vitamin E an increased number of strokes were observed in the vitamin E treatment group compared with the control group.[5]

IMMUNOAUGMENTATIVE THERAPY

As proposed by Burton, immunoaugmentative therapy (IAT) is based on balancing four protein components in the blood and relies on strengthening the patient's immune system.[54,145] The use of various organ extracts from cows and pigs is claimed to suppress tumors selectively, stimulate defense cells, and revitalize several tissues. No studies have shown clinical effectiveness.[8,56,384] Popularity of IAT has apparently declined.[56] Based on data from 79 patients who received IAT, the University of Pennsylvania Cancer Center researchers could not make meaningful comparisons between IAT patients and those treated with conventional treatment.[317] The FDA banned the import of IAT drugs in 1986.

Another approach may be to simply replace immune system function (immunotherapy) with T cells that are taken from each patient's tumor, grown in the laboratory, and then readministered with protein (interleukin-2 [IL-2]) for continued stimulation. The technique, known as *adoptive transfer*, has recently been shown in preliminary studies to shrink metastatic melanoma in a small number of patients.[87a]

MIND-BODY TECHNIQUES

A number of laboratories have documented that psychologic techniques have affected the immune system of specific people with a high absorption ability. The response purportedly is based on an ability to concentrate so intently that physiologic action results from mental events such as fantasies or memories.[370] Screening for these inclusionary personal characteristics may be helpful before prescribing a particular adjunctive technique, such as relaxation or imagery.[135]

Prayer, meditation, biofeedback, t'ai chi,[52] Qi Gong,[321,322,394] and yoga are all being used with increasing frequency in the treatment of cancer. Anecdotal cases of tumor regression in juxtaposition with *prayer* have been discussed, as has the role of prayer in lessening anxiety.[86] *Biofeedback* has been beneficial in treating cancer pain as well as in regaining both urinary and fecal continence after cancer surgery.[58,197,330] *Visualization* of the cancer so that the body can fight the disease may help patients regain control of their health care and may help with stress reduction,[337] but failure of the method to change the course of cancer puts the blame squarely on the patient's shoulders.

The use of mind-body approaches as a primary cancer treatment has not been studied in a controlled way. Anecdotal reports of response, for example, in "Bob Brody's Athlete's Edge against Cancer," implies that the mind of the athlete is particularly conducive to "fighting" against cancer and that others can learn to do this as well.[53]

DISTRACTION, COGNITIVE-BEHAVIORAL, AND GROUP THERAPY

Distraction therapies involve pleasant thoughts or activities that distract the patient from the unpleasant effects of cancer such as pain. *Cognitive-behavioral therapies* involve the patient making an active effort to view the cancer in the best possible light (e.g., "taking one day at a time"). Both forms of therapy may have a role in the overall care of the cancer patient.

A 1989 report showed a survival advantage for women who were randomly assigned to a weekly talk and support group, including training in self-hypnosis for pain, compared with control patients.[346] A second study failed to replicate such an advantage.[117] More recently, Goodwin et al.[128] reported that "supportive-expressive group therapy did not prolong survival in women with metastatic breast cancer," although it did improve mood and pain perception. These other end points in addition to survival (satisfaction with treatment, coping skills) are important when designing studies. Also, combining methods such as nutrition with relaxation or other mind-body therapies can lead to additive effects.[397] A greater self-awareness in one arena may potentiate good health practices in another area.

AROMATHERAPY

Aromatherapy is becoming more popular in the United States. Wilkinson[400] described 51 patients in a hospice who were divided into two massage therapy groups, one using standard massage oil alone and one group with 1% essential oil, Roman chamomile, added. Although both groups showed a decrease in anxiety, the experimental aromatherapy group exhibited even lower anxiety, fewer physical symptoms, and a better quality of life. Although no scientific evidence indicates that aromatherapy cures or prevents disease, a few clinical studies suggest aromatherapy may be a beneficial complementary therapy in reducing stress, pain, and depression as well as enhancing quality of life.[73,190,317]

MEDITATION

Transcendental meditators have been found to have higher daytime levels of the serotonin metabolite 5-hydroxyindole-3-acetic acid (5-HIAA) compared with control subjects, and these levels increased with meditation. *Serotonin* is a precursor of melatonin (see later discussion). Meditation and melatonin have some similar effects: analgesia, antistress effect, antiinsomnia/hypnotic effect, and decreased heart rate and blood pressure.[233]

MUSIC THERAPY

Some studies have found that music therapy can lower heart rate, blood pressure, and breathing; alleviate insomnia and depression; and relieve stress and pain.[45,115,317,343,393] Music therapy may help reduce pain and ease physical symptoms of chemotherapy-induced nausea and vomiting.[24,99]

HEAT THERAPY (HYPERTHERMIA)

Heat therapy involves exposing part or all of the body to high temperatures (up to 106° F). External and internal heating devices are used to enhance other treatments, such as radiation therapy, biologic therapy, and chemotherapy. A potential hypothesis is that heat may help shrink tumors by damaging cells or depriving them of substances they need to live. The effectiveness of laboratory and animal studies on heat therapy led to numerous clinical trials using whole-body heat therapy, and NCI is currently sponsoring several studies using whole-body heat therapy.[317,399] With the high mortality and labor-intensive methods associated with whole-body heat therapy, more research is needed before hyperthermia can be considered as a permanent element in a multi-modal therapeutic concept in cancer treatment[149,181] (see Chapter 2).

BIOELECTRIC TREATMENTS

Nordenström[272–274] described electric stimulation treatment for cancer. *Electroporation,* a new technique to enhance antitumor effects of chemotherapeutic agents, has been expounded recently by a number of researchers.[83,121,152,153] They report that electric current delivered to the tumor reversibly increases permeability of the cell membranes, allowing intracellular concentrations of chemotherapy to increase significantly, up to 700 times with some agents.

Chou et al.[68,69] reported beneficial treatment of fibrosarcomas in mice and rats with direct current (DC) through apoptosis. A number of reports on small studies indicate the potential of electrochemotherapy in several types of cancer, including salivary gland and breast,[85] lung,[417] hepatocellular carcinoma,[163,206] and others.[198,234,419]

A clinical study of two patients with basal cell carcinoma used untreated nodules as controls while applying DC to other nodules simultaneously with systemic bleomycin chemotherapy. Improvement with DC was significantly greater than with bleomycin alone. Mir et al.[246] found that the addition of IL-2 to bleomycin/electrochemotherapy increased cure rates in mice with subcutaneously implanted cancer.

Seven patients with squamous cell carcinoma of the head and neck were treated with electroporation and very low dose bleomycin.[245] Of the 34 treated nodules in these seven patients, 14 showed a complete remission and nine showed partial regression. Multiple nodular disease is an unusual presentation for head and neck carcinomas, and questions surround the natural history of these patients. The results indicate a need for randomized studies with clear measurements and follow-up.

HYDRAZINE SULFATE

Claims that hydrazine sulfate is a cure for cancer and a treatment of its devastating effects, including cachexia, have been made for several decades. The potential mechanism of action was said to be hydrazine's monoamine oxidase–like effect. Many anecdotal and some controlled studies were reported throughout the 1970s and 1980s indicating effectiveness of hydrazine as a cancer treatment[*] and as treatment for the abnormal glucose tolerance of cachectic cancer patients.[67] Other studies, however, failed to confirm these findings.[209,276,350]

Recently, several randomized, well-controlled studies showed no beneficial effect of hydrazine sulfate in lung cancer or colorectal cancer.[196,223,224] The double-blind study by Kosty et al.[196] included 291 newly diagnosed, untreated patients with non–small cell cancer of the lung randomly selected after optimal treatment with cisplatin and etoposide to receive hydrazine sulfate or placebo. There was no evidence of increased response rate or survival difference as a result of the hydrazine, but evidence did show a poorer quality of life in the treated group. There was no difference in the two groups of this double-blind study with regard to anorexia, weight gain, or nutritional status. In the study by Loprinzi et al.,[223] 127 assessable patients with advanced colorectal cancer were randomly selected to use hydrazine sulfate or placebo. The hydrazine-treated patients showed trends for poorer survival and poorer quality of life. There were no differences in the two arms of this randomized study relating to anorexia or weight loss. Chlebowski et al.[66] reported a randomized study of non–small cell lung cancer patients treated with bleomycin, vinblastine, and cisplatin followed by either observation or hydrazine sulfate. Neither response rate nor survival was statistically different in the two groups. Caloric intake and albumin maintenance levels were improved in the hydrazine-treated patients.

A further double-blind, randomized study of patients with colorectal cancer receiving hydrazine sulfate had to be discontinued early because the mortality in the treated arm was higher than predicted. However, proponents of hydrazine sulfate therapy continue to claim its value and report further noncontrolled studies to support their claims.[105] In the treatment of 200 patients with lung cancer and 55 patients with colorectal cancer, proponents claimed "positive" results when 6 of 740 patients were said to have a complete remission, although no clear evidence of measurable, biopsy-proven disease was provided.

Much discussion has surrounded the increased feeling of wellness and the improvement in cachexia of cancer patients.[65,67] Chlebowski and Grosvenor[64] described the abnormal glucose tolerance and increased glucose production frequently seen in cancer patients, as well as the improvement in these measurable parameters seen with hydrazine sulfate treatment, thought to result from the inhibition of gluconeogenesis. In the first of these "randomized" studies, however, the control group of 30 had an addition of 40 nonrandomized treated patients, a serious flaw in the study's design. Furthermore, the results of these studies were not confirmed in the well-designed study by Kosty et al.[196] and in the previously cited studies. A recent case study reported fatal hepatorenal failure in a 55-year-old man with maxillary sinus cancer resulting from self-medication with hydrazine sulfate.[140]

---

[*]*References 65–67, 103, 104, 119, 123–125, 289.*

AMYGDALIN (LAETRILE)

No discussion of CAM and cancer would be complete without a mention of the drug amygdalin (Laetrile), derived from apricot and other fruit pits. Although amygdalin had been used for centuries, it was elevated to new heights under the trade name Laetrile by Ernest Krebs, Jr., in 1952, and it totally eclipsed all other unorthodox treatments. A review was undertaken that revealed six cases in which there was a possible Laetrile effect. Based on these findings, Moertel et al.[249] treated 178 previously untreated patients with good performance status with Laetrile; vitamins A, C, E, and B complex; and minerals, as well as with pancreatic enzymes. Only one patient, who had a gastric carcinoma with cervical lymph node metastases, had a possible short-lived, partial remission of 10 weeks. All others showed no response. No evidence indicated stabilization of disease. Blood cyanide levels were high and often in the toxic range, at levels known to kill animals and humans. In addition, the Laetrile was generally available from Mexican suppliers and was found to be contaminated with infectious agents and endotoxin.

Deaths attributable to Laetrile have been reported.[32,41,155,319] Laetrile use is not approved in the United States.

MELATONIN

The pineal gland appears to have an important role in regulating the body's circadian rhythm. In animal studies, pinealectomy has been reported to cause a proliferation of cancers, and physiologic concentrations of melatonin, a hormone synthesized in the pineal gland, inhibit growth in vitro of some breast cancer cell lines.[312] *Epithalamin,* a low-molecular-weight, pineal-derived peptide, prolonged the life of various strains of mice and rats. Epithalamin decreased the incidence of spontaneous tumors and radiation-induced mammary carcinoma in rats, inhibited the growth of N-nitrosoethylurea (NEU)-induced transplacental carcinogenesis in rats, inhibited the growth of transplanted tumors and their metastases, and increased tumor sensitivity to cytotoxic therapies.[13] One explanation for these actions may be the observed increase in the night peak of melatonin with epithalamin treatment.

Melatonin levels rise to a plateau between midnight and 3 AM in people who have a standard work-sleep lifestyle, then fall to low levels after light appears. The pineal gland and melatonin are involved in regulation and timing of reproduction, in development, and in the aging process.[233] Possible mechanisms for melatonin activity are as (1) an anti–physical stress hormone, (2) an immunomodulatory agent through the release of opioid peptides and IL-2 by T helper cells, (3) a scavenger of endogenous hydroxyl radicals, (4) an oncostatic agent inhibiting proliferation of estrogen-responsive cells (e.g., MCF-7 human breast cancer cells), and (5) an endogenous antiestrogen inhibiting breast cancer growth in vivo and in vitro. Studies indicate that melatonin may act synergistically with tamoxifen.

Melatonin level has a suppressed nighttime rise in patients with breast cancer. Patients who exhibited a twofold rise in peak levels were associated with a low proliferative index, possibly indicating a more favorable outcome.[233] A depressed or absent nocturnal peak level has also been reported in men with prostate cancer when compared to men with benign prostatic hypertrophy or normal control subjects. Also, melatonin has resulted in a survival advantage and an improvement in quality of life indicators in patients with brain metastases from solid tumors.[217]

It has been suggested that melatonin is a gonadal inhibitor and that the loss of this function with the decrease of melatonin could be related to the development of hormonally sensitive cancers, such as those of the breast and prostate. Melatonin also appears to antagonize the immunosupressor effects of corticosteroids, to increase the cytotoxic activity of NK cells, and to interact reciprocally with beta-endorphins. There has been evidence of in vitro cytotoxic effects on cell culture preparations of breast, ovarian, and bladder cancers. Lissoni et al.[218] reported on preliminary work in which melatonin appeared to enhance the effect of IL-2 in patients with solid tumors other than renal cancer and to ameliorate the IL-2 toxicity. Evidence also indicates that melatonin blocks macrophage activation of IL-2, producing a possible beneficial effect in the treatment of cancer-related thrombocytopenia.[219,220]

The melatonin cycle may be abnormal in some cancer patients. High rather than low levels of melatonin have been reported in the morning in women with breast cancer. Abnormal levels in the cycle of melatonin have been reported in men with prostate cancer.[233]

Based on a very small, noncontrolled trial using subjective end points related to performance status, Braczkowski et al.[40] reported that "melatonin has to be considered as an essential drug in the curative or palliative therapy of human neoplasms and as a drug that plays an important role in reducing the administration toxicities of some cytokines." Further studies are needed to draw such a conclusion. Maestroni and Conti[228] reviewed the published literature on the effects of melatonin on tumor growth and quality of life. They concluded that "melatonin protects against IL-2 and synergizes with the IL-2 anticancer action. This combined strategy represents a well-tolerated intervention to control tumor growth. In most cases performance status and quality of life seem improved." However, these reviewed studies were noncontrolled and often anecdotal, with subjective measurements.

Lissoni et al.[220] reported a study of 100 people with solid tumors who were to have no further conventional chemotherapy and were randomly selected to receive either IL-2 plus melatonin or supportive care. There was no single drug arm of the study. The investigators found a 17% response rate in the immunotherapy group and the expected "no response" in the supportive therapy arm of the study. In addition, 1-year survival was significantly improved, as was the experimental arm's performance status.

The circadian timing of chemotherapy may play an important role.[161] The timing of the doxorubicin (Adriamycin) dose when given in combination with cisplatin in the treatment of 31 ovarian cancer patients was a determinant in the toxicity, with a morning dose being less toxic. This finding again points to a potential influence of the circadian rhythm system.

SHARK CARTILAGE

The use of shark cartilage as a potential treatment of cancer has become so well known that, according to one oncologist, 80% of cancer patients in that practice had asked about this treatment in the preceding several months.[231] The scientific basis for the use of shark cartilage is based on the findings that (1) sharks infrequently develop cancer (but in fact they have been shown to develop melanomas and brain malignancies[225]) and most of the shark's bulk is cartilage, which may be protective, and (2) cartilage from calves as well as other animals contains substances that decrease angiogenesis.[42,208] Cartilage itself is resistant to invasion by most tumors.[339] Cartilage is vascularized in its embryonal form, then loses this vascularization, which led Brem and Folkman[42] to postulate the production of a factor from cartilage that inhibits vascularization and that could inhibit tumor angiogenesis. Such a cartilage-derived factor has been discovered, purified, and found to be a protein with an approximate molecular weight of 24,000 and potent anticollagenase properties. This factor is very similar to a collagenase inhibitor isolated from cultured human skin fibroblasts.

McGuire et al.[238] reported that shark cartilage produced a concentration-dependent decline in endothelial cell ^{3}H-thymidine incorporation using a human umbilical vein cell proliferation assay. Gomes, Souto, and Felzenszwalb[127] reported that shark cartilage was instrumental in protecting cells against lesions induced by hydrogen peroxide in normal and low iron conditions, suggesting a possible scavenger role against free radicals.

A small study conducted in Cuba was reported in a segment of the television show "60 Minutes" in 1993. In 29 patients receiving shark cartilage, three of 15 "evaluable" patients were said to have responded to treatment. No further information was given regarding the types of cancer, the definition of response, or the reason for deeming the other patients not evaluable. A further study of 70 patients was reported as ongoing, but no results have been generated.[164]

Even if cartilage has antitumor properties, the likelihood of the ingested material reaching the tumor at all, and in an active state, would be unlikely.[231] Further, toxicity appears to be rare, although one case of presumed hepatitis attributable to shark cartilage has been reported.[14]

More recently a study concluded that orally administered liquid shark cartilage effectively inhibited the growth of new blood vessels in healthy men, suggesting that the active ingredients in liquid shark cartilage were available for use by the body.[29] On the basis of laboratory, animal, and human data, two randomized Phase III trials of shark cartilage along with conventional therapies have been approved by the FDA in patients with stage III non–small cell lung cancer and patients with metastatic renal cell carcinoma.

BOVINE TRACHEAL CARTILAGE

Bovine tracheal cartilage (BTC) is an acidic glycosaminoglycan complex containing 20% chondroitin sulfate and lesser quantities of dermatan sulfate, heparan sulfate, hyaluronic acid, and other polysaccharides. Human tumor stem cell assays have shown antitumor effect in vitro.[88] In 1985, Prudden[298] reported a significant response rate to BTC of 10% to 15% in various tumor types, including pancreatic, non–small cell lung, gastric, and colon cancers and glioblastoma, but with no follow-up series. In 1994, Puccio et al.[299] reported three responders in 20 patients with metastatic renal cell cancer receiving the same BTC agent. No toxicity has been reported.

HYPERBARIC OXYGEN THERAPY

Hyperbaric oxygen therapy (HBOT) is an emerging specialty of medicine that uses oxygen at greater (1.5 to 3 times) than atmospheric pressures. HBOT has been used as an additional therapy for the prevention and treatment of osteoradionecrosis and clostridial myonecrosis and for assisting skin graft and flap healing and other cancer treatment complications.[33,50,264] NCCAM is currently funding a specialized center to study the mechanisms of action, safety, and clinical efficacy of HBOT for head and neck tumors. HBOT side effects include claustrophobia, fatigue, headache, and myopia. Complications may result in convulsions and respiratory failure, as well as death from fires and explosions in hyperbaric chambers.

HOMEOPATHY

Homeopathy[30] is based on the assumption that a substance that causes symptoms of illness can relieve those same symptoms when used in very small amounts. German physician Samuel Hahnemann developed homeopathy in the 1800s. A randomized controlled study with 32 patients ages 3 to 25 years suggests that TRAUMEEL S may reduce the severity and duration of chemotherapy-induced stomatitis in children undergoing stem cell transplantation.[275] Additional studies with large sample sizes are needed to confirm this finding. Several reviews of homeopathy suggest that some individualized homeopathy remedies may have some effects over the placebo, possibly in palliative care.[77,98,100,213,324]

However, the evidence is not convincing because of methodologic shortcomings and inconsistencies, such as poor sampling and measurement techniques as well as no replication. Furthermore, studies with better methodologic quality tended to yield less positive results. Scheen and Lefebvre[324] even questioned the validity of a meta-analysis of controlled studies, concluding that the clinical effects of homeopathy are not completely caused by a placebo effect.[25] Therefore it is still questionable whether homeopathy has a role in palliative cancer care.

NEWCASTLE DISEASE VIRUS

Newcastle disease virus (NDV) is a paramyxovirus that causes Newcastle disease in a variety of birds but only minor illness in humans. The two strains of NDV are *lytic* and *nonlytic*. Lytic NDV is used for its ability to kill cancer cells directly, but both strains have been used to make vaccines to stimulate the immune system to fight cancer. Although several clinical studies report the benefit of NDV-based anticancer therapy, their results are questionable due to their poor designs, incomplete reporting, and small number of patients. Future studies should explore the possibility that the immune system may produce virus-neutralizing antibodies by repeated administration and may defeat the underlying vaccine mechanism.[286]

◣ Side Effects of Cancer and Cancer Treatment: Palliative and Supportive Care

Cancer and its treatment cause many types of symptoms. Pain, nausea, and weakness are all potentially disabling. Patients' perceptions of their discomfort are so different that health care providers must treat patients individually with varying methods. Physical suffering, or *pain*, is the most common and the most quantifiable, although imprecisely and subjectively, of these side effects (see Chapters 10 and 12).

Ahmedzai et al.[2] define *supportive care* for cancer patients as the "multi-professional attention to the individual's overall physical, psychosocial, spiritual and cultural needs, [which] should be available at all stages of the illness, for patients of all ages, and regardless of the current intention of any anti-cancer treatment." *Palliative care* is the achievement of the best possible "quality of life" for the patient. It focuses on the palliation of physical symptoms such as pain, nausea, vomiting, constipation, and fatigue as well as psychologic symptoms such as anxiety, depression, and spiritual distress.[409]

A nonrandomized controlled trial compared one group who heard a personal tape-recorded message from the patient's physician at chemotherapy with a control group who heard no recording. The study found a reduction in overall anxiety levels in patients who heard the personal message but found no difference in specific side effects of chemotherapy.[318]

An independent NIH panel found strong evidence for the use of *hypnosis* in reducing pain associated with cancer.[168] Wong et al.[406] provided preliminary evidence suggesting how Chinese medicine modalities such as herbs, acupuncture, meditation, Qi Gong, and t'ai chi can be integrated into the supportive cancer care. Ernst[95] provided some evidence indicating that complementary therapies such as acupuncture, acupressure, aromatherapy, massage, reflexology, and relaxation have potential in palliative and supportive cancer care. However, due to the lack of well-designed and large-scale studies, the evidence is still preliminary. More rigorous clinical research in these CAM modalities is required before they can be fully integrated into standard care of cancer patients.

BREATHLESSNESS

Breathlessness in cancer patients is a common finding and a late sign of disease. The first treatment is for the underlying disease entity, such as a mass lesion (primary lung cancer, metastasis from other cancers, finding of a pleural effusion), and if that fails, treatment of the symptom itself. Treatment is often chest physiotherapy (to remove secretions), bronchodilators, oxygen, and respiratory sedatives (e.g., opioids), frequently with little benefit. Other symptoms are controllable; pain generally improves, but breathlessness does not improve.[18]

Filshi et al.[106] found significant improvement in 14 of 20 patients with various cancer types who received treatment with sternal and hand *acupuncture*. This beneficial result lasted over the next $1\frac{1}{2}$ to 6 hours and was independent of the patient's anxiety index. The authors acknowledged that the placebo effect could have played a significant role and that a controlled study is needed. Bailey[18] discussed breathing control techniques and nursing therapy to alleviate loss of function and to ease the psychologic burden through an integrative model. The aims of these techniques are to promote a relaxed and gentle breathing pattern; minimize the work of breathing; establish a sense of control; improve ventilation at the bases of the lungs; increase the strength, coordination, and efficiency of the respiratory muscles; maintain mobility of the thoracic cage; and promote a sense of well-being. The authors reported preliminarily that their techniques are successful in enhancing a quality of life of patients with lung cancer experiencing breathlessness.

MUCOSITIS

A controlled clinical trial of 94 patients in the use of imagery and cognitive-behavioral training designed to reduce mucositis pain during cancer treatment was performed by Syrjala et al.[365] Four groups of patients who had undergone bone marrow transplantation were compared: (1) treatment as usual to act as controls, (2) therapist support, (3) relaxation and imagery training, and (4) training in a package of cognitive-behavioral coping skills that included relaxation and imagery. The authors concluded that relaxation and imagery training reduced the cancer treatment–related pain of mucositis relative to the control arm but that adding cognitive-behavioral skills did not enhance this improvement.

NAUSEA AND VOMITING

Keller[183] summarized several nonpharmacologic approaches to the treatment of nausea and vomiting resulting from cancer treatment in children. *Distraction,* including listening to music, was effective in decreasing the duration of the nausea but not its severity. Video games decreased both the anticipatory and the post treatment nausea. Hypnosis, used in children as young as 4 years old, resulted in decreased severity and duration of nausea. Progressive muscle relaxation with relaxation tapes appeared to decrease nausea. Diet modification also could be helpful. Acupuncture, acupressure, or transcutaneous electric stimulation of the P6 antiemetic acupuncture site seemed to have some effect, which was not found with treatment to a dummy acupuncture site.

Nausea resulting from chemotherapy can be ameliorated by *hypnosis.*[118] Jacknow et al.[170] reported a decrease in anticipatory nausea in children, a common and often treatment-limiting side effect of chemotherapy, that was sustained after only 2 months of treatment using self-hypnosis. Significantly fewer doses of as-needed antiemetics were used by the treatment group compared with a control group in this small, randomized study of 20 patients. Hypnosis also was found to improve coping skills in cancer patients, leading to decreased symptoms.[143]

RADIATION-INDUCED XEROSTOMIA

Xerostomia is a common toxic effect of radiation therapy. Acupuncture was given to 41 patients with varying degrees of xerostomia.[37] No explanation for the rationale for this treatment was given. Classic acupuncture was used as the treatment arm, and superficial, subcutaneous acupuncture 1 cm from the classic site was used as a control. No difference in results was seen between the two arms, although some improvement occurred in both groups. Whether this improvement was normal healing or a result of the acupuncture could not be determined. The authors concluded that acupuncture might be helpful in xerostomia and that superficial acupuncture should not be the control.

SUMMARY

CAM is widely used in the treatment of cancer by all types of people and more often by educated and affluent patients. As insurance companies increase coverage, CAM use will rise. It is important for health care providers to be knowledgeable about these treatments and to discuss them openly with patients.

Diet has been implicated as a means of preventing cancer. Low-fat, high-fiber diets are associated with lower risks of colon, breast, and aggressive prostate cancer. The use of antioxidants (e.g., vitamins A, C, and E) is controversial as preventive treatment. No diets or herbal treatments have been shown to reliably achieve responses for active cancer, although the polysaccharide agent PSK prolonged survival in Phase III trial patients when used as an adjuvant agent. Melatonin, *Chlorella*, PC SPES, and other herbal agents have shown indications of anticancer activity in preliminary studies and merit closer investigation. Even with well-designed studies, however, the products' contamination, such as PC SPES with warfarin, is still one of the major obstacles toward integrating herbal remedies into standard care of cancer patients.

An important use of CAM in cancer patients appears to be in the treatment of side effects of the cancer and its treatment. The value of acupuncture, even in the treatment of pain, is still controversial. Mind-body methods such as hypnosis, relaxation, and imagery techniques seem to benefit patients with pain, anxiety, and nausea.

All alternative therapies, including diet, herbal products, and electric stimulation, must be studied in controlled, preferably blinded, randomized trials to prove effectiveness and to be included in the general armamentarium of treatments for patients with cancer.

REFERENCES

1. Abrams DB, et al.: Cancer control at the workplace: the Working Well Trial, *Prev Med* 23(1):15, 1994.
2. Ahmedzai SH, Lubbe A, Van den Eynden B: Towards a European standard for supportive care of cancer patients. Final report for European Commission on behalf of EORTC Pain and Symptom Control Task Force, 2001.
3. Agha AM et al: Chemopreventive effect of *Ginkgo biloba* extract against benzo(a)pyrene-induced forestomach carcinogenesis in mice: amelioration of doxorubicin cardiotoxicity, *J Exp Clin Cancer Res* 20(1):39, 2001.
4. Akazaki K, Stemmermann GN: Comparative study of latent carcinoma of the prostate among Japanese in Japan and Hawaii, *J Natl Cancer Inst* 50:1137, 1973.
5. Albanes D et al: Effects of alpha-tocopherol and beta-carotene supplements on cancer incidence, *Am J Clin Nutr* 62(6 suppl):1427, 1995.

6. Alderman S et al: Cholestatic hepatitis after ingestion of chaparral leaf: confirmation by endoscopic retrograde cholangiopancreatography and liver biopsy, *J Clin Gastroenterol* 19(3):242, 1994.

7. Amagase H et al: Intake of garlic and its bioactive components, *J Nutr* 131(3 suppl):955, 2001.

8. American Cancer Society: Questionable methods of cancer management: immuno-augmentative therapy (IAT), *CA Cancer J Clin* 41:357, 1991.

9. American Cancer Society: Questionable methods of cancer management: "nutritional therapies," *CA Cancer J Clin* 43(5):309, 1993.

10. American Cancer Society: Questionable methods of cancer management: electronic devices, *CA Cancer J Clin* 44(2):115, 1994.

11. American Cancer Society: Psychic surgery, *CA Cancer J Clin* 40(3):18, 1990.

12. Anderson S, Lundeberg T: Acupuncture: from empiricism to science—functional background to acupuncture effects in pain and disease, *Med Hypotheses* 45(3):271, 1995.

13. Anisimov VN, Khavinson VKh, Morozov VG: Twenty years of study on effects of pineal peptide preparation: epithalamin in experimental gerontology and oncology, *Ann NY Acad Sci* 719:483, 1994.

14. Ashar B, Vargo E: Shark cartilage–induced hepatitis, *Ann Intern Med* 125(9):780, 1996.

15. Aulas JJ: Alternative cancer treatments, *Sci Am* 275(3):162, 1996.

16. Austin S, Dale EB, DeKadt S: Long term follow-up of patients using Contreras, Hoxsey, and Gerson therapies, *J Naturopath Med* 5:74, 1995.

17. Bagneal FS et al: Survival of patients with breast cancer attending Bristol Cancer Help Centre, *Lancet* 336:606, 1990.

18. Bailey C: Nursing as therapy in the management of breathlessness in lung cancer, *Eur J Cancer Care (Engl)* 4(4):184, 1995.

19. Banner RO, et al.: A breast and cervical cancer project in a native Hawaiian community: Wai'anae Cancer Research Project, *Prev Med* 24(5):447, 1995.

20. Barber DA, Harris SR: Oxygen free radicals and antioxidants: a review, *Am Pharm* NS34(9):26, 1994.

21. Barken I: Personal communication, 1997.

22. Barnes S: Effect of genistein on in vitro and in vivo models of cancer, *J Nutr* 125(3 suppl):777, 1995.

23. Batchelor WB, Heathcote J, Wanless JR: Chaparral-induced hepatic injury, *Am J Gastroenterol* 90(5):831, 1995

24. Beck SL: The therapeutic use of music for cancer-related pain, *Oncol Nurs Forum* 18(8):1327, 1991.

25. Beecher HK: The powerful placebo, *JAMA* 159:1602, 1995.

26. Begbie SD, Kerestes ZL, Bell DR: Patterns of alternative medicine use by cancer patients, *Med J Aust* 165(10):536, 1996.

27. Beisel WR: Single nutrients and immunity, *Am J Clin Nutr* 35:416, 1982.

28. Benmeir P et al: Giant melanoma of the inner thigh: a homeopathic life-threatening negligence, *Ann Plast Surg* 27:583, 1991.

29. Berbari P et al: Antiangiogenic effects of the oral administration of liquid cartilage extract in humans, *J Surg Res* 87(1):108, 1999.

30. Berkowitz CD: Homeopathy: keeping an open mind, *Lancet* 344:701, 1994.

31. Bernstein BJ et al: Prevalence of complementary and alternative medicine use in cancer patients, *Oncology (Huntingt)* 15(10):1267, 2001.

32. Betz JM et al: Determination of pyrrolizidine alkaloids in commercial comfrey products (*Symphytum* sp.), *J Pharm Sci* 83(5):649, 1994.

33. Bill TJ et al: Applications of hyperbaric oxygen in otolaryngology–head and neck surgery: facial cutaneous flaps, *Otolaryngol Clin North Am* 34(4):753, 2001.

34. Bin W: Effect of acupuncture on the regulation of cell-mediated immunity in the patients with malignant tumors, *Chen Tzu Yen Chiu* 20(3):67, 1995.

35. Bin W, Zhou RX, Zhou MS: Effect of acupuncture on interleukin-2 level and NK cell immunoactivity of peripheral blood of malignant tumor patients, *Chung Kuo Chung Hsi I Chieh Ho Tsa Chih* 14(9):537, 1994.

36. Blackburn GL: Fatty acids decrease colonic epithelial cell proliferation in high-risk bowel mucosa. Second International Congress of the International Society for the Study of Fatty Acids and Lipids (ISSFAL), Congress Program and Abstracts, Symposium H, Washington, DC, 1995.

37. Blom M et al: Acupuncture treatment of patients with radiation-induced xerostomia, *Eur J Cancer Oral Oncol* 32B(3):182, 1996.
38. Bold J, Leis A: Unconventional therapy use among children with cancer in Saskatchewan, *J Pediatr Oncol Nurs* 18(1):16, 2001.
39. Bounoux P et al: Alpha-linolenic acid content of adipose breast tissue: a host determinant of the risk of early metastasis in breast cancer, *Br J Cancer* 70:330, 1994.
40. Braczkowski R et al: Modulation of tumor necrosis factor, *Ann NY Acad Sci* 768:334, 1995.
41. Braico KT et al: Laetrile intoxication: report of a fatal case, *N Engl J Med* 300:238, 1979.
42. Brem H, Folkman J: Inhibition of tumor angiogenesis mediated by cartilage, *J Exp Med* 141:427, 1975.
43. Brigden ML: Unproven (questionable) cancer therapies, *West J Med* 163(5):463, 1995.
44. Buckner JC et al: Phase II study of antineoplastons A10 (NSC 648539) and AS2-1 (NSC 620261) in patients with recurrent glioma, *Mayo Clin Proc* 74(2):137, 1999.
45. Burns SJ et al: A pilot study into the therapeutic effects of music therapy at a cancer help center, *Altern Ther Health Med* 7(1):48, 2001.
46. Burzynski SR: Potential antineoplastons in disease of old age, *Drugs Aging* 7(3):157, 1995.
47. Bussing A et al: Induction of apoptosis in human lymphocytes treated with *Viscum album* L. is mediated by the mistletoe lectins, *Cancer Lett* 99(1):59, 1996.
48. Camp V: The place of acupuncture in medicine today, *Br J Rheumatol* 34(5):404, 1995.
49. Campion EW: Why unconventional medicine? *N Engl J Med* 328:282, 1993.
50. Carl UM et al: Hyperbaric oxygen therapy for late sequelae in women receiving radiation after breast-conserving surgery, *Int J Radiat Oncol Biol Phys* 49(4):1029, 2001.
51. Carey BM et al: Skeletal toxicity with isotretinoin therapy: a clinico-radiological evaluation, *Br J Dermatol* 119:604, 1988.
52. Cassileth BR: Evaluating complementary and alternative therapies for cancer patients, *CA Cancer J Clin* 49(6):362, 1999.
53. Cassileth BR, Chapman CC: Alternative cancer medicine: a ten-year update, *Cancer Invest* 14(4):396, 1996.
54. Cassileth BR, Chapman CC: Alternative and complementary cancer therapies, *Cancer* 77(6):1026, 1996.
55. Cassileth B et al: Contemporary unorthodox treatments in cancer medicine: a study of patients, treatments, and practitioners, *Ann Intern Med* 101:105, 1984.
56. Cassileth BR et al: Survival and quality of life among patients receiving unproven as compared with conventional cancer therapy, *N Engl J Med* 324:1180, 1991.
57. Cassileth BR et al: Alternative medicine use worldwide: the International Union against Cancer Survey, *Cancer* 91(7):1390, 2001.
58. Cavina E: Outcome of restorative perineal graciloplasty with simultaneous excision of the anus and rectum for cancer: a ten-year experience with 81 patients, *Dis Colon Rectum* 39(2):182, 1996.
59. Caygill CP, Charlett A, Hill MJ: Fat, fish, fish oil, and cancer, *Br J Cancer* 74(1):159, 1996.
60. Chan TY et al: Poisoning due to an over-the-counter hypnotic: Sleep-Qik (hyoscine, cyproheptadine, valerian), *Postgrad Med J* 71(834):227, 1995.
61. Chen CH, Yang SW, Shen YC: New steroid acids from *Antrodia cinnomomea*, a fungal parasite of *Cinnamomum micranthum*, *J Nat Prod* 58(11):1655, 1995.
62. Chen GO et al: In vitro studies on cellular and molecular mechanisms of arsenic trioxide As_2O_3 in the treatment of acute promyelocytic leukemia: As_2O_3 induces NB4 cell apoptosis with downregulation of Bci-2 expression and modulation of PML-RAR alpha/PML proteins, *Blood* 88(3):1052, 1996.
63. Chitturi S, et al.: Herbal hepatotoxicity: an expanding but poorly defined problem, *J Gastroenterol Hepatol* 15(10):1093, 2000.
64. Chlebowski RT, Grosvenor M: The scope of nutrition intervention with cancer-related endpoints, *Cancer* 74(suppl 91):273, 1994.
65. Chlebowski RT et al: Influence of hydrazine sulfate on abnormal carbohydrate metabolism in cancer patients with weight loss, *Cancer Res* 44:857, 1984.
66. Chlebowski RT et al: Hydrazine sulfate in cancer patients with weight loss, *Cancer* 59:406, 1987.
67. Chlebowski RT et al: Hydrazine sulfate influence on nutritional status and survival in non–small-cell lung cancer, *J Clin Oncol* 8:9, 1990.

68. Chou C-K, Ren R-L: Preclinical studies in complementary/alternative medicine. In Spencer JW, Jacobs JJ: *Complementary/alternative medicine: an evidence-based approach*, St Louis, 1999, Mosby, p 37.

69. Chou C-K et al: Electrochemical treatment of mouse and rat fibrosarcoma with direct current, *Bioelectromagnets* 18:14, 1997.

70. Chung CH, Go P, Chang KH: PSK immunotherapy in cancer patients: a preliminary report, *Chung Hua Min Kuo Wei Sheng Wu Chi Mien I Hseuh Tsa Chih* 20(3):210, 1987.

71. Clark L, Combs GF Jr, Turnbull BW: The nutritional prevention of cancer with selenium: 1983 to 1993—a randomized clinical trial, *FASEB J* 10:A550, 1996 (abstract).

72. Cohen LA, Rose DP, Wynder EL: A rationale for dietary intervention in postmenopausal breast cancer patients: an update, *Nutr Cancer* 19:1, 1993.

73. Cooke B et al: Aromatherapy: a systematic review, *Br J Gen Pract* 50(455):493, 2000.

74. Couet CE, Crews C, Hanley AB: Analysis, separation, and bioassay of pyrrolizidine alkaloids from comfrey (*Symphytum officinale*), *Nat Toxins* 4(4):163, 1996.

75. Couldwell WT et al: Hypericin: a potential antiglioma therapy, *Neurosurgery* 35(4):705, 1994; erratum, *Neurosurgery* 35(5):993, 1994.

76. Criss WE et al: Inhibition of tumor growth with low dietary protein and dietary garlic extracts, *Fed Proc* 41:281, 1982.

77. Cucherat M et al: Evidence of clinical efficacy of homeopathy: a meta-analysis of clinical trials, *Eur J Clin Pharmacol* 56(1):27, 2000.

78. Currier NL et al: *Echinacea purpurea* and melatonin augment natural-killer cells in leukemic mice and prolong life span, *J Altern Complement Med* 7(3):41, 2001.

79. D'Arcy PF: Adverse reactions and interactions with herbal medicines. I. Adverse reactions, *Adverse Drug React Toxicol Rev* 10:189, 1991.

80. Dady PJ: New Zealand cancer patients and alternative medicine, *NZ Med J* 100:110, 1987.

81. Das UN, Prasad VV, Reddy DR: Local application of gamma-linolenic acid in the treatment of human gliomas, *Cancer Lett* 94:147, 1995.

82. Dawson E, Nosovitch J, Hannigan E: Serum vitamin and selenium changes in cervical dysplasia, *Fed Proc* 46:612, 1984.

83. Dev SB, Hoffmann GA: Electrochemotherapy: a novel method of cancer treatment, *Cancer Treat Rev* 20(1):105, 1994.

84. DiPaola RS et al: State-of-the-art prostate cancer treatment and research: a report from the Cancer Institute of New Jersey, 98(2): 23, 2001.

85. Domenge C et al: Antitumor electrochemotherapy, *Cancer* 77:956, 1996.

86. Dossey L: *Healing words*, San Francisco, 1993, Harper.

87. Downer SM et al: Pursuit and practice of complementary therapies by cancer patients receiving conventional treatment, *Br Med J* 309(6947):86, 1994.

87a. Dudley ME et al: Cancer regression and autoimmunity following clonal repopulation with antitumor lymphocytes and non-myeloablative conditioning, *Science Express*, Sept 19, 2002.

88. Durie BG, Soehnlen B, Prudden JF: Antitumor activity of bovine cartilage extract (Catrix-S) in the human tumor stem cell assay, *J Biol Response Mod* 4(6):590, 1985.

89. Dwivedi C et al: Inhibitory effects of Maharishi-4 and Maharishi-5 on microsomal lipid peroxidation, *Pharmacol Biochem Behav* 39:649, 1991.

90. Early Breast Cancer Trialists' Collaborative Group: Systemic treatment of early breast cancer by hormonal, cytotoxic, or immune therapy—133 randomized trials involving 31,000 recurrences and 24,000 deaths among 75,000 women, *Lancet* 339:71, 1992.

91. Eggermont AM et al: European Organization for Research and Treatment of Cancer Melanoma Group trial experience with more than 2,000 patients, evaluating adjuvant treatment with low or intermediate doses of interferon alpha-2b. In Perry MC, editor: *Educational Book: 37th Annual Meeting of the American Society of Clinical Oncology*, Alexandria, Va, 2001.

92. Ernst E: Complementary medicine: changing attitudes, *Complement Ther Med* 2:121, 1994.

93. Ernst E: Complementary medicine: common misconceptions, *J R Soc Med*, 88(5):244, 1995 (editorial).

94. Ernst E: Complementary cancer treatments: hope or hazard? *Clin Oncol (R Coll Radiol)* 7(4):259, 1995.

95. Ernst E: Complementary therapies in palliative cancer care, *Cancer* 91(11):2181, 2001.

96. Ernst E: Heavy metals in traditional Chinese medicines: a systematic review, *Clin Pharmacol Ther* 70(6):497, 2001.
97. Ernst E: The risk-benefit profile of commonly used herbal therapies: ginkgo, St. John's wort, ginseng, echinacea, saw palmetto, and kava, *Ann Intern Med* 136(1):42, 2002. Also see http://www.cfsan.fda.gov/~dms/addskava.html.
98. Ernst E, Pittler MH: Efficacy of homeopathic arnica: a systematic review of placebo-controlled clinical trials, *Arch Surg* 133(11):1187, 1998.
99. Ezzone S et al: Music as an adjunct to antiemetic therapy, *Oncol Nurs Forum* 25:1551, 1998.
100. Ferley IP et al: A controlled evaluation of a homeopathic preparation in the treatment of influenza-like syndromes, *Br J Clin Pharmacol* 27:329, 1989.
101. Fields J et al: Oxygen free radical (OFR) scavenging effects of an anti-carcinogenic natural product, Maharishi Amrit Kalask (MAK), *Pharmacologist* 32:A155, 1990 (abstract).
102. Filiaci F et al: Local treatment of nasal polyposis with capsaicin: preliminary findings, *Allergol Immunopathol (Madr)* 24(1):13, 1996.
103. Filov VA et al: Hydrazine sulfate: experimental and clinical results, mechanisms of action. In Filov VA et al, editors: *Medical therapy of tumors*, Leningrad, 1983, USSR Ministry of Health, p 92.
104. Filov VA et al: Results of clinical evaluation of hydrazine sulfate, *Vopr Onkol* 36:721, 1990.
105. Filov VA et al: Experience of the treatment with Sehydrin (hydrazine sulfate, HS) in the advanced cancer patients, *Invest New Drugs* 13(1):89, 1995.
106. Filshi J et al: Acupuncture for the relief of cancer-related breathlessness, *Palliat Med* 10(2):145, 1996.
107. Fisher P, Ward A: Complementary medicine in Europe, *Br Med J* 309:107, 1994.
108. Food and Drug Administration safety information and adverse event reporting program, 2002 safety information summaries, http://www.fda.gov/medwatch/SAFETY/2002/safety02.htm.
109. Fotsis T et al: Genistein, a dietary ingested isoflavinoid, inhibits cell proliferation and in vitro angiogenesis, *J Nutr* 125(suppl 3):790, 1995.
110. Frame B et al: Hypercalcemia and skeletal effects in chronic hypervitaminosis A, *Ann Intern Med* 80:44, 1974.
111. Freedman LS et al: Dietary fat and breast cancer: where we are, *J Natl Cancer Inst* 85:764, 1994.
112. Friess H et al: Treatment of advanced pancreatic cancer with mistletoe: results of a pilot trial, *Anticancer Res* 16(2):915, 1996.
113. Fukushima M: Adjuvant therapy of gastric cancer: the Japanese experience, *Semin Oncol* 23(3):369, 1996.
114. Gabius HJ et al: The mistletoe myth: claims, reality, and provable perspectives, *Z Arztl Fortbild (Jena)*, 90(2):103, 1996.
115. Gallagher LM et al: Music therapy in palliative medicine, *Support Care Cancer* 9(3):156, 2001.
116. Garewal HS, Diplock AT: How safe are antioxidant vitamins? *Drug Saf* 13(1):8, 1995.
117. Gellert GA et al: Survival of breast cancer patients receiving adjunct psychosocial support therapy: a 10-year follow-up study, *J Clin Oncol* 11:66, 1993.
118. Genuis ML: The use of hypnosis in helping cancer patients control anxiety, pain, and emesis: a review of recent empirical studies, *Am J Clin Hypn* 37(4):316, 1995.
119. Gershanovich ML et al: Results of clinical study of antitumor action of hydrazine sulfate, *Nutr Cancer* 3:7, 1981.
120. Giovannucci E et al: A prospective study of dietary fat and risk of prostate cancer, *J Natl Cancer Inst* 85:1571, 1993.
121. Glass LF et al: Bleomycin-mediated electrochemotherapy of basal cell carcinoma, *J Am Acad Dermatol* 34(1):82, 1996.
122. Gohil K et al: mRNA expression profile of a human cancer cell line in response to *Ginkgo biloba* extract: induction of antioxidant response and the Golgi system, *Free Radic Res* 33(6):831, 2000.
123. Gold J: The use of hydrazine sulfate in terminal and preterminal cancer patients: results of investigational new drug (IND) study in 84 evaluable patients, *Oncology* 32:1, 1975.
124. Gold J: Anabolic profiles in late-stage cancer patients responsive to hydrazine sulfate, *Cancer* 3:13, 1981.
125. Gold J: Hydrazine sulfate: a current perspective, *Nutr Cancer* 9:59, 1987.
126. Goldin BR et al: The effect of dietary fat and fiber on serum estrogen concentrations in premenopausal women under controlled dietary conditions, *Cancer* 74:1125, 1994.

127. Gomes EM, Souto PR, Felzenszwalb I: Shark-cartilage–containing preparation protects cells against hydrogen peroxide–induced damage and mutagenesis, *Mutat Res* 367(4):204, 1996.

128. Goodwin PJ et al: The effect of group psychosocial support on survival in metastatic breast cancer, *N Engl J Med* 345(24):1719, 2001.

129. Goodwin WJ Jr, Lane HW, Bradford K: Selenium and glutathione peroxidase levels in patients with epidermoid carcinoma of the oral cavity and oropharynx, *Cancer* 51:110, 1983.

130. Gordon DW et al: Chaparral ingestion: the broadening spectrum of liver injury caused by herbal medications, *JAMA* 273(6):489, 1995.

131. Greenberg ER, Sporn MB: Antioxidant vitamins, cancer, and cardiovascular disease, *N Engl J Med* 334(18):1145, 1996.

132. Greenberg ER et al: A clinical trial of beta-carotene to prevent basal cell and squamous-cell cancers of the skin: the Skin Cancer Prevention Study Group, *N Engl J Med* 323(12):825, 1990.

133. Greenwald P: Preventive clinical trials: an overview, *Ann N Y Acad Sci* 768:129, 1995.

134. Greenwald P: The potential of dietary modification to prevent cancer, *Prev Med* 25(1):41, 1996.

135. Gregerson (Jasnoski) MB, Roberts I, Amiri M: Absorption and imagery locate immune responses in the body, *Biofeedback Self-Regul* 21(2):149, 1996.

136. Grobstein C: *Assembly of life sciences, National Academy of Sciences*, Committee on Diet, Nutrition and Cancer, National Academy of Science, Washington, DC, 1982, National Academy Press.

137. Grossgebauer K: The "cancell" theory of carcinogenesis: re-evolution of an ancient holistic neoplastic unicellular concept of cancer, *Med Hypotheses* 45(6):545, 1995.

138. Guengerich FP: Influence of nutrients and other dietary materials on cytochrome P-450 enzymes, *Am J Clin Nutr* 61(suppl 3):651, 1995.

139. Gupta S et al: Plasma selenium level in cancer patients, *Indian J Cancer* 31(3):192, 1994.

140. Hainer MI et al: Fatal hepatorenal failure associated with hydrazine sulfate, *Ann Intern Med* 133(11):877, 2000.

141. Hall CL et al: Overexpression of the hyaluron receptor RHAMM is transforming and is also required for H-ras transformation, *Cell* 82:19, 1995.

142. Hammar M et al: Acupuncture treatment of vasomotor symptoms in men with prostatic carcinoma: a pilot study, *J Urol* 161:853, 1999.

143. Handel DL: Complementary therapies for cancer patients: what works, what does not, and how to know the difference, *Tex Med* 97(2):68, 2001.

144. Harada M et al: Oral administration of PSK can improve the impaired anti-tumor CD4+-cell response in gut-associated lymphoid tissue (GALT) of specific-pathogen–free mice, *Int J Cancer* 70(3):362, 1997.

145. Hauser SP: Unproven methods in cancer treatment, *Curr Opin Oncol* 5(4):646, 1993.

146. Hawrylewica EJ, Zapata JJ, Blair WH: Soy and experimental cancer: animal studies, *J Nutr* 125 (suppl 31):698, 1995.

147. Hayakawa K et al: Effect of krestin (PSK) as adjuvant treatment on the prognosis after radical radiotherapy in patients with non–small cell lung cancer, *Anticancer Res* 13(5C):1815, 1993.

148. Hayashi I et al: Effects of oral administration of *Echinacea purpurea* (American herb) on incidence of spontaneous leukemia caused by recombinant leukemia viruses in AKR/J mice, *Nihon Rinsho Meneki Gakkai Kaishi* 24(1):10, 2001.

149. Hegewisch-Becker S et al: Addition of hyperthermia: heat potentiates cancer therapy, *MMW Fortschr Med* 143(25):28, 2001.

150. Heinonen OP et al: Prostate cancer and supplementation with alpha-tocopherol and beta-carotene: incidence and mortality in a controlled trial, *J Natl Cancer Inst* 90(6):440, 1998.

151. Helary SS: Unproven treatments in cancerology, *Bull Cancer (Paris)*, 78(10):915, 1991.

152. Heller R: Treatment of cutaneous nodules using electrochemotherapy, *J Fla Med Assoc* 82(2):147, 1995.

153. Heller R et al: Phase I/II trial for the treatment of cutaneous and subcutaneous tumors using electrochemotherapy, *Cancer* 77(5):964, 1996.

154. Henneckens CH et al: Lack of effect of long-term supplementation with beta-carotene on the incidence of malignant neoplasms and cardiovascular disease, *N Engl J Med*, 334(18):1146, 1996.

155. Herbert V: *Nutrition cultism: facts and fictions*, Philadelphia, 1981, Stickley.

156. Herbert V: The antioxidant supplement myth, *Am J Clin Nutr* 60(2):157, 1994.
157. Hijikata Y et al: Traditional Chinese medicines improve the course of refractory leukemic lymphoblastic lymphoma and acute lymphocytic leukemia: two case reports, *Am J Chin Med* 23(2):195, 1995.
158. Horie Y et al: Bu ji (hozai) for treatment of postoperative gastric cancer patients, *Am J Chin Med* 22(3/4):300, 1994.
159. Horowitz RS et al: The clinical spectrum of Jin Bu Huan toxicity, *Arch Intern Med* 156(8):899, 1996.
160. Hoshino T: Effects of garlic preparations on the gastrointestinal mucosa, *J Nutr* 131(3 suppl):1109, 2001.
161. Hrushesky WMJ: Circadian timing of cancer chemotherapy, *Science* 228:73, 1985.
162. Hsieh T et al: Regulation of androgen receptor (AR) and prostate specific antigen (PSA) expression in the androgen-responsive prostate LNCaP cells by ethanolic extract of the Chinese herbal preparation, PC SPES, *Biochem Mol Biol Int* 42(3):535, 1997.
163. Hua-ling W: Electrochemical therapy of 74 cases of liver cancer, *Eur J Surg* 574(suppl):55, 1994.
164. Hunt TJ, Connelly JF: Shark cartilage for cancer treatment, *Am J Health Syst Pharm* 52(16):1756, 1995.
165. Iino Y et al: Eight-year results of adjuvant immunochemotherapies vs. chemotherapy in the treatment of operable breast cancer. In *Proceedings of the 18th International Congress of Chemotherapy*, 1993, Stockholm, Sweden, p 162.
166. Iino Y et al: Immunochemotherapies versus chemotherapy as adjuvant treatment after curative resection of operable breast cancer, *Anticancer Res* 15(6B):2907, 1995.
167. Ikezoe T et al: Baicalin is a major component of PC-SPES, which inhibits the proliferation of human cancer cells via apoptosis and cell cycle arrest, *Prostate* 49(4):285, 2001.
168. Integration of behavioral and relaxation approaches into the treatment of chronic pain and insomnia, National Institutes of Health, Technology Assessment Conference Statement, 1995. http://odp.od.nih.gov/consensus/ta/017/017_statement.htm
169. Izzo AA, Ernst E: Interactions between herbal medicines and prescribed drugs, *Drugs* 61(15):2163, 2001.
170. Jacknow DS et al: Hypnosis in the prevention of chemotherapy-related nausea and vomiting in children: a prospective study, *J Dev Behav Pediatr* 15:258, 1994.
171. Jackson J: Unproven treatment in childhood oncology: how far should pediatricians co-operate? *J Med Ethics* 20(2):77, 1994.
172. Janne PA, Mayer RJ: Chemoprevention of colorectal cancer, *N Engl J Med* 342(26):1960, 2000.
173. Jordan KS, Mackey D, Garvey E: A 39-year-old man with acute hemolytic crisis secondary to intravenous injection of hydrogen peroxide, *J Emerg Nurs* 17:8, 1991.
174. Joshi BS et al: Alternative medicine: herbal drugs and their critical appraisal. Part I, *Prog Drug Res* 56:1, 2001.
175. Joyce CRB: Placebo and complementary medicine, *Lancet* 344:1279, 1994.
176. Jurkowski JJ, Cave WB: Dietary effects of menhaden oil on the growth and membrane lipids of rat mammary tumors, *J Natl Cancer Inst* 74(5):1145, 1985.
177. Kaegi E: Unconventional therapies for cancer. 6. 714-X. Task Force on Alternative Therapies, Canadian Breast Cancer Research, *CMAJ* 158(12):1621, 1998.
178. Kaegi E: Unconventional therapies for cancer. 1. Essiac. Task Force on Alternative Therapies, Canadian Breast Cancer Research, *CMAJ* 158(7):897, 1998.
179. Kaizer L et al: Fish consumption and breast cancer risk: an ecological study, *Nutr Cancer* 12:61, 1989.
180. Kalble T, Otto T: Unconventional methods in superficial bladder cancer, *Urologe A* 33(6):553, 1994.
181. Kang M et al: Treatment of pleural effusion caused by lung carcinoma with circular intrapleural hyperthermic perfusion and its mechanism, *Zhonghua Yi Xue Za Zhi* 81(19):1176, 2001.
182. Kaul PN: Alternative medicine: herbal drugs and their critical appraisal. Part II, *Prog Drug Res* 57:1, 2001.
183. Keller VE: Management of nausea and vomiting in children, *J Pediatr Nurs* 10(5):280, 1995.
184. Kelloff GJ et al: Mechanistic considerations in chemopreventive drug development, *J Cell Biochem Suppl* 20:1, 1994.
185. Kennedy AR: The evidence for soybean products as cancer preventive agents, *J Nutr* 126(2):582, 1996.
186. Kennedy CW, Donohue JJ, Wan XS: Effects of the Bowman-Birk protease inhibitor on survival of fibroblasts and cancer cells exposed to radiation and cis-platinum, *Nutr Cancer* 26(2):209, 1996.

187. Key TJA et al: Sex hormones in women in rural China and in Britain, *Br J Cancer* 62:631, 1990.

188. Khan S et al: Therapeutic plants of Ayurveda: a review of selected clinical and other studies for 166 species, *J Altern Complement Med* 7(5):405, 2001.

189. Kilcoyne RF et al: Minimal spinal hyperostosis with low-dose isotrentinoin therapy, *Invest Radiol* 21:41, 1986.

190. Kite SM et al: Development of an aromatherapy service at a Cancer Centre, *Palliat Med* 12(3):171, 1998.

191. Kleeberg UR et al: Adjuvant trial in melanoma patients comparing rIFN-alpha to rIFN-gamma to Iscador to a control group after curative resection of high-risk primary (> = 3 mm) or regional lymph node metastasis (EORTC 18871), *Eur J Cancer* 35(suppl 4):82, 1999.

192. Klepser TB et al: Unsafe and potentially safe herbal therapies, *Am J Health Syst Pharm* 56(2):125, 1999.

193. Ko RJ: Causes, epidemiology and clinical evaluation of suspected herbal poisoning, *Clin Toxicol* 37(6):697, 1999.

194. Koch E: Extracts from fruits of saw palmetto (*Sabal serrulata*) and roots of stinging nettle (*Urtica dioica*): viable alternatives in the medical treatment of benign prostatic hyperplasia and associated lower urinary tracts symptoms, *Planta Med* 67(6):489, 2001.

195. Konishi F et al: Antitumor effect induced by a hot water extract of *Chlorella vulgaris* (CE) resistant to meth-A tumor growth mediated by CE-induced polymorphonuclear leukocytes, *Cancer Immunol Immunother*, 19:73, 1985.

196. Kosty MP et al: Cisplatin, vinblastine, and hydrazine sulfate in advanced non–small cell lung cancer: a randomized placebo-controlled, double-blind Phase III study of the cancer and leukemia group B, *J Clin Oncol* 12:1113, 1994.

197. Kroesen AJ et al: Incontinence after ileo-anal pouch anastomosis: diagnostic criteria and therapeutic sequelae, *Chirurg* 66(4):385, 1995.

198. Kuanhong Q: Analysis of the clinical effectiveness of 144 cases of soft tissue and superficial malignant tumors treated with electrochemical therapy, *Eur J Surg* 574(suppl):37, 1994.

199. Kushi M: *The macrobiotic approach to cancer*, Wayne, NJ, 1982, Avery.

200. Kuttan G et al: Prevention of 20-methylcholanthrene–induced sarcoma by a mistletoe extract, Iscador, *Carcinogenesis* 17(5):1107, 1996.

201. Ladermann JP: Accidents of spinal manipulation, *Ann Swiss Chiropractors Assoc* 7:161, 1981.

202. Lai SS: Clinical observations: a Chinese herbal formula for the treatment of pain and associated symptoms of cancer, Conference of World Association of Chinese Medicine, Toronto, 1995.

203. Lamm DL et al: Megadose vitamins in bladder cancer: a double-blind clinical trial, *J Urol* 151:21, 1994.

204. Lamm DL et al: Enhanced immunocompetence by garlic: role in bladder cancer and other malignancies, *J Nutr* 131(3 suppl):1067, 2001.

205. Lamson DW et al: Natural agents in the prevention of cancer. Part 2. Preclinical data and chemoprevention for common cancers, *Altern Med Rev* 6(2):167, 2001.

206. Lao YH et al: Electrochemical therapy for intermediate and advanced liver cancer: a report of 50 cases, *Eur J Surg* 574(suppl):51, 1994.

207. Lavie G et al: The chemical and biological properties of hypericin: a compound with a broad spectrum of biological activities, *Med Res Rev* 15(2):111, 1995.

208. Lee A, Langer R: Shark cartilage contains inhibitors of angiogenesis, *Science* 221:1185, 1983.

209. Lerner HJ, Regelson W: Clinical trial of hydrazine sulfate in solid tumors, *Cancer Treat Rep* 60:959, 1976.

210. Lerner IJ: The physician and cancer quackery: the physician's role in promoting the scientific treatment of cancer and discouraging questionable treatment methods, *NY State J Med* 93(2):96, 1993.

211. Lerner IJ, Kennedy BJ: The prevalence of questionable methods of cancer treatment in the United States, *CA Cancer J Clin* 42:181, 1992.

212. Liberti LE et al: Evaluation of commercial ginseng products, *J Pharm Sci* 67(10):1487, 1978.

213. Linde K, Melchart D: Randomized controlled trials of individualized homeopathy: a state-of-the-art review, *J Altern Complement Med* 4(4):371, 1998.

214. Linde K, Mulrow CD: St John's wort for depression, Cochrane Review. In *The Cochrane Library*, Oxford (online: Update software, latest July 9, 1998).

215. Lipp FJ: The efficacy, history, and politics of medicinal plants, *Alternat Ther Health Med* 2(4):36, 1996.

216. Lippman SM et al: Retinoid chemoprevention studies in upper aerodigestive tract and lung carcinogenesis, *Cancer Res* 54(suppl 7):2025, 1994.

217. Lissoni P et al: A randomized study with the pineal hormone melatonin versus supportive care alone in patients with brain metastases due to solid neoplasms, *Cancer* 73:699, 1994.

218. Lissoni P et al: A randomized study with subcutaneous low-dose interleukin-2 alone vs. interleukin 2 plus the pineal neurohormone melatonin in advanced solid neoplasms other than renal cancer and melanoma, *Br J Cancer* 69(1):196, 1994.

219. Lissoni P et al: A biological study on the efficacy of low-dose subcutaneous interleukin 2 plus melatonin, *Oncology* 52(5):360, 1995.

220. Lissoni P et al: A randomized study of neuroimmunotherapy with low-dose subcutaneous interleukin-2 plus melatonin, *Support Care Cancer* 3(3):194, 1995.

221. Long K, Long R: Diet and development of cancer, *Nurse Pract Forum* 6(4):183, 1995.

222. Lopez-Carillo L, Hernandez Avila M, Dubrow R: Chili pepper consumption and gastric cancer in Mexico: a case-control study, *Am J Epidemiol* 139(3):263, 1994.

223. Loprinzi ChL et al: Randomized placebo-controlled evaluation of hydrazine sulfate in patients with advanced colorectal cancer, *J Clin Oncol* 12:1121, 1992.

224. Loprinzi ChL et al: Placebo-controlled trial of hydrazine sulfate in patients with newly diagnosed non–small-cell lung cancer, *J Clin Oncol* 12:1126, 1994.

225. Lowenthal RM: On eye of newt and bone of shark, *Med J Aust* 160(6):323, 1994.

226. Lowenthal RM: Alternative cancer treatments, *Med J Aust* 165(10):536, 1996.

227. MacGregor et al: Hepatotoxicity of herbal remedies, *Br Med J* 299:1156, 1989.

228. Maestroni GJ, Conti A: Melatonin in human breast cancer tissue: association with nuclear grade and estrogen receptor status, *Lab Invest* 75(4):557, 1996.

229. Maione TE, Sharpe RJ: Development of angiogenesis inhibitors for clinical applications, *Trends Pharmacol Sci* 11:457, 1990.

230. Malpas JS: Oncology, *Postgrad Med J* 69(808):85, 1993.

231. Markman M: Shark cartilage: the Laetrile of the 1990s, *Cleve Clin J Med* 63(3):179, 1996.

232. Marnett LJ, Honn KV: Overview of articles on eicosanoids and cancer, *Cancer Metastasis Rev* 13(3/4):237, 1994.

233. Massion AO et al: Meditation, melatonin and breast/prostate cancer: hypothesis and preliminary data, *Med Hypotheses* 44(1):39, 1995.

234. Matsushima Y et al: Clinical and experimental studies of anti-tumoral effects of electrochemical therapy (ECT) alone or in combination with chemotherapy, *Eur J Surg Suppl* 574:59, 1994.

235. Matthew B: Evaluation of chemoprevention of oral cancer with *Spirulina fusiformis*, *Nutr Cancer* 24:197, 1995.

236. McCarthy MF: Fish oil may impede tumor angiogenesis and invasiveness by down-regulating protein kinase C and modulating eicosanoid production, *Med Hypotheses* 46(2):107, 1996.

237. McGinnis LS: Alternative therapies: 1990—an overview, *Cancer* 67(suppl 6):1788, 1991.

238. McGuire TR et al: Antiproliferative activity of shark cartilage with and without tumor necrosis factor-alpha in human umbilical vein endothelium, *Pharmacotherapy* 16(2):237, 1996.

239. McIntyre M: A review of the benefits, adverse events, drug interactions and safety of St. John's wort (*Hypericum perforatum*): the implications with regard to the regulation of herbal medicines, *J Altern Complement Med* 6(2):115, 2000.

240. McLarty JW et al: Beta-carotene, vitamin A, and lung cancer chemoprevention: results of an intermediate endpoint study, *Am J Clin Nutr* 62(suppl 6):1431, 1995.

241. Merchant RE, Rice CD, Young HF: Dietary *Chlorella pyrenoidosa* for patients with malignant glioma: effects on immunocompetence, quality of life, and survival, *Phytother Res* 4:220, 1990.

242. Messina MJ et al: Soy intake and cancer risk: a review of the in vitro and in vivo data, *Nutr Cancer* 2(2):113, 1994.

243. Metz JM et al: Cancer patients use unconventional medical therapies far more frequently than standard history and physical examination suggest, *Cancer J* 7(2):149, 2001.

244. Milas L, Hanson WR: Eicosanoids and radiation, *Eur J Cancer* 31A(10):1580, 1995.

245. Mir LM et al: Electrochemotherapy, a novel antitumor treatment: first clinical trial, *C R Acad Sci Paris* 313:613, 1991.

246. Mir LM et al: Systemic antitumor effects of electrochemotherapy combined with histocompatible cells secreting interleukin-2, *J Immunother Emphasis Tumor Immunol* 17(1):30, 1995.
247. Misra UK et al: Consequences of neck manipulation performed by a non-professional, *Spinal Cord* 39(2):112, 2001.
248. Miyazawa Y et al: Immunomodulation by a unicellular green algae (*Chlorella pyrenoidosa*) in tumor-bearing mice, *J Ethnopharmacol* 24:135, 1994.
249. Moertel CG et al: A clinical trial of amygdalin (Laetrile) in the treatment of human cancer, *N Engl J Med* 306:201, 1982.
250. Molteni A, Brizio-Molteni L, Persky V: In vitro hormonal effects of soybean isoflavones, *J Nutr* 125(suppl 3):751, 1995.
251. Monaco GP, Green S: Recognizing deception in the promotion of untested and unproven medical treatments, *NY State J Med* 93(2):88, 1993.
252. Montbriand MJ: Decision heuristics and patients with cancer: alternate and biomedical choices, Unpublished doctoral dissertation, College of Medicine, University of Saskatchewan, 1993.
253. Montbriand MJ: An overview of alternative therapies chosen by patients with cancer, *Oncol Nurs Forum* 21(9):1547, 1994.
254. Moon RC: Vitamin A, retinoids and breast cancer, *Adv Exp Med Biol* 364:101, 1994.
255. Morant R et al: Warum Benutzen Tumorpatienten alternativemedizin? *Schweiz Med Wochenschr* 121:1029, 1991.
256. Morimoto T et al: Anti-tumor–promoting glyceroglycolipids from the green alga, *Chlorella vulgaris, Phytochemistry* 40:1433, 1995.
257. Morimoto T et al: Postoperative adjuvant randomized trial comparing chemoendocrine therapy, chemotherapy, and immunotherapy for patients with stage II breast cancer: 5-year results from the Nishinihon Cooperative Study Group of Adjuvant Chemoendocrine Therapy for Breast Cancer (ACETBC) of Japan, *Eur J Cancer* 32A(2):235, 1996.
258. Morre DJ et al: Capsaicin inhibits plasma membrane NADH oxidase and growth of human and mouse melanoma lines, *Eur J Cancer* 32A(11):1995, 1996.
259. Munstedt K et al: Unconventional cancer therapy: survey of patients with gynecological malignancy, *Arch Gynecol Obstet* 258(2):81, 1996.
260. Naidu MRS, Das UN, Kishan A: Intratumoral gamma-linolenic acid therapy of human gliomas, *Prostagland Leukot Essent Fatty Acids* 45:181, 1992.
261. Nakadaira H et al: Distribution of selenium and molybdenum and cancer mortality in Niigata, Japan, *Arch Environ Health* 50(5):374, 1995.
262. Nakazato H et al: Efficacy of immunochemotherapy as adjuvant treatment after curative resection of gastric cancer: Study Group of Immunochemotherapy with PSK for Gastric Cancer, *Lancet* 343(8906):1122, 1994.
263. Nanji AA et al: Dietary saturated fatty acids down-regulate cyclooxygenase-2 and tumor necrosis factor alfa and reverse fibrosis in alcohol-induced liver disease in the rat, *Hepatology* 26(6):1538, 1997.
264. Narozny W et al: Hyperbaric oxygen therapy as a method of treatment of laryngeal and pharyngeal radionecrosis, *Otolaryngol Pol* 55(1):57, 2001.
265. National Research Council: *Diet and health: implications for reducing chronic disease risk,* 1989, Washington, DC, National Academy Press.
266. Nesher G, Zuckner J: Rheumatologic complications of vitamin A and retinoids, *Semin Arthritis Rheum* 24(4):291, 1995.
267. Niekerk VW: Cervical cytological abnormalities caused by folic acid deficiency, *Acta Cytol* 10:67, 1966.
268. Nio Y et al: Immunomodulation by orally administered protein-bound PSK in patients with gastrointestinal cancer, *Biotherapy* 4(2):117, 1992.
269. Nishino H et al: Anti-tumor promoting activity of garlic extracts, *Oncology* 46:277, 1989.
270. Niwa Y: Effect of Maharishi-4 and Maharishi-5 on inflammatory mediators with special reference to their free radical scavenging effect, *Indian J Clin Pract* 1:23, 1991.
271. Nomura AMY et al: The effect of dietary fat on breast cancer survival among Caucasian and Japanese women in Hawaii, *Breast Cancer Res Treat* 18:8135, 1991.
272. Nordenström BE: Electrostatic field interference with cellular and tissue function, leading to dissolution of metastases that enhances the effect of chemotherapy, *Eur J Surg Suppl* 574:121, 1994.

273. Nordenström BE: Survey of mechanisms in electrochemical treatment (ECT) of cancer, *Eur J Surg Suppl* 574:93, 1994.

274. Nordenström BE: The paradigm of biologically closed electric circuits (BCEC) and the formation of an international association (IABC) for BCEC systems, *Eur J Surg Suppl* 574:7, 1994.

275. Oberbaum M et al: A randomized, controlled clinical trial of the homeopathic medication TRAUMEEL S in the treatment of chemotherapy-induced stomatitis in children undergoing stem cell transplantation, *Cancer* 92(3):684, 2001.

276. Ochua M Jr et al: Trial of hydrazine sulfate (NSC-150014) in patients with cancer, *Cancer Chemother Rep* 59:1151, 1975.

277. Ogoshi K et al: Immunotherapy for esophageal cancer: a randomized trial in combination with radiotherapy and radiochemotherapy, *Am J Clin Oncol* 18(3):216, 1995.

278. Olson JA: Adverse effects of large doses of vitamin A and retinoids, *Semin Oncol* 10:290, 1983.

279. Omenn GS: What accounts for the association of vegetables and fruits with lower incidence of cancers and coronary heart disease? *Ann Epidemiol* 5(4):333, 1995.

280. Orr J et al: Nutritional status of patients with untreated cervical cancer, *Am J Obstet Gynecol* 151:632, 1985.

281. Pandey DK et al: Dietary vitamin C and beta-carotene and risk of death in middle-aged men: the Western Electric Study, *Am J Epidemiol* 142(12):1269, 1995.

282. Parkin DM: Cancer in developing countries, *Cancer Surv* 19/20:519, 1994.

283. Pastorino U et al: Adjuvant treatment of stage I lung cancer with high-dose vitamin A, *J Clin Oncol* 11:1216, 1993.

284. Patel VK et al: Reduction of metastases of Lewis lung carcinoma by an Ayurvedic food supplement in mice, *Nutr Res* 12:667, 1992.

285. Pawlicki M et al: Results of delayed treatment of patients with malignant tumors of the lymphatic system, *Pol Tyg Lek* 46(48/49):922, 1991.

286. PDQ (Physician Data Query), National Cancer Institute database: http://www.cancer.gov/cancer_information/pdq/.

287. Pennes DR et al: Evolution of skeletal hyperostoses caused by 13-cis-retinoic acid therapy, *Am J Roentgenol* 151:967, 1988.

288. Petterson M: The camptothecin tree: harvesting a Chinese anticancer compound, *Altern Ther Health Med* 2(2):23, 1996.

289. Piantadosi S: Hazards of small clinical trials, *J Clin Oncol* 8:1, 1990.

290. Pinn G: Herbal medicine in oncology, *Aust Fam Physician* 30(6):575, 2001.

291. Pisani P, Parkin DM, Ferlay J: Estimates of the worldwide mortality from eighteen major cancers in 1985: implications for prevention and projections of future burden, *Int J Cancer* 5:891, 1993.

292. Piscitelli SC et al: Disposition of phenylbutyrate and its metabolites, phenylacetate and phenylglutamine, *J Clin Pharmacol* 35(4):368, 1995.

293. Pisters KM et al: Phase I trial of oral green tea extract in adult patients with solid tumors, *J Clin Oncol* 19(6):1830, 2001.

294. Pittsley RA, Yoder FW: Retinoid hyperostosis: skeletal toxicity associated with long-term administration of 13-cis-retinoic acid for refractory ichthyosis, *N Engl J Med* 308:1012, 1983.

295. Prasad KN et al: Ayurvedic agents induce differentiation in murine neuroblastoma cells in culture, *Neuropharmacology* 31:599, 1992.

296. Prentice RL et al: Dietary fat reduction and plasma estradiol concentration in healthy postmenopausal women, *J Natl Cancer Inst* 82:129, 1990.

297. Primack A, Spencer J: *The collection and evaluation of clinical research data relevant to alternative medicine and cancer*, Bethesda, Md, 1996, Office of Alternative Medicine, National Institutes of Health.

298. Prudden JF: The treatment of human cancer with agents prepared from bovine cartilage, *J Biol Response Mod* 4(6):551, 1985.

299. Puccio C et al: Treatment of metastatic renal cell carcinoma with Catrix, *Proc Annu Meet Am Soc Clin Oncol* 13:A769, 1994.

300. Pyrhonen S et al: Randomized comparison of fluorouracil, epidoxorubicin and methotrexate (FEMTX) plus supportive care with supportive care alone in patients with non-resectable gastric cancer, *Br J Cancer* 71(3):587, 1995.

301. Recchia F et al: Beta-interferon, retinoids and tamoxifen as maintenance therapy in metastatic breast cancer: a pilot study, *Clin Ther* 146(10):603, 1995.

302. Reizenstein P, Modan B, Kuller LH: The quandary of cancer prevention, *J Clin Epidemiol* 47(6):575, 1994.

303. Revici E: *Research in physiopathology as the basis of guided chemotherapy with special application to cancer*, Princeton, NJ, 1961, Van Nostrand.

304. Rexnu G, Yuanming G: The treatment of pain in bone metastases of cancer with the analgesic decoction of cancer and the acupoint therapeutic approach, *J Tradit Chin Med* 15(4):262, 1995.

305. Reynolds T: News, *J Natl Cancer Inst* 83:594, 1991.

306. Richardson MA et al: Complementary/alternative medicine use in a comprehensive cancer center and the implications for oncology, *J Clin Oncol* 18:2505, 2000.

307. Richardson MA et al: Assessment of outcomes at alternative medicine cancer clinics: a feasibility study, *J Altern Complement Med* 7(1):19, 2001.

308. Risberg T et al: The use of non-proven therapy among patients treated in Norwegian oncological departments: a cross-sectional national multicenter study, *Eur J Cancer* 31A(11):1785, 1995.

309. Risberg T et al: Spiritual healing among Norwegian hospitalised cancer patients and patients' religious needs and preferences, *Eur J Cancer* 32A(2):274, 1996.

310. Rivlin RS: Misuse of hair analysis for nutritional assessment, *Am J Med* 75(3):489, 1983.

311. Romney SL et al: Nutrient antioxidants in the pathogenesis and prevention of cervical dysplasias and cancer, *J Cell Biochem Suppl* 23:96, 1995.

312. Ronco AL, Halberg F: The pineal gland and cancer, *Anticancer Res* 16(4A):2033, 1996.

313. Rose DP: Dietary fat and breast cancer: controversy and biological plausibility. In Weisburger EK, editor: *Diet and breast cancer*, New York, 1994, Plenum, p 1.

314. Rose DP: The mechanistic rationale in support of dietary cancer prevention, *Prev Med* 25(1):34, 1996.

315. Rose DP et al: Effect of a low-fat diet on hormone levels in women with cystic breast disease. I. Serum steroids and gonadotropins, *J Natl Cancer Inst* 78:623, 1987.

316. Rose DP et al: The effects of a low-fat dietary intervention and tamoxifen adjuvant therapy on the serum estrogen and sex hormone–binding globulin concentrations of post-menopausal breast cancer patients, *Breast Cancer Res Treat* 27:253, 1993.

317. Rosenthal DS: *American Cancer Society's guide to complementary and alternative cancer methods*, Atlanta, 2000, American Cancer Society.

318. Sabo CE, Michael SR: The influence of personal massage with music on anxiety and side effects associated with chemotherapy, *Cancer Nurs* 9(4):283, 1996.

319. Sadoff L, Fuchs K, Hollander J: Rapid death associated with laetrile ingestion, *JAMA* 239:1532, 1978.

320. Salerno JW, Smith DE: Selective growth inhibition of a human malignant melanoma cell line by sesame oil in vitro, *Prostagland Leukot Essent Fatty Acids* 46:145, 1992.

321. Sancier KM: Therapeutic benefits of qigong exercises in combination with drugs, *J Altern Complement Med* 5(4):383, 1999.

322. Sancier KM, Hu B: Medical applications of Qigong and emitted qi on humans, animals, cell cultures, and plants, *Am J Acupunct* 19:376, 1991.

323. Sawyer MG et al: The use of alternative therapies by children with cancer, *Med J Aust* 160:320, 1994.

324. Scheen A, Lefebvre P: Is homeopathy superior to placebo? Controversy apropos of a meta-analysis of controlled studies, *Bull Mem Acad R Med Belg* 154(7/9):295, 1999.

325. Schumacher U et al: Biochemical, histochemical and cell biological investigations on the actions of mistletoe lectins I, II and III with human breast cancer cell lines, *Glycoconj J* 12(3):250, 1995.

326. Scotia Pharmaceuticals: Dose/survival relationship in 48 patients with non-resectable pancreatic carcinoma treated with a single 10-day treatment course of IV LiGLA, Appendix I, Clinical Study Protocol ISN 930095, 1994.

327. Selvam R et al: The anti-oxidant activity of turmeric (*Curcuma longa*), *J Ethnopharmacol* 47(2):59, 1995.

328. Settheetham W, Ishida T: Study of genotoxic effects of antidiarrheal medicinal herbs on human cells in vitro, *Southeast Asian J Trop Med Public Health* 26(suppl 1):306, 1995.

329. Shafir Y, Kaufman BA: Quadriplegia after chiropractic manipulation in an infant with congenital torticollis caused by a spinal astrocytoma, *J Pediatr* 120:266, 1992.

330. Shamberger RC et al: Anorectal function in children after ileoanal pull-through, *J Pediatr Surg* 29(2):329, 1994.

331. Sharma HM, Dwivedi C, Satter BC: Antineoplastic properties of Maharishi-4 against DMBA-induced mammary tumors in rats, *Pharmacol Biochem Behav* 35:767, 1991.

332. Sharma RA et al: Familiar drugs may prevent cancer, *Postgrad Med J* 77:492, 2001.

333. Shekelle PG, Adam AH: Spinal manipulation, *Ann Intern Med* 117:590, 1992.

334. Shimizu H et al: Serum estrogen levels in postmenopausal women: comparison of American whites and Japanese in Japan, *Br J Cancer* 62:451, 1990.

335. Shinke SP, Moncher MS, Singer BR: Native American youths and cancer risk reduction, *J Adolesc Health* 15(2):105, 1994.

336. Silverstein DD, Spiegel AD: Are physicians aware of the risks of alternative medicine? *J Community Health* 26(3):159, 2001.

337. Simonton OC, Matthews-Simonton S, Creighton J: *Getting well again*, Los Angeles, 1978, Tarcher.

338. Simopoulos AP, Herbert V, Jacobson B: *Genetic nutrition: designing a diet based on your family medical history*, New York, 1993, Macmillan.

339. Sipos EP et al: Inhibition of tumor angiogenesis, *Ann NY Acad Sci* 732:263, 1994.

340. Slevin ML: Quality of life: philosophical question or clinical reality? *Br Med J* 305(6851):466, 1992.

341. Smit HF et al: Ayurvedic herbal drugs with possible cytostatic activity, *J Ethnopharmacol* 47(2):75, 1995.

342. Smith AY et al: Cystic renal cell carcinoma and acquired renal cystic disease associated with consumption of chaparral tea: a case report, *J Urol* 152(1):2089, 1994.

343. Smith M et al: Music as a therapeutic intervention for anxiety in patients receiving radiation therapy, *Oncol Nurs Forum* 28(5):855, 2001.

344. Soltysiak-Pawluczuk D, Burzynski SR: Cellular accumulation of antineoplaston AS21 in human hepatoma cells, *Cancer Lett* 88(1):107, 1995.

345. Song K, Milner JA: The influence of heating on the anticancer properties of garlic, *J Nutr* 131 (3 suppl):1054, 2001.

346. Spiegel D et al: Effect of psychosocial treatment on survival of patients with metastatic breast cancer, *Lancet* 2:888, 1989.

347. Spigelblatt L: The use of alternative medicine by children, *Pediatrics* 94:811, 1994.

348. Spigelblatt LS: Alternative medicine: should it be used by children? *Curr Probl Pediatr* 25(6):180, 1995.

349. Spiller HA et al: Retrospective study of mistletoe ingestion, *J Toxicol Clin Toxicol* 34(4):405, 1996.

350. Spremulli E et al: Clinical study of hydrazine sulfate in advance cancer patients, *Cancer Chemother Pharmacol* 3:121, 1979.

351. Stal P: Iron as a hepatotoxin, *Dig Dis* 13(4):205, 1995.

352. Steenblock D: *Chlorella*, El Toro, Calif, 1987, Aging Research Institute, p 7.

353. Stemmermann GN et al: Breast cancer in women of Japanese and Caucasian ancestry in Hawaii, *Cancer* 56:206, 1985.

354. Steuer-Vogt MK: The effect of an adjuvant mistletoe treatment programme in resected head and neck cancer patients: a randomised controlled clinical trial, *Eur J Cancer* 37(1):23, 2001.

355. Stich HF, Wei L, Whiting RF: Enhancement of the chromosome-demagascorbate by transition metals, *Cancer Res* 39:4145, 1979.

356. Stich HF et al: Mutagenic action of ascorbic acid, *Nature* 260:722, 1976.

357. Stickel F et al: Hepatotoxicity of botanicals, *Public Health Nutr* 3(2):113, 2000.

358. Strain JJ: Putative role of dietary trace elements in coronary heart disease and cancer, *Br J Biomed Sci* 51(3):241, 1994.

359. Sueoka N et al: A new function of green tea: prevention of lifestyle-related diseases, *Ann NY Acad Sci* 928:274, 2001.

360. Sugita Y et al: The effect of antineoplaston: a new antitumor agent on malignant brain tumors, *Kurume Med J* 42(3):133, 1995.

361. Sun HD et al: Ai-Lin I treated 32 cases of acute promyelocytic leukemia, *Chin J Integrat Chin Western Med* 12:170, 1992.

362. Surh Y: Molecular mechanisms of chemopreventive effects of selected dietary and medicinal phenolic substances, *Mutat Res* 428(1/2):305, 1999.

363. Surh YJ, Lee SS: Capsaicin, a double-edged sword: toxicity, metabolism, and chemopreventive potential, *Life Sci* 56(22):1845, 1995.
364. Suto T et al: Clinical study of biological response modifiers as maintenance therapy for hepatocellular carcinoma, *Cancer Chemother Pharmacol* 33(suppl):145, 1994.
365. Syrjala KL et al: Relaxation and imagery and cognitive behavior training reduce pain during cancer treatment: a controlled clinical trial, *Pain* 63(2):189, 1995.
366. Tagliaferri M et al: Complementary and alternative medicine in early-stage breast cancer, *Semin Oncol* 28(1):121, 2001.
367. Takeda T et al: Bryonolic acid production in hairy roots of *Trichosanthes kirilowii* max. var. *Japonica kitam* transformed with *Agrobacterium rhizogenes* and its cytotoxic activity, *Chem Pharm Bull (Tokyo)* 42(3):730, 1994.
368. Takezaki T et al: Dietary protective and risk factors for esophageal and stomach cancers in a low-epidemic area for stomach cancer in Jiangsu Province, China: comparison with those in a high-epidemic area, *Jpn J Cancer Res* 92(11):1157, 2001.
369. Tanaka K et al: Oral administration of *Chlorella vulgaris* augments concomitant antitumor immunity, *Immunopharmacol Immunotoxicol* 12:277, 1990.
370. Tellegen A, Atkinson G: Openness to absorbing the self-altering experience ("absorption"), a trait related to hypnotic susceptibility, *J Abnorm Psychol* 83:268, 1974.
371. Thibault A et al: Phase I study of phenylacetate administered twice daily to patients with cancer, *Cancer* 75(12):2932, 1995.
372. Torisu M et al: Significant prolongation of disease-free period gained by oral polysaccharide K (PSK) administration after curative surgical operation of colorectal cancer, *Cancer Immunol Immunother* 31:261, 1990.
373. Torun M et al: Serum beta-carotene, vitamin E, vitamin C, and malondialdehyde levels in several types of cancer, *J Clin Pharm Ther* 20(5):259, 1995.
374. Trawick W: An Ayurvedic theory of cancer, *Med Anthropol* 13(1/2):121, 1991.
375. Tsubono Y et al: Green tea and the risk of gastric cancer in Japan, *N Engl J Med* 344(9):632, 2001.
376. Tsuda H et al: Toxicological study on antineoplaston A-10 and AS2-1 in cancer patients, *Kurume Med J* 42(4):241, 1995.
377. Tsuda H et al: Inhibitory effect of antineoplaston A10 and AS2-1 on human hepatocellular carcinoma, *Kurume Med J* 43(2):137, 1996.
378. Tsukagoshi S et al: Krestin (PSK), *Cancer Treat Rev* 11(2):131, 1984.
379. Tsur M: Inadvertent child health neglect by preference of homeopathy to conventional medicine, *Harefuah* 122:137, 1992.
380. Tyler VE: *The new honest herbal: a sensible guide to herbs and related remedies*, Philadelphia, 1987, Stickley.
381. Tyson JE: Use of unproven therapies in clinical practice and research: how can we better serve our patients and their families? *Semin Perinatol* 19(2):98, 1995.
382. Ulett GA: Conditioned healing with electroacupuncture, *Altern Ther Health Med* 2(5):56, 1996.
383. Umezawa I et al: An acidic polysaccharide, chlon A, from *Chlorella pyrenoidosa*, *Chemotherapy* 30(9):1041, 1982.
384. US Congress Office of Technology Assessment: Immuno-augmentative therapy. In *Unconventional cancer treatments*, Pub No OTA-H-405, Washington, DC, 1990, US Government Printing Office, p 129.
385. US Congress Office of Technology Assessment: Herbal treatment. In *Unconventional cancer treatments*, Pub No OTA-H-405, Washington, DC, 1990, US Government Printing Office, p 75.
386. US Department of Health and Human Services, Public Health Service: *The Surgeon General's report on nutrition and health*, Pub No NIH-88- 50210, Washington, DC, 1988, US Government Printing Office.
387. Van der Merwe CF, Booyens J: Oral gamma-linolenic acid in 21 patients with untreatable malignancy: an ongoing pilot open clinical trial, *Br J Clin Pract* 41:907, 1987.
388. Van der Zouwe N et al: Alternative treatments in cancer: extent and background of utilization, *Ned Tijdschr Geneeskd* 138(6):300, 1994.
389. Van Zandwijk N: *N*-acetylcysteine (NAC) and glutathione (GSH): antioxidant and chemopreventive properties, with special reference to lung cancer, *J Cell Biochem Suppl* 22:24, 1995.

390. Vanchieri C: Alternative therapies getting notice through Best Case Series Program, *J Natl Cancer Inst* 92(19):1558, 2000.

391. Vermeil C, Morin O: *Role experimental des algues unicellulaires* Protheca *et* Chlorella *(Chorellaceae) dans l'immunogenese anticancereuse (sarcome murin BP 8)*, Societe de Biologie de Rennes, Seance du 21, 1976, Avril.

392. Vogler BK et al: The efficacy of ginseng: a systematic review of randomised clinical trials, *Eur J Clin Pharmacol* 55(8):567, 1999.

393. Waldon EG: The effects of group music therapy on mood states and cohesiveness in adult oncology patients, *J Music Ther* 38(3):212, 2001.

394. Wang XM, Yu RC, Wang YT: Study on advanced non-small cell lung cancer patients with Qi deficiency and blood stasis syndrome, *Chung Kuo Chung Hsi I Chieh Tsa Chih* 14(12):724, 1994.

395. Wang ZY, Nixon DW: Licorice and cancer, *Nutr Cancer* 39(1):1, 2001.

396. Wargovich MJ: Diallyl sulfide, a flavor component of garlic (*Allium sativum*), inhibits dimethyl-hydrazine-induced colon cancer, *Carcinogenesis* 8:487, 1987.

397. Warpeha A, Harris J: Combining traditional and nontraditional approaches to nutrition counseling, *J Am Diet Assoc* 93(7):797, 1993.

398. West DW et al: Adult dietary intake and prostate cancer risk in Utah: a case-control study with special emphasis on aggressive tumors, *Cancer Causes Control* 2:85, 1991.

399. Westermann AM et al: A pilot study of whole body hyperthermia and carboplatin in platinum-resistant ovarian cancer, *Eur J Cancer* 37(9):1111, 2001.

400. Wilkinson S: Aromatherapy and massage in palliative care, *Int J Palliat Nurs* 1(1):21, 1995.

401. Willett WC: Diet and health: what should we eat? *Science* 264(5158):532, 1994.

402. Willey LB et al: Valerian overdose: a case report, *Vet Hum Toxicol* 37(4):364, 1995.

403. Wilson DJ et al: Skeletal hyperostosis and extraosseous calcification in patients receiving long term etretinate (Tigason), *Br J Dermatol* 119:597, 1988.

404. Woerdenbag HJ et al: Isolation of two cytotoxic dipertenes from the fern *Pteris multifada*, *Z Naturforsch C* 51(9/10):635, 1996.

405. Wong GH et al: Strategies for manipulating apoptosis for cancer therapy with tumor necrosis factor and lymphotoxin, *J Cell Biochem* 60(1):56, 1996.

406. Wong GH et al: Integration of Chinese medicine into supportive cancer care: a modern role for an ancient tradition, *Cancer Treat Rev* 27(4): 235, 2001.

407. Woolf GM et al: Acute hepatitis associated with the Chinese herbal product Jin Bu Huan, *Ann Intern Med* 121(10):729, 1994.

408. World Health Organization: *Prevention of cancer*, Technical Report Series No 276, Geneva, 1964, WHO.

409. World Health Organization: *Cancer pain relief and palliative care*, Technical Report Series No 804, Geneva, 1990, WHO.

410. Wynder EL: Cancer prevention: optimizing life-styles with special reference to nutritional carcinogenesis, *Monogr Natl Cancer Inst* 12:87, 1992.

411. Wynder EL, Rose DP, Cohen LA: Diet and breast cancer in causation and therapy, *Cancer* 58:1804, 1986.

412. Wynder EL et al: Comparative epidemiology of cancer between the United States and Japan: a second look, *Cancer* 67:746, 1991.

413. Ye WC et al: Triterpenoids from *Pulsatilla chinensis*, *Phytochemistry* 42(3):799, 1996.

414. Yeoh C, Kiely E, Davies H: Unproven treatments, *J Med Ethics* 20(2):75, 1994.

415. Yoon TJ et al.: Inhibitory effect of Korean mistletoe (*Viscum album coloratum*) extract on tumor angiogenesis and metastasis of haematogenous and non-haematogenous tumor cells in mice, *Cancer Lett* 97(1):83, 1995.

416. You W-C et al: Allium vegetables and reduced risk of stomach cancer, *J Natl Cancer Inst* 81:162, 1989.

417. Yu-ling X, Deruo L: Electrostatic therapy (EST) of lung cancer and pulmonary metastasis: report of 15 cases, *Eur J Surg* 574(suppl):91, 1994.

418. Yun T-K, Choi SY: Preventive effect of ginseng intake against various human cancers: a case-control study on 1987 pairs, *Cancer Epidemiol Biomark Prev* 4(4):401, 1995.

419. Yunqin S et al.: Electrochemical therapy in the treatment of malignant tumors on the body surface, *Eur J Surg* 574(suppl):41, 1994.

SUGGESTED READINGS

American Cancer Society's handbook of complementary and alternative cancer methods, Atlanta, 2002, American Cancer Society.

American Cancer Society's guide to pain control: powerful methods to overcome cancer pain, Atlanta, 2001, American Cancer Society.

Dunlop R, Rubens R, editors: *Cancer: palliative care,* New York, 1998, Springer.

Simpson KH, Budd K, editors: *Cancer pain management: a comprehensive approach,* Oxford, 2000, Oxford University Press.

CHAPTER 5

Atherosclerotic Vascular Disease

WILLIAM L. HASKELL, FREDERIC M. LUSKIN, and
FARSHAD F. MARVASTI, *with assistance from*
KATHRYN A. NEWELL, ELLEN M. DINUCCI, and
MICAH HILL

Atherosclerotic vascular disease (AVD) is the major cause of death and disability in most technologically advanced societies and will soon become the leading cause of death worldwide. As underdeveloped societies adopt the lifestyle typified in "advanced westernized cultures," the incidence of AVD greatly increases, with substantial evidence that personal choices regarding lifestyle are more important determinants of disease risk than heredity.[118]

Two important features of AVD have become apparent in the past 30 years: (1) the disease process is multifactorial, with many personal characteristics and habits influencing disease initiation, progression, stabilization, or regression, and (2) AVD is preventable or can be delayed to very old age in many people. Although pharmacologic and surgical procedures have dominated therapy for AVD in the United States, prevention of the underlying disease or its clinical manifestations requires the effective management of personal health-related behaviors.[119]

Given the complex nature of the AVD process, a number of therapies now considered complementary or alternative may be effective in preventing AVD, managing patients' clinical status, or assisting patients in coping with their disease. This chapter provides an overview of select complementary and alternative medicine (CAM) therapies that have been proposed as potentially beneficial in the prevention or management of AVD, including coronary heart disease, peripheral vascular disease, and stroke (cerebrovascular accident). This review focuses on CAM therapies currently being promoted and receiving the most research or clinical attention in the United States.

N Pathophysiology

Atherosclerotic deposits, or plaques, develop in select arteries when the amount of *low-density lipoprotein cholesterol* (LDL-C) entering the subintimal space exceeds that removed, resulting in the accumulation of LDL-C droplets in the form of cholesterol esters. The *response to injury theory* proposes that mechanical or chemical injury to the endothelium increases its permeability and exposes the subintimal and medial layers of the artery wall to the infiltration of LDL-C, monocytes, platelets, and other vasoactive factors.[61] The accumulation of LDL-C in the subintimal space increases the tendency for monocytes to adhere to the endothelium and migrate into this space, where monocytes take up the extracellular lipid as they become macrophages. Modification of LDL-C by oxidation and other processes facilitates its uptake by macrophages.

Continued accumulation of lipid by macrophages leads to their conversion to *foam cells,* the major constituent of fatty streaks and the early lipid-filled plaque. The *lipid filtration hypothesis* assumes that at increased concentrations of LDL-C in the blood, LDL-C filtrates through the endothelium into the subintimal space, followed by infiltration by monocytes, which produces a series of events similar to that proposed by the response to injury theory.[24] Conversion of the plaque from being mainly lipid filled to a complex structure involving smooth muscle cells, platelets, inert lipid crystals, calcification, and formation of a fibrous cap is the result of events currently under intense investigation.[61] Platelets, macrophages, and modified (oxidized) LDL-C all release a variety of chemoattractants and growth factors, resulting in the migration and proliferation of smooth muscle cells, which contribute to the formation of raised lesions.

Many clinical cardiac events, including myocardial infarction (MI), cardiac arrest, and unstable angina pectoris, occur when a plaque ruptures. Platelet aggregation factors are released into the artery lumen, stimulating the formation of a blood clot that can rapidly occlude the artery.[34] These "culprit lesions" that rupture tend to be the early, lipid-filled plaques rather than the more advanced, complex lesions. Thus clinical cardiac events may be prevented by (1) reduction of new lesion formation, (2) stabilization of existing lesions, (3) reduction in the rate of existing lesion growth or progression, (4) decrease in lesion size or regression, and (5) decrease in platelet aggregation or increase in fibrinolysis.

Given the complex multifactorial nature of the pathobiologic events that contribute to the development, progression, regression, and stabilization of atherosclerotic lesions and thrombosis, a variety of mechanisms exist by which therapies could cause a reduction in AVD morbidity and mortality. Select therapies might reduce the occurrence or severity of clinical cardiac events by their effects on the myocardium instead of the coronary arteries, including reduction of myocardial work at rest and during exercise, an increase in myocardial electrical stability, or enhancement of intrinsic myocardial contractility.

N Epidemiology

AVD, clinically evident as coronary heart disease, peripheral vascular disease, or stroke, occurs most frequently in technologically advanced societies that consume a diet high in calories, animal products, and salt and low in plant-based foods. Reduced levels of energy expenditure are caused by a relatively low level of habitual physical activity.[119] As people from primitive, low-mechanized cultures with a predominantly plant-based diet acculturate to a more "westernized" way of life, the occurrence of AVD rapidly increases and becomes the primary cause of death within several generations.[116] Approximately as many women as men die from AVD; however, women tend to develop AVD 10 to 15 years later than men, with their early protection believed to result primarily from the effects of endogenous estrogens.

A select genetic predisposition for developing AVD has been identified, but environmental factors explain more of the intergroup and individual differences in AVD morbidity and mortality than heredity. Major factors found to be causally linked to AVD include (1) abnormal lipoprotein profiles (elevated levels of LDL-C and low levels of high-density cholesterol), (2) elevated blood pressure, (3) cigarette smoking, (4) obesity, and (5) sedentary lifestyle. Strongly associated with an increased risk of AVD are (1) diabetes mellitus; (2) a diet low in fruits, vegetables, and grains and high in animal fats; (3) elevated levels of homocysteine in the blood; (4) indicators of compromised immune function; and (5) chronically high levels of psychologic stress, depression, and hostility. Thus substantial opportunities exist to alter the basic disease process or clinical manifestations of AVD using various complementary or alternative therapies.

N Prevention and Treatment

Many different CAM therapies have been promoted as beneficial for the prevention and treatment of AVD, including vegetarian diets, dietary supplements, herbal remedies, stress reduction/relaxation, both Western and Eastern approaches to exercise, and chelation therapy. Also, entire traditional medical systems, such as traditional Chinese medicine (TCM) and Ayurveda, have been proposed as being effective in both the prevention and the treatment of AVD. Although many claims have been made and numerous clinical observations or case studies reported, few therapies have been rigorously tested by appropriately conducted randomized trials that demonstrate a reduction in clinical AVD events as the primary outcome.[63]

Claims regarding the beneficial effects of CAM therapies on AVD have been based on the influence of therapy on (1) one or more AVD risk factors (e.g., elevated cholesterol, hypertension, high level of stress); (2) the basic disease processes of atherosclerosis and thrombosis; (3) clinical events, including angina pectoris, MI, and sudden cardiac death; and (4) psychologic status, especially depression, anxiety, hostility, and health-related quality of life.

N Chelation Therapy

Introduced as a treatment for AVD in 1955, chelation therapy is the repeated administration of the amino acid *ethylenediaminetetraacetic acid (EDTA)*.[38] Typically, 3 g Na_2 EDTA or 50 mg/kg body weight of EDTA is infused through a vein over 4 hours several times per week, up to a total of 20 infusions over 10 to 12 weeks. Because of its poor absorption by the gastrointestinal (GI) tract, EDTA is administered intravenously. Also, EDTA is often given with multivitamin and mineral supplementation because it tends to remove a variety of micronutrients from the body.

The original clinical rationale provided by those in support of chelation therapy is that EDTA has a high affinity for divalent ions, in particular *calcium*, which EDTA binds and which is then eliminated by the kidneys in a nonmetabolized form. In theory, the calcium deposits found in many advanced atherosclerotic plaques are removed, thus reducing their size and helping to increase blood flow through the artery. No study has been reported using techniques (e.g., electron beam computed tomography, intravascular ultrasound) that can detect calcium deposits in atherosclerotic plaques. More recently, claims have been made that chelation therapy reduces oxidation of lipoproteins, possibly by removal of copper from the blood, and increases the dilating capacity of arteries.

A number of clinical observations and anecdotal reports have been cited, many unpublished, supporting the effectiveness of chelation therapy to reduce progression of atherosclerosis in coronary and peripheral arteries, enhance disease regression, or improve clinical cardiovascular status.[38] These reports lack the scientific rigor required to attribute a causal benefit to chelation therapy. This type of reporting by proponents of chelation therapy leads to a selection bias favoring a beneficial effect. An even greater problem in the proper interpretation of these data are studies that do not have a randomized/control or stratified group(s), because other AVD risk reduction therapies are often initiated with chelation therapy. Many patients undergoing chelation therapy are advised to make changes in their diet and exercise, take dietary supplements, and participate in a program of stress reduction. Thus, in studies without randomized control groups, there is no way to assign improvement in patient status to just the chelation therapy.

Only a few randomized, placebo-controlled trials testing chelation therapy have been published. The first two randomized trials reported a beneficial effect of chelation therapy, but conclusions from these studies are limited because of poor study design. In a double-blind study, Kitchell et al.[49] administered EDTA to four patients and placebo to five patients with angina pectoris. Two of the patients receiving EDTA "improved" compared with none who received placebo. In another small trial, Olszewer, Sabbag, and Carter[78] attempted a randomized placebo-controlled trial in 10 subjects with peripheral vascular disease but aborted the trial because of refusal of patients to be randomized; the authors reported a "profound improvement" in patients receiving EDTA. In a randomized trial of active versus placebo chelation therapy in patients with documented coronary artery disease (CAD) and angina during exercise, 33 treatment sessions over 27 weeks of active chelation did not produce a greater increase in exercise time to ischemia than placebo chelation.[50]

Two well-designed placebo-controlled randomized trials involving patients with peripheral arterial disease failed to demonstrate any net benefit of chelation therapy. Guldager et al.[39] randomized 153 patients with stable intermittent claudication to either EDTA or saline (20 infusions over 5 to 7 weeks). Vitamins, minerals, and trace elements were added to the EDTA. Pain-free treadmill walking distance, maximal walking distance, ankle/brachial blood pressure index, and patient symptoms were assessed before and 3 and 6 months after the infusions. Angiography of the lower limbs was performed in a subset of patients.[102] No treatment differences were observed at either 3 or 6 months. Also, van Rij et al.[111] did not find any benefit of EDTA infusions on walking distance, ankle/brachial index, cardiac function, hematology, blood glucose and lipids, and symptoms in patients with intermittent claudication up to 3 months after 20 infusions of either EDTA (15 patients) or normal saline (17 patients).

Under experienced medical supervision, including the use of generally accepted exclusion criteria, administration of EDTA appears relatively safe but does not provide any biologic, chemical, or symptomatic benefit to patients with AVD.[30] Given the lack of benefit, the low but real risk for some patients, and the significant cost, chelation therapy should be discarded in favor of therapies that have been proven to have major beneficial effects on AVD.

◼ Behavioral and Mind-Body Therapies

Behavioral and mind-body therapies have been a component of non-Western medical systems for centuries. Techniques such as yoga, meditation, and t'ai chi exercise and systems of social support function to promote health and longevity by using the connection between mind and body. However, research into the effectiveness of these therapies is often sketchy, and further work using randomized controlled trials is necessary. Nonetheless, a body of research offers some indication as to the effectiveness of the mind-body approaches to the prevention and management of AVD.

One of the primary links creating the need for mind-body therapies is the insidious effect of *stress* on cardiovascular function and health. Stress and anxiety have been shown to increase blood pressure, contribute to the development of atherosclerosis, and predispose to arrhythmias that can lead to sudden death.[76,86] Mind-body therapies are designed to work with both the cognitive and the physiologic aspects of the development and amelioration of the stress response.[83]

MEDITATION

Meditation practice may be the most basic of the mind-body approaches. Meditation is a cognitive tool used to develop focused attention through concentration on a specified thought or object. Research has shown that meditation can lead to a healthy relaxation state by dampening sympathetic response and decreasing respiration rate, heart rate, plasma cortisol, and blood pressure.[95] In a well-designed randomized single-blind trial, the blood pressure–lowering effects of transcendental meditation were compared with a program of progressive muscle relaxation and a health education control over 3 months in 111 older African American men and women with moderate hypertension.[90] After controlling for age and baseline blood pressure, the meditation program produced significantly greater reduction in blood pressure than either the health education control or the program of progressive muscle relaxation (Figure 5-1). The blood pressure–lowering effects were similar in men and women and subjects at high or low risk for developing cardiovascular disease.[5]

The practice of meditation has been shown to have a salutary effect on risk factors of AVD, including hypertension,[96,114] elevated cholesterol levels,[23] cigarette smoking,[23] oxidative stress,[91] and chronic stress.[108] The practice of meditation also creates the *relaxation response*, which is hypothesized to be the contrasting bodily mechanism to the *fight-or-flight response*.[11] Several studies have shown that meditation can also have a beneficial effect on patients with existing cardiovascular disease.[10,56,101] In one study, 21 patients with CAD who were taught to meditate displayed a significant improvement in exercise tolerance as well as a reduction in ischemia after 8 months of practice compared with a "wait-list" control group.[120] In another study, a 3-year follow-up showed that the effects of meditation significantly reduced measured levels of anxiety and depression and decreased medical treatment.[70]

GUIDED IMAGERY

Imagery is the use of imagination to invoke one or more of the senses. Imagery is hypothesized as a means of communication among emotion, perception, and bodily

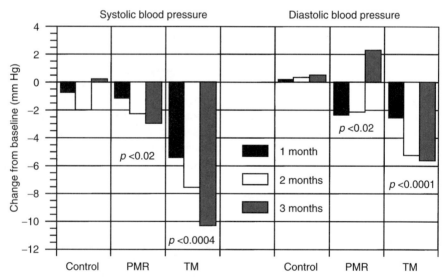

FIGURE 5–1. Change in mean blood pressure over 3 months in patients with moderate hypertension assigned to control (education class), progressive muscle relaxation (*PMR*), or transcendental meditation (*TM*) groups. The *p* values are for the differences in the change in blood pressure in each treatment group versus the control group using repeated analysis of variance (ANOVA).

change.[1] Laboratory experiments and controlled trials have shown imagery to be effective in reducing stress, heart rate reactivity, blood pressure, and resting heart rate.[21,29,71,80] It is speculated that the person's ability to "image" can become evident in an altered state of consciousness, as in hypnosis, and thus lead to physiologic changes, such as a reduction in sympathetic activity.[1]

In the "Ornish" multidisciplinary approach to AVD management, the practice of imagery was an important component.[79] Other studies have shown imagery to be effective in managing aspects of AVD. In one study, male autonomic defibrillator recipients were given audiotapes of guided imagery exercises for use at home.[105] The treatment group demonstrated lower state and trait anxiety after 1 month of practice. In another experiment, healthy subjects were trained in biofeedback-assisted imagery while experiencing a standard stressor.[97] This laboratory experiment showed significantly lower heart rate reactivity for the treatment group compared with control subjects that continued at 28 weeks' follow-up.

MUSIC THERAPY

Music therapy includes the active playing of instruments, singing, chanting, or drumming as well as the passive listening to live or prerecorded music.[4] Research has shown music therapy to influence risk factors for AVD, including blood pressure, heart rate, and anxiety.[73,92] A randomized controlled trial showed both music therapy and relaxation to be effective in reducing physiologic indicators of stress (e.g., peak heart rate, peripheral temperature) in patients with AVD.[40] However, some studies have shown little or no effect for similar interventions.[7] Patients with CAD exhibited no difference in recovery rate when assigned to one of three groups listening to either taped therapeutic suggestions, taped music, or a blank tape.[14]

EASTERN EXERCISE

Yoga and two forms of the martial arts, t'ai chi and Qi Gong, are culturally rooted in Eastern philosophic and medical systems. Each form of exercise is considered a mind-body therapy because of its multifaceted approach, which often includes imagery, meditation, and physical exercise. As with meditation, the cognitive goal of practice is to develop concentrated attention that creates certain physiologic correlates. Research has shown acute physiologic changes from practice, such as decreases in sympathetic activity, oxygen consumption, blood pressure, heart rate, and respiratory rates.[6,62,87,89,106]

Yoga

Yoga, a Sanskrit term meaning "union," has strong ties with spiritual and mystical traditions originating in India. The two primary forms practiced in the West are *hatha yoga* (physical postures and breathing) and *raja yoga* (the yoga of mental and spiritual mastery).[19] Yoga practice has been shown to reduce blood pressure and heart rate.[16,82] Studies have shown yoga to be valuable in promoting cardiovascular fitness in healthy subjects. A study involving 40 male high school students revealed higher cardiovascular endurance and anaerobic power in the yoga group compared with the control group after 1 year of practice.[12] Another study involved male physical education teachers who had an average of 8.9 years of physical activity before treatment.[106] After 3 months of yoga intervention the subjects showed a significant reduction in systolic and diastolic blood pressure, heart rate, and respiratory rate and a decrease in autonomic arousal. Studies of yoga practice conducted with healthy women have also shown a decrease in blood pressure and heart rate compared with controls.[89]

T'ai Chi

T'ai chi (t'ai chi ch'uan, tai chi, tai chi chuan), also known as "shadow boxing," originated in China hundreds of years ago and is a component of TCM.[54,117] Most studies on t'ai chi have limited generalizability because they did not use randomized trials with a control group. However, positive cardiovascular change has been demonstrated when comparing a participant's pretest and posttest performance. Reductions in heart rate, blood pressure, and urinary catecholamine levels have been shown.[48] T'ai chi may also promote cardiorespiratory functioning in elderly subjects[47,48,54] as well as enhance positive mood effects[47,48] and aerobic capacity.[121]

SOCIAL SUPPORT

A study on cardiovascular reactivity defines social support as the expression of positive affect, agreement, acknowledgment, and feelings through social encouragement.[36] Considered an independent risk factor for AVD, minimal social support has been associated with worse cardiovascular health in classic studies such as the Alameda County Study.[94] Other studies have shown a correlation between minimal social support and increased sympathetic response.[31] Also, patients who lacked social resources were more at risk for mortality independent of other accepted risk factors.[115] Uchino and Garvey[109] suggested that cardiovascular reactivity to acute psychologic stress may by reduced through the availability of social support. The specific social support mechanism of religious attendance resulted in improved cardiovascular status in 22 of 27 studies, as determined by such AVD indices as ischemic heart disease and hypertension.[57]

COGNITIVE-BEHAVIORAL THERAPY

Through the modification of certain thought processes and assumptions, cognitive-behavioral therapy strives to reduce AVD risk factors that are amenable to lifestyle change.[28] These factors include cessation of smoking, enhanced social relationships, reduced hostility, decreased "type A" behavior, increased treatment adherence, and improved nutrition.[95] Although group settings make it difficult for researchers to isolate the specific component of cognitive-behavioral therapy, many studies have documented its positive effect in reducing AVD risk factors. For example, hypertensive participants experienced a significant reduction in the need for medications.[57]

Eisenberg et al.[27] evaluated the effects of various cognitive-behavioral therapies (e.g., relaxation, meditation, biofeedback) on blood pressure levels in patients with hypertension through meta-analysis. They identified 26 randomized controlled trials involving 1264 patients that met their criteria of an acceptable research design, then analyzed the primary results for systolic and diastolic blood pressure (Figure 5-2). When cognitive therapies are compared with no treatment or a wait-list control, a significant effect of the therapy is observed, whether the baseline blood pressure value is for 1 day or less or longer than 1 day. However, if the "placebo effect" is taken into account and cognitive therapies are compared with a placebo treatment, the net blood pressure–lowering effect is smaller and not statistically significant.

SPIRITUAL CARE AND RELIGIOUS INVOLVEMENT

Spiritual care and religious involvement have long held an important role in medical care in diverse cultures and settings. Often, however, use of spiritual therapies is based

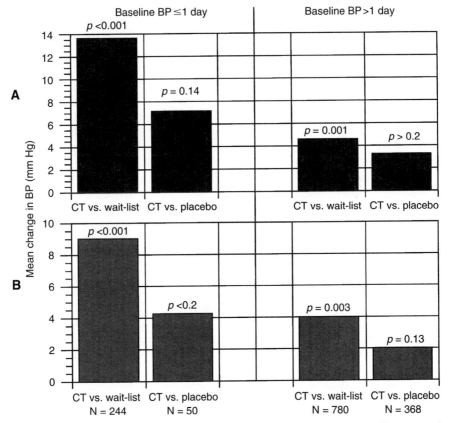

FIGURE 5–2. Difference in mean reduction in systolic (**A**) and diastolic (**B**) blood pressure between cognitive-behavioral therapy group and either wait-list (no treatment) control or placebo group. Data are presented for meta-analysis that grouped studies by length of baseline measurement period (>1 day vs. 1 day). The *p* values are for differences in the change in blood pressure between the treatment and control or placebo group. *CT*, Cognitive therapy.

on faith and not on scientifically documented effectiveness. Over the past 40 years a number of observational studies and a limited number of prospective trials have documented improvements in mortality, clinical status, and quality of life from the use of spiritual care or religious involvement. Although research shows that religious observance and spiritual care positively affect cardiovascular functioning, the reasons are complex and may include benefit from factors not directly related to religion or spirituality. For example, religious observance helps promote a healthy lifestyle, creates social support, and increases ability to cope with stress.[51,58,69]

The strongest evidence reveals that regular religious involvement extends life and decreases mortality from all causes. The most recent meta-analysis, which reviewed 42 independent samples representing 125,000 participants, showed that religious involvement was significantly associated with lower mortality (odds ratio = 1.29; 95% confidence interval [CI] = 1.20 to 1.39).[68] Previous work had demonstrated that religious involvement had a salutary effect on high blood pressure,[59] heart disease,[32] and stroke.[20] In a study examining the incidence of stroke, 7-year follow-up of 2812 people showed that religious attendance was a significant predictor of fewer strokes.

Religious involvement has been shown to have a positive impact on diverse aspects of AVD and recovery. Elderly patients were found to be up to 14 times less likely to die after elective heart surgery if they took comfort from their religious faith and were socially active.[81] Another study found that heart transplant patients who had stronger religious beliefs and involvement showed improved functioning, better treatment adherence, and fewer health concerns 1 year after surgery.[42] In a study of cardiac surgery patients, those with a higher degree of religious involvement had postoperative stays that were 20% shorter than those of less religiously involved patients.[56] A 2000 review linked religious involvement and spiritual care with cardiovascular disease.[65]

The most controversial aspect of spiritual care involves *intercessory prayer*, or praying for the well-being of others. A famous and controversial study in the late 1980s showed that in a randomized double-blind study of coronary care unit patients, those for whom others prayed had better outcomes. Treatment consisted of daily prayer of three to seven prayers until discharge. Patients who received prayers had fewer cases of heart failure, pneumonia, intubation, and cardiopulmonary arrest.[17] A second randomized trial of patients in a coronary care unit found an improved hospital course score in a prayer group versus usual care but no decreased length of hospital stay.[43] Two other randomized double-blind prayer studies showed modest effects on blood pressure.[13,72] Although this limited evidence suggests a link between prayer and cardiac health, no established mechanism explains the effect.

Clearly, more research is needed before prayer will be an accepted adjunct of healing. The entire field of spiritual care and religious involvement needs careful prospective studies to establish mechanisms of effect and to clarify the role of spiritual and religious factors in cardiovascular health and disease.

REDUCTION IN CLINICAL CARDIOVASCULAR EVENTS

Some evidence suggests that patients with AVD assigned to a mind-body therapy have a greater reduction in recurrent clinical events than patients assigned to usual medical care.[110] Freidman et al.[33] found that altering type A behavior through counseling over $4^1/2$ years in patients after MI significantly reduced the rate of nonfatal infarctions and cardiac death compared with patients assigned to a noncounseling control group. This large, well-designed multicenter study included 1013 patients, and the differences were clinically significant: 12.9% cardiac event rate for patients receiving counseling versus 21.8% and 28.2% in the control group.

A smaller study of stress reduction in patients with AVD reported a significant benefit of stress reduction compared with exercise rehabilitation on myocardial ischemia and cardiac events.[15] The stress reduction and exercise programs were conducted over 4 months, with patients followed an average of 38 months. Compared with a nonrandomized control group, patients in the stress reduction program had significantly fewer cardiac events during follow-up, as well as fewer episodes of ischemia. These studies, along with the large amount of data on the benefits of mind-body therapies on cardiovascular function and regulation, support their use in comprehensive programs of AVD prevention and management.

A meta-analysis of 37 studies examined the effects of *psychoeducational* (health education and stress management) programs for CAD patients. The results suggest that these programs yielded a 34% reduction in cardiac mortality, a 29% reduction in recurrence of MI, and significant ($p <.025$) positive effects on blood pressure, cholesterol, body weight, smoking behavior, physical exercise, and eating habits. No effects of psychoeducational programs were found in regard to coronary bypass surgery, anxiety, or depression.[26]

◪ Diet, Dietary Supplements, and Herbal Therapy

Substantial data from epidemiologic and experimental studies in animals and humans demonstrate that the consumption of foods or dietary supplements can have a major effect on AVD risk factors, disease progression, and clinical events.[98] Over the past several decades, therapies for AVD (e.g., plant-based diets, dietary fiber supplementation, antioxidant supplementation) previously considered "alternative" are now regarded as complementary or as part of standard medical practice for AVD risk reduction or treatment, along with low-saturated-fat diets, aerobic exercise, and stress reduction.

PLANT-BASED DIETS

Populations who consume diets low in animal products and high in a variety of vegetables, fruits, and grains have a lower mortality from AVD than populations who have a diet higher in animal products and processed foods.[35] Plant-based diets not only decrease LDL-C but also have been shown to reduce the rate of oxidation of LDL-C,[24] blood pressure,[76] and platelet aggregation.[53]

Rate of progression of coronary artery atherosclerosis may decrease while disease regression may increase in patients with AVD. Ornish et al.[79] reported these findings from a 1-year trial of a multifactorial risk reduction program featuring a plant-based diet very low in fat (less than 10% calories from fat, 15% to 20% from protein, 70% to 75% from predominantly complex carbohydrates). Other treatments included moderate-intensity aerobic exercise and stress reduction/relaxation. The rate of atherosclerosis was assessed by computer-based quantitative coronary arteriography at baseline and after 1 year. The 19 patients in the usual-care group demonstrated disease progression (from 42.7% to 46.1% closure of artery segments), whereas the 22 patients in the treatment group showed regression of their disease (from 40.0% to 37.8% closure of artery segments). In another angiographically based study, Schuler et al.[93] reported a decrease in coronary atherosclerotic progression during 1 year in patients with AVD who participated in a low-fat diet and exercise program compared with patients assigned to the usual care of their physicians.

Several studies have assigned patients with AVD to either a plant-based diet or a usual diet or another type of control diet and determined the development of nonfatal and fatal clinical events attributable to AVD. Singh et al.[100] randomly assigned 406 patients with MI or unstable angina pectoris to either a low-fat diet or a low-fat diet with increased emphasis on the intake of fruits, vegetables, nuts, and grains. After 1 year, patients assigned to the low-fat and plant-based diet had fewer cardiac events (50 vs. 82 patients; $p > .001$) and a lower total mortality (21 vs. 38 died; $p < .01$). Patients with MI who were then given a "Mediterranean diet" were compared with patients given the usual post-MI "prudent" diet (606 patients).[64] They were randomly assigned to one of the two diets and followed for up to 5 years, with the primary outcome being nonfatal MI or cardiac death. At a mean follow-up of 27 months, the patients assigned to the Mediterranean diet had had eight events, and patients consuming the prudent diet had had 33 events (risk ratio = 0.27; 95% CI = 0.12 to 0.82; $p = .02$).

Although no randomized trial of a lifestyle risk reduction program that features a plant-based diet has been conducted, patients treated at the Pritikin Longevity Center have been reported to do better clinically for up to 5 years.[8] The combined diet and exercise program significantly reduces adiposity, LDL-C, and blood pressure and the need for various cardiovascular medications during the 4-week inpatient program.[9]

DIETARY SUPPLEMENTS

Numerous attempts have been made to achieve the risk reduction benefits for AVD seen with plant-based diets by providing specific substances from plants in the form of a supplement. Of the many different substances found in plants, the most promising delivered as a supplement include water-soluble dietary fiber, antioxidants, folic acid, and plant estrogens.

Dietary Fiber

Some cholesterol that returns to the liver is delivered to the intestine as part of the bile acid secreted by the gallbladder. Water-soluble dietary fibers found in a number of plants reduce blood cholesterol concentrations by binding this cholesterol and excreting it from the body before it has a chance to be reabsorbed. Part of the decrease in cholesterol achieved by a plant-based diet is this effect of water-soluble fiber. A number of randomized controlled trials have shown that supplementation with water-soluble fiber (oats, guar gum, pectin, mixed fibers) in the range of 10 to 40 g/day results in a reduction of plasma cholesterol of about 10% (range, 0% to 17%).[46]

Antioxidants

Antioxidants appear to influence a number of processes in the body that may help reduce the rate of development of AVD. Of particular interest has been their potential role in reducing the oxidation of LDL-C that has found its way through the endothelium and into the artery wall. Oxidation of these particles is necessary before they can be taken up by macrophages and become part of the atherosclerotic plaque. The antioxidant vitamins A, C, and E and beta-carotene all appear to help protect the LDL particles against oxidation by free radicals.[24] Also, antioxidant vitamins have a favorable effect on the endothelium-mediated vasodilation, helping to restore a reduction in dilation caused by hypercholesterolemia and cigarette smoking.[44,60]

In population studies, people who report a greater antioxidant supplementation use have less AVD.[24] Results of trials attempting to document a causal relation between supplementation use and reduced clinical cardiovascular events have been mixed. Two prospective cohort studies reported a 35% to 40% reduction in the incidence of major coronary events in individuals in the highest quintile of vitamin E intake versus those in the lowest quintile.[85,103] The greatest benefit was in persons taking 100 to 250 IU/day. However, only one of five recently published randomized studies of antioxidant supplementation and AVD clinical events has demonstrated benefit.[38,45,104,107,112] In a study of heavy smokers who were treated with beta-carotene, vitamin E, both, or neither for 5 to 8 years, supplementation provided no benefit.[107] Deaths from AVD were not reduced in physicians receiving supplemental beta-carotene over 12 years.[45] In a randomized trial involving 2545 women and 6996 men at increased risk for cardiovascular clinical events, 400 IU of vitamin E daily did not decrease clinical events compared with the placebo group over 5 years. Also, in a randomized trial with men and women with recent MI, 300 mg/day of vitamin E did not provide protection against fatal and nonfatal AVD events over 3.6 years.[37] In contrast to these studies, patients with AVD treated with vitamin E (400 to 800 IU/day α-tocopherol) had a 77% reduction in clinical cardiac events compared with patients not receiving vitamin E over a median of 510 days.[104]

In addition to the antioxidant vitamins, other substances with antioxidant properties being promoted to help protect against AVD include various bioflavonoids, the trace mineral selenium, and coenzyme Q10 (Co-Q10). *Bioflavonoids* are found in fruits (large amounts in berries and grapes), vegetables, tea, and wine. These substances appear to reduce LDL-C oxidation and improve endothelial function and may be one factor in the low AVD rate in southern France (the so-called French paradox). *Selenium* is needed for the production of antioxidant enzymes, and thus deficiency can cause increased oxidation of LDL-C. Some studies have shown that low selenium blood levels are associated with increased risk of AVD, but no studies have shown that selenium supplementation reduces clinical AVD. *Coenzyme Q10* can be produced by the body and is available in U.S. diets (especially in meat and seafood) or as a supplement. Co-Q10 has been shown to help protect LDL-C against oxidation,[121] and several clinical trials have shown improved clinical status in patients with congestive heart failure.[74]

Folic Acid

Elevated blood levels of the amino acid *homocysteine* are strongly related to an increased risk of AVD, and this relationship is largely independent of other major risk factors.[75] The mechanism of action by which elevated homocysteine increases AVD has not been fully established, but it appears to influence endothelial toxicity, coagulation, and smooth muscle cell proliferation. Elevated homocysteine levels can be reduced by even moderate amounts (400 to 650 µg/day) of folic acid supplementation.[77] To date, no randomized trial has been conducted to test whether persons with elevated levels of homocysteine who take a folic acid supplement will have a reduction in the number of clinical events attributable to AVD.

Plant Estrogens

Many populations who consume a plant-based diet and have lower rates of AVD tend to have a much higher intake of various plant (or *phyto*) estrogens than populations who consume more animal products.[2] Various plant estrogens that have been identified are found in numerous food products, including many grains, beans, vegetables, and fruits. The highest concentrations are found in flax seed (*linseed*) and *soybeans*, whereas products with lower concentrations include sunflower seeds, cranberries, and Japanese green tea.[3] Plant estrogens appear to have an effect on a large number of biochemical mechanisms that impact AVD processes, including the lowering of LDL-C, inhibition of LDL-C oxidation, and the reduction of platelet adhesion and endothelial cell proliferation. No reported randomized studies have evaluated the effects of plant estrogen supplementation on clinical events attributable to AVD.

L-Arginine

The amino acid L-arginine is a precursor of endogenous-derived *nitric oxide* (NO), one of the most potent vasodilators produced in the body. NO produced by the endothelium (inner lining of arteries) plays an extremely important role in maintaining the health of the artery by triggering local dilation and reducing platelet aggregation. Substantial research over the past decade has shown that increasing L-arginine intake by supplementation can improve blood flow through arteries with AVD, increase exercise performance, and reduce symptoms in patients with peripheral vascular disease[67] or with CAD.[25] Daily supplementation with L-arginine has been shown to reduce the rate of progression of atherosclerosis in animals,[22] and depletion of available NO increases the rate of atherosclerosis.[18]

Studies to date have demonstrated that 3 to 9 g/day of L-arginine will significantly improve artery dilation and reduce symptoms in patients with AVD. The average daily intake of L-arginine for U.S. adults is 1 to 4 g; to reach a goal of 6 g or more usually requires a supplement.

HERBAL PRODUCTS

A major component of many native or traditional medical systems is the use of a wide variety of herbal products independently or in combination. In prevention/treatment systems such as TCM or Ayurveda, herbal therapies are important elements for AVD. For example, *curcumin* (a major component of the spice turmeric) possesses antiplatelet activities,[101] and MA-631, a complex herbal mixture, reduces LDL-C oxidation.[41] Both are herbal products used in Ayurveda. Another example is the use of green tea in TCM. One form of green tea has been shown to lower plasma cholesterol concentrations[52] and is claimed to reduce blood pressure.

Another herb considered as one of those that protect against some aspect of AVD is *garlic*. A number of trials have demonstrated that garlic supplementation reduces plasma cholesterol concentrations by 8% to 10%[113] and decreases lipoprotein oxidation susceptibility[84] but has only a minor blood pressure–lowering effect.[99] For the lowering of cholesterol, the active ingredient in garlic is thought to be *allicin*. The processing of garlic into tablets or capsules may substantially reduce the availability of allicin and thus reduce the cholesterol-lowering effects of processed versus natural garlic.[55]

Difficulties in the evaluation of herbal therapies used in traditional medical systems include (1) a number of potentially active ingredients in a single herb, (2) lack of standardization or quality control of the individual herbs, and (3) the use of a combination of herbs in a single preparation. As various herbs are evaluated, however, it is likely that a number of them will be shown to have active ingredients that are useful in AVD prevention or treatment. It is important to recognize that a substance being considered "natural" does not mean it is safe.[88] Herbs such Ma Huang can be cardiotoxic for some patients, and other herbs can interact with selected cardiac medications and negate or potentiate the drug effects.[66]

SUMMARY

Atherosclerotic vascular disease is a complex biologic process that can be favorably modified by a number of therapeutic approaches. Recent advances in preventive actions include stopping smoking, shifting to a diet lower in animal fat, managing pharmacologically various risk factors (reductions in cholesterol, blood pressure, and platelet aggregation), and surgical treatment (coronary artery bypass surgery, balloon angioplasty), including more aggressive patient management (treatment by paramedics and coronary care units). All have contributed to a significant reduction in age-adjusted mortality attributable to AVD in many countries.

However, AVD is still the major cause of mortality in most technologically advanced cultures and is a major economic burden. A number of therapies still considered alternative or complementary have the potential to reduce AVD significantly when effectively integrated into a comprehensive prevention/management program. Of particular promise are the increased consumption of a plant-based diet, selective dietary or herbal supplementation, and mind-body therapies that can be learned easily and done without supervision. All these therapies can be implemented as preventive measures for the general population or for patients with existing disease.

REFERENCES

1. Achterberg J: *Imagery in healing: shamanism in modern medicine*, Boston, 1985, Shambhala.
2. Adlercreutz H: Western diet and Western diseases: some hormonal and biochemical mechanisms and associations, *Scand J Clin Lab Invest* 50(suppl 201):3, 1990.
3. Adlercreutz H, Mazur W: Phyto-oestrogens and western diseases, *Ann Med* 29:95, 1997.
4. Aldridge D: The music of the body: music therapy in medical settings, *Advances* 9(1):17, 1993.
5. Alexander C et al: Trial of stress reduction for hypertension in older African Americans. II. Sex and risk subgroup analysis, *Hypertension* 28(2):228, 1996.
6. Ankun K, Chongxing W: Research on "anti-aging" effect of qigong, *J Tradit Chin Med* 11(2):153, 1991.
7. Bamason S, Zimmerman L, Nieveen J: The effects of music interventions on anxiety in the patient after coronary artery bypass grafting, *Heart Lung* 24(2):124, 1995.
8. Barnard RJ et al: Effects of an intensive, short-term exercise and nutrition program on patients with coronary heart disease, *J Card Rehabil* 2:995, 1981.
9. Barnard RJ et al: Effects of an intensive exercise and nutrition program on patients with coronary artery disease, *J Card Rehabil* 3:1830, 1983.
10. Benson H, Alexander S, Feldman C: Decreased premature ventricular contractions through use of the relaxation response in patients with stable ischemic heart disease, *Lancet* 2:380, 1975.
11. Benson H, Kotch J, Crasswelter K: The relaxation response: a bridge between psychiatry and medicine, *Med Clin North Am* 61(4):929, 1977.
12. Bera T, Rajapurkar M: Body composition, cardiovascular endurance and anaerobic power of yogic practitioner, *Indian J Physiol Pharmacol* 37(3):225, 1993.
13. Beutler JJ et al: Paranormal healing and hypertension, *Br Med J* 296:1491, 1988.
14. Blankfield R, Zyzanski S, Flocke S: Taped therapeutic suggestions and taped music as adjuncts in the care of coronary-artery-bypass patients, *Am J Clin Hypn* 37(3):32, 1995.
15. Blumenthal JA et al: Stress management and exercise training in cardiac patients with myocardial ischemia, *Arch Intern Med* 157:2213, 1997.
16. Brownstein A: Treatment of essential hypertension with yoga relaxation therapy in a USAF aviator: a case report, *Aviat Space Environ Med* 60:684, 1989.
17. Byrd RC: Positive therapeutic effects of intercessory prayer in a coronary care unit population, *South Med J* 81:826, 1988.
18. Cayette AJ et al: Chronic inhibition of nitric oxide production accelerates neointimal formation and impairs endothelial function in hypercholesterolemic rabbits, *Arterioscler Thromb* 14:746, 1994.
19. Christensen A: *The American Yoga Association wellness book*, New York, 1996, Kensington.
20. Colantino A, Kasl SV, Ostfeld AM: Depressive symptoms and other psychosocial factors as predictors of stroke in the elderly, *Am J Epidemiol* 136:884, 1992.
21. Collins JA, Rice VH: Effects of relaxation intervention in phase II cardiac rehabilitation: replication and extension, *Heart Lung* 26(1):31, 1997.
22. Cooke JP et al: Anti-atherogenic effects of L-arginine in the hypercholesterolemic rabbit, *J Clin Invest* 90:1168, 1994.
23. Cooper M, Aygen M: Effect of meditation on blood cholesterol and blood pressure, *J Isr Med Assoc* 95:1, 1978.
24. Diaz MN et al: Antioxidants and atherosclerotic heart disease, *N Engl J Med* 337:408, 1997.
25. Dubois-Rande JL, Zelinsky R, Chabrier PE, et al: L-Arginine improves endothelial-dependent relaxation of conductance and resistance coronary arteries in coronary artery disease, *J Cardiovasc Pharmacol* 20(suppl 12):211, 1992.
26. Dusseldorp E et al: A meta-analysis of psychoeducational programs for coronary heart disease patients, *Health Psychol* 18(5):506, 1999.
27. Eisenberg D et al: Cognitive behavioral techniques for hypertension: are they effective? *Ann Intern Med* 118:964, 1993.
28. Emmelkamp P, Van Oppen P: Cognitive interventions in behavioral medicine, *Psychother Psychosom* 59:116, 1993.
29. Eppley K, Abrams A, Shear J: Differential effects of relaxation techniques on trait anxiety: a meta-analysis, *J Clin Psychol* 45(6):957, 1989.

30. Ernst E: Chelation therapy for peripheral artery occlusive disease: a systematic review, *Circulation* 96:1031, 1997.
31. Fontana A et al: Support, stress and recovery from coronary heart disease: a longitudinal causal model, *Health Psychol* 8:175, 1989.
32. Friedlander Y, Kark JD, Stein Y: Religious orthodoxy and myocardial infarction in Jerusalem: a case control study, *Int J Cardiol* 10:33, 1986.
33. Friedman M et al: Alteration in type A behavior and its effect on cardiac recurrences in post-myocardial infarction patients: summary results of the Recurrent Coronary Prevention Project, *Am Heart J* 12:653, 1986.
34. Fuster V et al: The pathogenesis of coronary artery disease and the acute coronary syndromes, *N Engl J Med* 326:241, 1992.
35. Gardner CD: The role of plant-based diets in the treatment and prevention of coronary artery disease, *Coron Artery Dis* 12:553, 2001.
36. Germ W et al: Social support in social interaction: a moderator of cardiovascular reactivity, *Psychosom Med* 54(3):324, 1992.
37. GISSI Prevention Trial Investigators: Dietary supplementation with n-3 polyunsaturated fatty acids and vitamin E after myocardial infarction: results of the GISSI Prevention Trial, *Lancet* 354:447, 1999.
38. Grier MT, Meyers DG: So much writing, so little science: a review of 37 years of literature on edetate sodium chelation therapy, *Ann Pharmacother* 27:1504, 1993.
39. Guldager B et al: EDTA treatment of intermittent claudication: a double blind placebo-controlled study, *J Intern Med* 231:261, 1992.
40. Guzzetta C: Effects of relaxation and music therapy on patients in a coronary care unit with the presumptive diagnosis of acute myocardial infarction, *Heart Lung* 18:609, 1989.
41. Hanna AN et al: In vitro and in vivo inhibition of microsomal lipid peroxidation by MA-631, *Pharmacol Biochem Behav* 48:505, 1994.
42. Harris RC, Dew MA, Lee A: The role of religion in heart transplant recipient's long-term health and well-being, *J Relig Health* 34(1):17, 1995.
43. Harris WS et al: A randomized, controlled trial of the effects of remote, intercessory prayer on outcomes in patients admitted to the coronary care unit, *Arch Intern Med* 159:2273, 1999.
44. Heitzer T, Just H, Munzel T: Antioxidant vitamin C improves endothelial dysfunction in chronic smokers, *Circulation* 94:6, 1996.
45. Hernnekens CH et al: Lack of effect of long-term supplementation with beta carotene on the incidence of malignant neoplasm and cardiovascular disease, *N Engl J Med* 334:1145, 1996.
46. Jensen C, Haskell WL, Whittum JH: Long-term effects of water-souble dietary fiber in the management of hypercholesterolemia in healthy men and women, *Am J Cardiol* 79:34, 1997.
47. Jin P: Changes in heart rate, noradrenaline, cortisol and mood during tai chi, *J Psychosom Res* 33:197, 1989.
48. Jin P: Efficacy of tai chi, brisk walking, meditation, and reading in reducing mental and emotional stress, *J Psychosom Res* 36:361, 1992.
49. Kitchell JR et al: The treatment of coronary artery disease with disodium EDTA, *Am J Cardiol* 11:501, 1963.
50. Knudtson ML et al: Chelation therapy for ischemic heart disease: a randomized controlled trial, *JAMA* 287:481, 2001.
51. Koenig HG et al: *Handbook of religion and health*, Oxford, 2001, Oxford University Press.
52. Kono S et al: Green tea consumption and serum lipid profiles: a cross-sectional study in northern Kyushu, Japan, *Prev Med* 31:526, 1992.
53. Kwon JS et al: Effects of diets high in saturated fatty acids, canola oil, or safflower oil on platelet function, thromboxane B2 function and fatty acid composition of plasma phospholipids, *Am J Clin Nutr* 54:351, 1991.
54. Lai J-S, Lan C: Two-year trends in cardiorespiratory function among older tai chi chuan practitioners and sedentary subjects, *J Am Geriatr Soc* 43:1222, 1995.
55. Lawson L: Garlic powder for hypercholesterolemia: analyses of recent negative results, *Q Rev Nat Med* Fall 1998, p 187.

56. Lesennan J et al: The efficacy of the relaxation response in preparing for cardiac surgery, *Behav Med* 15:111, 1989.

57. Levin J: Religion and health: is there an association, is it valid, is it causal? *Soc Sci Med* 38(11):1475, 1994.

58. Levin J: *God, faith and health: exploring the spirituality-healing connection*, New York, 2001, Wiley.

59. Levin JS, Vanderpool HY: Is religion therapeutically significant for hypertension? *Soc Sci Med* 29:69, 1989.

60. Levine GN et al: Ascorbic acid reverses endothelial vasomotor dysfunction in patients with coronary artery disease, *Circulation* 93:1107, 1996.

61. Libby P: Current concepts of the pathogenesis of the acute coronary syndromes, *Circulation* 194:365, 2001.

62. Lim Y, Boone T: Effects of qigong on cardiorespiratory changes: a preliminary study, *Am J Chin Med* 21(1):106, 1993.

63. Lin MC et al: State of complementary and alternative medicine in cardiovascular, lung and blood research: executive summary of a workshop, *Circulation* 103:2038, 2001.

64. Logeril M-D et al: Mediterranean diet, traditional risk factors, and the rate of cardiovascular complications after myocardial infarction. Final report of the Lyon Diet Heart Study, *Circulation* 99:779, 1999.

65. Luskin F: Review of the effects of spiritual and religious factors on mortality and morbidity with a focus on cardiovascular and pulmonary disease, *J Cardiopulm Rehabil* 20:8, 2000.

66. Mashour N, Lin G, Fishman W: Herbal medicine for the treatment of cardiovascular disease, *Arch Intern Med* 158:2225, 1998.

67. Maxwell A, Anderson B, Cooke JP: Nutritional therapy for peripheral artery disease: a double-blind, placebo-controlled randomized trial of HeartBar, *Vasc Med* 5:1:11, 2000.

68. McCullough ME et al: Religious involvement and mortality: a meta-analytic review, *Health Psychol* 19(3):211, 2000.

69. McSherry E et al: Spiritual resources in older hospitalized men, *Soc Compass* 35(4):515, 1987.

70. Miller J, Fletcher K, Kabat-Zinn J: Three-year follow-up and clinical implications of a mindfulness meditation-based stress reduction intervention in the treatment of anxiety disorders, *Gen Hosp Psychiatry* 17:192, 1995.

71. Miller K, Perry P: Relaxation technique and postoperative pain in patients undergoing cardiac surgery, *Heart Lung* 19(2):136, 1990.

72. Miller RN: Study on the effectiveness of remote mental healing, *Med Hypotheses* 8:481, 1982.

73. Mockel M, Rocker L, Stork T: Immediate physiological responses of healthy volunteers to different types of music: cardiovascular, hormonal, and mental changes, *Eur J Appl Physiol Occup Physiol* 68(6):451, 1994.

74. Morisco C, Trimarco B, Condorelli M: Effect of coenzyme Q10 therapy in patients with congestive heart failure: a long-term multicenter randomized study, *Clin Invest* 71(suppl):134, 1993.

75. Morrison HI et al: Serum folate and risk of fatal coronary heart disease, *JAMA* 275:1893, 1996.

76. National High Blood Pressure Education Program Working Group: Report on primary prevention of hypertension, *Arch Intern Med* 153:186, 1993.

77. O'Keefe CA et al: Controlled dietary folate affects folate levels in nonpregnant women, *J Nutr* 125:2717, 1995.

78. Olszewer E, Sabbag FC, Carter JP: A pilot double-blind study of sodium-magnesium EDTA in peripheral vascular disease, *J Natl Med Assoc* 82:173, 1989.

79. Ornish D et al: Can lifestyle changes reverse coronary artery disease? *Lancet* 336:129, 1990.

80. Osborne R, Brajkovich C: Brief imagery training: effects of psychological, physiological and neuroendocrinological measures of stress and pain, *Dissertat Abstr Int* 53(9):4938-B, 1993.

81. Oxman TE, Freeman DH, Manheimer ED: Lack of social participation or religious strength of comfort as risk factors for death after cardiac surgery in the elderly, *Psychosom Med* 57:5, 1995.

82. Patel C: Yoga and bio-feedback in the management of hypertension, *Lancet* 7837:1053, 1973.

83. Pelletier K: Friends can be good medicine. In *Sound mind, sound body*, New York, 1994, Simon & Schuster.

84. Phelps S, Harris WS: Garlic supplementation and lipoprotein oxidation susceptibility, *Lipids* 28:475, 1993.

85. Rimm EB et al: Vitamin E consumption and the risk of coronary disease in men, *N Engl J Med* 328:1450, 1993.
86. Rozanski A, Bairey N, Krantz D: Mental stress and the induction of silent myocardial ischemia in patients with coronary artery disease, *JAMA* 318(6):1005, 1988.
87. Sachdeva U: The effect of yogic lifestyle on hypertension. CIANS-ISBM Satellite Conference Symposium: lifestyle changes in the prevention and treatment of disease, 1992, Hannover, Germany, *Homeost Health Dis* 5(4/5):264, 1994.
88. Samenuk D et al: Adverse cardiovascular events temporally associated with Ma Huang, an herbal source of ephedrine, *Mayo Clinic Proc* 77:12, 2002.
89. Schell F, Allolio B, Schonecke O: Physiological and psychological effects of hatha-yoga exercise in healthy women, *Int J Psychsom* 41:46, 1994.
90. Schneider R et al: A randomized controlled trial of stress reduction for hypertension in older African Americans, *Hypertension* 26:820, 1995.
91. Schneider R et al: Lower lipid peroxide levels in practitioners of the transcendental meditation program, *Psychosom Med* 60:38, 1998.
92. Schroeder-Sheker T: Music for the dying: a personal account of the new field of music thanatology: history, theories, and clinical narratives, *Advances* 9(1):36, 1993.
93. Schuler G et al: Regular physical exercise and low-fat diet: effects on progression of coronary artery disease, *Circulation* 86:1, 1992.
94. Seeman TE: Health promoting effects of friends and family on health outcomes in older adults, *Am J Health Promot* 14(6): 362, 2000.
95. Shapiro D: Meditation. In Strohecker J et al, editors: *Alternative medicine: the definitive guide,* Fife, Wash, 1995, Future Medicine.
96. Shapiro D et al: Reduction in drug requirements for hypertension by means of a cognitive behavioral intervention, *Am J Hypertens* 10:9, 1997.
97. Sharpley C: Maintenance and generalizability of laboratory-based heart rate reactivity control training, *J Behav Med* 17(3):309, 1994.
98. Shrapnel WS et al: Diet and coronary heart disease, *Med J Aust* 156:1, 1992.
99. Silagy CA, Neil AW: A meta-analysis of the effect of garlic on blood pressure, *J Hypertens* 12:463, 1994.
100. Singh RB et al: An Indian experiment with nutritional modulation in acute myocardial infarction, *Am J Cardiol* 69:879, 1992.
101. Sirvastava KC: Extracts from two frequently consumed spices—cumin (*Cuminum ciminum*) and turmeric (*Curcuma longa*)—inhibit platelet aggregration and alter eicosanoid biosynthesis in human platelets, *Prostagland Leukot Essent Fatty Acids* 37:57, 1989.
102. Sloth-Nielson J et al: Arteriographic findings in EDTA chelation therapy on peripheral arteriosclerosis, *Am J Surg* 162:122, 1991.
103. Stampfer MJ et al: Vitamin E consumption and the risk of coronary disease in women, *N Engl J Med* 328:1444, 1993.
104. Stephens NG et al: Randomized controlled trial of vitamin E in patients with coronary disease: Cambridge Heart Antioxidant Study (CHOS), *Lancet* 347:781, 1996.
105. Stockdale L: The effects of audiotaped guided imagery relaxation exercises on anxiety levels in male automatic implantable cardioverter defibrillator recipients, *Dissertat Abstr Int* 51(9):4270-B, 1991.
106. Telles S et al: Physiological changes in sports teachers following 3 months of training in Yoga, *Indian J Med Sci* 47(10):235, 1993.
107. α-Tocopherol, β-Carotene Cancer Prevention Study Group: The effect of vitamin E and beta carotene on the incidence of lung cancer and other cancers in male smokers, *N Engl J Med* 330:1029, 1994.
108. Traver M: Efficacy of short-term meditation as therapy for symptoms of stress, *Dissertat Abstr Int* 50(12):5897-B, 1989.
109. Uchino BN, Garvey TS: The availability of social support reduces cardiovascular reactivity to acute psychological stress, *J Behav Med* 20(l):15, 1997.
110. Van Dixhoon W: Effect of relaxation therapy on cardiac events after myocardial infarction: a 5 year follow-up study, *J Cardiopulm Rehabil* 19:178, 1999.
111. Van Rij AM et al: Chelation therapy for intermittent claudication: a double-blind randomized controlled trial, *Circulation* 90:1194, 1994.

112. Vitamin E supplementation and cardiovascular events in high-risk patients. Heart Outcomes Prevention Evaluation Study, *N Engl J Med* 342:154, 2000.

113. Warshafsky S, Kamer RS, Sivak SL: Effect of garlic on total serum cholesterol: a meta-analysis, *Ann Intern Med* 119:599, 1995.

114. Wenneberg S et al: A controlled study of the effects of the transcendental meditation program on cardiovascular reactivity and ambulatory blood pressure, *Int J Neurosci* 89:15, 1997.

115. Williams R, Barefoot J, Califf R: Prognostic importance of social and economic resources among medically treated patients with angiographically documented coronary artery disease, *JAMA* 267:520, 1992.

116. Worth RM et al: Epidemiologic studies of coronary heart disease and stroke in Japanese men living in Japan, Hawaii and California: mortality, *Am J Epidemiol* 102:481, 1975.

117. Yan J: The health and fitness benefits of tai chi, *J Physical Educ Health Recreat* 87:61, 1995.

118. Yusuf S et al: Global burden of cardiovascular diseases. Part I. General considerations, the epidemiologic transition, risk factors, and impact on urbanization, *Circulation* 104:2746, 2001.

119. Yusuf S et al: Global burden of cardiovascular diseases. Part II. Variations in cardiovascular disease by specific ethnic groups and geographic regions and prevention strategies, *Circulation* 104:2855, 2001.

120. Zamarra JW et al: Usefulness of the transcendental meditation program in the treatment of patients with coronary artery disease, *Am J Cardiol* 77(10):867, 1996.

121. Zhuo D et al: Cardiorespiratory and metabolic response during tai chi chuan exercise, *Can J Sport Sci* 9:7, 1984.

SUGGESTED READINGS

Cooke JP: *Cardiovascular cure,* New York, 2002, Broadway Books.

Goldstrich JD: *Healthy heart, longer life,* Santa Monica, Calif, 1996, Ultimate Health.

Miller M, Vogel RA: *The practice of coronary disease prevention,* Baltimore, 1996, Williams & Wilkins.

Robbins J: *The food revolution,* Berkeley, Calif, 2001, Conari.

CHAPTER 6

Diabetes Mellitus

ANGELE V. MCGRADY and JAMES F. KLESHINSKI

$\mathbf{D}$iabetes mellitus (DM) is a chronic disease that becomes evident as hyperglycemia and affects all aspects of metabolism. About 6 million people in the United States have the diagnosis of diabetes. The two major types of DM are type 1, formerly called "insulin-dependent" diabetes or type I, and type 2, previously termed "non-insulin-dependent" diabetes or type II. *Type 1* DM occurs when the pancreatic beta (B) cells are injured or destroyed by autoimmune processes or infection and become incapable of producing insulin. Symptoms develop rapidly in individuals under the age of 30 years.

Type 2 DM, the most common form, is diagnosed in about 90% of diabetic individuals. Type 2 develops slowly, is usually associated with obesity, begins after age 30, and is characterized by tissue insulin resistance. The prevalence of type 2 DM is steadily increasing in the United States, and the age at diagnosis is concomitantly decreasing.[111] Essential hypertension and hyperlipidemia are often comorbid conditions with type 2 diabetes. The most common acute complication is *hypoglycemia*, which can occur in both types of diabetes but is more frequent in type 1 DM. Long-term complications include microvascular deterioration and neuropathy.[7,57,64]

◤ Standard Medical Treatment

Blood glucose (BG) values are expressed in milligrams per deciliter (mg/dl) or in millimoles (mmol). Diagnostic standards exist to guide the physician in identifying the prediabetic or at-risk person and to diagnose both types of DM. Physicians monitor disease status by reviewing their patients' records of daily average BG values, *fasting blood glucose* (FBG), and by a biologic assay, *glycohemoglobin*, which represents the average BG value for the previous 2 to 3 months.

Treatment recommendations for patients with type 1 DM are based on provision of exogenous insulin by injection. Patients are strongly advised to monitor BG several times a day with a glucometer, exercise regularly, and follow the diet recommended by the American Diabetes Association (ADA). For patients with type 2 DM, the physician initially recommends diet, weight loss if appropriate, and exercise. Education is usually provided by a diabetes educator, based on ADA guidelines.[7] If this regimen does not produce *euglycemia* (BG level within the normal range), oral medication is prescribed. Oral hypoglycemic agents stimulate the pancreas to make more insulin, decrease the production of glucose, or decrease tissue resistance to insulin. Many type 2 patients are now treated with insulin in addition to oral hypoglycemics.[64]

SELF-CARE

In both types of diabetes, self-care is the cornerstone of management.[20,37,60,77] At diagnosis the patient is informed that *self-monitoring of blood glucose* (SMBG) and regular checkups are necessary. Nutrition and exercise recommendations are sometimes conflicting and often complicated. Acute illness challenges BG control, requiring adjustments in diet and dosage of hypoglycemic agents. The physician caring for patients with diabetes may emphasize the seriousness of the disease to promote better self-care and foster adherence while compromising empathy in the physician-patient relationship.

The importance of patient self-care was emphasized by a former ADA president: "We [physicians] are finally accepting the central role of the person with diabetes in making daily decisions."[13] Two major clinical trials comparing usual care with intensive monitoring and insulin dosing showed conclusively that the latter decreased the incidence of long-term complications, particularly retinopathy. However, the Diabetes Control and Complications Trial (DCCT) regimen was much more demanding of patients with type 1 DM than usual care.[23] Similarly, the large-scale diabetes trial performed in the United Kingdom (UKPDS) compared intensive therapy to conventional management in type 2 DM. This study also reported decreased complications with intensive therapy.[98] Thus patient behavior, motivation for change, psychosocial factors, and variables related to adherence should be emphasized to practitioners caring for diabetic patients.

The adolescent who is diagnosed with DM has particular challenges. The social environment, peer acceptance, and family support can all play important roles in helping the adolescent maintain BG control. Supportive, cohesive families promote better metabolic control, particularly during the early years after diagnosis. Open, empathetic communication fosters good adherence. Developmental issues must be considered in adolescents who are trying to learn about their disease and take responsibility for its control.[16]

A model has been developed to explain the interplay among support, perceived threat, and depression in diabetic patients. "Threat" is defined as the impact of diabetes on self-esteem, happiness, or life satisfaction. Lower levels of depression were associated with higher perceived support of family and friends. Patients who saw diabetes as very threatening were less satisfied with their life and had a higher incidence of depressive disorder.[18]

PERSONALITY, CULTURE, AND BELIEFS

The sense of locus of control is important in patients' views of the physician and their willingness to accept the physician's advice. *Locus of control* refers to a concept embodying whether patients believe that outcomes (e.g., BG control) depend on their own decisions or those of "powerful others" or whether outcomes occur largely by chance. Some patients believe they have diabetes because it is "God's will" or because DM is a "punishment."[110] In general, patients with a belief in powerful others have less knowledge of diabetes and poorer glycemic control than patients who believe that they have a significant amount of control over the outcome of their diabetes.[56]

Culture and race affect the person's perception of disease and the sick role, thereby affecting self-care. Is an individual with diabetes "sick" in the sense of feeling unwell, held blameless for the condition, or permitted to decrease responsibilities?[86] In general, persons with type 1 or type 2 DM are expected to incorporate their self-care into their usual responsibilities of occupation and family, but individuals react differently to these demands. Self-care was the most significant factor predicting dietary adherence in African Americans, whereas social support was the best predictor for whites.[27] *Culture* may be particularly influential in the acceptance of mind-body therapies because patients' views of the mind-body connection are often influenced by their personal value system and religious beliefs. Assessment and treatment of the patient from a biopsychosocial framework improve the physician-patient relationship and facilitate treatment.

A British survey on the impact of beliefs on adherence found that patients with poorer glycemic control are not only at greater risk for complications but are also more likely to have psychiatric conditions such as eating, mood, and anxiety disorders. Patients who frequently miss their medical appointments and are poorly adherent to their prescribed regimen are more likely to be living in families with high levels of conflict.[43] Negative life events and frequent conflicts are associated with disease onset and severity and diabetic patients' quality of life.[107]

Because of the chronic nature of diabetes, impact of DM on quality of life, possibility of severe complications, and requirements for self-care, diabetic patients may seek complementary and alternative medicine (CAM) therapies. This chapter discusses the role of the CAM therapies in type 1 and type 2 DM based on outcome studies only on human subjects. The final section offers recommendations for physicians providing treatment to diabetic patients who use CAM.

■ Role of CAM Therapies

In type 1 DM there are few or no functioning beta cells, and no proven substitutes exist for insulin. However, CAM therapies may be very useful adjuncts to insulin, may enhance the effect of injected insulin, and may lower BG levels. The type 2 diabetic patient may seek CAM therapies to lower BG levels, to decrease dosage of oral hypoglycemic medication, and to decrease insulin resistance. For both types of patients at any stage of the disease, quality of life issues are important because the demands of the daily routine may compromise quality of life.[35] CAM therapies may also decrease the impact of complications from DM, such as acupuncture for pain control (see Chapter 10). Acupuncture may be indicated for the diabetic patient with neuropathy.

Nonetheless, SMBG and biologic assay are the only ways to test the efficacy of both standard and complementary interventions. The goal of the CAM therapies must be to obtain preprandial BG levels between 80 and 120 mg/dl or glycosylated hemoglobin (Hb A$_{1c}$) values less than 7%.[7] To be accepted by the ADA, an unproved therapy must meet specific criteria. Efficacy must be supported by data generated from well-controlled studies. The research must meet the goals of reducing BG, lessening the incidence of complications, and maintaining euglycemia, without increasing the frequency of dangerous hypoglycemic episodes.[6] It is important to be aware that recommendations to the lay public by self-proclaimed "experts" in CAM do not always follow the ADA guidelines.

◼ Diet and Nutritional Supplements

PRITIKIN, LOW-CALORIE, ORNISH, AND OSLO DIETS

The *Pritikin diet* is a largely vegetarian diet, high in complex carbohydrates and fiber and containing less than 10% fat. The diet is usually combined with aerobic exercise. Studies of the Pritikin diet in type 2 DM showed significantly improved BG levels and decreased hypoglycemic dosage. Patients with newly diagnosed diabetes were the best responders; many were able to decrease or eliminate oral hypoglycemic agents. In type 2 patients requiring insulin, results were less striking, although decreased BG was achieved in more than one third of these patients as well.[10,11]

The effect of a *very-low-calorie diet*—400 to 600 kcal/day with most calories in the form of high-quality protein—was tested in 36 type 2 DM patients. A 20-week behavioral program was combined with 1200 to 1500 kcal/day, or the same behavioral program was provided with 8 weeks of the very-low-calorie diet. Results showed that the combination of low-calorie diet and behavior modification was effective in lowering BG levels.[108]

The *Ornish diet*, originally designed as therapy to reverse cardiovascular disease, is also applicable to patients with diabetes, since many patients with long-term diabetes develop hypertension and heart disease. The Ornish diet consists of a low-fat, high-fiber, basically vegetarian diet with 75% of the calories from carbohydrates. Critical components of the Ornish plan, including exercise, yoga, and relaxation, are combined with the diet. In a group of type 2 patients requiring insulin who adhered to the Ornish plan, 60% no longer required insulin at the end of the study.[73,74]

The *Oslo diet*, featuring increased intake of fish and reduced fat intake, was tested by a randomized trial in 219 persons with neither hypertension nor diabetes. Although it is not directly relevant to this chapter, the findings of significant decreases in insulin resistance suggest a potential avenue toward prevention of type 2 DM.[103]

Importantly, these "diets" are actually broad-based *lifestyle change programs* and comprise multiple modules of exercise, stress management, and sometimes group therapy. Although these programs are effective for normalizing BG, further research is needed to distinguish the specific effects of each component of these programs and to explore long-term adherence.

SUPPLEMENTS

An excellent review of micronutrients in diabetes management summarizes the clinical trials on the effects of chromium, vanadium, magnesium, and nicotinamide.[15] Of the four, evidence indicates positive effects of chromium on FBG and glycohemoglobin.

Chromium functions as a cofactor for insulin action, thus regulating the activity of insulin; it sensitizes glucoreceptors in the brain, suppressing appetite. No recommended daily allowance exists for chromium.[15] One study suggested that chromium supplementation prevents type 2 DM, rather than acting as a cure or a replacement for insulin or oral hypoglycemic agents.[8] The major controlled studies of chromium in type 2 DM, although successful, were done in China and thus are potentially limited to non-U.S. populations. Prestudy deficiency of chromium and bioavailability of the chromium preparation are major considerations. It is likely that only patients whose impaired glucose metabolism is related to dietary chromium will respond to supplementation, but most U.S. diabetic patients are not chromium deficient.[26] Side effects from taking chromium supplements are possible, in particular severe hypoglycemia.

No reproducible, significant benefits were found for *nicotinamide* on FBG or glycohemoglobin. The studies on *vanadium*, although small scale, suggest mild effects on glucose utilization and insulin sensitivity; but the authors caution that long-term use of small doses has the potential for serious side effects.[72] Low serum *magnesium* level is associated with a number of diabetic complications, especially retinopathy and cardiovascular disease. According to an ADA panel, supplementation with magnesium is recommended for diabetic persons at risk for these complications or documented with hypomagnesemia.[106]

N Traditional Chinese Medicine

Traditional Chinese medicine (TCM) consists of many diagnostic procedures and forms of treatment. "Disease" is conceptualized as resulting from an imbalance between *yin* and *yang*, causing a disturbance in vital energy (*Qi*). In a recent text on the practice of TCM, diabetes is briefly mentioned under the heading of "tiredness" or "exhaustion."[62] Treatment recommendations are based on restoring energy to the patient; however, documentation of BG levels or other indicators of disease is sparse.

More than 800 elderly Chinese diabetic patients were given treatment within the TCM conceptual framework, which included (1) "regular life," (2) "rational diet," (3) hypoglycemic agents including insulin, (4) working within the "patients' power," and (5) physical exercise. The study reported that 12.5% of participants obtained "clinical alleviation" (FBG levels less than 110 mg/dl), 40% showed marked improvement (FBG levels less than 130 mg/dl), 44% had some improvement, and no effects were observed in 3%.[61] Detailed information about these interventions was not described. Also, results in the 85 patients with the most severe diabetes and late complications (classified as having "yin, yang, and Qi failure") were not reported.

QI GONG

Qi Gong, a component of TCM for centuries, has been reported to produce healing in many disorders, some of which are considered to be incurable within the realm of Western medicine. One year of daily Qi Gong practice decreased FBG and serum insulin levels in a group of 31 type 2 diabetic patients. These changes were statistically and clinically significant.[65]

ACUPUNCTURE

A paucity of sound clinical data exists supporting the use of acupuncture in the treatment of DM. One comprehensive review of the literature over the past 40 years purports acupuncture's effectiveness in the treatment of diabetes.[46] The authors cite several studies with positive effects, but none reports any control groups, and little detail is provided regarding study design and length of treatment. Specific study references could not be verified because they were listed in Chinese.

Acupuncture was compared with a TCM remedy in 60 patients with DM.[22] Thirty-eight diabetic patients (8 classified with type 1, 30 with type 2) were treated with acupuncture for 30 days, and 22 diabetic patients (classification not given) were administered "pills of consumptive thirst," 4 to 10 pills daily for 30 days; the specific ingredients of these pills were not identified. BG levels dropped significantly in both groups after treatment ($p < .001$ in acupuncture group), without significant differences between the two groups. Six of the eight type 1 DM patients in the acupuncture group were able to reduce their insulin doses after completion of the acupuncture regimen, but no other information was given with regard to follow-up in these patients.

In one observational study, acupuncture combined with modified diet was tested in 26 patients, 21 with type 2 and five with type 1 DM. FBG and postprandial BG levels were significantly reduced in the type 2 patients ($p < .001$), but no positive effects were observed in the type 1 patients. No information was given about the exact content of the diet, and no control group was included. Effectiveness rates between 60% and 88% from other studies are referenced in this report, but again, little benefit was noted in type 1 DM patients.[51]

In 1997 an expert panel convened at the National Institutes of Health (NIH) to prepare a consensus statement on the appropriate use of acupuncture. Although the panel found evidence suggesting beneficial effects from acupuncture for adult postoperative and chemotherapy nausea and vomiting, as well as for other conditions (e.g., myofascial pain, headache, addiction, stroke rehabilitation), diabetes was not included as a condition for which acupuncture would be useful as "an adjunct treatment or an acceptable alternative or . . . in a comprehensive management program."[71] The panel acknowledged the need for more rigorously designed studies in the future to help elucidate the effectiveness of acupuncture in various medical conditions.

◪ Herbal Medicine

TCM uses plant extracts in combination, not as single agents. Herbal therapies may demonstrate inconsistency in their preparation or combination of herbs, and may vary in composition among different cultural groups.[87] In many cultures, herbal medicine is incorporated into comprehensive diabetic therapy, including diet, exercise, and depending on the culture, Qi Gong, meditation, or relaxation.[17] Thus, although herbal medicine is listed as part of TCM, some of the plants described in the next section are also components of other treatment models, such as ayurvedic medicine. In fact, after an extensive literature search, which included assistance in India to identify pertinent literature, a recent report by the Agency for Healthcare Research and Quality (AHRQ) mentions a number of ayurvedic herbals, including *Coccinia indica*, *Gymnema sylvestre*, and fenugreek (*Trigonella foenum graecum*), that warrant additional investigation in larger, controlled studies of adequate duration.[2]

The risk/benefit ratio must always be considered when testing adjunctive therapies, as in U.S. Food and Drug Administration (FDA)–sponsored Phase I, II, or III clinical trials. Patients may be put at considerable risk by discontinuing their hypoglycemic medication to test a new substance. For example, an herbal substance was tested in 67 persons, some with type 1 and others with type 2 DM. A hypoglycemic effect was claimed, but very high BG values were listed after patients were withdrawn from their medication. Final BG levels remained greater than 200 mg/dl.[84]

Several hundred plant treatments for diabetes have been recorded; only a few have been evaluated in human studies, and fewer are reported as outcome studies on BG. Some of the herbs are useful for their effects on complications of diabetes, but there is no evidence of positive effects on BG. *Ginkgo biloba*, for example, has documented ability to improve circulation and may be beneficial for patients with peripheral neuropathy and retinopathy.[48]

Research on plant substances as hypoglycemic agents has been conducted on individuals with diabetes using a control group (Table 6-1). Other herbals used for diabetes lack controlled human trials (Box 6-1).

COCCINIA INDICA

Coccinia indica, also known as *ivy gourd*, is used in ayurvedic medicine as a treatment for DM. In a randomized double-blind placebo-controlled trial, 16 type 2 DM patients taking 3 tablets (containing 300 mg of *C. indica* leaf powder) twice a day for 6 weeks were compared to 16 patients taking placebo.[52] Ten of 16 patients in the treatment group, but none of the control subjects, showed marked improvement in glucose tolerance. Also, in the treatment group at the study's conclusion, FBG as well as BG levels at 1 hour and 2 hours after an oral glucose tolerance test (OGTT) were significantly reduced compared with pretreatment values. No changes in electrolytes, liver function tests, or hematologic parameters were noted. Glycohemoglobin levels were not reported.

TABLE 6–1. **EFFECTS OF PLANT SUBSTANCES ON BLOOD GLUCOSE (BG) IN PATIENTS WITH DIABETES MELLITUS**

Substance	Study	Patients	Length	Dosage	Documented Effect
Allium sativum (garlic)	Double-blind randomized placebo-controlled[96]	33 type 2	1 mo	350 mg twice daily	No decreased BG versus placebo
Coccinia indica (leaves)	Double-blind randomized placebo-controlled[52]	32 type 2	6 wk	900 mg leaf powder twice daily	Decreased BG (fasting and after OGTT)
Ginseng					
• Type not specified	Double-blind randomized placebo-controlled[97]	36 type 2	8 wk	100 or 200 mg daily	Decreased BG (100 mg) Decreased Hb A_{1c} (200 mg)
• American (*Panax quinquefolius*)[105]	Randomized placebo-controlled	9 type 2 10 nondiabetic	2 hr	3 g	Decreased BG
Gymnema sylvestre (leaf extract)	Controlled[12]	47 type 2	18-20 mo	400 mg daily	Decreased BG Decreased Hb A_{1c}
Momordica charantia (polypeptide-p)	Controlled[91] Controlled[53]	64 type 1 11 type 1 8 type 2	6-30 mo 12 hr	400 mg daily 10-30 units polypeptide-p*	Decreased Hb A_{1c} at 6-8 mo Decreased BG
Ocimum species (holy basil leaves)					
• Specific species not identified	Single-blind crossover randomized placebo-controlled[3]	40 type 2	8 wk	2.5 g fresh leaf daily	Decreased BG
• *Ocimum sanctum*	Controlled[79]	37 type 2	30 days	1 g leaf powder daily	Decreased BG Decreased Hb A_{1c}
Opuntia streptacantha lemaire (nopal)	Controlled[30] Controlled[31]	32 type 2 14 type 2 14 healthy volunteers	3 hr 3 hr	500 g broiled stems 500 g grilled stems	Decreased BG (type 2) No significant changes in healthy volunteers
Silybum marianum (milk thistle)	Randomized controlled open-label[104]	60 insulin-treated type 2	12 mo	200 mg three times daily	Decreased BG Decreased Hb A_{1c}
Trigonella foenum graecum					
• Fenugreek seed powder	Randomized controlled[92]	10 type 1	10 days (2 periods)	100 g daily	Decreased BG
• Fenugreek	Placebo-controlled[14]	80 type 2	1 mo	5 g daily	Decreased BG (mild type 2) No significant changes (severe type 2)

*Depending on BG levels.

OGTT, Oral glucose tolerance test; Hb A_{1c}, glycosylated hemoglobin (glycohemoglobin).

BOX 6–1. Herbals with No Controlled Human Trials Supporting Purported Glycemic Benefits

Alfalfa (*Medicago sativa*)
Aloe (*Aloe barbadensis,* also known as *Aloe vera*)
Bilberry (*Vaccinium myrtillus*)
Couch grass (*Elymus repens*)
Dandelion root (*Taraxacum officinale*)
Divi-divi (*Caesalpinia bonducella*)
Eucalyptus (*Eucalyptus globulus*)
German sarsaparilla (*Carex arenaria*)
Goat's rue (*Galega officinalis*)
Mountain ash berry (*Sorbus aucuparia*)
Nettle (*Urtica dioica*)
Reed herb (*Phragmites communis*)
Spanish needles (*Bidens pilosa*)
Wormwood (*Artemisia herba alba*)
Yellow bells (*Tecoma stans*)

FENUGREEK

Fenugreek seed powder (*Trigonella foenum graecum*) is a common spice used in India. To date, few human trials have been carried out examining fenugreek's benefits in the diabetic population.

In a small randomized, controlled trial of 10 type 1 DM patients, 100 g/day of fenugreek seed powder was added to a standard diet over 10 days. Results showed significantly reduced mean FBG levels compared with control patients.[92] A placebo-controlled study found that fenugreek administered in doses of 5 g/day for 1 month significantly reduced FBG and postprandial BG levels in 80 patients with mild type 2 DM.[14] However, few details were provided with regard to study design, patient characteristics, and criteria used to determine disease severity. In those with severe type 2 DM, no statistically significant changes in BG levels were observed. In another study of 60 type 2 patients taking fenugreek seed powder in a prescribed diet (25 g/day) for 24 weeks, decreases in glycosylated hemoglobin, FBG, and insulin levels were noted.[93]

GARLIC

The one human study performed examining the effect of garlic on glucose control in diabetic patients did not show a significant decrease in BG or in total insulin response in those patients taking garlic compared with the placebo group.[96]

GINSENG

A number of ginseng preparations exist, often leading to confusion for consumers. One variety, *Panax ginseng,* is also known as Asian, Chinese, or Korean ginseng. Others include *Panax quinquefolius,* identified as "American ginseng," and *Eleutherococcus senticosus,* recognized as "Siberian ginseng." Often referred to as an "adaptogen," ginseng's purported effects include enhancing physical and mental stamina as well as increasing resistance to stress. Many of these claims have not been substantiated by rigorous scientific studies.

The use of ginseng has been evaluated in two studies in patients with type 2 DM. In one randomized double-blind placebo-controlled study, 36 newly diagnosed type 2 diabetic patients were given placebo, 100-mg ginseng tablets, or 200-mg ginseng tablets daily for 8 weeks (after an 8-week run-in period monitoring patient physical activity).[97] At the study's conclusion, mean FBG concentrations were significantly reduced in the 100-mg/day group (p <.05), and Hb A$_{1c}$ values were significantly reduced in the 200-mg/day group (p <.05). The particular type of ginseng preparation administered in this study was not identified.

Another recent study compared the postprandial glycemic effect of American ginseng (*P. quinquefolius*) with that of placebo in 10 nondiabetic patients and 9 type 2 diabetic patients.[105] Patients received placebo or 3 g of American ginseng either 40 minutes before or at the time of a 25-g OGTT. Blood samples measuring glucose concentrations were taken up to 120 minutes after the glucose challenge. In the diabetic patients, significant reductions in postprandial BG levels were noted when ginseng was given both 40 minutes before and at the time of OGTT. In the nondiabetic group, significant reductions in postprandial BG levels were seen when the ginseng was administered 40 minutes before the glucose challenge, but not when given together with OGTT.

GYMNEMA SYLVESTRE (GURMAR)

Gymnema sylvestre is a plant native to the tropical forests of Africa and Asia, also important in ayurvedic medicine as a treatment for DM. *G. sylvestre* is known as the "destroyer of sugar" from historical observations that chewing its leaves desensitizes the tongue to the taste of sweetness.[41] An active ingredient, *gymnemic acid,* has postulated mechanisms of action that include inhibition of glucose uptake in the intestine and direct stimulation of pancreatic beta cells.[76,94]

A small number of trials have studied the leaf extract of *G. sylvestre* in both type 1 and type 2 DM patients. In a study involving 47 type 2 patients taking sulfonylureas, 22 received 400 mg/day of leaf extract for 18 to 20 months, and 25 were maintained on oral sulfonylureas alone.[12] Statistically significant reductions in FBG and Hb A$_{1c}$ levels were observed in those patients taking the leaf extract (p <.001). During the study period, five patients in this group were able to discontinue their oral hypoglycemic medication, 16 were able to decrease their dose, and one patient remained on the same dose. No significant changes were noted in the FBG and Hb A$_{1c}$ in the group taking sulfonylureas alone. Another small study included six type 2 DM patients and 10 healthy volunteers taking *G. sylvestre* leaf powder at a dose of 2 g three times daily for 10 to 15 days. Statistically significant reductions in mean fasting blood glucose were noted in both groups.[54] In addition, statistically significant reductions in mean blood glucose levels were observed in the diabetic subjects during the follow-up glucose tolerance test at both 30 minutes and 2 hours.

In a controlled trial of 64 type 2 DM patients, 27 were given 400 mg/day of *G. sylvestre* leaf extract in addition to their daily insulin dose for 6 to 30 months; 37 patients were followed with insulin therapy alone. Statistically significant reductions in Hb A$_{1c}$ values were noted in the leaf extract group after 6 to 8 months ($p < .001$).[91] Unfortunately, no p values were given for the 8-month to 30-month time frame with respect to Hb A$_{1c}$. In addition, despite declines in daily mean insulin dose and FBG values over the entire study, p values also were not given for these parameters.[90]

HOLY BASIL LEAVES (*OCIMUM*)

Holy basil leaves (genus *Ocimum*) come from plants found mainly in tropical regions of the world, particularly India.

During an 8-week randomized placebo-controlled crossover single-blind trial, 40 patients with type 2 DM were studied to evaluate the effects of holy basil leaves versus placebo on both FBG and postprandial BG levels.[3] Mean FBG levels during treatment with holy basil leaves were 17.6% lower ($p < .001$) than during treatment with placebo. Also, mean postprandial BG levels were 7.3% lower ($p < .02$) during treatment with holy basil leaves than during placebo treatment. No adverse effects were noted with holy basil leaves. No details were provided on the standardization and specific species of the preparation. Another small controlled trial of 27 type 2 DM patients utilizing *Ocimum sanctum* leaf powder also showed reductions in mean FBG and glycosylated serum proteins.[79]

MILK THISTLE

Indigenous to Europe, milk thistle (*Silybum marianum*) receives it name from the milky sap that leaks from its leaves when they are broken open.[95] Because of its purported hepatoprotective effect, *S. marianum* has traditionally been used in cases of mushroom poisoning and in patients with chronic liver disease, including alcoholic cirrhosis and viral hepatitis. Milk thistle contains a component called *silymarin*, which is found in the fruit, seeds, and leaves of the plant. Silymarin is made up of several active constituents, including silybin, silychristine, and silydianin.[28] A typical product purchased over the counter is standardized to a milk thistle seed extract containing 70% to 80% silymarin.

A randomized open controlled, 12-month human clinical trial of 60 diabetic patients with alcoholic cirrhosis found that silymarin improved glycemic control, resulting in decreased exogenous insulin requirements.[104] Thirty patients received silymarin (600 mg/day) in addition to their standard insulin regimen, whereas 30 patients in the control group received their standard insulin therapy alone. A stable insulin regimen for at least 2 years, negative hepatitis serology, history of DM for at least 5 years treated only with insulin, and biopsy-proven liver cirrhosis were some of the major inclusion criteria. At the study's conclusion, FBG, mean daily BG, and Hb A$_{1c}$ levels and mean daily insulin requirements were significantly lower ($p < .01$) in the silymarin-treated group compared with the control group. Also, no increases in hypoglycemic episodes were observed in the silymarin-treated group.

MOMORDICA CHARANTIA

Also known by such names as "bitter melon" or "karolla," *Momordica charantia* is grown in South America, India, and other parts of Asia, where it is used medicinally as a hypoglycemic agent. The fruit and seeds of *M. charantia* contain several active components, including charantin, momordicin, and an insulin-like polypeptide called *polypeptide-p* or p-insulin, believed to account for its beneficial glycemic effect.[53] Bitter melon is ingested in both capsule and tincture form.

Few controlled trials with *M. charantia* have been performed. One study involving 19 diabetic patients (11 type 1, 8 type 2) evaluated the hypoglycemic effect of polypeptide-p.[51] Depending on the BG range, 10 to 30 units of polypeptide-p were given subcutaneously to 11 subjects (5 type 1, 6 type 2) with eight patients (6 type 1, 2 type 2) in the control group. BG values were drawn periodically up to 12 hours after injection. Of the type 1 diabetic patients injected with polypeptide-p, significant decreases in mean BG values were observed beginning at $1^1/_2$ hours and lasting up to 12 hours when compared to their fasting values. Significant decreases in mean BG values were also noted beginning at 1 hour and lasting up through 12 hours compared with type 1 patients in the control group. Of the type 2 diabetic subjects injected with polypeptide-p, no significant changes in mean BG were noted compared with their fasting values. When compared to the control group, significant decreases in mean BG were observed at 1 hour and 6 hours after injection. Other experimental studies have also found improvement in BG values in type 2 DM patients after ingestion of *M. charantia* (powder and juice form), although these investigations lacked control groups.[4,5]

NOPAL (*OPUNTIA*)

Nopal (*Opuntia* species) is a member of the cactus family and has traditionally been used in the Mexican culture for the treatment of DM. Currently, many questions exist about the appropriate dose, plant part (stem vs. leaf), method of preparation (broiled vs. raw), and species (*Opuntia streptacantha* vs. other species) necessary for glycemic control.[70,90] Most trials in the English language are of very short length and provide little information about randomization or blinding.

Of the studies reviewed, the longest study was 10 days in duration.[29] In this trial, 100 g of broiled nopal leaves (specific species not mentioned) were administered three times a day to 7 patients with type 2 DM and 22 nondiabetic individuals. A significant reduction in FBG was seen in the diabetic ($p < .001$) as well as the nondiabetic ($p < .05$) group. Other studies with type 2 patients have also shown statistically significant decreases in BG levels at 60, 120, and 180 minutes after nopal ingestion compared with control subjects.[30,31]

▨ Homeopathy

Currently, evidence is insufficient to support that homeopathic remedies are efficacious in DM, and the research data supporting use in diabetes are sparse.

One meta-analysis of 107 controlled trials in humans evaluating the efficacy of homeopathy was performed.[55] Using a point scale, the methodologic quality of every study was assessed using criteria such as patient number, randomization, double-blindness, adequately described patient characteristics, and well-described interventions and measurement of effect. One trial in this review involved patients with diabetes. Although a positive result was reported, details of the results were not presented because it was not considered one of the best trials with respect to the methodologic criteria. Another review of 40 randomized trials on the value of homeopathy revealed no studies in diabetic patients.[44] One later study in Russian did report that homeopathic treatments used in 68 patients resulted in statistically significant reductions in hyperglycemia and glucosuria, although a control group was not mentioned.[63]

◼ Mind-Body Therapies

EMOTIONAL AND SPIRITUAL FACTORS

The basic tenet underlying the mind-body therapies is that cognitive, emotional, and spiritual factors affect physiology in health and disease. As used by diabetic patients, mind-body interventions may include supportive counseling, specific treatments targeting BG and glycohemoglobin, and therapies to complement medical management of complications (Table 6-2).

Psychologic care of patients with type 1 or type 2 DM is suggested as an integral part of the lifetime management of the disease. Different types of mental and emotional support are appropriate (1) at diagnosis, (2) for management of day-to-day challenges, and (3) for complications. Adjustment problems often accompany the

TABLE 6–2. **EFFECTS OF MIND-BODY THERAPIES ON BLOOD GLUCOSE (BG) IN DIABETIC PATIENTS**

Intervention	Study	Patients	Documented Effect
Yoga	Controlled; plus diet[50]	140 type 2	Improved glucose tolerance Decreased drug dosage
	Case series[85]	4 type 1 31 type 2	Decreased FBG and postprandial BG
Coping skills training (CST)	Controlled; plus intensive therapy[39,40]	65 type 1 77 type 1	Decreased Hb A$_{1c}$
Cognitive-behavioral training	Controlled[42]	15 type 1	None
Biofeedback/relaxation	Controlled[99]	12 type 2	Improved glucose tolerance
	Case series[25]	20 type 1	None
	Controlled[59]	38 type 2	None
	Controlled[102]	108 type 2	Decreased Hb A$_{1c}$
	Controlled[67,68]	18 type 1 16 type 1	Decreased BG and FBG
	Controlled[69]	19 type 1	None
Hypnosis	Case series[80]	7 type 1	Decreased Hb A$_{1c}$ and FBG

FBG, Fasting blood glucose; Hb A$_{1c}$, glycohemoglobin.

early months after diagnosis of diabetes. Long-term consistent self-care is often diffi-cult to maintain, and up to 30% of DM patients will develop depressive symptoms.[9] When complications develop, patients need assistance in coping with the loss of some of their abilities. Family members should be considered an important part of the sup-port system throughout the life span of the diabetic patient.[45,49]

Spiritual well-being may affect adjustment to living with a chronic illness such as diabetes. Individuals with a greater sense of spiritual well-being reported less uncer-tainty and psychologic distress and were better adjusted to living with diabetes.[58] In a well-designed study of therapeutic touch and intercessory prayer, a majority of the participants decreased insulin use; however, there were no significant differences between groups. Patients reported a greater sense of calm and peacefulness, both of which are positive psychologic benefits in terms of quality of life.[109]

YOGA

Yoga as practiced for thousands of years in India is considered a way of life. As such, yoga comprises diet, supplements, meditation, physical exercise, and adherence to ethical principles. The practice of yoga in the Western world is usually more limited, consisting only of breathing exercises, static postures, and simple relaxation.[1]

A controlled study tested the effects of 40 days of yoga and a vegetarian diet in 140 hospitalized patients with type 2 DM. Outcome measures were an OGTT and the number of hypoglycemic medications. Results showed that the duration of disease was related to response. Patients with less than 10 years of diabetes showed improve-ments in glucose tolerance and decreased dosage of hypoglycemic agents.[50] The regu-lar practice of yoga decreased FBG and postprandial BG levels, improved insulin kinetics, and enhanced the sense of well-being in both type 1 and type 2 patients.[85] Yoga may be a useful low-risk adjuvant to traditional diabetes therapy.[34]

BIOFEEDBACK

A mind-body therapy often used for stress-related disorders in Western medicine is relaxation combined with biofeedback. *Electromyography* (EMG) and *thermal biofeedback*, recommended therapies for muscle contraction and migraine headaches respectively, are applicable to assist patients in managing their BG level.[89] Patients with diabetes can be treated safely with biofeedback-assisted relaxation as long as daily SMBG is maintained and medication changes are not made without physician consul-tation.[66]

In most stress-related disorders for which biofeedback is recommended, passive or active relaxation therapy is used concomitantly. *Passive relaxation* involves concen-tration on words or phrases designed to produce the state of relaxation, whereas *pro-gressive relaxation* or *active relaxation* consists of sequential tensing and relaxation of specific muscle groups.[21] Often, counseling or psychotherapy, particularly of the cog-nitive-behavioral type, is incorporated into a biofeedback-assisted relaxation proto-col. *Hypnosis* combined with relaxation was explored in a small study of seven type 1 DM patients. Decreased FBG and Hb A$_{1c}$ values were reported.[80]

The basic premise underlying the use of relaxation therapies in diabetes is that *psychologic stress* has an influence on BG levels. The relationship between stressful life events and BG may worsen existing hyperglycemia in diabetic persons or hasten the onset of diabetes. This hypothesis has been explored on a theoretic basis and through laboratory testing of diabetic individuals. A detailed analysis of this concept is beyond the scope of this chapter, but several references are provided for the interested reader.[19,20,36,77,100,101]

Biofeedback and relaxation therapies have been tested in controlled studies in type 1 and type 2 DM with varying results. In these studies, patients' medical management regimens were maintained. An early study compared the effects of progressive relaxation and EMG biofeedback in six type 2 patients to usual care in another six patients.[99] Glucose tolerance, but not insulin sensitivity, improved. In a study of patients with poorly controlled type 1 DM, 10 patients received EMG biofeedback and progressive relaxation, whereas 10 others received no additional treatment.[25] Treatment was provided in a hospital setting, followed by home practice of relaxation. Neither Hb A_{1c} level nor total insulin dose changed in either group. However, a recent large, well-controlled study of stress management in type 2 DM showed positive results in glycohemoglobin values. Surwit et al.[102] provided five sessions of diabetes education with or without stress management. The latter consisted of active relaxation, cognitive-behavioral skill building, guided imagery, and education on the effects of psychologic stress. Compared with diabetes education alone, the stress management group achieved small but significant decreases in the biologic indicator glycohemoglobin.

In another study carried out in Greece, statistically significant decreases in BG and Hb A_{1c} were reported in a relaxation group compared with an untreated control group. Both type 1 and type 2 patients participated in this study.[75] Thirty-eight patients with type 2 DM were given treatment with intensive diabetes therapy. Half the patients also received EMG biofeedback-assisted relaxation. Significant improvements in glycohemoglobin levels were observed in both groups, but no additional benefit came with the biofeedback-assisted relaxation. The patients who did benefit from the relaxation treatment were those with higher "trait anxiety" whose BG levels appeared to be stress sensitive.[59] Another study of type 2 DM patients also reported no advantage for the patients given treatment with EMG biofeedback and progressive relaxation.[47]

A preliminary short-term study of six type 2 diabetic patients in our laboratory has shown some improvement in BG with 10 sessions of EMG, thermal biofeedback, and passive relaxation. A problem-solving approach has been incorporated into the biofeedback sessions. The use of the feedback to gain control of facial muscle tension is used as a demonstration of the possibility of better control of the physiologic response to stress and in turn hyperglycemia (unpublished results).

Cognitive restructuring and problem solving were presented to eight adolescents with poorly controlled type 1 DM in a group format. Glycohemoglogin values in the treatment group were compared with those in the usual care control group. Analysis showed improvements on measures of anxiety and coping but no parallel decreases in glycohemoglobin.[42] Coping skills training was tested in two groups of patients with type 1 DM. Skill building was added to intensive therapy and compared with intensive therapy alone. The former group showed significant decreases in Hb A$_{1c}$ values.[39,40]

McGrady and colleagues tested the effects of a biofeedback and passive relaxation protocol in a total of 34 patients (17 experimental, 17 control) with type 1 DM in three separate studies.[67-69] Both EMG and thermal feedback were used, with passive relaxation and home practice of relaxation. Patients continued under the care of their own physician, and no changes in insulin dosage were done without physician permission. Patients monitored BG daily and met with a nurse weekly to discuss BG and insulin data. Average BG value, percentage of BG values greater than 200 mg/dl, and percentage of FBG values greater than 120 mg/dl were all significantly reduced in the treated groups compared with control subjects. Results were documented for average BG value and percentage of FBG values greater than 120 mg/dl in the first study.[67] Furthermore, in the second study, glycohemoglobin values were correlated with self-reported BG values at pretest, suggesting that the self-reported values were accurate.[68]

The third study from our laboratory investigated the impact of patients' *moods* on their responses to biofeedback-assisted relaxation therapy.[69] The protocol was similar to earlier studies, except that the baseline was extended to 6 weeks to allow for additional education about diabetes, with follow-up extended to 3 months to explore changes in glycohemoglobin values. In contrast to our two earlier reports, we found no significant differences between the experimental and control groups in average BG value or any other related variable, although five of nine individuals did show decreases in BG and glycohemoglobin versus one of eight control subjects. Analysis of the mood data was of interest in that the successful patients reported lower levels of depression, anxiety, and daily conflicts at baseline. The patients who failed treatment were more depressed and anxious and took longer to complete the protocol. Statistically significant correlations were found between the indicators of mood, particularly depression and anxiety, and BG values.

The relatively high incidence of *depression* in diabetic patients has been consistently documented.[9,32] Depressed diabetic patients are at greater risk of hyperglycemia because, enveloped in a negative mood and sense of failure, they may fail to use SMBG or to administer hypoglycemic agents appropriately. In the context of mind-body interventions, depressed patients may not practice relaxation as recommended or, when doing so, may lack sufficient concentration to realize its full benefit. Recently the serotonin reuptake inhibitors (SSRIs) have been shown to have BG-lowering effects in depressed diabetic patients.[38]

Other applications of biofeedback may exist in ameliorating symptoms of complications of diabetes. For example, thermal biofeedback helped 40 diabetic patients to voluntarily increase the temperature of their hands and feet, thereby improving circulation.[81] The higher temperatures in the feet were associated with decreased pain and faster healing of ulcers; the response was limited by degree of neuropathy.[82] An additional case study reported decreased symptoms of intermittent claudication in one patient provided with thermal biofeedback training.[88]

FUTURE STUDIES

The mind-body therapies hold promise for incorporation into diabetes management. Although some studies show no effects on BG indicators, other large studies have reported significant therapeutic effects. It appears, however, that relaxation or psychotherapy alone does not confer added benefit, but that multimodal programs, one component of which is skill building, have the potential to help patients lower BG and Hb A_{1c} values. Risk associated with these therapies is very low, as long as patients continue SMBG, consult with their physicians, and take their medication as prescribed. In addition, even in the studies with no effects on BG, patients expressed satisfaction with what they learned and reported improved quality of life.

Two areas require further study: predicting who will respond to mind-body therapies and the consistency of short-term benefits. Data on long-term maintenance of improved BG in those patients who have undergone mind-body therapy are limited but extremely important. A key question is, how much continued practice is necessary once active treatment is complete? Regarding prediction of short-term success or failure, important factors are patient mood and adherence to treatment recommendations. In particular, depressive symptoms and mood disorder may prevent acquisition of the relaxation response[69] and may predict poorer self-care.[18,32,38]

CAM Therapies: Patient Usage and Physician's Role

"Diabetes is a nearly pure example of behavioral medicine; it is an outcome of the interplay among the underlying disease process, the environment and the behavior and psychological state of the affected individual."[78] Many of the CAM therapies discussed here also require personal effort and commitment over the patient's lifetime.

Ryan, Pick, and Marceau[83] recently reported that approximately one third of surveyed diabetic patients were taking alternative medicines. Most diabetic patients seem to use alternative medications in combination with their standard regimen rather than in place of traditional treatment. Also, 61% of diabetic patients using alternative medications thought that the therapies were of significant benefit. No difference in use was found between type 1 and type 2 diabetic patients.

Information about patients' use of CAM therapies is critical to determining the potential impact of the CAM therapy on BG level and the interaction between the CAM therapy and the patient's prescribed regimen. The therapeutic physician-patient relationship is enhanced by careful questioning of patients about their self-care practices and usage of CAM therapies and by a review of safety and efficacy issues.[24] There is cause for concern if proper monitoring is not performed and physicians are not informed of the patient's actions.[33] Because a patient's decision to miss insulin shots or eliminate oral medicine will have rapid, life-threatening consequences, open communication is crucial.

Present and future physicians providing treatment for patients with diabetes must be informed about some forms of CAM. First, a source of basic information about diabetes should be recommended to newly diagnosed patients (see Suggested Readings). Second, the crucial role of the patient's behavior and the physician-patient partnership must be emphasized to patients. Third, the diabetologist should be updated about the mind-body therapies, phytomedicine, diet programs, and some areas of traditional Chinese medicine as adjunctive therapies to control BG. Fourth, alternative methods of pain control for management of diabetic complications should be used. Fifth, the patient's culture, available social support, and quality of life must be considered in making treatment decisions.

SUMMARY

Diabetes mellitus is a chronic disorder of metabolism that is characterized by hyperglycemia and can progress to serious complications over the person's life span. The two predominant types of DM are type 1 and type 2. Treatment is directed at decreasing elevated blood glucose levels by means of oral hypoglycemic agents or by injected insulin. Outcome of therapy is determined by BG values and biologic assay. Self-care on the part of the patient is critical to day-to-day management. Social support, mood, and locus of control affect adherence to prescribed therapy, and depression especially seems to have a impact. The most common types of CAM applicable to patients with DM are mind-body, herbal, and diet therapies.

Although scientific literature on many CAM therapies is difficult to obtain, this chapter provides support for relaxation, biofeedback, yoga, and structured diet. Present evidence does not support the use of acupuncture or homeopathy in the treatment of diabetes. Several phytotherapies have promise, but it is too early to recommend them in the comprehensive treatment plan of diabetic patients until larger, more rigorous clinical trials have been done. Questions regarding appropriate preparation and dosing remain.

REFERENCES

1. Achterberg J et al: Mind-body intervention. In *Alternative medicine: expanding medical horizons*, Washington, DC, 1992, US Government Printing Office.
2. Agency for Healthcare Research and Quality: *Ayurvedic interventions for diabetes mellitus: a systematic review*, Summary, Evidence Report/Technology Assessment No 41, AHRQ Pub Nos 01-039, Rockville, Md, 2001, The Agency.
3. Agrawal P, Rai V, Singh RB: Randomized placebo-controlled, single blind trial of holy basil leaves in patients with noninsulin-dependent diabetes mellitus, *Int J Clin Pharmacol Ther* 34(9):406, 1996.
4. Ahmad N et al: Effect of *Momordica charantia* (Karolla) extracts on fasting and postprandial serum glucose levels in NIDDM patients, *Bangladesh Med Res Counc Bull* 25(1):11, 1999.
5. Akhtar MS: Trial of *Momordica charantia* linn (Karela) powder in patients with maturity-onset diabetes, *J Pak Med Assoc* 8:106, 1982.
6. American Diabetes Association: Unproven therapies, *Diabetes Care* 20(1):S60, 1997.
7. American Diabetes Association: Standards of medical care for patients with diabetes mellitus, *Diabetes Care* 24(suppl 1):33, 2001.
8. Anderson RA: Chromium, glucose tolerance and diabetes, *Biol Trace Elem Res* 32:19, 1992.

9. Anderson RJ et al: The prevalence of comorbid depression in adults with diabetes, *Diabetes Care* 24:1069, 2001.

10. Barnard RJ et al: Response of noninsulin-dependent diabetic patients to an intensive program of diet and exercise, *Diabetes Care* 5:370, 1982.

11. Barnard RJ et al: The role of diet and exercise in the management of hyperinsulinemia and associated atherosclerosis risk factors, *Am J Cardiol* 69:330, 1992.

12. Baskaran K et al: Antidiabetic effect of a leaf extract from *Gymnema sylvestre* in non–insulin-dependent diabetes mellitus patients, *J Ethnopharmacol* 30:295, 1990.

13. Bernstein RK: *Dr. Bernstein's diabetes solution*, Boston, 1997, Little, Brown.

14. Bordia A, Verma SK, Srivastava KC: Effect of ginger (*Zingiber officinale* Rosc.) and fenugreek (*Trigonella foenum graecum* L.) on blood lipids, blood sugar and platelet aggregation in patients with coronary artery disease, *Prostaglandins Leukot Essent Fatty Acids* 56(5):379, 1997.

15. Boucher JI, Shafer KJ, Chaffin JA: Weight loss, diets and supplements: does anything work? *Diabetes Spectrum* 14(3):169, 2001.

16. Burroughs TE et al: Research on social support in adolescents with IDDM, *Diabetes Educator* 23(4):438, 1997.

17. Burton Group: *Alternative medicine*, Fife, Wash, 1993, Future Medicine.

18. Connell CM et al: Impact of social support, social cognitive variables and perceived threat on depression among adults with diabetes, *Health Psychol* 13(3):263, 1994.

19. Cox DJ, Gonder-Frederick LA: The role of stress in diabetes mellitus. In McCabe PM et al, editors: *Stress, coping, and disease*, Hillsdale, NJ, 1991, Lawrence Erlbaum Association.

20. Cox DJ, Gonder-Frederick LA: Major developments in behavioral diabetes research, *J Consult Clin Psychol* 60(4):628, 1992.

21. Davis M, Eshelman ER, McKay M: *The relaxation and stress reduction workbook*, ed 4, Oakland, Calif, 1995, New Harbinger.

22. Decheng C, Dianqin G, Yao Z: Clinical and experimental studies in treating diabetes mellitus by acupuncture, *J Tradit Chin Med* 14(3):163, 1994.

23. Diabetes Control and Complications Trial Research Group: The effect of intensive treatment of diabetes on the development and progression of long-term complications in insulin-dependent diabetes mellitus, *N Engl J Med* 329(14):977, 1993.

24. Eisenberg DM: Advising patients who seek alternative medical therapies, *Ann Intern Med* 127:61, 1997.

25. Feinglos MN, Hastedt P, Surwit RS: Effects of relaxation therapy on patients with type I diabetes mellitus, *Diabetes Care* 10(1):72, 1987.

26. Finney LS, Gonzalez-Campoy JM: Dietary chromium and diabetes: is there a relationship? *Clin Diabetes* 15(1):6, 1997.

27. Fitzgerald JT et al: Differences in the impact of dietary restrictions on African Americans and Caucasians with NIDDM, *Diabetes Educator* 23(1):41, 1997.

28. Flora K et al: Milk thistle (*Silybum marianum*) for the therapy of liver disease, *Am J Gastroenterol* 93(2):139, 1999.

29. Frati-Munari AC et al: Effects of nopal (*Opuntia* sp.) on serum lipids, glycemia and body weight, *Arch Invest Med Mex* 14:117, 1983.

30. Frati-Munari AC et al: Hypoglycemic effect of *Opuntia streptacantha lemaire* in NIDDM, *Diabetes Care* 11(1):63, 1988.

31. Frati AC et al: Influence of nopal intake upon fasting glycemia in type II diabetics and healthy subjects, *Arch Invest Med* 22:51, 1991.

32. Gavard JA, Lustman PJ, Clouse RE: Prevalence of depression in adults with diabetes, *Diabetes Care* 16:1167, 1993.

33. Gill GV et al: Diabetes and alternative medicine: cause for concern, *Diabet Med* 11(2):210, 1994.

34. Gimbel MA: Yoga, meditation, and imagery: clinical applications, *Nurse Pract Forum* 9(4):243, 1998.

35. Glasgow RE et al: Behavioral science in diabetes, *Diabetes Care* 22(5):832, 1999.

36. Goetsch V: Stress and blood glucose in diabetes mellitus: a review and methodological commentary, *Ann Behav Med* 11(3):102, 1989.

37. Goodall T, Halford NK: Self-management of diabetes mellitus: a critical review, *Health Psychol* 10(1):1, 1991.

38. Goodnick PJ, Henry JH, Buki VM: Treatment of depression in patients with diabetes mellitus, *J Clin Psychiatry* 56(4):128, 1995.

39. Grey M et al: Short-term effects of coping skills training as adjunct to intensive therapy in adolescents, *Diabetes Care* 21(6):902, 1998.

40. Grey M et al: Coping skills training for youths with diabetes on intensive therapy, *Appl Nurs Res* 12(1):3, 1999.

41. *Gymnema, http://www.naturalDatabase.com*, 2002 (monograph).

42. Hains AA et al: A stress management intervention for adolescents with type 1 diabetes, *Diabetes Educator* 26(3):417, 2000.

43. Hawthorne K, Mello M, Tomlinson S: Cultural and religious influences in diabetes care in Great Britain, *Diabet Med* 10(1):8, 1993.

44. Hill C, Doyon F: Review of randomized trials of homeopathy, *Epidemiol Sante Publ* 38:139, 1990.

45. Holmes DM: The person and diabetes in psychosocial context, *Diabetes Care* 9(2):194, 1986.

46. Hui H: A review of treatment of diabetes by acupuncture during the past forty years, *J Tradit Chin Med* 15(2):145, 1995.

47. Jablon SL et al: Effects of relaxation training on glucose tolerance and diabetic control in type II diabetes, *Appl Psychophysiol Biofeedback* 22(3):155, 1997.

48. Jacobs J et al: Herbal medicine. In *Alternative medicine: expanding medical horizons*, Washington, DC, 1992, US Government Printing Office.

49. Jacobson AM: The psychological care of patients with insulin-dependent diabetes mellitus, *N Engl J Med* 334(19):1249, 1996.

50. Jain SC et al: A study of response pattern of non–insulin dependent diabetics to yoga therapy, *Diabetes Res Clin Pract* 19(1):69, 1993.

51. Jianfei C, Jia W: Changes of plasma insulin level in diabetics treated with acupuncture, *J Tradit Chin Med* 5(2):79, 1985.

52. Khan AKA, Akhtar S, Mahtab H: *Coccinia indica* in the treatment of patients with diabetes mellitus, *BMRC Bull* V(2):60, 1979.

53. Khanna P, Jain SC: Hypoglycemic activity of polypeptide-p from a plant source, *J Nat Prod* 44(6):648, 1981.

54. Khare AK, Tondon RN, Tewari JP: Hypoglycaemic activity of an indigenous drug (*Gymnema sylvestre*, "Gurmar") in normal and diabetic persons, *Indian J Physiol Pharmacol* 27:257, 1983.

55. Kleijnen J, Knipschild P, Riet GT: Clinical trials of homoeopathy, *BMJ* 302:316, 1991.

56. Kohlmann CW et al: Associations between type of treatment and illness-specific locus of control in type 1 diabetes patients, *Psychol Health* 8(5):383, 1993.

57. Krall LP, Beaser RS: *Joslin diabetes manual*, ed 12, Philadelphia, 1989, Lea & Febiger.

58. Landis BJ: Uncertainty, spiritual well-being and psychosocial adjustment to chronic illness, *Issues Ment Health Nurs* 17(3):217, 1996.

59. Lane JD et al: Relaxation training for NIDDM: predicting who may benefit, *Diabetes Care* 16(8):1087, 1993.

60. Lebovitz HE, editor: *Therapy for diabetes mellitus and related disorders*, ed 3, Alexandria, Va, 1998, American Diabetes Association.

61. Lu R: Treatment of diabetes in the elderly: an analysis of 885 cases, *J Tradit Chin Med* 13(2):83, 1993.

62. Maciocia G: *The practice of Chinese medicine*, Edinburgh, 1994, Churchill Livingstone.

63. Mamchenko GF, Kolesova GP: The use of homeopathy in treating diabetics, *Lik Sprava* (Index for Medline) 11-22:74-76, 1992.

64. Margolis S, Saudek CD: Diabetes mellitus. In *The Johns Hopkins white papers*, Baltimore, 1997, Johns Hopkins University.

65. McGee CT, Sancier K, Chow EPY: Qigong in traditional Chinese medicine. In Micozzi MS, editor: *Fundamentals of complementary and alternative medicine*, New York, 1996, Churchill Livingstone.

66. McGrady A, Bailey B: Biofeedback-assisted relaxation and diabetes mellitus. In Schwartz MS: *Biofeedback: a practitioner's guide*, ed 2, New York, 1995, Guilford.

67. McGrady A, Bailey B, Good M: A controlled study of biofeedback-assisted relaxation in type I diabetes, *Diabetes Care* 14(5):360, 1991.

68. McGrady A, Graham G, Bailey B: Biofeedback-assisted relaxation in insulin dependent diabetes: a replication and extension study, *Ann Behav Med* 18(3):185, 1996.

69. McGrady A, Horner J: Role of mood in outcome of biofeedback assisted relaxation therapy in insulin dependent diabetes mellitus, *Appl Psychophysiol Biofeedback* 24(1):79, 1999.

70. Medical implications of prickly pear cactus, *http://www.tamuk.edu*, 2001.

71. National Institutes of Health: Acupuncture. Consensus statement, 15(5):1, 1997.

72. O'Connell BS: Select vitamins and minerals in the management of diabetes, *Diabetes Spectrum* 14(3):133, 2001.

73. Ornish DM: *Dr. Dean Ornish's program for reversing heart disease*, New York, 1990, Random House.

74. Ornish DM et al: Can lifestyle changes reverse coronary heart disease? *Lancet* 336:129, 1990.

75. Paschali A, Karamanos B, Griggiths I: Effect of relaxation therapy on the control of diabetes mellitus. In Christodoulou GN: *Psychosomatic medicine: past and future*, New York, 1987, Plenum.

76. Persaud SJ et al: *Gymnema sylvestre* stimulates insulin release in vitro by increased membrane permeability, *J Endocrinol* 163:207, 1999.

77. Peyrot M, McMurray JF Jr, Kruger DF: A biopsychosocial model of glycemic control in diabetes: stress, coping and regimen adherence, *J Health Soc Behav* 40(2):141, 1999.

78. Pohl SL, Gonder-Frederick LC, Daniel J: Diabetes mellitus: an overview, *Behav Med Update* 6(1):3, 1984.

79. Rai V, Mani UV, Iyer UM: Effect of *Ocimum sanctum* leaf powder on blood lipoproteins, glycated proteins and total amino acids in patients with non-insulin-dependent diabetes mellitus, *J Nutr Environ Med* 7:113, 1997.

80. Ratner H et al: A hypnotherapeutic approach to the improvement of compliance in adolescent diabetes, *Am J Clin Hypn* 32(3):154, 1990.

81. Rice BI, Schindler JV: Effects of thermal biofeedback-assisted relaxation training on blood circulation in the lower extremities of a population with diabetes, *Diabetes Care* 15(7):853, 1992.

82. Rice BI et al: Effect of biofeedback-assisted relaxation training on foot ulcer healing, *J Am Podiatr Med Assoc* 91(3):132, 2001.

83. Ryan EA, Pick ME, Marceau C: Use of alternative medicines in diabetes mellitus, *Diabet Med* 18:242, 2000.

84. Sadhukhan B et al: Clinical evaluation of a herbal antidiabetic product, *J Indian Med Assoc* 92(4):115, 1994.

85. Sahay BK: Yoga and diabetes, *J Assoc Physicians India* 34(9):645, 1986.

86. Salloway JC: Medical sociology. In Sierles F, editor: *Behavioral science*, Baltimore, 1993, Williams & Wilkins.

87. Sanders D, Kennedy N, McKendrick MW: Monitoring the safety of herbal remedies: herbal remedies have a heterogeneous nature, *BMJ* 311(7019):1569, 1995.

88. Saunders JT et al: Thermal biofeedback in the treatment of intermittent claudication in diabetes: a case study, *Biofeedback Self-Regul* 19(4):337, 1994.

89. Schwartz MS: *Biofeedback: a practitioner's guide*, ed 2, New York, 1995, Guilford.

90. Shane-McWhorter L: Biological complementary therapies: a focus on botanical products in diabetes, *Diabetes Spectrum* 14(4):199, 2001.

91. Shanmugasundaram ERB et al: Use of *Gymnema sylvestre* leaf extract in the control of blood glucose in insulin-dependent diabetes mellitus, *J Ethnopharmacol* 30:281, 1990.

92. Sharma RD, Raghuram TC, Sudhakar RN: Effect of fenugreek seeds on blood glucose and serum lipids in type I diabetes, *Eur J Clin Nutr* 44:301, 1990.

93. Sharma RD et al: Use of fenugreek seed powder in the management of non-insulin dependent diabetes mellitus, *Nutr Res* 16(8):1331, 1996.

94. Shimizu K et al: Suppression of glucose absorption by some fraction extracted from *Gymnema sylvestre* leaves, *J Vet Med Sci* 59(4):245, 1997.

95. *Silybum marianum* (milk thistle), *http://www.thorne.com*, 2001 (monograph).

96. Sitprija S et al: Garlic and diabetes mellitus Phase II clinical trial, *J Med Assoc Thailand* 70(2):223, 1987.

97. Sotaniemi EA, Haapakoski E, Rautio A: Ginseng therapy in non-insulin dependent diabetic patients, *Diabetes Care* 18(10):1373, 1995.

98. Stratton IM et al: Association of glycemia with macrovascular and microvascular complications of type 2 diabetes (UKPDS 35): prospective observational study, *BMJ* 321:405, 2000.

99. Surwit RS, Feinglos MN: The effects of relaxation on glucose tolerance in noninsulin dependent diabetes, *Diabetes Care* 6(2):176, 1983.

100. Surwit RS, Schneider MS: Role of stress in the etiology and treatment of diabetes mellitus, *Psychosom Med* 55(4):380, 1993.

101. Surwit RS, Schneider MS, Feinglos MN: Stress and diabetes mellitus, *Diabetes Care* 15(10):1413, 1992.

102. Surwit RS et al: Stress management improves long-term glycemic control in type 2 diabetes, *Diabetes Care* 25(1):30, 2002.

103. Torjesen PA et al: Lifestyle changes may reverse development of the insulin resistance syndrome, *Diabetes Care* 20(1):26, 1997.

104. Velussi M et al: Long-term (12 months) treatment with an anti-oxidant drug (silymarin) is effective on hyperinsulinemia, exogenous insulin need and malondialdehyde levels in cirrhotic diabetic patients, *J Hepatol* 26:871, 1997.

105. Vuksan V et al: American ginseng (*Panax quinquefolius* L) reduces postprandial glycemia in nondiabetic subjects and subjects with type 2 diabetes mellitus, *Arch Intern Med* 160:1009, 2000.

106. White JR, Campbell RK: Magnesium and diabetes: a review, *Ann Pharmacother* 27:775, 1993.

107. Wilkerson G: The influence of psychiatric, psychological and social factors on the control of insulin-dependent diabetes mellitus, *J Psychosom Res* 31(3):277, 1987.

108. Wing RR: Very low calorie diets in the treatment of type II diabetes: psychological and physiological effects. In Wadden TA, Vanitallie TB, editors: *Treatment of the seriously obese patient,* New York, 1992, Guilford.

109. Wirth DP, Mitchell BJ: Complementary healing therapy for patients with type I diabetes mellitus, *J Sci Explor* 8(3):367, 1994.

110. Zaldivar A, Smolowitz J: Perceptions of the importance placed on religion and folk medicine by non–Mexican American Hispanic adults with diabetes, *Diabetes Educator* 20(4):303, 1994.

111. Zimmet PZ, McCarty DJ, deCourten MP: The global epidemiology of non-insulin-dependent diabetes mellitus and the metabolic syndrome, *J Diabetes Complications* 11:60, 1997.

SUGGESTED READINGS

American Diabetes Association: *Complete guide to diabetes,* ed 2, 2000, Bantam Books.

Beaser RS: *The Joslin guide to diabetes,* New York, 1995, Simon & Schuster.

Guthrie DW, Guthrie RA: *The diabetes sourcebook,* ed 5, 2002, NTC Publishing Group.

CHAPTER 7

Neurologic Disorders

SAMUEL C. SHIFLETT and ANN C. COTTER

$\mathbf{D}$isorders of the central nervous system (CNS) affect the lives of hundreds of thousands of individuals each year, resulting in impairments in areas such as memory, attention, movement, sensation, mood, personality, and physiologic regulation. Neurologic disorders may become evident as acute, nonprogressive events or may follow a progressive, insidious course, inflicting an uncertain future on the lives of patients and families. Although modern medicine has made great strides in the management of acute trauma to the CNS, its success with the chronic aftermath may be less impressive. Consequently, increasing numbers of individuals survive neurologic disorders only to find themselves with enduring and at times profoundly debilitating impairments. For this reason, patients with neurologic disorders increasingly look to complementary and alternative medicine (CAM) in the hope of finding relief for their conditions.

Many CAM therapies have been used to treat CNS disorders, but the research validating their effectiveness is often limited or nonexistent. The purpose of this chapter is to identify CAM techniques that are typically used or suggested in treating neurologic sequelae and to summarize the adequacy of the research evidence for their effectiveness. After a brief description of some of the most common CAM therapies used, etiology and sequelae of particular neurologic disorders are described, along with evidence for the effectiveness of CAM treatments. Six specific neurologic disorders are discussed: stroke, brain injury, spinal cord injury (SCI), multiple sclerosis, Parkinson's disease, and epilepsy.

N Categories of CAM Therapies

Literally hundreds of CAM therapies are currently used in the treatment of "abnormal" conditions of the physical body. In an effort to narrow and focus the field, the treatments of relevance to CNS disorders have been generally categorized according to their mechanism of application in medical conditions, as ascertained by current research evidence (Table 7-1). A few therapies represent "alternative" uses of techniques or medications already used in conventional medicine. These therapies may not adhere to conventional concepts of alternative medicine but are important to mention.

Text continued on p. 200.

TABLE 7–1. **COMPLEMENTARY AND ALTERNATIVE MEDICINE (CAM) FOR NEUROLOGIC DISORDERS**

CAM Therapy	Research Studies	Neurologic Condition(s)
ALTERNATIVE SYSTEMS OF MEDICAL PRACTICE		
Homeopathy	Two meta-analyses across diagnoses with encouraging findings[90,102] Two controlled studies for stroke[32,161] Preliminary study for TBI[218]	Some use for stroke and TBI
Ayurvedic medicine	Uncontrolled study of hemiplegia showed decreased cholesterol levels and improved motor functioning[188]	Designed to treat wide spectrum of physical and psychologic disorders
NONCONVENTIONAL BODYWORK		
Acupressure (shiatsu)	Uncontrolled study on use as adjunct to stroke rehabilitation showed improvement[69] Clinical observation in clinical birth injury showed improvement in 89% of children treated[208]	Some application in stroke and TBI
Acupuncture*	Extensive literature on variable quality; less than 20 well-controlled studies, many showing positive effects; controversy over interpretation of results in some recent studies	Most research on stroke
Alexander technique	Uncontrolled pilot study for Parkinson's disease showed improvement in motor functioning, daily activities, and depression[171]	Primarily used for postural difficulties and back/neck pain
Chiropractic*	Controlled study of "whiplash"[52] Case study on SCI with recovery of function[217] Uncontrolled study of posttraumatic brain injury headache[81]	Limited application; used most often for musculoskeletal problems
Craniosacral therapy*	Case reports of efficacy in cerebral palsy and Erb's palsy[210] Anecdotal reports of good effects in TBI and SCI	Used for pain conditions and functional problems; potential applicability in CNS trauma
Massage therapy*	Two controlled studies on SCI with encouraging findings[55,196] Case series showed improvement in pressure ulcers[26]	Applicability as adjunctive treatment; often used for musculoskeletal or stress-related conditions
Reflexology	Case series on stroke patients[222] Three case reports on SCI[93]	Stroke, brain injury, SCI, childhood developmental disorders
Feldenkrais method	Mostly anecdotal information Reduced stress and mood symptoms but not somatic symptoms in MS[83a]	Applied to cerebral palsy, MS, arthritis
Pilates method	Anecdotal information only	SCI, MS, arthritis

Trager psychophysical integration	Case reports on MS note improved strength, flexibility, balance, and energy	Parkinson's disease, MS; most often used for painful musculoskeletal conditions
Therapeutic horseback riding (hippotherapy)	Reduces shoulder pain associated with wheelchair overuse in SCI[48]	Used to improve physical and emotional functioning of children and adults with disabilities†
	Case series of para/tetraplegia found decreased spasticity, easier catheterization, and improved bowel function, mood balance, and sleep[50]	

MIND-BODY INTERVENTIONS

Hypnosis*	Case reports on stroke, SCI, and TBI note improvement in physical and emotional functioning[38,70,101,104,175]	Applied as adjunct; often used for pain reduction and behavior modification
Meditation*	Studies report relevance in stroke reduction[13,36,62,161,203]	Used for stress management, health promotion, and hypertension reduction, with possible application to stroke prevention
	Anecdotal report of physical improvement after stroke[221]	
	Study on relaxation in SCI, equivalent to control group[204]	
Music therapy	Three controlled trials[40,98,185]	Used after stroke and brain injury to encourage verbal and nonverbal communication, improve muscle coordination, and minimize stress and anxiety
	Seven pre/posttherapy studies with objective measures; many anecdotal and case reports	
	As adjunct in neurologic rehabilitation, findings are encouraging for improved motor, speech, and emotional functioning	
T'ai chi*	Two controlled studies showed improved cardiorespiratory function, psychological function, strength, and balance and reduced falls in healthy elderly patients[215,216]	Applicability to neurologic disorders; used to improve strength, balance, coordination, and concentration
Yoga*	Minimal controlled research	Used for stress and health promotion, with possible neurologic application
	Reports of symptom improvement in MS[45]	

ENERGY HEALING TECHNIQUES

Qi Gong*	Animal studies in China report positive findings[205]	Substantial use in China for paralysis
	Small U.S. study showed no effect in hemiplegia[23]	
Reiki	Anecdotal information	Adjunct healing technique with range of diagnoses
	Controlled stroke study showed no effect[167]	
Therapeutic touch	No controlled neurologic studies	Simple adjunct in rehabilitation; taught at more than 30 U.S. nursing schools
	Controlled studies on wound healing with mixed results;[213] may be applicable to pressure ulcers in SCI	

Continued

TABLE 7–1. **COMPLEMENTARY AND ALTERNATIVE MEDICINE (CAM) FOR NEUROLOGIC DISORDERS—cont'd**

CAM Therapy	Research Studies	Neurologic Condition(s)
PHYTOTHERAPIES		
Ginkgo biloba*	More than 20 controlled human trials, more than 20 animal/in vitro studies; results encouraging for cognitive deficits common in stroke and TBI	Used for 25-35 years in Europe for impaired memory/attention and other disorders‡
Hydergine (ergot preparation)	Three controlled studies on stroke with mixed results[6,17,157]	FDA-approved for age-related cognitive decline; possible applicability to stroke prevention
Asian herbs	Large body of mostly Chinese literature; few controlled studies with individual herbs	Used for many disorders Practitioners prescribe different herb combinations based on symptoms and TCM
PHARMACOLOGIC AND BIOLOGIC THERAPIES		
Bee venom	Case reports of MS symptom relief Studies in MS treatment under way	Arthritis, MS
Dimethyl amino ethanol (DMAE)	Pilot study showed elimination of Parkinson's disease–related dyskinesia in 8 of 11 patients[114] Pilot study on Huntington's chorea showed improvement in 5 of 7 patients[201]	Available as nutritional supplement; used to enhance cognitive functioning (memory, concentration); possible applicability to epilepsy
Dimethyl sulfoxide (DMSO)*	Substantial research in 1970s–1980s with some encouraging findings for stroke and other brain injury; less research now	Used after stroke and head injury; appears to lower ICP, stabilize BP, and increase blood flow to injured areas
EDTA chelation*	Uncontrolled study of stroke showed decrease in cerebral artery stenosis[109] Case series without objective outcome measures reported "good recovery" from stroke for 60% of sample[131]	Conventional use in lead poisoning; use in cardiovascular disease controversial Recommended in MS and Parkinson's disease§
Hyperbaric oxygen*	Controlled study[129] and uncontrolled studies[78,127] of stroke report some positive outcomes Study on stroke was discontinued[4] Two controlled studies of TBI reported mixed results[149,150] More than 10 animal studies showed suggestive findings	Conventionally used to treat decompression sickness and air embolism; use in stroke controversial
Melatonin*	Suggested role in stroke, Parkinson's disease, MS, and epilepsy No controlled studies	Sleep disturbances, depression; available in health food stores

Piracetam	Four double-blind placebo-controlled studies of dementia: two showed significant improvement in memory and cognitive functioning,[51,169] two showed no difference[39,145]	Reported to enhance integrative brain mechanisms (memory, learning, problem solving)
ELECTROTHERAPY		
Bioelectro-magnetics	Conventional use: functional electromagnetic stimulation[28] and electromagnetic biofeedback[10] Studies report positive findings for wound healing, including pressure sores in SCI[153,198]	Used to treat skin lesions, edema, and muscle weakness, pain, and spasticity and to accelerate wound healing
Magnetic stimulation	Animal studies suggest applicability of pulsed electromagnetic fields to stroke[58] Most controlled studies are for diagnosis rather than treatment	Diagnostic and treatment tool for evaluating activity in corticospinal tracts in MS, Parkinson's disease, stroke, others

*See text for additional information.
†Cerebral palsy, MS, spinal deformities, paraplegia, muscular dystrophy, lumbago.
‡Cerebral ischemia, vascular insufficiency, sequelae of stroke, tinnitus.
§Because some believe MS and Parkinson's disease are caused by heavy metal intoxication, EDTA chelation therapy has been recommended. However, no research has shown that this therapy is effective, or even that heavy metals are implicated, in these conditions.

TBI, Traumatic brain injury; *SCI*, spinal cord injury; *CNS*, central nervous system; *MS*, multiple sclerosis; *FDA*, U.S. Food and Drug Administration; *TCM*, traditional Chinese medicine; *ICP*, intracranial pressure; *BP*, blood pressure; *EDTA*, ethylenediamine-tetraacetic acid.

A few words of caution regarding the state of scientific evidence are warranted. Although a number of techniques have scientific evidence for effectiveness, lack of scientific evidence does not mean that the technique is not effective. Rather, the lack of evidence simply indicates that (1) no research has been conducted or published on a particular technique as applied to a particular medical condition, or (2) research articles have not been located in the highly diverse, often diffuse, and difficult-to-access alternative medicine literature.

In many cases the lack of evidence may result from the attempt to include only articles that are *peer reviewed* and have at least a minimally adequate research design, consisting of an experimental and control group, objective and valid outcome measures, a well-defined sample, and evidence of randomization and blinding. With a few notable exceptions, however, strict application of these criteria results in the elimination of whatever research evidence is available for most of the techniques. On the other hand, even the techniques that have been subjected to substantial research still lack the definitive degree of confidence that only large, multisite, double-blind studies bring to bear. Two CAM therapies, acupuncture and *Ginkgo biloba*, have received the greatest amount of research scrutiny and are discussed here in detail.

The following descriptions of CAM methods are not meant to provide a comprehensive list of definitions of all therapies used for neurologic conditions; such definitions are provided elsewhere in this textbook. Rather, therapies discussed in more detail here are used most frequently to treat neurologic conditions or have the most substantive research support.

ALTERNATIVE SYSTEMS OF MEDICAL PRACTICE

All the "traditional" medical practices of varying cultures fall in the category of alternative systems of medical practice. These traditions include such systems as Ayurveda, traditional Chinese medicine (TCM), and shamanism, as well as several of the Western systems, such as naturopathy and homeopathy. Alternative healing systems usually involve a large set of diverse practices and remedies that involve a number of different methods. These systems are based on an underlying model of the healing process that may or may not correspond to conventional medical models. Consequently, it is difficult to evaluate the entire system in a single study or even a large research program. Specific aspects of TCM, for example, are discussed in this chapter within sections on bodywork (acupuncture and massage), bioenergy (Qi Gong), and phytotherapies (*Ginkgo biloba*).

NONCONVENTIONAL BODYWORK

Research involving the use of manipulative techniques to influence neurologic conditions has focused more on soft tissue than on articulatory techniques. This is a reasonable approach because dysfunction in CNS conditions stems from abnormal muscle tonus and motor control, not vertebral malalignment and peripheral nerve compression. Of the neuromuscular soft tissue techniques, *proprioceptive neural facilitation* is investigated most often. Although well reported in the physical therapy literature (and thus not regarded as "complementary" by some rehabilitation practitioners), this technique is included here because it serves as a model that may elucidate the underlying mechanism of other soft tissue neuromuscular techniques that have been less thoroughly researched.

Few articles in the chiropractic literature address treatment of traumatic brain injury (TBI).[41] Research on osteopathic manipulation and craniosacral therapy is sparse. A few case studies involve other neurologic conditions, such as cerebral palsy, Erb's palsy, and learning disorders, but none exists for SCI, stroke, brain injury, or multiple sclerosis. *Craniosacral therapy* is sometimes used as part of a multidisciplinary treatment approach for spinal cord and brain injuries. Although no scientific studies have been conducted on this multidisciplinary approach, anecdotal evidence from the Upledger Institute's Brain and Spinal Cord Dysfunction Program indicates its effectiveness with these conditions.[194] However, when craniosacral therapy is used in combination with other therapies, it is difficult to isolate its specific action and efficacy. Anecdotal evidence also exists for the effectiveness of craniosacral therapy in treating symptoms of a concussion, including loss of clarity of thinking, loss of equilibrium, and eye pain.[34]

A number of case reports of injuries attributed to *chiropractic manipulation* have been published in the medical literature. Certain types of manipulation may produce greater risk than other types. Of 49 cases of stroke (cerebrovascular accident [CVA]) after chiropractic manipulation in which the technique was described, rotational manipulation of the upper cervical spine had been performed in 45 patients.[105] It should be noted, however, that complications arising from chiropractic manipulation occur less frequently than those observed in more common interventions.[57,111,209]

Although craniosacral therapy is asserted to be virtually risk free,[195] *adverse effects* or *events* (AEs) have been reported in a small number of individuals with TBI. In a study of craniosacral manipulation using the cranial osteopathy approach with 55 TBI patients,[59] several subjects reported mild headaches after treatment. Three subjects demonstrated more severe reactions, however, including exacerbation of vertiginous symptoms; visceral symptoms involving the cardiac, respiratory, and gastrointestinal systems; psychologic disturbances necessitating psychiatric institutional care; and severe total body spasticity. Such reactions are uncommon, however, and occurred in only 5% of the subjects in this study. Practitioners, particularly those treating TBI patients, are advised to be prepared to deal with this small but potential risk of serious AEs.

Acupuncture

Acupuncture is not a unitary method, and techniques vary. For example, some methods involve the use of low-voltage electric current across the needles to strengthen the effects of the needles, and laser acupuncture uses a high-wavelength, low-energy laser.[122] Other forms include TCM, five elements, scalp, Korean hand, and auricular acupuncture. The use of burning herbs (*moxa*) on acupoints and creation of a vacuum over a small section of the skin (*cupping*) are integral parts of many forms of acupuncture, both Eastern and Western.

Research on the effectiveness of acupuncture is abundant, although many reports involve case studies rather than controlled research protocols, and much of the literature is in Chinese. A number of systematic reviews of acupuncture research involving pain management exist, but quality evidence regarding treatment of neurologic disorders is still sparse. Nevertheless, several reasonably well-controlled studies report that acupuncture has shown efficacy in the treatment of some neurologic conditions.[108]

Evidence is clearly encouraging in the use of acupuncture in the treatment of stroke; however, the evidence is currently so limited that it can only be considered as suggestive. The research of Naeser et al.[120,122] is important because it suggests that major limiting factors in acupuncture effectiveness are the nature and extent of cerebral damage. Although treatment of TBI is common among acupuncturists trained in traditional Oriental methods, and the limited evidence for the treatment of stroke is encouraging with respect to treatment of cerebral trauma, no reports of controlled research involve acupuncture in TBI. Similarly, except for a few research projects involving animal models, no evidence exists for the utility of acupuncture in the treatment of SCI. Acupuncture has shown potential for managing some symptoms in multiple sclerosis, epilepsy, and Parkinson's disease, but the research methodology is so poor that no firm conclusions can be drawn.

PHYTOTHERAPY

Herbal medicine involves the use of whole-plant material, such as the root, stem, flower, or extract. Plant materials are the oldest form of medication and are part of virtually all indigenous medical traditions. Plant materials can be directly ingested, inhaled, or applied topically. As with conventional pharmaceutic drugs, herbal medicine is believed to work either because of the action of a specific chemical in the herb or because of the synergistic interaction between various components of the plants. Numerous medications and pharmaceutic compounds originate in substances originally isolated from plants.

Some herbs and plant materials appear to have useful medicinal effects that may be of relevance to rehabilitation. For example, herbs have been reported to exert effects on vascular elasticity, act as antiplatelet activating factors, exhibit antiedemic properties, and improve cognitive functioning. Despite being "natural," not all plants and herbs are safe for human consumption, however, and such medicines should only be used with full knowledge of the nature and effects of the plant component in question and their possible interactions with a patient's medications.

Chinese herbs and other plants have been used in medical treatments for thousands of years. Hundreds of natural substances are currently available for use, and most TCM herbal prescriptions contain up to 15 ingredients, which makes it difficult to identify the specific components that exert a treatment effect. A number of botanic extracts have been identified as beneficial in the treatment of cerebral ischemia, cerebral thrombosis, and stroke. These substances are generally used as elements of complex decoctions. No controlled clinical trials of their efficacy have been located; however, some may exist in Chinese or Japanese scientific literature not yet translated in English. Shiflett et al.[168] discuss Chinese herbs applied to CNS trauma.

Ginkgo biloba

The leaf of the ginkgo tree has been part of the traditional Chinese pharmacopoeia for 5000 years. Standardized extracts of the ginkgo leaf are widely used in Asia, Germany, and France and are increasingly being used in the United States. *Ginkgo* shows promise in the treatment of some of the most salient and debilitating symptoms associated with stroke, TBI, cerebrovascular insufficiency, senile dementia, and normal and pathologic aging.[45a] For example, *Ginkgo biloba* extract (GBE) has been used in the treatment of stroke,[103] ischemia (inadequate oxygenation/reperfusion),[21] impairments in memory/information processing (in older people, patients with Alzheimer's disease and other types of dementia),[65,89,141,184,181,200] vestibular disorders,[63] and tinnitus.[113]

A placebo-controlled study of EGb 761, the GBE produced by Schwabe in Germany, examined efficacy in a sample of 202 patients with Alzheimer's disease or multiinfarct dementia.[95] Patients treated with GBE showed modest but significantly greater improvements on the cognitive subscale of the Alzheimer's disease assessment scale (ADAS-COG) and on a geriatric assessment scale completed by relatives (Figure 7-1). There were no differences between groups in the incidence or severity of AEs.

Although the duration of treatment with EGb 761 and the window of time required to demonstrate efficacy have varied across studies, improvement generally has been observed within 4 to 12 weeks.[117,214] No serious side effects have been observed in clinical trials; rarely, however, patients have shown allergic skin reactions, headache, and mild gastrointestinal upset. Despite that patients taking GBE are often receiving a variety of medications, there are no known drug interactions.[88]

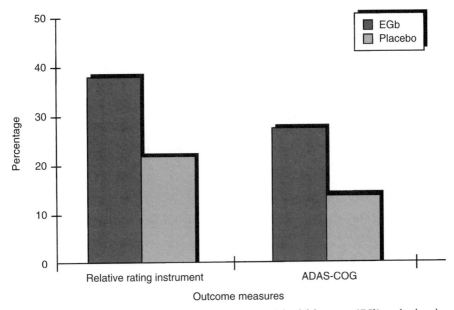

FIGURE 7–1. Percentage of patients with dementia receiving *Ginkgo biloba* extract (*EGb*) or placebo who demonstrated statistically significant improvement on two outcome measures. *ADAS-COG*, Cognitive subscale of Alzheimer's disease assessment scale. (*Data from Le Bars PL et al: JAMA 278[16]:1327, 1997.*)

Overall, GBE (most notably, EGb 761) has been cited in at least 130 publications, with approximately one third of the reports published in non-English journals. An analysis derived from a subset of 65 studies using experimental, quasi-experimental, or observational methods showed that 16 studies used in vitro methods, 14 involved animal models, and 35 reports were based on human models. The animal models that have been used to assess the activity of GBE have used rigorous laboratory-based techniques. For example, animal models of ischemia using carotid artery clamping procedures have been used to examine the mechanisms underlying GBE's purported antiplatelet activating factor properties and its ability to confer protection against ischemia/reperfusion damage.[130] Animal models using both histologic and behavioral delayed-spatial alternation paradigms have also examined the effectiveness of GBE in treating the cerebral injury and edema often observed in the acute stages of TBI.[173]

Almost 75% of the evaluated studies were based on experimental or quasi-experimental and observational methods. In 94% of the human studies, subjects were randomly assigned and control groups were used. A review of representative clinical studies published in peer-reviewed journals since 1990 shows that most of these studies employed randomized placebo-controlled double-blind procedures. Almost 97% of human studies used objective or standardized outcome measures. Many studies used universally recognized tests of neurobehavioral function, although some descriptions of the outcome measures lacked sufficient detail to enable adequate evaluation. Many outcome studies that evaluated activities of daily living were administered to geriatric patients and were largely based on self-report measures.

One of the major weaknesses or ambiguities in some studies, particularly those in the German literature, is the vaguely defined diagnostic category "vascular insufficiency."[45a] Although patients included in this category tend to be geriatric and display slower processing and memory impairments, the precise correspondence of this diagnostic category to diagnostic categories used in the United States is uncertain. Although most published studies on *G. biloba* have reported positive effects, not all studies have confirmed such efficacy. For example, Hartmann and Frick[65] evaluated 52 ambulatory patients with a diagnosis of vascular dementia. GBE was administered over 3 months in a drinking solution, 20 ml three times daily, equivalent to a 150-mg daily dosage. Because of an unexpectedly strong placebo effect, patients treated with GBE displayed marginally but not significantly better results than placebo on psychometric performance.

NONCONVENTIONAL USES OF PHARMACOLOGIC AND CONVENTIONAL THERAPIES

The category discussed in this section refers to a broad group of drugs and conventional treatments approved for one type of medical condition but believed to have beneficial effects on other conditions for which they are not approved by the U.S Food and Drug Administration (FDA), such as the common use of anticonvulsants for the treatment of pain or depression. Even though these alternative uses of conventional medical treatments are available under a physician's supervision, these CAM therapies may be difficult to obtain because so few physicians know about or are willing to prescribe such treatments.

Melatonin

Melatonin is a hormone produced continuously throughout the life cycle by the pineal gland. However, its production may progressively decline with age. Melatonin secretion exhibits cyclic variation, with humans producing 5 to 10 times more melatonin at night than during the day. Melatonin has been reported to exert an inhibitory effect on the production of free radicals and thus limit the resulting damage, exhibiting antioxidant effects. In one experiment in which a dilute solution of hydrogen peroxide was exposed to ultraviolet light, melatonin reportedly was effective in reducing the number of free radicals.[61] The pineal gland's activity is mediated by melatonin and appears to exert a depressive influence on CNS excitability. Evidence supports a role for melatonin in the regulation of the gamma-aminobutyric acid (GABA) or benzodiazepine receptor complex, as a potentiator of this inhibitory neurotransmitter system.

SAFETY. Melatonin may play a role in other conditions, including sleep disorders, chronic fatigue syndrome, fibromyalgia, depression, and Alzheimer's disease. Because of melatonin's apparent role in a number of medical conditions, there is a popular movement to self-administer melatonin in a "hormone replacement" or "hormone supplementation" program, since melatonin levels are generally believed to decline with age. This approach raises the urgent issue of safety, as addressed by several studies. In a 1960 study, 200 mg of melatonin was injected into human subjects with skin disorders, and no negative side effects were reported.[96]

In healthy volunteers who were injected with a synthetic version of melatonin of varying doses, the hormone was found to have tranquilizing properties.[5] Subjects injected with 75 mg of melatonin showed slower brain wave patterns, lower heart rates, and muscle relaxation, with no carryover fatigue or negative effects on memory performance. A similar pattern of response was observed in elderly subjects administered 50 mg/day. Despite the apparent safety of melatonin use over a short period, there is no evidence regarding the long-term effects of melatonin supplementation, so caution is necessary in its use. Melatonin at least should be administered under physician supervision.

ELECTROMAGNETIC THERAPIES

A number of electromagnetic therapies that might be considered alternative in many medical fields are used conventionally in rehabilitation. These therapies include *functional neuromuscular stimulation* (FNS) and biofeedback. FNS is a form of electrical stimulation in which muscles are activated sequentially to allow performance of motor tasks. Chae et al.[28] discuss FNS as applied to spinal cord injury (SCI), stroke-related hemiplegia, and other types of paralysis.

Biofeedback generally involves the use of equipment to measure internal physiologic events, make patients aware of their occurrence, and teach them to manipulate these events.[10] In the treatment of neurologic disorders the most frequently used form of biofeedback is *myoelectric*, or *electromyographic* (EMG), which is based on electrical signals from muscles and can be used to regulate body positions, movement, blood pressure, and sphincter control. EMG biofeedback is used in the treatment of stroke, SCI, cerebral palsy, TBI, multiple sclerosis, and dyskinesias. Basmajian[10] examines EMG biofeedback in the treatment of neurologic disorders.

◼ Stroke (Cerebrovascular Accident)

Stroke, or CVA, is associated with an interruption of blood flow to some portion of the brain or brain stem as a result of hemorrhage or arterial blockage by thrombi or emboli. The immediate results are the classic symptoms of a stroke, which include numbness, weakness, or paralysis of face, arm, or leg, especially on one side of the body. The person may have difficulty speaking or understanding simple statements. The individual may experience sudden or decreased vision in one or both eyes, dizziness, loss of balance, or loss of coordination. Other symptoms may include sudden, unexplainable, and intense headache; sudden nausea, fever, and vomiting; and brief loss of consciousness or a period of decreased consciousness, such as fainting, confusion, convulsions, or coma.[156] Because cerebral metabolism depends on a fairly constant supply of blood and oxygen, deprivation of oxygen in the brain can result in extensive damage within 10 to 20 seconds and irreversible damage after 3 to 10 minutes.[163] The four major types of stroke are as follows:

1. *Cerebral occlusion,* or *thrombotic stenosis,* when a clot forms in an artery supplying blood to the brain, totally obstructing blood flow, and *cerebral stenosis,* when an artery is partially obstructed
2. *Embolic stroke,* when a clot from a region outside the brain breaks loose and is carried in the bloodstream to an artery in the brain, plugging a blood vessel and cutting off the brain's blood supply
3. *Lacunar stroke,* when multiple small cerebral infarcts affect subcortical regions
4. *Hemorrhagic stroke,* when a hemorrhage results in blood spilling into brain tissue or into the area surrounding the brain

Stroke ranks third among all causes of death in the United States, and over the course of a lifetime four of five families will be affected by stroke. Stroke is a major cause of long-term disability, with 550,000 Americans annually experiencing a stroke and almost two thirds of the survivors demonstrating some form of impairment.[106] There is a clear difference in racial/ethnic mortality. Ayala et al.[7] recently reported that mortality rates for ischemic, intracerebral, and subarachnoid strokes were higher for blacks and Asian/Pacific Islanders than for whites between ages 25 and 44 years. These disparities in different ethnic groups need careful tracking and awareness on the part of the health care provider.

Several well-recognized deficit patterns are associated with lesion site. *Anterior cerebral artery* stroke is associated with contralateral lower extremity and sometimes upper extremity paresis and hypesthesia as well as impaired judgment. *Middle cerebral artery* infarct may be accompanied by contralateral upper and lower extremity paresis and hypesthesia, visual field deficits, agnosia, and aphasias. *Posterior cerebral artery* lesions may result in visual deficits, deficits in memory and cognition, alexia, agraphia, and balance problems. *Cerebellar* infarcts involve coordination and motor planning and execution. *Brain stem* lesions may involve any of these conditions, as well as vegetative functions such as respiration and autonomic regulation. Other sources provide more detailed descriptions of anatomic localization of deficits.[151] Any of these lesions may be accompanied by long-term sequelae of seizures, spasticity, dysphagia, incontinence, depression, memory/learning impairment, peripheral nerve injury, reflex sympathetic dystrophy, and sexual impairment.[54]

ACUPUNCTURE

In general, acupuncture has been reported to work best when used as early as possible on stroke patients. Acupuncture appears to be more effective with stroke patients if their lesions are singular, shallow, and with a small focus, instead of large, bilateral lesions with deep multiple foci.[32] Researchers at the University of Lund, Sweden, hypothesized that the sensory stimulation of traditional acupuncture points with needles and electrostimulation may promote the restructuring and consolidation of coordinated motor function of affected limbs in the stroke patient, thus serving to enhance the recovery of postural control.[102]

In a well-controlled study, 40 hemiparetic male and female patients who received 10 weeks of acupuncture, along with standard physical therapy (PT) and occupational therapy (OT) beginning 10 days after stroke, recovered faster and had significant improvements in activities of daily living (Barthel index), quality of life (Nottingham Health Profile), and balance/mobility (idiosyncratic motor function assessment scale) compared with a control group of 38 patients who received only PT and OT.[83] A drawback to this study was the lack of a sham acupuncture condition; positive results could also be attributable to general sensory stimulation of the muscles surrounding the acupuncture point rather than to acupuncture per se. In a follow-up of the 48 survivors in this study, conducted approximately 3 years after original treatment,[102] subjects received *perturbations* (vibratory stimulation to the calf muscle or galvanic stimulation of the vestibular nerves) in three different tests, each with eyes open and closed. Significantly more of the treatment group (17 of 21) than the control group (9 of 25) could maintain stance on all six tests ($p < 0.0025$).

More recently, Johansson et al.[82] evaluated acupuncture and transcutaneous electrical nerve stimulation (TENS) in a randomized controlled trial (Figure 7-2).[82] While they concluded that there was no effect from acupuncture in aiding functional recovery, it has been suggested that their statistical analysis did not treat the data adequately.[166] Among various problems mentioned, the failure to correct for baseline deficit was most telling. Figure 7-2 shows a simple linear correction to the data published by Johansson et al. It is clear that, for this sample at least, acupuncture had a substantial positive effect on recovery of activities of daily living compared with the two control conditions. Since the raw data are not available, it is not possible to calculate a significance level, but it seems apparent that there is a high probability that acupuncture would be shown to be more effective if an appropriate statistical test, such as repeated measures analysis of variance, were performed. In any case, we choose to interpret their findings as strongly supportive of the effectiveness of acupuncture in this situation.

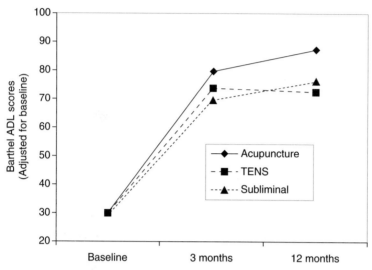

FIGURE 7–2. Functional outcome according to Barthel index on activities of daily living (*ADL*) for stroke patients receiving acupuncture, transcutaneous electrical nerve stimulation (*TENS*), or subliminal therapy. (*From Johansson BB et al: Stroke 32[3]:707, 2001.*)

A very recent study[180] seems to have a similar problem in dealing with baseline impairment in terms of statistical treatment. In a prospective randomized controlled trial on 106 stroke patients, with treatments begun 3 to 15 days after stroke, the control group consisted of standard of care, including physical, occupational, and speech therapy, and the experimental group received acupuncture in addition to standard of care. Observations on functional independence measures were made just prior to commencing treatment, at 5 weeks into treatment, and when treatment was completed at week 10.[63a,102a] This procedure differs in a very important way from other similar studies in that the measurements are made *during* and immediately after the treatment period, rather than after treatment is completed with one or more longer-term follow-ups, at 3, 6, and/or 12 months, as in most other studies of this type. Using the Mann-Whitney U statistical test, it was concluded that there was no difference in the groups, despite the obvious positive effect acupuncture was having in their sample, based on visual inspection of the reported data. Yet visual inspection of the results indicates that acupuncture combined with standard of care was clearly superior to standard of care alone. This conclusion that acupuncture had failed to improve recovery over standard of care resulted in the researchers' decision not to perform the follow-up evaluations, despite the fact that nearly all of the studies with longer term measurements found increasing differences over time between the control and acupuncture groups, always in favor of acupuncture. Thus there was no opportunity to observe longer-term improvements, and a low-power statistical test (relative to analysis of variance) may have caused an erroneous conclusion to be drawn.

A research program directed by Naeser and colleagues at the Boston University Medical Center and Boston Veterans Administration (VA) hospital provides some evidence for the efficacy of acupuncture in the treatment of stroke under certain limiting conditions. In a study comparing real versus sham acupuncture in the treatment of paralysis in acute stroke patients, 16 patients with right-side paralysis who had left-hemisphere ischemic infarction were randomly assigned to receive either 20 real acupuncture treatments (11 points, some with electrical stimulation) or 20 sham acupuncture treatments (nonacupoints with no electrical stimulation) over 1 month beginning 1 to 3 months after stroke onset.[120] The outcome measure was "good" versus "poor" response on the Boston Motor Inventory for upper and lower extremities. Results indicated that significantly more patients had a good response after real acupuncture than sham acupuncture when a computed tomography (CT) scan indicated that there was a lesion in half or less than half of the motor pathways involving the periventricular white matter ($p < 0.013$). A follow-up study demonstrated similar results with laser acupuncture;[122] however, five of the seven patients in this study had been subjects in the 1992 acupuncture study.[120]

In a study of both chronic and acute stroke patients, eight chronic stroke patients were treated with acupuncture beginning 6 months to 8 years after stroke, and three acute stroke patients were treated with acupuncture beginning 2 months after stroke onset.[121] Patients received 20 or 40 acupuncture treatments over 2 to 3 months. All patients had a good response, defined as improvement on at least four of six hand tests that was sustained for at least 2 months after completion of the acupuncture treatments. The researchers concluded that acupuncture may be an additional beneficial treatment method for stroke patients with hand paresis, even when started as late as 5 to 8 years after stroke. Although there was no control condition in this study, chronic patients were their own controls in the sense that their condition had been stable for 6 months or more before treatment. This same study also reported that patients exhibiting a beneficial response to treatment had damage to less than half of the motor pathway areas, as seen on CT scans.

Two other randomized controlled trials of acupuncture treatment of stroke support the previously described findings. In a study of ischemic stroke conducted in Taiwan, when compared with subjects receiving standard rehabilitation only, subjects receiving acupuncture in addition to standard care had significantly better functional outcomes as measured by the Barthel index at 1 month and 3 months after stroke.[72] Subjects began receiving treatment within 36 hours after stroke and received 12 treatments over 4 weeks. Subjects with poor neurologic scores responded better to acupuncture than did control subjects, whereas no difference was found in subjects with good neurologic scores. This finding suggests that acupuncture has an incrementally helpful effect only when the condition is serious enough that full recovery is not likely through spontaneous recovery or standard rehabilitation. In a Norwegian study, 45 patients with cerebral infarction or cerebral hemorrhage were randomly entered into either a standard rehabilitation condition or the acupuncture plus standard rehabilitation condition.[55] Six weeks after treatment, individuals receiving acupuncture had significantly better outcomes in activities of daily living and on the motor assessment scale and Nottingham Health Profile.

One study questioned acupuncture's value to standard poststroke rehabilitation.[180] Groups were stratified and randomized; 14 patients dropped out and one AE was recorded. Also, a systematic review evaluating the effectiveness of acupuncture for stroke described the majority of studies as "average-poor" with many confounding variables, including etiology, location of lesions, degree of neural damage, sample size, blinding, treatment scheduling, needle insertion, and inadequate outcome measures.[137]

GINKGO BILOBA

Research into the mechanisms of action of *Ginkgo biloba* suggests that it may improve cognitive function by altering arterial and vascular elasticity.[33] In addition, evidence derived from animal models and clinical studies supports the idea that *G. biloba* acts as an antiplatelet activating factor.[21] Taken together, these findings suggest that *G. biloba* can play a role in treating the symptoms of cerebrovascular disease during both the acute and the chronic stages. *Ginkgo* has shown efficacy in the treatment of stroke in clinical investigations. For example, Maier-Hauff[103] reported that in 50 subarachnoid hemorrhage patients who had been administered GBE (L1 1370) in a placebo-controlled double-blind study, GBE was effective in countering the effects of cerebral insufficiency, with significant improvements noted in attention and verbal short-term memory. These results may support early initiation of *G. biloba* therapy to treat the varied metabolic changes that may accompany cerebral ischemia, such as free-radical production and electrolyte shifts (e.g., increases in extracellular K^+ and intracellular Ca^{2+}, lactic acidosis), as well as increased release of free fatty acids, prostaglandins, and excitatory neurotransmitters.[42]

Hofferberth[68] conducted a double-blind placebo-controlled trial to examine the effects of EGb 761 on neurophysiologic and psychometric parameters in patients with cerebrovascular disease. Of the 36 patients in the study, half received EGb 761 (120 mg/day) for 8 weeks, and half were given a placebo. A high proportion of slow-wave activity in the electroencephalogram (EEG) spectrum generally indicates neurologic damage. After 4 to 8 weeks of therapy the proportion of theta waves (i.e., slow-wave activity) in the EEG spectrum was reduced in the patients given EGb 761. The neurophysiologic changes were evident as an increase in the relative power of the alpha component of the cortical EEG, which suggests that EGb 761 may have a therapeutic role in treating cerebrovascular disease (i.e., stroke).[42]

HOMEOPATHY

The research evidence on the use of homeopathic remedies for neurologic conditions is sparse. *Arnica montana* is an herb that is popular in the mountainous areas of Europe for the treatment of acute traumatic injuries, and it is a frequently used homeopathic remedy. Savage and Roe[158] studied 40 inpatients within 7 days after a stroke in a double-blind study with random assignment to either treatment or control group. Twenty of the patients received *A. montana*, and the 20 patients in the control condition received an equivalent dose of an unmedicated lactose powder similar in appearance to *A. montana*. The authors found no differences between the groups in mortality, survival, and functioning over a 3-month period. The investigators conducted a second study in 1978 with *A. montana* of a different dilution. Results replicated the early study, and no beneficial effect of the herb was found after stroke. Several case studies exist involving stroke, each using a different homeopathic remedy, and not surprisingly, report improvements in the patient's condition.[44,164]

MASSAGE AND OTHER MANUAL MANIPULATION

Massage has been suggested to be a valuable adjunct in treatment regimens for hemiplegia.[212] Soothing massage before performing exercises can help reduce spasticity, and in patients with flaccid paralysis, more stimulating massage can help stimulate nerves and increase circulation.

Investigators of *proprioceptive neural facilitation* (PNF) have studied both laboratory measures of nervous system excitability and clinically relevant parameters, such as hemiplegia. It is thought that contraction of antagonist muscle groups invokes a neurally mediated decrease in tone by way of inhibition of motoneurons through centrally mediated reflexes.[182] Entyre and Abraham[49] found that use of the *contract-relax-antagonist-contract* (CRAC) technique significantly decreased motor pool excitability during performance of PNF. Wang[206] found that in patients with hemiplegia of both long and short duration, gait speed and cadence improved in a cumulative manner after 12 sessions of PNF. On the other hand, when PNF used alone was compared with EMG muscle stimulation in hemiplegic patients, PNF produced less improvement than electrical stimulation.[92]

HYPNOSIS

In case reports, patients treated with hypnosis after stroke have shown increased movement in hemiplegic limbs, improved ambulation, and return of normal speech.[38,70,103] However, findings from these case studies are confounded because they occurred during the first year after the accident, a period during which spontaneous recovery is still probable.

MEDITATION

With regard to stroke prevention, the most robust finding is the success of meditation in reducing *hypertension*.[13,62,161,203] Evidence also indicates a reduction in cholesterol level.[36] Given the success of meditation for reducing hypertension, and because hypertension is a predisposing factor for CVA and its recurrence, it seems reasonable to conclude that meditation may be effective in reduction of risk for stroke.

No studies were found that specifically address the issue of stroke prevention. In a well-controlled, randomized study comparing several relaxation techniques, however, regular practice of transcendental meditation (TM) by elderly nursing home residents was associated with significantly reduced systolic blood pressure and significantly increased 3-year survival rate compared with the simple relaxation and no-treatment conditions.[3] After 3 years, 100% of the TM group were alive versus 68% of the no-treatment group.

BOTANICALS

Ischemic reoxygenation plays an important role in the pathogenesis of stroke and brain trauma. Some non-Chinese herbs can exert a protective effect, shielding cells from the pathologic effects of ischemic reoxygenation. This protective effect may be mediated by antioxidant and free-radical scavenging properties, which suggests a role for herbal therapies in the treatment of stroke and neurotrauma.[176]

Uchida et al.[192] reported that in stroke-prone, spontaneously hypertensive rats, the herb *Persimmon tannin* appeared to have helped increase the rat's life span, in addition to reducing the severity of damage resulting from brain hemorrhage and infarction. *Kampo* herbal formulations, which contain several ingredients and are available in various forms, have been reported to reduce the complications resulting from ischemia.[53] Through in vitro experimentation using an electron spin resonance technique, Kampo formulations and components have shown radical scavenging activity, which suggests that Kampo, when used in treatment of brain damage, could play a preventive role in reducing the ischemic complications after TBI. Similarly, the extract *Kava* (*Piper methysticum*) and its constituents have also displayed anti-ischemic properties in rodent models. The kava constituents were found to display protective and anticonvulsive effects in two models of focal ischemia.[9]

ENERGY HEALING

McGee and Chow[110] relate a number of case studies on the success of *Qi Gong* for many different medical conditions, including stroke, paralysis, and cerebral palsy. A randomized controlled trial of Reiki on subacute stroke inpatients showed no improvement over a sham treatment.[167] However, truly rigorous research is sparse and definitely needed, given the popularity of these techniques today.

DIET AND NUTRITION

Epidemiologic studies have suggested that a daily diet of fruits and vegetables has a protective effect against stroke. Ness and Powles[125] conducted a review of studies published between 1966 and 1995 on the protective action of fruits and vegetables against cardiovascular disease. Nine of 14 studies on stroke showed that the consumption of fruits and vegetables had a significant protective association with stroke. Similar results were found in a 17-year follow-up of 11,000 subjects who consumed a vegetarian diet.[87] The authors found that daily consumption of fresh fruit was associated with significantly reduced mortality from cerebrovascular disease and ischemic heart disease.

The protective action of fruits and vegetables is attributed to dietary antioxidant vitamins (beta-carotene and vitamin C) and flavonoids. This hypothesis was examined in a 15-year follow-up of 552 males.[86] The investigators found an inverse relation between the intake of dietary antioxidants and stroke incidence. Antioxidants prevent low-density lipoprotein (LDL) oxidation and therefore reduce its absorption by macrophages and the subsequent formation of atherosclerotic plaques. Support for the protective antioxidant action of *vitamin C* was found in a review of the research literature between 1966 and 1996.[126] The review indicated a protective association of measures of vitamin C intake or blood levels of vitamin C and cardiovascular disease. Although evidence was limited, there was support for the premise that vitamin C had a protective effect against stroke. Research suggests that *garlic* has the ability to provide some protection against atherosclerosis, coronary thrombosis, and stroke, effects believed to be directly related to its ability to inhibit aggregation of blood platelets.[190] Further, *alcohol* intake in moderation may decrease the incidence of stroke, although binge drinking or high intake of alcohol may increase the risk of stroke 10-fold.[148]

Nutritional supplementation has been suggested to reduce the risk of a subsequent occurrence of CVA. Although these recommendations are often based on a presumed protective mechanism of action within the body based on the biochemistry of the substance, little research directly relating these substances to effective treatment of neurologic conditions exists. When the limited studies are examined closely, there is often contradictory information. For example, the belief that *fish* consumption reduces risk of stroke is supported by several retrospective studies,[79,85] but a recent population-based retrospective study not only failed to support these earlier findings, but also tended to contradict them, finding a slightly higher level of stroke in men with the highest level of reported fish consumption.[132]

MELATONIN

It has been proposed that the nocturnal rise in melatonin level observed in humans may mediate the lower nocturnal risks for heart attack and stroke. When human blood platelets are incubated in a melatonin solution, the hormone reduces platelets' tendency to clump by as much as 85%.[118] Some research also suggests a link between melatonin and cholesterol; studies have shown that melatonin partially blocks cholesterol production, thus reducing LDL accumulation.[119]

A circadian rhythm involving melatonin is suggested by studies showing that during stroke a major metabolite, *urinary sulfatoxymelatonin* (6-SMT), is delayed in its excretion during the early poststroke period when compared to levels at day 10.[12] Interestingly, the observations were most obvious in the more extensive cortical lesions.

CHELATION

Although chelation therapy is recommended for the treatment and prevention of cerebrovascular disorders, no controlled trials substantiate its use.

In an uncontrolled trial, cerebral arterial occlusion was measured in 57 patients before and after treatment with 10 to 46 sessions of ethylenediaminetetraacetic acid (*EDTA*) chelation therapy; 88% improved (criteria for improvement not stated), and cerebral arterial stenosis reportedly was reduced from a mean 28% to 10%.[109] A retrospective analysis was conducted in Brazil of 2870 patients who were treated with EDTA chelation therapy between 1983 and 1985.[131] These patients had a variety of vascular and degenerative diseases, with about 18% of the patients (504) diagnosed with cerebrovascular disease or degenerative CNS disease. The investigators reported "marked recovery" in 24% of the patients and "good recovery" in 60%. Animal studies with another chelating agent, *deferoxamine*, showed that the hypoxic-ischemic injury is reduced if deferoxamine is administered soon after the injury.[8,75,135]

HYPERBARIC OXYGEN

A problem for stroke patients is the deprivation of oxygen in key brain areas resulting from an interruption of blood flow. Hyperbaric oxygen (HBO) therapy has been advocated in these patients because it may enhance neuronal viability by its ability to increase the amount of dissolved oxygen in the blood without changing blood viscosity.[116]

In a large study by Neubauer and End,[127] 122 patients with thrombotic stroke were treated with HBO in addition to standard treatment. In the bedridden group, 64% of the patients improved by showing ability to use a wheelchair or to walk with or without aids. In the wheelchair group, 71% of the patients showed improved ambulation. In the group categorized as walking with aids, 56% of the patients improved enough to walk independently. However, in a study of HBO therapy for acute ischemic stroke in patients with middle cerebral artery occlusion, the results were mixed.[129] In addition, although there have been a number of animal studies and isolated small clinical/case-based studies, no major study has showed the benefit of HBO for wide-scale application. In general, existing research suggests that HBO therapy in patients with stroke may be beneficial, but additional research is clearly needed.

Also, it is useful to continue to review and evaluate the role of modification of body temperature (*hypothermia*) and stroke prognosis, especially with a focus toward the potential for neural protectiveness.[37]

Safety

Issues of safety and toxicity have been a major concern surrounding HBO therapy. AEs such as increased free-radical production and peroxidation have been reported.[151] However, serious side effects have been virtually eliminated by keeping pressures at 1.5 to 2 atmospheres (atm), limiting exposure time, and following more rigorous procedures during compression and decompression.[128]

◼ Brain Injury

Brain injury refers to damage to the brain caused by either external trauma (e.g., motor vehicle accidents, gunshot wounds) or internal lesions (e.g., tumors, anoxic injuries). TBI is of two major types: the more common, *closed-head injuries*, in which rapid movement of the brain within the skull results in global deficits, and *open-head injuries*, which involve penetration of the skull and localized damage. *Mild* TBI refers to brain injury that may produce no obvious problems, signs, or symptoms and may go unexamined and untreated. However, increasing evidence suggests that mild TBI, such as that incurred in a single episode or in repeated episodes in contact sports (e.g., football), can result in permanent damage.

Of the numerous causes of TBI, the most common are *motor vehicle accidents* (MVAs), which account for 50% of all injuries. Falls account for 21% of injuries, firearms for 12%, and sports/recreational accidents for 10%. Each year, 373,000 Americans are hospitalized as a result of TBI. Of these, 99,000 have severe lifelong disabilities. Males in the 14- to 24-year-old age group are at the greatest risk for TBI, and more than 30,000 children are permanently disabled each year.[19] In terms of emergency room (ER) visits, Guerrero, Thurman, and Sniezek[60] reported that the mean incidence of TBI is more than 1 million per year in the United States. Children up to age 14 account for the largest percentage of patients with TBI, and falls are the primary reason for the ER visit. Other major reasons can include MVAs and "being struck by an object."

The AEs of TBI vary widely, ranging from mild concussive syndromes that may result in little to mild loss of function, to moderate and severe head injuries that may leave patients with long-term impairments and disabilities. After acute effects of TBI are stabilized, patients with moderate and severe injuries usually require long-term care for treatment and rehabilitation of conditions such as seizure, spasticity, movement disorder, neuroendocrine dysfunction, cranial and sensory nerve impairment, and significant cognitive deficit and mood disturbance.

GINKGO BILOBA

GBE has reportedly shown efficacy in improving outcomes in animal models of TBI. For example, EGb 761 enhances recovery in rats with bilateral frontal damage after 30 days of treatment. When administered GBE before injury, rats have shown decreased activity and sensitivity to light and noxious stimuli, along with improved performance on a delayed spatial-alternation learning task.[173] Improved motor function was also found in an experimental model of cortical hemiplegia. Brailowsky et al.[18] administered EGb 761 using two rat models of hemiplegia, one induced by aspiration and a second group subjected to reversible inactivation of motor cortex through GABA infusion. Rats given the GBE exhibited a faster, more complete recovery from motor deficits, with histologic analysis also showing that EGb 761–treated rats had significantly smaller ventricular diameters than untreated rats (given only saccharin solutions). One explanation for these results is that EGB 761 possesses an antioxidant that includes ginkgolide and flavonoid components.[43]

HOMEOPATHY

Chapman et al.[29] found that using a pre/posttherapy, randomized double-blind placebo-controlled design, 50 patients with mild TBI and an average of almost 3 years since injury were responsive to homeopathic medication. Although more cognitive types of testing (e.g., speech, language, memory) did not change, social functioning (e.g., participating in daily activities) and handling "difficult situations" (e.g., eating in a restaurant) were improved and predictive of change. With one reported AE, the authors suggest the findings are "clinically significant." Additional larger scale research should evaluate the relevance of variables such as potency of homeopathic medication and the duration of treatment as factors influencing outcome.

HYPNOSIS

In a study without a control condition, hypnosis was used in the treatment of headache or vertigo after TBI in a sample of 155 patients. Almost half the patients reported resolution of symptoms, and another 20% had significant symptom reduction.[27] Outcome was best for those who had been injured less than 6 months before treatment. In two case reports of young people with TBIs, hypnotic treatment was followed by increased social interaction, improved mood, increased participation in treatment, and substantial gains in physical therapy.[38]

HYPERBARIC OXYGEN

Research on the use of HBO in TBI still requires further analysis. HBO may have beneficial effects for reducing brain edema after head injury without impairing tissue oxygen delivery.[177] In general, the limited research suggests that HBO therapy may accelerate the healing process and lower the mortality rate but may not substantially improve functioning.[35,128,149,150]

One recent report in the Chinese literature found HBO to be useful for improving severe TBI.[147] The 35 patients showed improvement in motor behavior and Glasgow Coma Scale scores (good-mild disability range) and a decrease in "abnormal" EEG patterns.

Animal studies have shown that the administration of HBO at 2.5 atm absolute (ATA) after experimentally delivered blunt trauma helped to improve balance and motor skills, but with no identifiable change in underlying neural pathology (change in pyramidal cells in the CA3 region of the hippocampus), 10 days after contusion.[187] Further studies might evaluate other cortical and subcortical motor regions where cell change might occur.

Patients with TBI appear to be responsive to *cognitive rehabilitation*, which focuses on memory failures and psychologic issues of anxiety, self-concept, and relationships. More studies that focus on long-term effects of various rehabilitation therapies and include measurable outcomes are needed, along with control groups and more patients.[25]

A new therapy may hold some promise for treating several types of disorders, including TBI. The *Flexyx Neurotherapy System* uses EEG frequencies as feedback.[162] The basic assumption is that brain injury is associated not only with behavioral-cognitive dysfunction and emotional trauma, but also with underlying brain neural dysfunction. By using photic stimulation, EEG frequencies, as a neural measure, become "entrained or reset" over time to the frequency of the particular light stimulation so that brain pathways and large populations of cells are being constantly restabilized. Shoenberger et al.[162] report that this therapy resulted in improvements in "social and cognitive functioning" as well as depression and fatigue. Although the mechanism is unclear, this "normalizing" of EEG activity merits more evaluation.

N Spinal Cord Injury

SCI refers to the loss of neurologic function after traumatic injury to the spinal cord. At present, approximately 250,000 spinal cord–injured individuals are living in the United States, and on average, 11,000 new SCIs are reported each year. Traumatic MVAs cause 48% of SCIs; falls constitute 21%, violence 15%, and sports 14%. The location and severity of injury determine how the individual with SCI is affected; 55% of SCIs result in *tetraplegia*, with the remaining 45% resulting in *paraplegia*.[170]

If the spinal cord is only *partially transected* (approximately 54% of cases), some nerve impulses will be transmitted accompanied by incomplete loss of function. However, *total transection* of the spinal cord results in complete loss of function below the level of the lesion (i.e., complete injury). Level of injury corresponds with severity of neurologic deficit. Patients usually require surgical spinal stabilization followed by long-term intensive rehabilitation by a team of professionals. Depending on the level of injury, patients may have respiratory problems requiring support, chronic pulmonary conditions, cardiac and autonomic abnormalities, loss of bowel and bladder control, muscle weakness, spasticity, changes in body composition and regulation, sexual dysfunction, and skin breakdown.

Persons who survive SCI frequently have chronic medical problems that may be amenable to CAM interventions. For example, in a recent telephone survey of CAM usage by 77 SCI patients,[124] acupuncture was the most used therapy but also the least in terms of satisfaction for relief of pain. Massage was rated the highest for pain relief. Variables predicting CAM usage included income and coverage by insurance. Strong, positive outcomes of other CAM therapies appeared problematical, indicating the need for more complete and controlled studies. Also, the issue of neuropathic pain often related to SCI should focus on strong measurements of multiple aspects of functioning, including quality of life, social support, work productivity, and change in medication usage.[66]

ACUPUNCTURE

Research using animal models has suggested that acupuncture may be effective in inducing regeneration in nerve tissue. Rats given treatment with electroacupuncture exhibited spontaneous sprouting of severed sciatic nerve tissue, with a 14% to 30% increase in regeneration rate compared with the no-treatment group.[14] Additional results from animal models using induced spinal cord contusion suggest that electroacupuncture applied 1 hour after SCI decreased posttraumatic sequelae.[139] One uncontrolled study of the use of acupuncture in the treatment of SCI patients reported improvements in functioning and decrease in paresthesias.[211] However, the study did not report results on any quantifiable outcomes or involve comparisons with a control group. Therefore, because of the absence of comparison controls and quantifiable measures of pain or mobility, it is difficult to draw any definite conclusions about the efficacy of treatment.

More recent work indicates the potential usefulness of acupuncture in treatment of SCI. Honjo et al.[71] reported that a quality of life issue, urinary incontinence, can be modified with the use of acupuncture. In eight patients with lesions at the cervical or thoracic level, 10 minutes of manually rotated acupuncture at BL-33 (Zhongliao) points for 4 weeks totally controlled incontinence in 38% of the patients and partially in another 38%. There was a significant increase in bladder capacity, but pressure was not changed. A larger number of patients evaluated would have been helpful, as well as other sham control sites. Dyson-Hudson et al.[48] compared acupuncture and *Trager psychophysical integration*, a form of manual therapy with mental exercises, over a 5-week period. Both groups reported a decrease in shoulder pain that was maintained throughout the posttreatment period.

Longer term follow-up and larger samples are needed. When patients are given acupuncture using a longer assessment period of 3 months, about half report continued improvement in pain relief.[123] Interestingly, expectation of treatment outcome by the patient (assessed through survey) was not predictive of pain relief. Again, the importance of control/comparison groups must be emphasized, with consideration of patient groups who have more individualized treatments compared with "standardized groups." More appropriate representation of the clinical situation can then be made.

Yamashita et al.[219] reviewed the issue of AEs with acupuncture and found that in 124 reported cases, the second most common AE was SCI (18 patients, 14.5%). Needle breakage was responsible for more than a third of the reported SCIs, indicating the importance of and need for strong and focused training.

MASSAGE

A few studies address the use of massage therapy in the treatment of CNS problems, with the majority of the published articles in Russian or German. Of the small number of English-language studies reviewed to date, most pertain to the use of massage therapy in the treatment of SCI, in terms of reflex responses and circulatory difficulties.

One study examined the effect of a 3-minute therapeutic massage of the triceps surae muscle group for its effect on the H-reflex amplitude in 10 individuals with SCI.[55] Although a decrease in mean peak-to-peak amplitude in the H-reflex occurred during massage, no long-term effects were noted. In another study, massage therapy with elastic stocking compression was used to treat thrombophlebitis in individuals with SCI.[196] Twenty-six subjects with complete paraplegia or tetraplegia were given massage and permanent elastic stocking compression, in addition to active and passive mobilization of the extremities. A control group of 15 paraplegic and tetraplegic patients were given treatment with only mobilization of the extremities. No evidence of thrombophlebitis or pulmonary embolism was observed in any of the massage/compression subjects, compared with a 40% incidence of thrombophlebitis and a 13% incidence of pulmonary embolism in the control group.

Casady and Curry[26] discussed the benefits of light sacral massage for pressure ulcer prevention in SCI patients when used in the immediate postinjury period. In a retrospective review of medical records of 49 acutely injured SCI patients, the authors found that length of immobilization was significantly associated with subsequent decubitus ulcer formation and therefore suggested that of pressure-relieving therapies such as massage should be used in the early stages of acute SCI. A description of the proper application of massage to pressure areas can be found in Tappan.[183] For the immobilized patient, massage therapy can be useful in alleviating muscular tightness in the back or neck caused by the long-term maintenance of a particular body position. It can also facilitate relaxation and sleep for a patient who may be tense or in an uncomfortable position. Massage has been suggested for spastic and flaccid paralysis after stroke,[212] indicating its potential applicability to treat paralysis in the SCI population as well.

CHIROPRACTIC

A few studies have examined chiropractic manipulation for SCI patients. In a randomized double-blind study of 30 patients who experienced pain 12 weeks after "whiplash" trauma sustained in MVAs, chiropractic (including "phasic neck exercises" to treat eye-head-neck-arm–coordinated movements) produced significant reduction in neck pain.[52] In a case study an 11-year-old boy who had a diagnosis of incomplete tetraplegia below the seventh cervical vertebra (C7) experienced little change during 3 months of conventional treatment but demonstrated substantial improvement in motor functioning after 2 weeks of spinal manipulation (in addition to a rehabilitation program that continued for 2 months).[217] In another case study a man who sought medical attention for post-MVA paralysis of both arms and legs caused by a dislocation of C5 was given a relaxant, anesthesia, and treatment with closed manipulation, which reportedly resulted in a rapid and full recovery.[47]

HYPNOSIS

After hypnosis and self-hypnosis, a spinal cord–injured patient reported decreased "phantom pain" in his paralyzed arm, allowing a return to work.[175] Another SCI patient showed improved strength, decreased pain, and increased functional use of his arms.[101] Attempts to treat spasticity have apparently been less successful.[30]

ENERGY HEALING

Two studies from China evaluated paralysis and SCI. In one study, 43 paralysis patients (19 hemiplegic, 24 paraplegic) were treated with emitted qi from several Qi Gong masters.[73] Treatment also included massage of certain acupoints and performance of Qi Gong exercises that had been adjusted for physical limitations attributable to the paralysis. Results indicated that there were improvements in various functional indicators, including range of motion, walking, and activities of daily living, and in various psychosomatic symptoms. In an animal study, young pigs with surgically induced SCI received either Qi Gong or no treatment.[205] After 3 months, 91% of the pigs receiving Qi Gong could walk, whereas 0% of pigs in the control group could walk.

The quality of these two studies is not known because the information is based only on brief abstracts of conference presentations. In addition to the limited research evidence, a number of practitioners and at least one hospital in China specialize in the use of Qi Gong to treat paralysis and other neurologic disorders. Walker[202] claimed that thousands of paralysis patients have been treated at the Army General Qi Gong Hospital in Beijing, with 90% showing some improvement and 46% experiencing complete recovery from their paralysis. On the other hand, Brown[23] reported that a well-known Qi Gong master from China was unable to improve functioning in post-stroke hemiplegia patients in a controlled demonstration study conducted in the United States.

HYPERBARIC OXYGEN

Ishihara et al.[77] reported that in 22 patients who had received HBO, a significant correlation was found between HBO and recovery rate of motor scores on discharge, as measured by the American Spinal Cord Association index.

◤ Multiple Sclerosis

Multiple sclerosis (MS) is a chronic disease of the CNS white matter, the cause of which is unknown. MS is the third most common cause of significant disability in young to middle-age adults, exceeded only by trauma and arthritis.[160] MS is characterized by diffuse lesions or plaques, with the highest incidence of lesions occurring in the periventricular white matter. This degeneration is primarily caused by scattered neuronal demyelination and oligodendrocyte loss throughout the CNS.[114,152] Recent clinical data implicate autoimmune mechanisms, perhaps triggered by an unknown infectious agent or environmental factors encountered early in life.[184] The disruption in neurotransmission mainly results from the destruction and scarring of myelin.[193]

Magnetic resonance imaging (MRI) studies involving MS have reported breakdowns in the blood-brain barrier and abnormal autoimmune response, possibly of viral cause. In addition to producing a marked decrease in life expectancy, $9^1\!/_2$ years in men and 14 years in women, MS can produce profound and adverse effects on an individual's physical, mental, and social well-being.[184]

The earliest symptoms of MS are usually somatosensory, including tingling and burning sensations, tightness of the extremities, and less often, severe neuralgic pains. Numbness or absence of sensory symptoms occurs less often. Vision is often impaired in MS because of the optic nerve's susceptibility to MS plaques, and symptoms include nystagmus, impairment in ocular motility, blurred or double vision, and optic neuritis involving unilateral dimming of vision, accompanied by photophobia and pain on eye movement. Motor symptoms include stiffness and heaviness in the extremities (usually lower) and cramps, spasms, or pain, with patients often having tonic "seizures" or dystonic posturing of parts of the body.*

---

*References 15, 67, 84, 107, 133, 189.

Symptoms may evolve into an abnormal reflex activity and tremors, which then progress to severe spastic paraparesis. It is now well known that cognitive impairments exist in individuals with MS, with prevalence rates ranging from 43% to 65%.[138] MS is a disease characterized most often by exacerbation and remission of symptoms, with each period of remission ending with a lower level of functional status. The other most common course is that of steady progression of symptoms.

The age of onset of MS ranges from 15 to 50 years. It is most often seen in young adults, with one third of all cases occurring before age 20 years.[2] The prevalence of MS is reported to be 6 to 14 per 100,000 population in the southern United States and southern Europe, increasing in the more temperate latitudes to 30 to 80 per 100,000 in Canada, northern Europe, and the northern United States. Immigration studies suggest that predisposing conditions for MS may be critical before age 15 years.

At present, no specific treatments can prevent or reverse the course of demyelination during MS progression.[193] The focus of current major treatment procedures is primarily symptomatic, with the goals of alleviating the associated complications as well as lessening the length and severity of exacerbations. Similarly, most rehabilitative procedures have not been very successful at significantly altering the course of MS. Thus MS patients often have long-term deficits and may benefit from interventions that support overall health and well-being to offset a usually progressive condition.

ACUPUNCTURE

Acupuncture shows promise as a diagnostic tool for detecting MS before its clinical manifestations are expressed.[174] For example, even early in the course of the disease, it has been reported that in individuals with MS, acupuncture points show heightened sensitivity. Furthermore, MS patients who were administered a combination of traditional acupuncture ("Tien-Hsin Twelve Points" or "Ma Dan Yang's Points") and cerebral acupuncture showed more rapid improvement, which may suggest that *combination* acupuncture may be more effective than traditional acupuncture alone. In a case study, Rampes[144] reported symptomatic improvement from the pain associated with trigeminal neuralgia. In a small study, Miller[115] reported that acupuncture was effective in reducing spasticity.

BOTANICALS

Evening primrose oil has been reported to slow the progression of MS.[190] However, it should not be assumed that botanicals are harmless simply because they are natural, or that they have positive effects in some conditions. Tyler,[191] for example, indicated that *echinacea*, a popular "immune enhancer," should not be used by persons with systemic disorders, including MS.

DIET AND NUTRITION

Several diets, high in vegetables and cereal and low in animal and butter fat, are recommended to prevent MS and prevent relapses in patients with MS. One of the most consistent epidemiologic findings in MS is the higher prevalence of MS in populations who consume diets rich in *animal fats*.[11] Swank and Dugan[178] reviewed several surveys conducted in different parts of the world and found a significant correlation between dietary fats of animal origin and incidence of MS. A case-controlled matched study of 155 patients with MS and 155 healthy control subjects showed that of several environmental risk factors considered, the MS group had a predominantly meat (verus vegetable) diet during childhood. Swank and Dugan[179] also studied the effect of low-fat diet on patients with MS with various degrees of disease severity (minimum, moderate, severe). They followed patients for 34 years and found that the greatest benefit in survival rate and activity level was seen in those with minimum disability at the onset of the trial.

Because women have a higher incidence of MS, their nutritional intake has been the subject of study.[186] Older women diagnosed with MS consumed fewer calories and less total fat. Insufficient intake was recorded involving carbohydrates, vitamin E, calcium, and zinc for women as a group.

MELATONIN

The pineal gland has been implicated in the pathogenesis of MS. Researchers studied nocturnal plasma melatonin levels and the presence of pineal calcification (PC) on CT scan in a cohort of 25 patients (age range, 27 to 72 years) admitted to a hospital for exacerbation of symptoms. They found a positive correlation between melatonin levels and age of onset of symptoms and an inverse correlation with the duration of illness. Abnormal alpha–melatonin-stimulating hormone (MSH) levels were found in more than 70% of patients. These findings support the hypothesis that MS may be associated with pineal dysfunction and suggest that alterations in the secretion of alpha-MSH may occur during exacerbation of symptoms.[24,156]

The decrease in melatonin secretion during the prepubertal period (which may disrupt pineal-mediated immunomodulation) may either stimulate the reactivation of the infective agent or increase the susceptibility to infection during the pubertal period. Similarly, the rapid fall in melatonin secretion just before delivery may account for the frequent occurrence or relapse in MS patients during the postpartum period. In contrast, pregnancy (which is associated with high melatonin concentrations) is often accompanied by remission of symptoms. Thus the presence of high melatonin levels may provide a protective effect, whereas a decline in melatonin secretion may increase the risk for the development and exacerbation of MS.[136]

MIND-BODY TECHNIQUES

T'ai chi has been used in a program designed to evaluate its usefulness in treating patients with MS.[76] A nonrandomized noncontrolled pilot study reported that walking speed increased and social functioning improved. However, with more quantifiable evaluations using systematic reviews of CAM treatments for MS,[20,74] negligible if any strong evidence exists for their use. Recently, a study of Feldenkrais, a gentle body movement technique, on MS symptoms found that subjects receiving Feldenkrais showed improvements in stress-related and mood variables when compared with a sham intervention but no change in somatic symptoms.[83a] More studies are clearly needed for this devastating medical condition.

◼ Parkinson's Disease

Parkinson's disease (PD) is a neurodegenerative movement disorder affecting approximately 1% of the population, mostly 65 years of age and older.[22] The likelihood of developing PD increases with age, a history of depression, or severe extrapyramidal manifestations. The average age of onset is around 55 years in both genders, with the range of onset showing a wide distribution of 20 to 80 years of age.[151] Men appear to be more susceptible than women, with a male/female ratio of 3:2. The mean prevalence rate of PD is approximately 160 per 100,000 population; by age 70 years, however, the rate has increased to 550 per 100,000.

The etiology of PD is believed to be a combination of factors, such as accelerated aging, toxin exposure, genetic predisposition, and oxidative stress,[80] although the cause of PD is still a matter of speculation. The most prominent symptoms of PD are tremors, bradykinesia, rigidity, and postural instability. Another common characteristic feature of PD is "freezing," a transient inability to perform active movement, especially affecting the legs, but also the eyelids, arms, and facial muscles.[46,151] Other prominent symptoms include hypokinesia and difficulty in changing direction, as well as disorders in swallowing, speech, and writing.[46] Patients with PD also typically display fatigue and dementia. Tremor is one of the first symptoms to appear and is recognized in 70% of patients.[151] Most symptoms begin unilaterally but often become bilateral as the disease progresses. Many of these impairments are probably attributable to basal ganglia involvement, which plays an important role in motor planning and programming.[46]

ACUPUNCTURE

Electroacupuncture stimulation of the fibula at low frequencies of 4 to 8 Hz reportedly resulted in reduced tremor and muscle tone in PD patients.[97] Furthermore, a complete or partial resolution of muscle rigidity or tremor was noted in 94% of 63 patients after a combination treatment involving acupuncture and herbs, with the goal of enhancing the regenerative process in the disease site at the substantia nigra–corpus striatum tract.[207]

A study reported from China evaluated 29 PD patients.[223] Acupuncture reduced medication dosages of L-dopa by as much as 30%, and 52% of subjects rated the treatments as "markedly or effectively" improving symptoms. Small samples and no controls limit the usefulness of the conclusions, as does the great variance in the duration of the disease course.

MUSIC THERAPY

Several studies have reported that active music therapy can be a useful adjunct in treating PD.[64,134] Variables such as motor movements (balance, gait), speech intelligibility, and vocal intensity were improved.

BRAIN STIMULATION

Because L-dopa may have side effects, other procedures have been used to treat PD, including deep brain stimulation. Although this procedure requires further study, several groups have reported that stimulation of the subthalamic nucleus or the internal pallidum leads to improvement in parkinsonian symptomatology (e.g., dyskinesia) and reduction in medication by as much as 65%.[100,199] More monitoring and evaluation for long-term safety are required, but results are encouraging.

MELATONIN

Melatonin may be implicated in PD. *Melatonin inhibitory factor 1 (MIF-1)*, a synthetic tripeptide, has been reported to improve symptoms of PD, attenuate L-dopa–related dyskinesias, and diminish the dyskinetic movement of patients with tardive dyskinesia. Evidence suggests that MIF-1 increases nigrostriatal dopaminergic activity, but its ability to improve these symptoms cannot be explained solely on the basis of the drug's effect on striatal dopaminergic neurons. MIF-1 has been reported to potentiate the melanocyte-whitening effect of melatonin in rats, and it produces mood elevation in patients with PD and tardive dyskinesia. Therefore the effects of MIF-1 in movement disorders may be associated with increased melatonin secretion. Hypothalamic MIF may modulate nigrostriatal dopaminergic functions in part through pineal melatonin, which would constitute a novel mechanism by which hypothalamic peptides act to modulate the expression of movement disorders.[154]

◼ Epilepsy

Epilepsy affects about 40 million people worldwide. Epileptic seizures are the result of a temporary dysfunction of the brain caused by an abnormal hypersynchronous electrical discharge of neurons in the cortex. Currently, no medical treatments are able to cure or induce permanent remission of epileptic symptoms. Treatment has three main goals: (1) elimination of seizures or reduction in their frequency, (2) avoidance of side effects associated with long-term treatments, and (3) prediction and eventual prevention of epileptogenesis.

A typical epileptic syndrome is characterized by a cluster of signs and symptoms occurring at the same time.[151] Syndromes are characterized by type, family history, presence of abnormal neurologic findings, age of onset, and patient response to medication. Epilepsy can be categorized as arising from a known versus an idiopathic or cryptogenic origin. The classification of epilepsies is largely empiric and is usually not based on pathologic or etiologic origin. The most prominent forms of epilepsy involving complex partial seizures are as follows:

1. *Temporal lobe epilepsy*, the most common syndrome observed in adults, which mainly involves the hippocampus, amygdala, and parahippocampal gyrus
2. *Frontal lobe epilepsy*, characterized by bizarre motor and vocal manifestations and showing almost no abnormality on EEG recordings

3. *Epilepsia partialis continua* (EPC), involving unremitting motor seizures that may involve part or all of the body
4. *Posttraumatic epilepsy,* which occurs after brain injury and is usually observed in the first year after the accident

Seizures in generalized epilepsy are subdivided to include such types as *absence* seizures, *tonic-clonic* seizures, and "benign convulsions" and "neonatal seizures" (mainly occurring in children and infants).[151]

ACUPUNCTURE

Acupuncture has been used to treat epilepsy both during an acute attack and after the attack during remission. When applied during an attack, acupuncture has been used to stop the convulsions, clear the phlegm, and open the orifices.[220] In a study using scalp acupuncture involving 24 acupoints with electrical stimulation duration of 0.2 second at 6 Hz, 90% of 98 subjects showed improvement.[165] On the other hand, in an animal model of epilepsy, Chen and Huang[31] concluded that acupuncture had no therapeutic effects on experimentally induced epilepsy and may even aggravate the condition. Two more recent human studies also failed to find that acupuncture either significantly reduced seizures or had any effect on quality of life.[91,172]

YOGA

Panjwani et al.[136] reported that, based on assessments made of seizure control and EEG alterations in 32 patients with idiopathic epilepsy, yoga meditation could play a beneficial role in the management of patients with epilepsy. In this study, yoga helped 4 of 10 patients to remain seizure free 6 months after treatment, with 9 of 10 patients 50% seizure free and a decline in the mean number of attacks per month. This is the only study to meet inclusion criteria in a 2000 Cochrane Collaboration review.[143]

Future yoga-epilepsy studies need to address methodologic design issues of (1) potential interactions with medication, (2) the wide variety of seizures seen in epilepsy, (3) the wide range of yoga procedures that can be used, and (4) most important, the actual make-up of a control group.[142] It will be useful to compare (through randomization) yoga with another type of CAM therapy so as to potentially reduce the control problem and provide for more clinically driven, practical analyses.

MELATONIN

Researchers have found that melatonin lowers the excitability of individual neurons and acts as a mild anticonvulsant. Patients with epilepsy whose brain wave patterns were evaluated both before and after injection of melatonin displayed normalized brain waves after injection. Recent data from biochemical and electrophysiologic studies support the concept that the anticonvulsant and depressive effects of melatonin on neuron activity may depend on its antioxidant and anti-excitotoxic roles, that is, acting as a free-radical scavenger and brain glutamate receptor regulator.[1,146]

PSYCHOLOGIC TREATMENT

A Cochrane review group recently evaluated psychologic interventions such as biofeedback, relaxation, and cognitive therapy for the treatment of epilepsy. Although a few studies have reported that anxiety and depression were reduced, most of the research has not been well done or is incomplete, and conclusive evidence is not available.

SURGICAL INTERVENTION

A systematic review of 126 articles on the control of seizures through the use of *temporal lobectomy* found that about 70% (median) of studies reported positive effects (i.e., seizure free).[112] The best outcome was reported with more recent studies. *Vagus nerve stimulation* for partial seizures seems to produce some efficacious results and is well tolerated with a low incidence of AEs, primarily hoarseness.[140]

SUMMARY

Alternative treatments used as complementary tools show promise in helping to treat a variety of the signs and symptoms in patients with neurologic disorders. Impairments resulting from neurologic injury may manifest across multiple functional domains and may affect such diverse areas as cognition, affect, sensation, motor activity/control, proprioception, and regulation of autonomic, autoimmune, and vascular function. Thus, given the complexity of the systemic dysregulation that may follow neurologic injury, functional activities are often affected in an equally variable manner. CAM therapies provide an equally diverse spectrum of techniques that may expand the clinician's range of options.

Neurologic disorders, however, do not merely represent clusters of signs and symptoms, but rather manifest in the struggles and challenges faced by patients, families, and society. These patients reflect a growing cultural, religious, and ethnic diversity—a diversity that embraces many of the concepts and practices of CAM. It is from this social context that alternative therapies may represent socially, medically, and economically viable complementary options for treating acute and chronic neurologic impairments. For example, depressed mood, motivation, and feelings of self-efficacy, which may influence the course and effectiveness of mainstream medicine, may be treated with *hypnotherapy*. *Craniosacral therapy* may be a useful supplemental approach in multidisciplinary programs for the treatment of spinal cord and brain injuries.

The emotional and psychologic impact of neurologic disorders can be devastating to patients and families. Thus the integration of *religion* and *spirituality* treatment methods into mainstream medicine may offer a solace that could be beneficial to them. *Massage* therapy has reportedly shown efficacy in the prevention of thrombophlebitis and pulmonary embolism in SCI patients with paraplegia, as well as in the treatment of symptoms arising from stroke. *Acupuncture* has been used to treat pain, dysphasia, and disorders of motor control, sensation, and cognition. *Bioelectromagnetic techniques* have shown promise in the treatment of skin wounds, pain, depression, and cognitive impairments, as well as in the diagnosis and assessment of motor/nerve pathway function. *Herbal* and *pharmacologic* treatments have been used to treat a variety of neurologic signs and symptoms. For example, GBE has shown antiplatelet properties and vascular regulatory activity and has also been used to treat disorders of memory, affect, and information processing.

If the efficacy of various CAM therapies is validated in well-designed clinical trials, will mainstream medicine use them? In surveys evaluating the attitudes of North American physicians toward "alternative" therapies, 50% to 70% of physicians have recommended that their patients see a specialist in some form of CAM.[16,56,197] However, many physicians have reported little understanding of alternative techniques.[56,94] In a Canadian study, 56% of general practitioners thought that concepts and methods of CAM could be of benefit in conventional medical practice.[197] In a survey of U.S. physicians, 70% of the respondents expressed an interest in training in various areas of CAM.[16] Overall, a growing number of physicians seem to view CAM as offering potential treatment benefits that could enrich mainstream medicine and the health and well-being of their patients.

REFERENCES

1. Acuna-Castroviejo D et al: Cell protective role of melatonin in the brain, *J Pineal Res* 19(2):57, 1995.
2. Adams RD, Victor M: *Principles of neurology*, ed 5, New York, 1993, McGraw-Hill.
3. Alexander CN et al: Transcendental meditation, mindfulness, and longevity: an experimental study with the elderly, *J Pers Soc Psychol* 57(6):950, 1989.
4. Anderson DC et al: A pilot study of hyperbaric oxygen in the treatment of human stroke, *Stroke* 22(9):1137, 1991.
5. Anton-Tay F, Diaz JL, Fernandez-Guardiola A: On the effect of melatonin upon human brain: its possible therapeutic implications, *Life Sci* 10(15):841, 1971.
6. Arrigo A et al: Effects of intravenous high dose co-dergocrine mesylate ("Hydergine") in elderly patients with severe multi-infarct dementia: a double-blind, placebo-controlled trial, *Curr Med Res Opin* 11(8):491, 1989.
7. Ayala C et al: Racial/ethnic disparities in mortality by stroke subtype in the United States, 1995–1998, *Am J Epidemiol* 154(11):1057: 2001.
8. Babbs CF: Role of iron ions in the genesis of reperfusion injury following successful cardiopulmonary resuscitation: preliminary data and a biochemical hypothesis, *Ann Emerg Med* 14(8):777, 1985.
9. Backhaub C, Krieglstein J: Extract of kava (*Piper methysticum*) and its methysticin constituents protect brain tissue against ischemic damage in rodents, *Eur J Pharmacol* 215(2/3):265, 1992.
10. Basmajian JV: Biofeedback in physical medicine rehabilitation. In DeLisa JA, Gans BM, editors: *Rehabilitation medicine: principles and practice*, ed 3, Philadelphia, 1998, Lippincott-Raven.
11. Bates D: Dietary lipids and multiple sclerosis, *Upsala J Med Sci* 48(suppl):173, 1990.
12. Beloosesky Y et al: Melatonin rhythms in stroke patients, *Neurosci Lett* 319(2):103, 2002.
13. Benson H: Systemic hypertension and the relaxation response, *N Engl J Med* 296:1152, 1977.
14. Bensoussan A: Does acupuncture therapy resemble a process of physiological relearning? *Am J Acupunct* 22:137, 1994.
15. Berger JR, Sheremat WA, Melamed E: Paroxysmal dystonia as the initial manifestation of multiple sclerosis, *Arch Neurol* 41:747, 1984.
16. Berman BM et al: Physicians' attitudes toward complementary or alternative medicine: a regional survey, *J Am Board Fam Pract* 8:361, 1995.
17. Bochner F, Eadie MJ, Tyrer JH: Use of an ergot preparation (Hydergine) in the convalescent phase of stroke, *J Am Geriatr Soc* 21(1):10, 1973.

18. Brailowsky S et al: Effects of *Ginkgo biloba* extract on cortical hemiplegia in the rat. In Christen Y, Costentin J, Lacour M, editors: *Effects of* Ginkgo biloba *extract (EGb 761) on the central nervous system,* Paris, 1992, Elsevier, p 95.

19. Brain Injury Association: *Fact sheet: traumatic brain injury,* Washington, DC, 1995, Brain Injury Association.

20. Branas P et al: Treatments for fatigue in multiple sclerosis: a rapid and systematic review, *Health Technol Assess* 4(27):1, 2000.

21. Braquet P et al: Is there a case for PAF antagonists in the treatment of ischemic disease? *Trends Pharmacol Stud* 10:23, 1989.

22. Broe GA et al: Neurological disorders in the elderly at home, *J Neurol Neurosurg Psychiatry* 39(4):362, 1976.

23. Brown DA: Qigong master fails to substantiate claims during demonstration project, *MISAHA Newslett* 14/15:7, 1997.

24. Cahill GM, Grace MS, Besharce JC: Rhythmic regulation of retinal melatonin: metabolic pathways, neurochemical mechanisms, and the ocular circadian clock, *Cell Molecular Neurobiol* 11(5):529, 1991.

25. Carney N et al: Effect of cognitive rehabilitation on outcomes for persons with traumatic brain injury: a systematic review, *J Head Trauma Rehabil* 14(3):277, 1999.

26. Casady L, Curry K: The relationship between extended periods of immobility and decubitus ulcer formation in the acutely spinal cord-injured individual, *J Neurosci Nurs* 24(4):185, 1992.

27. Cedercreutz C, Lahteenmaki R, Tulikoura J: Hypnotic treatment of headache and vertigo in skull injured patients, *Int J Clin Exp Hypn* 24(3):195, 1976.

28. Chae J et al: Functional neuromuscular stimulation. In DeLisa JA, Gans BM, editors: *Rehabilitation medicine: principles and practice,* ed 3, Philadelphia, 1998, Lippincott-Raven.

29. Chapman EH et al: Homeopathic treatment of mild traumatic brain injury: a randomized, double-blind, placebo-controlled clinical trial, *J Head Trauma Rehabil* 14(6):521, 1999.

30. Chappell DT: Hypnosis and spasticity in paraplegia, *Am J Clin Hypn* 7(1):33, 1964.

31. Chen R-C, Huang Y-H: Acupuncture on experimental epilepsies, *Proc Natl Sci Counc* 8(1):72, 1984.

32. Chen Y-M, Fang Y-A: 108 cases of hemiplegia caused by stroke: the relationship between CT scan results, clinical findings and the effect of acupuncture in treatment, *Acupunct Electro-Ther Res* 15:9, 1990.

33. Christen Y, Costentin J, Lacour M: Effects of *Ginkgo biloba* extract (Egb 761) on the central nervous system. Paper presented at IPSEN Institute International Symposium, Montreaux, Switzerland, 1991.

34. Churchill PS, Dail NW: Massage/bodywork. Paper presented at Alternative Medicine: Implications for Clinical Practice, Harvard Medical School, Boston, 1996.

35. Clifton GL: Hypothermia and hyperbaric oxygen as treatment modalities for severe head injury, *New Horizons* 3(3):474, 1995.

36. Cooper MJ, Aygen MM: A relaxation technique in the management of hypercholesterolemia, *J Hum Stress* 5:24, 1979.

37. Correia M, Silva M, Veloso M: Cooling therapy for acute stroke, *Cochrane Library* 1, 2002 (online: *update software,* May 1999).

38. Crasilneck HB, Hall JA: The use of hypnosis in the rehabilitation of complicated vascular and post-traumatic neurological patients, *Int J Clin Exp Hypn* 18(3):145, 1970.

39. Croisile B et al: Long-term and high-dose piracetam treatment of Alzheimer's disease, *Neurology* 43(2):301, 1993.

40. Cross P et al: Observations on the use of music in rehabilitation of stroke patients, *Physiother Can* 36(4):197, 1984.

41. Dalby BJ: Chiropractic diagnosis and treatment of closed head trauma, *J Manipulative Physiol Ther* 19(6):392, 1993.

42. DeFeudis FV: *Ginkgo biloba* extract (EGb 761): pharmacological activities and clinical applications. In Christen Y, Costentin J, Lacour M, editors: *Effects of* Ginkgo biloba *extract (Egb 761) on the central nervous system,* Paris, 1992, Elsevier.

43. DeFeudis FV, Drieu K: *Ginkgo biloba* extract (EGb 761) and CNS functions: basic studies and clinical applications, *Curr Drug Target* 1(1):25, 2000.

44. Desai M: Paralysis, *Indian J Homeopathic Med* 23(2):109, 1988.

45. Despres L: Yoga and MS, *Yoga J* 135:94, 1997.
45a. Diamond BJ et al: Ginkgo biloba extract: mechanisms and clinical indications, *Arch Phys Med Rehabil* 81:668, 2000.
46. Dombovy ML: Rehabilitation concerns in degenerative movement disorders of the central nervous system. In Brandom RL, editor: *Physical medicine and rehabilitation*, Philadephia, 1996, WB Saunders.
47. Duke RF, Spreadbury TH: Closed manipulation leading to immediate recovery from cervical spine dislocation with paraplegia, *Lancet* 2(8246):577, 1981 (letter).
48. Dyson-Hudson TA et al: Acupuncture and Trager psychophysical integration in the treatment of wheelchair user's shoulder pain in individuals with spinal cord injury, *Arch Phys Med Rehabil* 82(8):1038, 2001.
49. Entyre BR, Abraham LD: H-reflex changes during static stretching and two variations of proprioceptive neuromuscular facilitation techniques, *Electroencephalogr Clin Neurophysiol* 63:174, 1986.
50. Exner G et al: Basic principles and effects of hippotherapy within the comprehensive treatment of paraplegic patients, *Rehabilitation* 33(1):39, 1994.
51. Ferris SH et al: Combination choline/piracetam treatment of senile dementia, *Psychopharmacol Bull* 18:84, 1982.
52. Fitz-Ritson D: Phasic exercises for cervical rehabilitation after "whiplash" trauma, *J Manipulative Physiol Ther* 18(1):21, 1995.
53. Fushitani S et al: [Studies on attenuation of post-ischemic brain injury by Kampo medicines: inhibitory effects of free radical production. I.], *Yakugaku Zasshi* 114(6):388, 1994.
54. Garrison SJ, Rolak LA: Rehabilitation of the stroke patient. In DeLisa JA, Gans BM, editors: *Rehabilitation medicine: principles and practice*, ed 2, Philadelphia, 1993, Lippincott.
55. Goldberg J et al: The effect of therapeutic massage on H-reflex amplitude in persons with a spinal cord injury, *Phys Ther* 74(8):728, 1994.
56. Goldszmidt M et al: Complementary health care services: a survey of general practitioners' views, *Can Med Assoc J* 153(1):29, 1995.
57. Gorman RF: Vertebral artery occlusion following manipulation of the neck, *NZ Med J* 90(640):76, 1979 (letter).
58. Grant G, Cadossi R, Steinberg G: Protection against focal cerebral ischemia following exposure to a pulsed electromagnetic field, *Bioelectromagnetics* 15:205, 1994.
59. Greenman PE, McPartland JM: Cranial findings and iatrogenesis from craniosacral manipulation in patients with traumatic brain syndrome, *J Am Osteopath Assoc* 95(3):182, 191, 1995.
60. Guerreo JL, Thurman DJ, Sniezek JE: Emergency department visits associated with traumatic brain injury: United States, 1995–1996, *Brain Inj* 14(2):181, 2000.
61. Gutteridge JM: Ageing and free radicals, *Med Lab Sci* 49(4):313, 1992.
62. Hafner RJ: Psychological treatment of essential hypertension: a controlled comparison of meditation and meditation plus biofeedback, *Biofeedback Self Regul* 7:305, 1982.
63. Hamann KF: Physikalische Therapie des vestibulären Schwindels in Verbindung mit *Ginkgo-biloba*-Extrakt, *Therapiewoche* 35:4586, 1985.
63a. Hamilton BB et al: A uniform national data system for medical rehabilitation. In Fuhrer MJ, editor: *Rehabilitation outcomes: analysis and measurement*, Baltimore, 1987, Brookes.
64. Haneishi MM: Effects of a music therapy voice protocol on speech intelligibility, vocal acoustic measures, and mood of individuals with Parkinson's disease, *J Music Ther* 38(4):273, 2001.
65. Hartmann A, Frick M: Wirkung eines *Ginkgo*-Spezialextraktes auf psychometrische Parameter bei Patienten mit vaskulär bedingter Demenz, *Munchener Medizinisch Wochenschrift* 133(suppl 1):23, 1991.
66. Haythornthwaite JA, Benrud-Larson LM: Psychological assessment and treatment of patients with neuropathic pain, *Curr Pain Headache Rep* 5(2):124, 2001.
67. Heath PD, Nightingale S: Clusters of tonic spasms as an initial manifestation of multiple sclerosis, *Ann Neurol* 12:494, 1986.
68. Hofferberth B: Einfluß von *Ginkgo biloba*-Extrakt auf neurophysiologische und psychometrische Meßergebnisse bei Patienten mit hirnorganischem Psychosyndrom, *Arzneimittel-Forschung* 39(8):918, 1989.

69. Hogg PK: The effects of acupressure on the psychological and physiological rehabilitation of the stroke patient, *Dissert Abstr Int* 47(2B):841, 1986.

70. Holroyd J, Hill A: Pushing the limits of recovery: hypnotherapy with a stroke patient, *Int J Clin Exp Hypn* 37(2):120, 1989.

71. Honjo H et al: Acupuncture for urinary incontinence in patients with chronic spinal cord injury: a preliminary report, *Nippon Hinyokika Gakkai Zasshi* 89(7):665, 1998.

72. Hu HH et al: A randomized controlled trial on the treatment for acute partial ischemic stroke with acupuncture, *Neuroepidemiology* 12:106, 1993.

73. Huang M: Effect of emitted qi combined with self-practice of Qigong in treating paralysis. First World Conference for Academic Exchange of Medical Qigong, Beijing, 1988 (abstract).

74. Huntley A, Ernst E: Complementary and alternative therapies for treating multiple sclerosis symptoms: a systematic review, *Complement Ther Med* 8(2):97, 2000.

75. Hurn PD et al: Deferoxamine reduces early metabolic failure associated with severe cerebral ischemic acidosis in dogs, *Stroke* 26(4):688, 1995.

76. Husted C et al: Improving quality of life for people with chronic conditions: the example t'ai chi and multiple sclerosis, *Altern Ther Health Med* 5(5):70, 1999.

77. Ishihara H et al: Prediction of neurologic outcome in patients with spinal cord injury by using hyperbaric oxygen therapy, *J Orthop Sci* 6(5):385, 2001.

78. Jain KK: Effect of hyperbaric oxygenation on spasticity in stroke patients, *J Hyperbar Med* 4(2):55, 1989.

79. Jamrozik E et al: The role of lifestyle factors in the etiology of stroke: a population-based case-control study in Perth, Western Australia, *Stroke* 25(1):51, 1994.

80. Jankovic J: Theories on the etiology and pathogenesis of Parkinson's disease, *Neurology* 43(suppl 1):29, 1993.

81. Jensen OK, Nielsen FF, Vosmar L: An open study comparing manual therapy with the use of cold packs in the treatment of post-traumatic headache, *Cephalalgia* 10(5):241, 1990.

82. Johansson BB et al: Acupuncture and transcutaneous nerve stimulation in stroke rehabilitation: a randomized, controlled trial, *Stroke* 32(3):707, 2001.

83. Johansson BB et al: Can sensory stimulation improve the functional outcome in stroke patients? *Neurology* 43:2189, 1993.

83a. Johnson SK et al: A controlled investigation of bodywork in multiple sclerosis, *J Altern Complement Med* 5:237, 1999.

84. Joynt RJ, Green D: Tonic seizures as a manifestation of multiple sclerosis, *Arch Neurol* 6:293, 1962.

85. Keli SO, Feskens EJM, Kromhout D: Fish consumption and risk of stoke: the Zutphen study, *Stroke* 25(2):328, 1994.

86. Keli SO et al: Dietary flavonoids, antioxidant vitamins, and incidence of stroke: the Zutphen study, *Arch Intern Med* 156:637, 1996.

87. Key TJ et al: Dietary habits and mortality in 11,000 vegetarians and health-conscious people: results of a 17-year follow-up, *Br Med J* 313(7060):775, 1996.

88. Kleijnen J, Knipschild P: *Ginkgo biloba*, *Lancet* 340:1136, 1992.

89. Kleijnen J, Knipschild P: *Ginkgo biloba* for cerebral insufficiency, *Br J Clin Pharmacol* 34:352, 1992.

90. Kleijnen J, Knipschild P, ter Riet G: Clinical trials of homeopathy, *Br Med J* 302:316, 1991.

91. Kloster R: The effect of acupuncture in chronic intractable epilepsy, *Seizure* 8(3):170, 1999.

92. Kraft GH, Fitts SS, Hammond MC: Techniques to improve function of the arm and hand in chronic hemiplegia, *Arch Phys Med Rehabil* 73:220, 1992.

93. Kunz K, Kunz B: The paralysis report, *J Reflexol Res Rep* 8:1, 1987.

94. LaValley JW, Verhoef MJ: Integrating complementary medicine and health care services into practice, *Can Med Assoc J* 153(1):45, 1995.

95. Le Bars PL et al: A placebo-controlled, double-blind, randomized trial of an extract of *Ginkgo biloba* for dementia, *JAMA* 278(16):1327, 1997.

96. Lerner AB, Case JD: Melatonin, *Fed Proc* 19(2):590, 1960.

97. Li S: A new method of acupuncture in treatment of Parkinson's syndrome, *Int J Clin Acupunct* 6(2):193, 1995.

98. Li S-J et al: Music and medicine in China: the effects of music electro-acupuncture on cerebral hemiplegia. In Maranto CD, editor: *Applications of music in medicine*, Washington, DC, 1991, National Association for Music Therapy, p 191.

99. Linde K et al: Are the clinical effects of homeopathy placebo effects? A meta-analysis of placebo-controlled trials, *Lancet* 350(9081):834, 1997.

100. Lopiano L: Deep brain stimulation of the subthalamic nucleus: clinical effectiveness and safety, *Neurology* 56(4):552, 2001.

101. Lucas D, Stratis DJ, Deniz S: From the clinic: hypnosis in conjunction with corrective therapy in a quadriplegic patient: a case report, *Am Correct Ther J* 35(5):116, 1981.

102. Magnusson M, Johansson K, Johansson BB: Sensory stimulation promotes normalization of postural control after stroke, *Stroke* 25(6):1176, 1994.

102a. Mahoney FI, Barthel DW: Functional evaluation: the Barthel index, *Md State Med J* 14:61, 1965.

103. Maier-Hauff K: LI 1370 nach zerebraler Aneurysma-Operation, *Munchener Medizinishe Wochenschrift* 133(suppl 1):34, 1991.

104. Manganiello AJ: Hypnotherapy in the rehabilitation of a stroke victim: a case study, *Am J Clin Hypn* 29(1):64, 1986.

105. Martienssen J, Nilsson N: Cerebrovascular accidents following upper cervical manipulation: the importance of age, gender and technique, *Am J Chiropract Med* 2(4):160, 1989.

106. Matchar DB et al: The stroke prevention patient outcomes research team: goals and methods, *Stroke* 24(12):2135, 1993.

107. Matthews WB: Tonic seizures in disseminated sclerosis, *Brain* 81:193, 1958.

108. Mayer DJ: Acupuncture: an evidence-based review of the clinical literature, *Annu Rev Med* 51:49, 2000.

109. McDonagh EW, Rudolph CJ, Cheraskin E: An oculocerebrovasculometric analysis of the improvement in arterial stenosis following EDTA chelation therapy. In Cranton EM, editor: *A textbook on EDTA chelation therapy*, New York, 1989, Human Sciences Press, p 155.

110. McGee CT, Chow EPY: *Miracle healing from China... Qigong*, Coeur d'Alene, Idaho, 1994, MediPress.

111. McGregor M, Haldeman S, Kohlbeck FJ: Vertebrobasilar compromise associated with cervical manipulation, *Top Clin Chiropract* 2(3):63, 1995.

112. McIntosh AM et al: Seizure outcome after temporal lobectomy: current research practice and findings, *Epilepsia* 42(10):1288, 2001.

113. Meyer B: A multicenter randomized double-blind study of *Ginkgo biloba* extract versus placebo in the treatment of tinnitus. In Fünfgeld EW, editor: Rökan, Ginkgo biloba: *recent results in pharmacology and clinic*, Berlin, 1988, Springer-Verlag.

114. Miller E: Deanol in the treatment of levodopa-induced dyskinesias, *Neurology* 24:116, 1974.

115. Miller RE: An investigation into the management of the spasticity experienced by some patients with multiple sclerosis using acupuncture based on traditional Chinese medicine, *Complement Ther Med* 4:58, 1996.

116. Mink RB, Dutka AJ: Hyperbaric oxygen after global cerebral ischemia in rabbits does not promote brain lipid peroxidation, *Crit Care Med* 23(8):1398, 1995.

117. Mouren X, Caillard P, Schwartz F: Study of the anti-ischemic action of Egb 761 in the treatment of peripheral arterial occlusive disease by TcPo2 determination, *Angiology* 45:13, 1994.

118. Muller JE et al: Circadian variation in the frequency of onset of acute myocardial infarction, *N Engl J Med* 313(21):1315, 1985.

119. Muller-Wieland D et al: Melatonin inhibits LDL receptor activity and cholesterol synthesis in freshly isolated mononuclear leukocytes, *Biochem Biophys Res Comm* 203(1):416, 1994.

120. Naeser MA et al: Real versus sham acupuncture in the treatment of paralysis in acute stroke patients: a CT scan lesion site study, *J Neurol Rehabil* 6:163, 1992.

121. Naeser MA et al: Acupuncture in the treatment of hand paresis in chronic and acute stroke patients: improvement observed in all cases, *Clin Rehabil* 8:127, 1994.

122. Naeser MA et al: Laser acupuncture in the treatment of paralysis in stroke patients: a CT scan lesion site study, *Am J Acupunct* 23(1):13, 1995.

123. Nayak S et al: Is acupuncture effective in treating chronic pain after spinal cord injury? *Arch Phys Med Rehabil* 82(11):1578, 2001.

124. Nayak S et al: The use of complementary and alternative therapies for chronic pain following spinal cord injury: a pilot survey, *J Spinal Cord Med* 24(1):54, 2001.

125. Ness AR, Powles JW: Fruit and vegetables, and cardiovascular disease: a review, *Int J Epidemiol* 26(1):1, 1997.

126. Ness AR, Powles JW, Khaw KT: Vitamin C and cardiovascular disease: a systematic review, *J Cardiovasc Risk* 3(6):513, 1996.

127. Neubauer RA, End E: Hyperbaric oxygenation as an adjunct therapy in strokes due to thrombosis: a review of 122 patients, *Stroke* 11(3):297, 1980.

128. Neubauer RA, Gottlieb SF, Pevsner H: Hyperbaric oxygen for treatment of closed head injury, *South Med J* 87(9):933, 1994.

129. Nighoghossian N et al: Hyperbaric oxygen in the treatment of acute ischemic stroke, *Stroke* 26(8):1369, 1995.

130. Oberpichler H et al: PAF antagonist ginkgolide B reduces postischemic neuronal damage in rat brain hippocampus, *J Cereb Blood Flow Metab* 10(1):133, 1990.

131. Olszewer E, Carter JP: EDTA chelation therapy in chronic degenerative disease, *Med Hypotheses* 27(1):41, 1988.

132. Orencia AJ et al: Fish consumption and stroke in men: 30-year findings of the Chicago Western Electric Study, *Stroke* 27(2):204, 1996.

133. Osterman PO, Westerberg CE: Paroxysmal dysarthria and other transient neurological disturbances in disseminated sclerosis, *J Neurol Neurosurg Psychiatry* 29:323, 1966.

134. Pacchetti C et al: Active music therapy in Parkinson's disease: an integrative method for motor and emotional rehabilitation, *Psychosom Med* 62(3):386, 2000.

135. Palmer C, Roberts RL, Bero C: Deferoxamine posttreatment reduces ischemic brain injury in neonatal rats, *Stroke* 25(5):1039, 1994.

136. Panjwani U et al: Effect of sahaja yoga practice on seizure control and EEG changes in patients of epilepsy, *Indian J Med Res* 103:165, 1996.

137. Park J et al: Effectiveness of acupuncture for stroke: a systematic review, *J Neurol* 248:558, 2001.

138. Peyser JM et al: Guidelines for neuropsychological research in multiple sclerosis, *Arch Neurol* 47(1):94, 1990.

139. Politis MJ, Korchinski MA: Beneficial effects of acupuncture treatment following experimental spinal cord injury: a behavioral morphological and biochemical study, *Acupunct Electro-Ther Res* 15(1):37, 1990.

140. Privitera MD et al: Vagus nerve stimulation for partial seizures, Cochrane Database System Review 1, CD 002896, 2002.

141. Rai GS, Shovlin C, Wesnes KA: A double-blind, placebo controlled study of *Ginkgo biloba* extract ("Tanakan") in elderly outpatients with mild to moderate memory impairment, *Curr Med Res Opin* 12:350, 1991.

142. Ramaratnam S: Yoga for epilepsy: methodological issues, *Seizure* 10(1):3, 2001.

143. Ramaratnam S, Sridharan K: Yoga for epilepsy, Cochrane Database System Review 2, CD 001524, 2000.

144. Rampes H: Treatment of trigeminal neuralgia with electro-acupuncture in a case of multiple sclerosis, *Acupunct Med* 12(1):45, 1994.

145. Reisberg B et al: Piracetam in the treatment of cognitive impairment in the elderly, *Drug Dev Res* 2:475, 1982.

146. Reiter RJ et al: A review of the evidence supporting melatonin's role as an antioxidant, *J Pineal Res* 18(1):1, 1995.

147. Ren H, Wang W, Ge Z: Glasgow Coma Scale, brain electric activity mapping and Glasgow Outcome Scale after hyperbaric oxygen treatment of severe brain injury, *Chin J Traumatol* 4(4):239, 2001.

148. Renaud SC: Diet and stroke, *J Nutr Health Aging* 5(3):167, 2001.

149. Rockswold GL, Ford SE: Preliminary results of a prospective randomized trial for treatment of severely brain-injured patients with hyperbaric oxygen, *Minn Med* 68:533, 1985.

150. Rockswold GL et al: Results of a prospective randomized trial for treatment of severely brain-injured patients with hyperbaric oxygen, *J Neurosurg* 76:929, 1992.

151. Rowland LP: *Merritt's textbook of neurology*, ed 9, Baltimore, 1995, Williams & Wilkins.

152. Sallstrom S: Acupuncture in the treatment of stroke patients in the subacute stage: a randomized, controlled study, *Complement Ther Med* 4:193, 1996.

153. Salzberg CA et al: The effects of non-thermal pulsed electromagnetic energy (Diapulse) on wound healing of pressure ulcers in spinal cord-injured patients: a randomized, double-blind study, *Wounds* 7(1):11, 1995.

154. Sandyk R: MIF-induced augmentation of melatonin function: possible relevance to mechanisms of action of MIF-1 in movement disorders, *Int J Neurosci* 52(1/2):79, 1990.

155. Sandyk R: Multiple sclerosis: the role of puberty and the pineal gland in its pathogenesis, *Int J Neurosci* 68(3/4):209, 1993.

156. Sandyk R, Awerbuch GI: Nocturnal plasma melatonin and alpha-melanocyte stimulating hormone levels during exacerbation of multiple sclerosis, *Int J Neurosci* 67(1/2):173, 1992.

157. Santambrogio S et al: Is there a real treatment for stroke? Clinical and statistical comparison of different treatments in 300 patients, *Stroke* 9(2):130, 1978.

158. Savage RH, Roe PF: A double blind trial to assess the benefit of *Arnica montana* in acute stroke illness, *Br Homeopath J* 66:207, 1977.

159. Savage RH, Roe PF: A further double blind trial to assess the benefit of *Arnica montana* in acute stroke illness, *Br Homeopath J* 67:210, 1978.

160. Scheinberg L, Smith CR: Rehabilitation of patients with multiple sclerosis, *Neurol Clin* 5(4):585, 1987.

161. Schneider RH, Alexander CN, Wallace RK: In search of an optimal behavioral treatment for hypertension: a review and focus on transcendental meditation. In Gentry WD, Julius S, editors: *Personality, elevated blood pressure, and essential hypertension*, Washington, DC, 1992, Hemisphere.

162. Schoenberger N et al: Flexyx Neurotherapy System in the treatment of traumatic brain injury: an initial evaluation, *J Head Trauma Rehabil* 16(3):260, 2001.

163. Sessler GJ: *Stroke: how to prevent it/how to survive it*, Englewood Cliffs, NJ, 1981, Prentice-Hall.

164. Sherr J: A case of hemiplegia, *Homeopathy Links* 7(1):27, 1994.

165. Shi Z et al: The efficacy of electro-acupuncture on 98 cases of epilepsy, *J Tradit Chin Med* 7(1):21, 1987.

166. Shiflett SC: Acupuncture and stroke rehabilitation, *Stroke* 34:1934, 2001.

167. Shiflett SC et al: Effect of Reiki treatments on functional recovery in post-stroke rehabilitation patients: a pilot study, *J Altern Complement Med* (in press).

168. Shiflett SC et al: Complementary and alternative medicine. In DeLisa JA, Gans BM, editors: *Rehabilitation medicine: principles and practice*, ed 3, Philadelphia, 1998, Lippincott.

169. Smith RC et al: Pharmacologic treatment of Alzheimer's-type dementia: new approaches, *Psychopharmacol Bull* 20:542, 1984.

170. Staas WE et al: Rehabilitation of the spinal cord-injured patient. In DeLisa JA, Gans BM, Editors: *Rehabilitation medicine: principles and practice*, ed 2, Philadelphia, 1993, Lippincott.

171. Stallibrass C: An evaluation of the Alexander technique for the management of disability in Parkinson's disease: a preliminary study, *Clin Rehabil* 11:8, 1997.

172. Stavem K et al: Acupuncture in intractable epilepsy: lack of effect on health-related quality of life, *Seizure* 9(6):422, 2000.

173. Stein DG, Hoffman SW: Chronic administration of *Ginkgo biloba* extract (EGb 761) can enhance recovery from traumatic brain injury. In Christen Y, Costentin J, Lacour M, editors: *Effects of* Ginkgo biloba *extract (EGb 761) on the central nervous system*, Paris, 1992, Elsevier.

174. Steinberger A: Specific irritability of acupuncture points as an early symptom of multiple sclerosis, *Am J Chin Med* 14(3/4):175, 1986.

175. Sthalekar HA: Hypnosis for relief of chronic phantom pain in a paralysed limb: a case study, *Aust J Clin Hypnother Hypn* 14(2):75, 1993.

176. Stolc S: [Hypoxia-reoxygenation damage to the nervous system: perspectives in pharmacotherapy], *Ceskoslovenska Fystolog* 44(1):8, 1995.

177. Sukoff MH, Ragatz RE: Hyperbaric oxygenation for the treatment of acute cerebral edema, *Neurosurgery* 10(1):29, 1982.

178. Swank RL, Dugan BB: *The multiple sclerosis diet book: a low-fat diet for the treatment of MS*, New York, 1987, Doubleday.

179. Swank RL, Dugan BB: Effect of low saturated fat diet in early and late case of multiple sclerosis, *Lancet* 336(8706):37, 1990.

180. Sze FK et al: Does acupuncture have additional value to standard poststroke motor rehabilitation? *Stroke* 33(1):186, 2002.

181. Taillandier J et al: *Ginkgo biloba* extract in the treatment of cerebral disorders due to aging: longitudinal, multicenter, double-blind study versus placebo. In Fünfgeld EW, editor: Rökan, Ginkgo biloba: *recent results in pharmacology and clinic,* Berlin, 1988, Springer-Verlag.

182. Tanigawa MC: Comparison of the hold-relax procedure and passive mobilization on increasing muscle length, *Phys Ther* 52:725, 1972.

183. Tappan FM: *Healing massage techniques: holistic, classic, and emerging methods,* Norwalk, Conn, 1988, Appleton & Lange.

184. Taylor RS: Rehabilitation of persons with multiple sclerosis. In Brandom RL, editor: *Physical medicine and rehabilitation,* Philadelphia, 1996, Saunders.

185. Thaut MH et al: Effect of rhythmic auditory cueing on temporal stride parameters and EMG patterns in hemiplegic gait of stroke patients, *J Neurol Rehabil* 7:9, 1993.

186. Timmerman GM, Stuifbergin AK: Eating patterns in women with multiple sclerosis, *J Neurosci Nurs* 31(3):152, 1999.

187. Tinianow CL, Tinianow TK, Wilcox M: Effects of hyperbaric oxygen on focal brain contusions, *Biomed Sci Instrum* 36:275, 2000.

188. Tripathi SN, Upadhyaya BN, Dwivedi LD: Management of hemiplegia with gum guggulu, *Rheumatism* 25(3):155, 1990.

189. Twomey JA, Espir MLE: Paroxysmal symptoms as the first manifestations of multiple sclerosis, *J Neurol Neurosurg Psychiatry* 43:296, 1980.

190. Tyler VE: *The honest herbal,* ed 3, New York, 1993, Pharmaceutical Products Press.

191. Tyler VE: *Herbs of choice,* New York, 1994, Pharmaceutical Products Press.

192. Uchida S et al: Prolongation of life span of stroke-prone spontaneously hypertensive rats (SHRSP) ingesting *Persimmon tannin, Chem Pharm Bull* 38(4):1049, 1990.

193. Umphred DA: *Neurological rehabilitation,* ed 2, St Louis, 1990, Mosby.

194. Upledger JE: *Your inner physician and you,* Berkeley, Calif, 1991, North Atlantic Books.

195. Upledger JE: Craniosacral therapy, *Phys Ther* 75(4):328, 1995 (letter).

196. Van Hove E: Prevention of thrombophlebitis in spinal injury patients, *Paraplegia* 16:332, 1978.

197. Verhoef MJ, Sutherland LR: Alternative medicine and general practitioners: opinions and behaviour, *Can Fam Physician* 41:1005, 1995.

198. Vodovnik L, Karba R: Treatment of chronic wounds by means of electric and electromagnetic fields. Part 1. Literature review, *Med Biol Eng Comput* 30(3):257, 1992.

199. Volkmann J: Safety and efficacy of pallidal or subthalamic nucleus stimulation in advanced PD, *Neurology* 56(4):548, 2001.

200. Vorberg G: *Ginkgo biloba* extract (GBE): a long-term study of chronic cerebral insufficiency in geriatric patients, *Clin Trials J* 22(2):149, 1985.

201. Walker JE et al: Dimethylaminoethanol in Huntington's chorea, *Lancet* 1(7818):1512, 1973.

202. Walker M: The healing powers of Qigong (Chi kung), *Towsend Letter for Doctors,* 1994.

203. Wallace RK et al: Systolic blood pressure and long-term practice of the transcendental meditation and TM-Sidhi program: effects of TM on systolic blood pressure, *Psychosom Med* 45:41, 1983.

204. Walter A: An evaluation of meditation as a stress reduction technique for persons with spinal cord injury, *Dissert Abstr Int* 46(11):3251, 1986.

205. Wan S et al: Repeated experiments by using the emitted qi in treatment of spinal cord injury. Paper presented at Second World Conference on Academic Exchange of Medical Qigong, San Clemente, Calif, 1994, China Healthways Institute (Abstract).

206. Wang RY: Effect of proprioceptive neuromuscular facilitation on the gait of patients with hemiplegia of long and short duration, *Phys Ther* 74:1108, 1994.

207. Wang X: Combination of acupuncture, Qigong and herbs in the treatment of parkinsonism, *Int J Clin Acupunct* 4(1):1, 1993.

208. Wang Z: Sequelae of cerebral birth injury in infants treated by acupressure, *J Tradit Chin Med* 8(1):19, 1988.

209. Watson NA: Acute brain stem stroke during neck manipulation, *Br Med J* 288:641, 1984.

210. Weiselfish S: An overview of Erb's palsy with case history documenting treatment with manual and craniosacral therapy, *Phys Ther Forum* 9:12, 1990.

211. Wen HL: Acute central cervical spinal cord syndrome treated by acupuncture and electrical stimulation (AES), *Comp Med East West* 6(2):131, 1978.

212. Westcott EJ: Traditional exercise regimens for the hemiplegic patient, *Am J Phys Med* 46(1):1012, 1967.

213. Wirth DP: Complementary healing intervention and dermal wound reepithelialization: an overview, *Int J Psychosom* 42(1-4):48, 1995.

214. Witte S, Anadere I, Walitza E: Improvement of hemorrheology with *Ginkgo biloba* extract: decreasing a cardiovascular risk factor, *Fortschr Medizin* 110:247, 1992.

215. Wolf SL et al: The effect of tai chi and computerized balance training on postural stability in older subjects, *Phys Ther* 77(4):371, 1997.

216. Wolfson LW, Whipple R, Derby C: Balance and strength training in older adults: intervention gain and t'ai chi maintenance, *J Am Geriatr Soc* 44:498, 1996.

217. Woo C-C: Post-traumatic myelopathy following flopping high jump: a pilot case of spinal manipulation, *J Manipulative Physiol Ther* 16(5):336, 1993.

218. Woo E et al: Homeopathic treatment of mild traumatic brain injury. Grant Application Submitted to Office of Alternative Medicine, National Institutes of Health, 1993.

219. Yamashita H et al: Systematic review of adverse events following acupuncture: the Japanese literature, *Complement Ther Med* 9(2):98, 2001.

220. Yang J: Treatment of status epilepticus with acupuncture, *J Tradit Chin Med* 10(2):101, 1990.

221. Yoffe E: Meditate away paralysis, *Nat Health* 50, 1995.

222. Zhao Z: Effect of foot reflexology on the hemiplegia by cerebral vascular thrombosis. In China Reflexology Symposium Report, China Reflexology Association, 1994.

223. Zhuang X, Wang L: Acupuncture treatment of Parkinson's disease: a report of 29 cases, *J Tradit Chin Med* 20(4):255, 2000.

SUGGESTED READINGS

Basmajian JV, Nyberg R, editors: *Rational manual therapies*, Baltimore, 1993, Williams & Wilkins.

DeLisa JA, Gans BM, editors: *Rehabilitation medicine: principles and practice*, ed 4, Philadelphia, 2003, Lippincott-Raven.

Fünfgeld EW, editor: Rökan, Ginko biloba: *recent results in pharmacology and clinic*, Berlin, 1988, Springer Verlag.

Pomeranz B, Stux G: *Scientific bases of acupuncture*, New York, 1989, Springer.

CHAPTER 8

Psychiatric Disorders

DAVID A. BARON and ANDREW BARON

This chapter reviews the extant literature on the use of several complementary and alternative medicine (CAM) treatment strategies in the treatment of psychiatric illnesses, along with an analysis of CAM usage by patients with psychiatric disorders. Database materials and methods commonly available to practitioners and one specialty database for CAM have been used in this review. The goal is to provide an overview of potentially efficacious complementary medical treatments often used in psychiatric disorders. Some portions of the CAM literature are not yet included in electronic databases; therefore the chapter is not an exhaustive review on the subject. It is hoped that the reader will gain insight into the breadth of CAM practices and the types of patients seeking these therapies for their mental health concerns.

Public interest in CAM therapies continues to grow. Between 1990 and 1997, the percentage of patients using CAM treatments rose from 33.8% to 42.1%.[46] Of the patients using CAM therapies, 53.7% were not supervised by a health care provider, and only 38.5% told their physician, despite 96% having seen their personal physician within the past year. In 2000, users of CAM treatments in the United States spent $21.2 to $32.7 billion in out-of-pocket expenses, compared with $29.3 billion paid for standard medical care.[25] Mental health concerns were among the most common conditions reported by patients seeking CAM treatment, with insomnia, depression, and anxiety the primary psychiatric complaints.[46]

In addition to addressing these provocative facts, this chapter reviews the study selection method and findings in database material available to practitioners. The epidemiology and clinical characteristics of the primary psychiatric disorders are also reviewed. Research findings are summarized, and promising CAM therapies that would benefit from further study are discussed.

◥ CAM Therapies and Psychiatric Research

Historically, research on the effectiveness of psychiatric treatments was similar to the existing data on alternative medicine. Both fields relied primarily on single-case reports, based on the belief that the detailed description and analysis of an individual case provided a more appropriate source of clinical data. Psychoanalytic treatment was difficult to evaluate using a double-blind placebo-controlled research design. Psychiatric treatment research has evolved from these early perceptions and now embraces controlled trials using appropriate statistical analysis. This approach has improved the taxonomy of psychopathology, improved treatment outcomes research, and demanded greater scientific rigor. Current psychiatric literature relegates case reports and small pilot studies to the "letters to the editor" section of journals.

The existing CAM treatment literature faces many of the same challenges that the early psychoanalytic papers had to overcome. For alternative practitioners to champion their efforts into the mainstream of care, they must employ standard research design when possible and openly challenge their own assertions.[7]

A number of conventional psychiatric treatments are also considered as CAM interventions. For example, relaxation training techniques such as biofeedback and hypnosis are accepted treatments for stress reduction in both fields. The psychiatric disorders reviewed in this chapter are those having the greatest impact on society; the CAM treatments are those with the greatest number of published reports, not necessarily the most efficacious, and those most widely used.

SCIENTIFIC EVALUATION

The studies reviewed here have met the standard of scientific merit if they satisfy the following conditions[153]:
1. The disease or syndrome of interest is clearly (operationally) defined.
2. The study includes controls consistent with the intention and design.
3. When possible, placebo controls are used (or active controls are used).
4. The study uses random sampling and random allocation.
5. When possible, blinding techniques are used.
6. Sample size is adequate to control for type 1 and type 2 errors and is appropriate for the statistics presented.
7. When possible, the study is prospective and has crossover conditions.

Other studies are reviewed based on their availability or when few studies meet the established standard.

CLINICALLY SIGNIFICANT PSYCHIATRIC DISORDERS

This chapter is limited to disorders of major clinical importance. The importance of a psychiatric disorder is derived from the following characteristics: *significant prevalence* (number of people affected), *severity* (impact on daily functioning), and *cost* (to the individual or society). Four psychiatric disorders—major depressive disorder, anxiety disorder, primary insomnia, and schizophrenia—and one psychiatric-related condition, stress, have been chosen. Each satisfies one or more of the three characteristics and is often seen in clinical practice.

Mood and anxiety disorders are common disabling conditions that generate significant costs to society. Schizophrenia, with its lifelong course and negative impact on daily functioning, is one of the most expensive illnesses to treat, despite its lower incidence. Emotional stress is pervasive in society and negatively affects overall health. These disorders all demonstrate the severity and social costs requisite for inclusion here. Sleep disturbance is a common complaint reported by patients in health care settings and, when persistent, can be disabling and extremely costly to society as well.

RELEVANT CAM PROCEDURES

The alternative medical procedures relevant to psychiatric disorders include Ayurveda, acupuncture, Qi Gong, chelation, chiropractic, craniosacral, nutritional, homeopathic, hypnosis, massage, naturopathic, herbal (e.g., *Hypericum*, kava, saunzaoretang), prayer, eye movement desensitization and reprocessing, and yogic therapies. Studies from other methods were evaluated if determined to be of potential impact. The methods reviewed were chosen based on two important factors: (1) the procedures given are the most frequently used approaches to date, and (2) the reviewable literature most available is found in medical journals.

Methodology for Identifying Research Studies

For conventional practitioners to consider the use of CAM procedures or to respond to questions about the practices of alternative therapy providers, they need to know how to obtain reliable information about these treatments and their effectiveness. The normal sources, such as specialty peer-reviewed journals, U.S. Food and Drug Administration (FDA) information, and referenced scientific publications provide, at best, limited information for those seeking to evaluate the CAM literature. Other increasingly important sources of information are electronic databases. The starting point for this review was the National Medical Library's *MEDLARS*, the most accessible and comprehensive medical database.

A MEDLARS search was conducted to identify articles for review and to determine the volume of published manuscripts. Each alternative form of treatment was entered, along with the word "research" and the specific disorder (e.g., "Ayurveda" and "research" and "anxiety"). All identified abstracts were reviewed. The abstracts generated from this search were evaluated using inclusion-exclusion criteria. The exclusion criteria were designed to remove articles not related to the diagnostic category (e.g., anxiety related to medical illness would not be counted) and those having total sample sizes less than 10. This method resulted in 14 articles that satisfied these criteria, highlighting the difficulties encountered by nonalternative health care providers in obtaining and evaluating the scientific merit of CAM treatments. By comparison, a search on "depression" and "research" identified 3225 citations, but when "acupuncture" (the most prevalent of the alternative methods identified) was added, the result was three citations.

To provide a more informative review, the search was expanded and Psychlit indices were added. In addition, a DataStar *Allied and Alternative Medicine* (AMED) database covering CAM from 1985 to the present was searched.[103] These sources were further augmented by discussions with CAM practitioners.

Mental Disorders and CAM Usage

U.S. government statistics confirm high rates of mental disorders in American citizens and that many patients do not receive proven effective mental health treatment.[117] In addition, persons suffering from mental illness are frequent consumers of general medical services.[162] Until recently, very little was known or reported about the use of CAM in people with mental illness. Unutzer et al.[172] surveyed 9585 adults who met established criteria for mental disorders to determine their use of CAM. They discovered a high rate of use of CAM interventions in study subjects who met criteria for common psychiatric disorders. These results were consistent with findings of Eisenberg et al.,[46] who reported that 40.9% of adults with depression and 42.7% of those with anxiety used CAM treatment in the previous year.

Depression

Depression is a psychopathologic condition with *disturbance in mood* as its hallmark. Being "depressed" can be a symptom of a transient mood state, a personality trait, or a major mood disorder. As a *transient mood state*, depression presents as a time-limited, subjective sense of feeling "low" or "blue." These feelings are often associated with real or perceived loss. A *depressed personality style* is characterized as the person who always "sees the glass half empty" (i.e., is overly pessimistic, with a limited capacity to experience joy). *Major depressive disorder* (MDD) is defined by the *Diagnostic and Statistical Manual of Mental Disorders* (fourth edition; *DSM*-IV) as one of the mood disorders and is operationally defined as experiencing at least five of the following symptoms or conditions:

- Feeling sad or "blue" most of the day, almost every day for at least 2 weeks
- Losing interest in past pleasurable activities
- Experiencing changes in weight and sleep patterns
- Experiencing loss of energy
- Feeling worthless, hopeless, and helpless
- Having poor concentration
- Having thoughts of not wanting to go on living

MDD is only one of the *DSM* depressive disorders. *Dysthymic disorder* is a condition similar to MDD but with less intense symptoms, no suicidal ideation, and a duration of at least 2 years. "Depressive disorder not otherwise specified" includes disorders with depressive symptoms that do not meet criteria for MDD. Other mood disorders include *bipolar disorders* (types I and II, cyclothymic disorder, "bipolar disorder not otherwise specified"), mood disorder attributable to a medical condition, substance-induced mood disorder, and "mood disorder not otherwise specified."[3]

Mood disorders may coexist with other psychiatric disorders or with nonpsychiatric medical disorders, or they may occur as a side effect of medications or illegal drug use. MDD may begin at any age but most often presents in the mid-20s through the 40s. Symptoms tend to develop gradually over days to weeks and are often attributed to stressful life events. Although some patients experience only a single episode that may remit without treatment, more than half of patients will have another depressive episode and may be at risk to develop bipolar disorder. The clinical course of recurrent major depression is highly variable and is difficult to predict. As the number of depressive episodes increases, the greater is the likelihood of additional episodes and the greater the risk of a suicide attempt.

PREVALENCE AND ECONOMIC IMPACT

The lifetime risk for experiencing a major depressive disorder is 7% to 12% for men and 20% to 25% for women. The increased incidence in women is not a function of more frequent help-seeking behavior.[138] Apart from gender differences, prevalence rates are unrelated to race, education level, income, or civil status. Recent data have demonstrated that the age at onset has decreased in many Western cultures. Post et al.[134] reported that psychosocial stressors may play little or no role in the onset of subsequent depressive episodes, contrary to conventional wisdom. A series of reports issued jointly by the Harvard School of Public Health and the World Health Organization (WHO) entitled *Global Burden of Disease and Injury Series* provides a comprehensive picture of health in eight worldwide demographic regions.[75] The results included the following conclusions:

1. In both developing and developed regions worldwide, depression is the leading cause of disease burden for women.
2. MDD was responsible for the fourth highest disease burden worldwide in 1990 and is expected to be second only to ischemic heart disease by 2020.
3. MDD was the number-one cause of disability in the world in 1990. In the United States the estimated cost of depression annually is $43.7 billion.

ETIOLOGY OF DEPRESSIVE DISORDERS

Depression, as with most psychiatric diseases, is a *genetic complex trait,* meaning many genes are likely to be responsible for the illness. The etiology of the depressive disorders is a complex interplay of genetic and environmental factors, with no single factor solely responsible. Depression is a biopsychosocial phenomenon with a number of causative factors, including biochemical, genetic, social, and psychologic. Medical illnesses, including stroke, thyroid disease, cancer, heart disease, and hepatitis, along with a long list of medications, have been associated with the development of depression.

Theories of etiology are often developed after a reported successful treatment strategy is discovered. Given the current popularity of biologic intervention for the treatment of depression, it is no surprise that genetic predisposition, monoamine synaptic transmission abnormalities, and psychologic trauma are viewed as important factors in the development of these disorders. Cultural variations in etiologic theory are often based on religious or cultural tenets, such as the yin and yang in the Asian culture and Pratyaksha-Gyan, Anuman, Yukti, and Sakhya in Indian Ayurveda.

Current conventional treatment strategies vary with the form of depression being treated. Diagnostic specificity is of utmost importance in determining appropriate treatment selection. MDD is most often treated with a combination of pharmacotherapy and psychotherapy (talk therapy). For severe, treatment-refractory depression, electroconvulsive therapy (ECT) may be used. Dysthymic disorder (DD), or less severe chronic depression, is usually treated with psychotherapy alone.[144] ECT is not indicated for DD, although antidepressant medication may be effective. Bipolar disorder is usually treated in the United States with a mood stabilizer such as lithium, valproic acid, or carbamazepine. In 2001 the FDA approved the use of olanzapine for the treatment of acute mania. Given its favorable side effect profile and ease of prescribing, olanzapine is becoming a drug of choice for many psychiatrists.

Treatment for depression resulting from a medical disease should focus on treating the underlying medical condition. For a review of current conventional treatments, the reader should consult a standard psychiatric textbook.

ADVANCES IN NEUROSCIENCE

Recent advances in neuroscience in general and specifically in neuroimaging for the first time have provided a technology to observe changes in brain function in patients with depression. Computer-analyzed electroencephalogram (CEEG), single-photon emission computed tomography (SPECT), and functional magnetic resonance imaging (FMRI) are proving to be valuable tools in identifying the neuroanatomy and neurophysiology of depression.[65] In addition to providing a better understanding of the etiology of the mood disorders, this technology may assist in monitoring the impact of current treatments and provide valuable information needed to develop and refine new therapeutic interventions.

Any treatment that results in a sustained improvement in mood and behavior should be considered biologic. "The outdated and false distinction between organic and functional psychiatric diseases (and treatments) may ultimately be abandoned."[66] Similarly, as current CAM treatments demonstrate efficacy in large, well-designed clinical trials, their distinction from conventional treatment will become blurred. Many of the therapies reviewed, although currently considered alternative, may prove in the future to be primary treatments or augmentative therapies to existing "mainstream" clinical interventions.

CAM TREATMENT STRATEGIES

The following literature review is not intended to be an endorsement or an indictment of CAM treatments for depression or any of the other mental disorders discussed. The standard used to evaluate the published studies reviewed is derived from a Western cultural perspective. Study designs that are flawed from this perspective do not necessarily invalidate the technique or procedure, but flawed designs do raise concern over claims of efficacy. With a placebo response rate as high as 50% in persons with depression, open-label trials, regardless of size, are at best suspect and difficult to generalize to a larger patient population.

In a number of areas, alternative and conventional treatment strategies overlap. Establishing and maintaining a healthful lifestyle and reducing psychologic stress are viewed as important adjuncts to treatment in both schools of thought.

ORTHOMOLECULAR THERAPY

Pauling[130,131] defines orthomolecular psychiatric therapy as the treatment of mental disease by providing the optimal molecular environment for the brain, especially the optimal concentrations of substances normally present in the human body. Pauling asserted that mental disease results from low concentrations in the brain of any one of the following vitamins: thiamine (B_1), nicotinic acid (B_3), pyridoxine (B_6), cyanocobalamin (B_{12}), biotin (H), ascorbic acid (C), and folic acid. In addition to vitamin deficiency, low molecular concentrations of essential fatty acids may also cause psychiatric symptoms.

Bell et al.[12] studied 16 nonalcoholic inpatient volunteers who met *DSM* criteria[2] for major depression ($n = 14$) or bipolar disorder ($n = 2$) by evaluating the effect of vitamins B_1, B_2, and B_6 augmentation of tricyclic antidepressant treatment in geriatric depression with cognitive dysfunction. The results, although statistically nonsignificant, did suggest a trend in improvement in affective and cognitive symptoms in the active treatment group compared with those receiving placebo. The proposed theory for the mechanism of action is that vitamin B augmentation stimulates synthesis of neurotransmitters[15] and that B complex vitamins act synergistically with tricyclics to produce enhanced clinical improvement.[33,69] The data presented in this small pilot study warrant additional, larger-scale trials to determine potential efficacy in geriatric and other depressed patients.

Based on Pauling's hypotheses that mental disease is caused by abnormal biochemical reaction rates, as determined by diet and abnormal molecular concentrations of essential substances such as *5-hydroxytryptophan* (5-HT), an endogenous serotonin precursor, studies assessing supplementation have been conducted to determine antidepressant effects. Byerley et al.[19] published an extensive review of antidepressant efficacy and adverse effects of 5-HT. In addition to providing an overview of serotonergic brain mechanisms, the study reviewed seven open-label studies of 5-HT in the treatment of depression.[173] Sano[150] studied 107 patients with endogenous depression and reported that 74 (69%) were either cured or showed dramatic improvement after 5-HT treatment. Fujiwara and Otsuki,[59] following a similar design, reported marked improvement in four and improvement in 6 of 20 endogenously depressed patients. Matussek et al.[114] found that 7 of 24 depressed study subjects were either symptom free or had a "good improvement" with 5-HT supplementation. Similarly, Takahashi, Kondo, and Kato[166] reported that 7 of 24 moderately to severely depressed inpatients had a "clear-cut" recovery when treated with 5-HT. Nakajima, Kudo, and Kaneko[125] reported a favorable response in 40 of 59 (67.8%) depressed patients. Kaneko et al.[86] reported improvement in 10 of 18 patients with endogenous depression. In all, 148 of 251 (59%) patients given treatment with 5-HT were reported as improved (Table 8-1).

TABLE 8–1. **SEROTONIN (5-HT) IN TREATMENT OF DEPRESSION***

Study	N	Improvement
Sano[150]	107	69%
Fujiwara, Otsuki[59]	20	50%
Matussek et al.[114]	24	29%
Takahashi et al.[166]	24	29%
Nakajima et al.[125]	59	68%
Kaneko et al.[86]	18	56%

*All studies open-label design, with imprecise diagnosis.

All these trials were open-label trials, lacked diagnostic rigor in identifying their study populations, and were limited by a study period of only 3 to 4 weeks. In addition to the open-label trials, five double-blind controlled studies were reported.[3,108,116,174,175] The results of the double-blind trials revealed an initial efficacy but a reduction of effectiveness over time, possibly reflecting a placebo effect. 5-HT may potentiate the effectiveness of *monoamine oxidase inhibitors* (MAOIs).[108] The study of Mendlewicz and Youdin[116] was the only one that did not demonstrate 5-HT to be more effective than placebo. Byerley et al.,[19] after reviewing all the studies, concluded that 5-HT has antidepressant properties; however, double-blind, placebo-controlled investigations with large sample sizes of well-defined patients are clearly indicated to assess effectiveness definitively. Final conclusions should be reserved until data from larger, better-controlled trials are analyzed.

Rosenbaum et al.[143] conducted an open-label pilot study of oral *S*-adenosylme Thionine (SAM) in the treatment of major depression. SAM is synthesized from L-methionine and adenosine triphosphate by methionine adenosyltransferase.[21,67] Reynolds and Stramentinoli[139] demonstrated that SAM is directly involved in the metabolism of folate. This compound is widely marketed in Europe for the treatment of osteoarthritis and a number of hepatic conditions.[111,119] SAM is also reported to have potent antiinflammatory properties, with fewer side effects than ibuprofen.[111] Fazio et al.[51] tested the efficacy of SAM in treating schizophrenia and noted an improvement in mood only. In a follow-up open trial with depressed patients, they reported remission in 14 of 35 patients. Using intravenous (IV) SAM in single-blind studies, independent investigators reported the compound to be an effective antidepressant with a more rapid onset of action and far fewer side effects than tricyclic antidepressants.[4,106] Rosenbaum et al.[143] reviewed six double-blind, placebo-controlled studies that demonstrated increased effectiveness when compared with placebo (Table 8-2). Consistent study design flaws were a lack of diagnostic homogeneity, varying degrees of symptom severity in the study population, and small sample size. Carney, Chary, and Bottiglieri[22] reported that 3 of 12 (25%) positive responders to IV SAM had a "switch state" to mania or hypomania.

SAM appears to have putative antidepressant effects. Its possible mechanism of action is unknown but may be related to an increase in serotonin turnover,[2] inhibition of norepinephrine reuptake, or increase in folate activity. Despite promising preliminary results and the call for additional large-scale efficacy trials, recent research with

TABLE 8–2. *S*-ADENOSYLMETHIONINE (SAM) IN TREATMENT OF DEPRESSION

Study	N	Results	Design
Fazio et al.[51]	35	40% improved	Open label
Carney et al.[22]	12	25% improved	Open label
Angoli et al.[4]	14	Effective	Single blind
Rosenbaum et al.[143]	6	Effective	Double blind
Lipinski et al.[106]	14	Effective	Single blind

this compound could not be identified. Additional studies exploring SAM's effectiveness as monotherapy or as an augmentation antidepressant are indicated.

Alpha-methyltryptophan (AMPT), a precursor of alpha-methylserotonin (AM5HT), is a synthetic analog of the endogenous amino acid *tryptophan*.[141] Sourkes[163] described AM5HT as a "substitute neurotransmitter" that metabolizes slowly and is present in the system for long periods (no actual time was reported) after a single dose. In the 1991 concept report, Sourkes proposed that alpha-methyltryptophan may be effective in treating depression and sleep disorders. No clinical trial data were presented.

Using 5-HT alone and in combination with a peripheral decarboxylase inhibitor in the treatment of depression, an open-label study of 25 depressed patients found therapeutic efficacy to be equal to that of traditional antidepressants, with a more rapid onset of action.[191] This study, however, had serious methodologic flaws. In 18 of the 25 patients there were no fixed trial conditions, and clinical evaluations were determined from a retrospective analysis of case records.

In addition to reviewing the use of L-tryptophan as an antidepressant/hypnotic and its metabolic activity, Boman[14] provides an extensive review of the published clinical trials on the use of L-tryptophan for depression and sleep disorders. He pointed out the frequent flaws in methodology but was able to identify a large ($n = 115$) 12 week double-blind, placebo-contolled study.[170] The findings were that tryptophan and amitriptyline were of equal antidepressant potency and that the combination of the two compounds was superior to either drug used alone. All active medication groups were significantly more effective than placebo. Although the research design was acceptable, the identification of depressed study subjects was poorly defined, and the issue of diagnostic homogeneity was not addressed. No mention was made of attempts to control for other clinical variables. Better-controlled trials are warranted, particularly in the use of L-tryptophan as an augmentation agent with an MAOI.

HYPERICUM (ST. JOHN'S WORT)

Plant extracts have been used for centuries to treat a wide variety of illnesses. *Hypericum perforatum*, a member of the Hypericaceae family, commonly known as St. John's wort, is a botanical indicated for the treatment of anxiety, depression, and insomnia. This compound has been licensed in Germany since 1984 and is reported to be a popular remedy for mood symptoms.

In an overview and meta-analysis of randomized clinical trials of St. John's wort for depression, Linde et al.[105] reported that the *Hypericum* extracts contain at least

10 active components that may contribute to its pharmacologic effects (Table 8-3). They include flavonoids, naphthodianthrones, xanthones, and bioflavonoids. Holzl[80] claimed that the mechanism of action as an antidepressant is unclear. Bisset et al.,[13] however, reported that *hypericin,* one of the active constituents, is an experimental MAOI and claimed that an average daily dose of 2 to 4 g (equal to 0.2 to 1.0 mg of hypericin) may be effective in treating psychogenic disturbances, depressive states, anxiety, or nervous excitement. Wagner and Bladt[178] challenged this assertion on the basis that it has not been confirmed in adequately controlled trials.

In their meta-analysis, Linde et al.[105] searched Medline Silver Platter CD-ROM (1983 to 1994), Psychlit and PsychIndex (1987 to 1994), Medline (1966 to 1996), and Phytodok and Embase (1974 to 1996) with no language restrictions and identified 23 randomized trials, which included 1757 outpatients with mild to moderately severe depression. Fifteen trials were placebo controlled, and eight compared *Hypericum* with another drug treatment. All the trials were conducted outside the United States and were assessed by at least two reviewers. Had the search been restricted to English-language publications, no studies would have been identified. Their results showed that *Hypericum* extracts were significantly superior to placebo and comparably effective to standard antidepressants. Their primary criticisms were the lack of well-defined groups of patients, varying extract concentrations, and use of doses ranging from 300 to 1000 mg/day.

Linde et al.[105] also noted that unpublished trials and multiple publications from the same data set could have led to an artificially inflated number of subjects who participated in published trials. Concerning adverse side effects, their review found a low incidence of reported problems with tolerance. Phototoxicity was reported in animals taking high doses of *Hypericum.* No data were provided regarding long-term safety in humans.

Gelenberg[64] reviewed the literature on St. John's wort. In addition to clarifying that the word "Wort" is Old English for "plant," Gelenberg reviewed Ernst's literature search on *Hypericum.*[48] He identified 14 studies comparing *Hypericum* with placebo and four comparing *Hypericum* with conventional antidepressant medications. The majority of the studies were conducted within the last few years, written in German, and published in journals unfamiliar to an international audience. Eight of the trials were placebo controlled and met conventional methodologic standards. All eight studies concluded that St. John's wort produced minimal adverse side effects and was superior to placebo. Gelenberg concluded, "The fact that a product is natural does not

TABLE 8–3. *HYPERICUM* **(ST. JOHN'S WORT): MECHANISM OF EFFECT**

Study	Results
Linde et al.[105]	At least 10 active components
Holzl[80]	Unclear mechanism
Bisset et al.[13]	MAOI-like effect
Wagner, Bladt[178]	Unknown, but not MAOI

MAOI, Monoamine oxidase inhibitor.

mean that it is either safe or efficacious. By the same token, there is no reason why an herb or other plant product cannot have healing powers."[64]

Hubner, Lande, and Podzuweit[84] conducted a randomized placebo-controlled, double-blind trial on the effects of *Hypericum* treatment on 39 patients with mild depression and somatic symptoms. Symptoms were monitored using the Hamilton Depression (HAMD) scale, the von Zerssen Health Complaint Survey, the Clinical Global Impressions (CGI) scale, and questions on somatic symptoms. The authors reported that 70% of patients treated with *Hypericum* were symptom free after 4 weeks and had significantly improved ($p < .05$) HAMD scores compared with the placebo group (Figure 8-1). These results, according to the authors, support the effectiveness of *Hypericum* in mild depression.

Woelk, Burkard, and Grunwald[187] conducted a drug-monitoring survey study of 663 private practitioners on the effectiveness of *Hypericum* extract LI 160 in 3250 patients. Their results suggested its effectiveness and tolerability in the reduction of physical symptoms associated with mild and moderate depression, as measured by the depression scale of von Zerssen (Figure 8-2). Adverse side effects were reported by 79 patients (2.4% of the sample), and 48 (1.5%) discontinued treatment during the trial. The authors concluded that 30% of the study patients "normalized or improved" during *Hypericum* treatment. Although this large sample size suggests safety, conclusions supporting effectiveness are questionable due to the lack of randomization of subjects and absence of placebo controls.

Medicine is an empiric science; some purported remedies have been found to be ineffective or even hazardous when subjected to systematic study, but others have "stood the test of time and science."[64] Despite preliminary results warranting larger

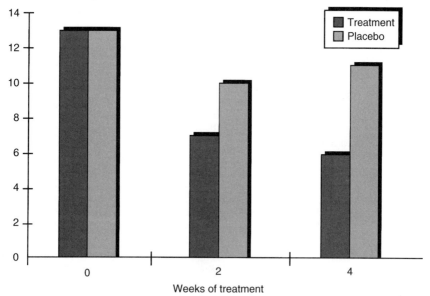

FIGURE 8–1. Improvement after 4 weeks of *Hypericum* treatment (St. John's wort) compared with placebo. *(Modified from Hubner WD, Lande S, Podzuweit H: J Geriatr Psychiatr Neurol 7[suppl 1]:12, 1994.)*

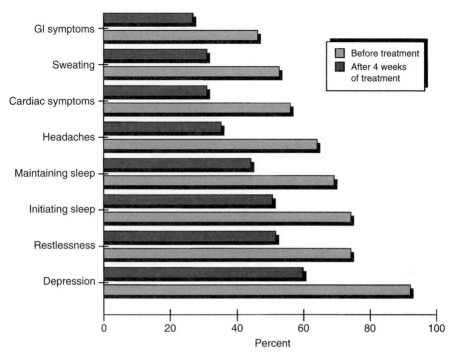

FIGURE 8–2. Percentage of 3250 patients displaying symptoms before and after treatment with *Hypericum* extract. GI, Gastrointestinal. *(Modified from Woelk H, Burkard G, Grunwald J: J Geriatr Psychiatr Neurol 7[suppl 1]:34, 1994.)*

trials, Gelenberg[64] recommended against the use of St. John's wort in 1997 because of an absence of data regarding long-term safety, efficacy, and product purity of non-FDA-regulated nutritional supplements. Interestingly, no review of the other single or multicenter trials reported on the possible use of St. John's wort as an adjunctive agent with standard antidepressant treatments.[72,112,155,186] Given the supplement's well-documented lack of side effects, this may be a reasonable area for future clinical trials (Table 8-4).

One methodologic problem in all the studies reviewed was the lack of diagnostic rigor used to identify a homogeneous depressed patient population. The operational definition of depression varies greatly in the studies; some used highly reliable measures, and others appeared to allow for the inclusion of patients with other forms of psychopathology. To compare results in depression treatment studies accurately, it is important for the study design to control for patient variables such as age, gender, and most important, type of depression.

A more recent study identified 200 adult outpatients with major depression confirmed by four standard psychometric instruments. Using a randomized double-blind placebo-controlled design, Shelton et al.[159] concluded that St. John's wort was not effective in treating major depression. However, *Hypericum* may be effective in mild to moderate depression in some patients or as adjunctive therapy.

TABLE 8–4. *HYPERICUM* **(ST. JOHN'S WORT) IN TREATMENT OF DEPRESSION**

Study	Results	Design
Linde et al.[105]	Superior to placebo	Meta-analysis: 23 randomized trials
Gelenberg[64]	Superior to placebo	Comparison: 18 trials (8 controlled)
Hubner et al.[84]	Effective: minor depression	Double blind, placebo (n = 39)
Woelk et al.[187]	Effective, low side-effects	Survey: 663 practitioners Nonrandomized, no controls
Schmidt, Sommer[155]	Effective: moderate depression	Multicenter, no controls
Martinez et al.[112]	Effective: moderate depression	Multicenter, nonrandomized
Witte et al.[186]	Effective: moderate depression	Multicenter, open
Shelton et al.[159]	Not effective	Randomized controlled meta-analysis, 200 confirmed patients

Finally, in response to the growing popularity of St. John's wort for the over-the-counter treatment of depressions, the National Center for Complementary and Alternative Medicine (NCCAM), the National Institute of Mental Health (NIMH), and the Office of Dietary Supplements (ODS) funded one of the first large-scale, multisite clinical trials of the compound in the United States.[84a] This randomized double-blind, placebo-controlled trial included 340 study subjects from multiple clinical sites across the country and was headed by Jonathan Davidson, M.D., professor of psychiatry at Duke University Medical Center. In addition to St. John's wort, the study design included the use of the FDA-approved antidepressant sertraline (Zoloft) to assess the sensitivity of the trial in detecting antidepressant drug effects.

The study included two phases: the acute phase and the continuation phase. The acute phase measured the antidepressant response during the first 8 weeks on St. John's wort, placebo, or Zoloft. This was the primary focus of the study. The continuation phase, or follow-up, offered positive responders to Phase 1 (acute) treatment the option to continue on their study drug for an additional 18 weeks. Continuation phase data were designed to evaluate longer-term use of the treatments.

The results of the study demonstrated that St. John's Wort treatment did improve depression rating scores, but no more than placebo treatment. In fact, placebo treatment was slightly better. Zoloft improved depression-rating scores more than either placebo or St. John's wort, but only minimally. In addition, 24% of patients taking St. John's wort reported a complete remission of symptoms, compared with 32% and 25% on Zoloft.

Does this mean St. John's wort is not effective in treating depression? Not necessarily. The fact that it was no better than placebo confirms that placebo treatment can be effective therapy, particularly in the early phases of treatment. The importance of the placebo response has been well documented by Benson and others, reviewed in this text.

The results of this trial underscore the need for well-designed, methodologically sound clinical studies to help determine the effectiveness of any compound that claims to treat depression.

HERBAL TREATMENTS

Saiko-ka-ryukotsu-borei-to, an Oriental compound, is reported to be effective in treating anxiety and depression.[151] Saki and Pogady,[149] reporting on the use of herbal drugs to treat resistant depression, claimed that saiko-ka-ryukotsu-borei-to can be used in patients unable to tolerate conventional anxiolytics and antidepressants. They advocated the use of this agent in combination with low doses of standard medications. Presenting data on the biochemical properties of several herbal preparations, the author concluded that the efficacy of herbal medicines has not yet been demonstrated in double-blind controlled studies and that the effective components are still unknown. The same plant might contain varying levels of bioactive components depending on the stage of plant growth, plant location, and environmental conditions in different years.[149]

Although weak with regard to clinical application, this study demonstrates that an accurate analysis of herbal compounds is attainable and is an important first step in assessing the role of these compounds in treating depression.

Kampo, traditional Asian medicine, is a combination compound used to treat physical and psychiatric disorders. Tanra et al.[167] described a new kampo compound, *TJS-010*, as having possible antidepressant or anxiolytic effects. TJS-010 is composed of seven herbal ingredients. No human trials were cited, although animal (rat) laboratory data were presented. The animal experiments were well controlled and demonstrated biologic activity. Before making assumptions about efficacy of TJS-010 in humans, Phase I (clinical safety in normal control subjects), Phase II (effectiveness in identified patients), and Phase III (multicenter trials with large numbers of patients) clinical trials are needed.

ACUPUNCTURE

Acupuncture has been used for centuries to treat virtually all forms of pain and disease. Xiujuan[188] reported on 20 cases of "mental depression" treated at the Institute of Mental Health at Beijing Medical University by inserting needles into extrachannel points. Study subjects were compared with 21 control cases medicated with amitriptyline. Results, as measured by HAMD scale ratings, revealed no significant differences in therapeutic effects. A detailed description is provided on how and where the needles were applied. Study patients were described as manic depressive, involutional depressive, and depressive neurotic. Neither the determination of diagnosis nor the control (or lack) of other clinical variables was described. A literature search revealed two other published clinical trials confirming Xiujuan's results.[28,142]

In a series of three case reports, Kurland[96] used acupuncture augmented by electrical stimulation of the needles (*Acu-EST*). He concluded that Acu-EST was less effective than ECT but did assist in reducing symptoms of depression without producing memory impairment; "Acu-EST was a reasonable alternative to ECT." This statement cannot be supported by a case series of three but does warrant a well-controlled clinical trial.

HOMEOPATHY

Reilly et al.[135] claimed homeopathic treatment may be used as primary therapy in combination with conventional interventions. Davidson et al.,[36] reporting on homeopathic treatment of depression and anxiety, described a case of a 47-year-old woman whose depressive and anxious symptoms improved after receiving fluoxetine (Prozac) and calcarea carbonica (a homeopathic remedy). It is difficult to evaluate efficacy based on single case reports, and no other controlled trials could be identified. Larger, well-controlled trials are warranted.

AYURVEDA

Ayurveda, according to Hindu mythology, is the "medicine of the gods." This ancient Indian treatment has its roots in religion and metaphysics. Ayurvedic treatment of mental illness includes herbal preparations and various forms of psychotherapy. Clinical trials using Ayurveda for the treatment of depression appear to be lacking, although Dube[44] describes the nosology and therapy of mental illness in Ayurveda. Others provide comprehensive overviews of psychiatric training, therapies, and theory in the ayurvedic tradition.[45,128]

T'AI CHI CHUAN

An ancient Chinese proverb, "Stagnant water is putrid," is interpreted to emphasize the importance of regular exercise in promoting good physical and mental health.[93] Specific forms of sitting, stretching, and squatting to promote health date back to 770 BC in China. T'ai chi chuan (t'ai chi) is traditional Chinese shadow boxing and is now commonly used to promote health. A review of the literature on exercise in the treatment of depression concluded that regular exercise reduces the stress often associated with depression and the intensity of mood symptoms.[113,140]

AROMATHERAPY

Aromatherapy is the use of distinct fragrances to treat disease. Rovesti and Colombo[145] divided several fragrances with purported psychotropic effects into two categories, nerve sedative and nerve stimulant.

In a report on the effects of citrus fragrance on immune function and depressive states, using an open-label design, Komori et al.[94] studied 20 depressed male inpatients who met *DSM* criteria for MDD[2] and 20 age-matched normal controls. In addition to monitoring depression ratings, extensive neuroimmunologic parameters were followed. Results revealed that depressed patients improved with citrus fragrance and tricyclic antidepressant. Immunologic measures showed a dramatic improvement with citrus therapy. In addition, citrus fragrance allowed reductions in the antidepressant dose. However, the initial dose reduced with citrus fragrance was below the normal therapeutic range initially. No serum level determinations of tricyclics were reported, making this reported finding difficult to interpret.

Komori et al.[94] concluded that the use of citrus fragrance in treating depressed patients could be of psychoneuroimmunologic benefit. The data presented would appear to confirm their claim. However, as the authors accurately point out, caution must be exercised in interpreting the findings due to a small sample size, lack of blinding in the study design, and very low dosing with tricyclic antidepressants in the active control group. Stimulation of the olfactory system can trigger a wide range of emotional responses through paired association as well as trigger cravings in patients with a substance abuse disorder. Despite the lack of well-controlled data, exploration into the role of aromatherapy in treating depression is warranted.

PRAYER

Few outcome studies review the effects of prayer in the treatment of mental illness. This is somewhat curious because the therapeutic role of "hopefulness" is well known, and prayer is intuitively correlated with hopefulness.

Larson[97] reviewed the effects of religiosity on several psychiatric conditions; 87% of research reports examining religious involvement as a variable report a positive therapeutic effect, with the remaining 13% reporting a negative impact on mental health. Galanter, Larson, and Rubenstone[61] surveyed 193 psychiatrists who were members of the Christian Medical and Dental Society. Respondents rated the Bible and prayer as potential interventions for those with suicidal intent, grief reaction, sociopathy, and alcoholism. Survey results indicated that for prayer to be an effective therapeutic modality, the patient needs to have strong religious beliefs.

Despite limited research in this area, religious conviction appears to improve mental health. Controlled trials of the therapeutic effect of prayer as a treatment modality are warranted. Caution should be taken to avoid overestimation of the positive effects of prayer independent of other components of living a religious life.

◼ Anxiety

Pathologic anxiety is different from stress in its intensity and effects on functioning. *DSM* anxiety disorders include panic disorder, specific and social phobias, obsessive-compulsive disorder, posttraumatic stress disorder, acute stress disorder, generalized anxiety disorder, and anxieties related to other conditions and substance abuse. The cost of anxiety disorders is unclear, but "more than 23 million Americans with anxiety disorders face much more than just normal stress."[1]

The lifetime prevalence of *panic disorder* (with or without agoraphobia) is between 1.5% and 3.5%, with 1-year prevalence rates of 1% to 2%.[3] Panic displays a bimodal distribution, with peaks in late adolescence and in the mid-30s. Close biologic family members of individuals with panic disorder have a four to seven times greater risk of developing this disorder. *Panic* is an intense fear or discomfort in which four (or more) of the following symptoms have a rapid onset and crescendo in 10 minutes: (a) palpitations, (b) sweating, (c) shaking, (d) shortness of breath, (e) choking, (f) chest pain, (g) nausea, (h) feeling faint, (i) derealization or depersonalization,

(j) fear of "going crazy," (k) fear of dying, (l) tingling sensations and chills, (m) or hot flashes in the absence of a disease causing these symptoms.

The estimated lifetime prevalence of *obsessive-compulsive disorder (OCD)* is 2.5%. It generally consists of a 1-year prevalence of 1.5% to 2.1%, making it an uncommon disorder.[3] OCD usually becomes evident first in adolescence or early adulthood, although it may begin in childhood, with the age of onset being earlier in males than in females. Patients with OCD have waxing and waning courses, with flare-ups that are related to stress. OCD presents with symptoms of either obsessions or compulsions. *Obsessions* are recurrent and persistent thoughts (not simply worries), impulses, or images that are intrusive and inappropriate and result in distress. Through active or passive means, patients attempt to relieve the thoughts, understanding that the thoughts are from their own mind. *Compulsions* are repetitive behaviors or mental activities driven to reduce obsessions and distress. The obsessions or compulsions resulting in distress are time-consuming and interfere with daily functioning.

Reports that anxiety runs in families have been inconsistent for *generalized anxiety disorder* (GAD). Individuals with GAD describe feeling anxious and nervous all of their lives. Onset in childhood or adolescence and after age 20 years are both common, with more cases starting early.[3] The course is chronic and variable and may intensify with stress. GAD becomes evident with excessive worry lasting more days than not for at least 6 months about a number of events. The worry is beyond the person's control, and three (or more) of six symptoms are present: (1) restlessness, (2) easy fatigability, (3) difficulty concentrating, (4) irritability, (5) muscle tension, and (6) sleep problems. In addition, these symptoms must have affected daily functioning.

MUSIC THERAPY

The use of music to alter mood and anxiety dates back to the Greeks. Springe[165] explored the anxiolytic effect of music on anxious mood generated by dental surgery procedures. Subjects were divided into two groups of 50, with one group choosing to listen to music of their selection. The other group was exposed to white noise preoperatively until sedated. The subjects' anxiety was measured using a variety of physiologic measurements. Significant measurements included pulse rate, mean arterial blood pressure, and plasma adrenocorticotropic hormone (ACTH) value.

This study's findings indicated the effectiveness of music in reducing acute anxiety. Unfortunately, the selection and assignment process was not discussed, and inclusion of a psychometric measure of anxiety would have improved the study. However, the study's size and the physiologic data indicate the effectiveness of music. Other areas to develop include the strength of music therapy over time and realistic limits for its use. Although effective in an anxiety-provoking situation, music may be ineffective in panic states.

MASSAGE THERAPY

Field et al.[54] studied massage for the reduction of diagnosable anxiety in a child psychiatry inpatient setting. They exposed 72 adolescents and children with depression and adjustment disorder to a daily, 30-minute back massage for 5 days. The patients were randomly stratified to either the massage group or a group watching a restful video. Patient responses to treatment were measured using State Anxiety Inventory for Children (STAIC), Profile of Mood States (POMS), behavior and activity observation ratings, pulse rate, saliva cortisol and 24-hour urine cortisol values, and nighttime sleep recording. The findings reported a reduction of anxiety and fidgeting ratings, decrease in saliva cortisol temporal to the massage, improvements in sleep, and reduction in STAIC values for those children with depression during the treatment phase. Longer-term effects were reduced depression for both depressed and adjustment-disordered children and improved anxiety and fidgeting ratings for both groups. The biochemical effects of treatment diminished over the 5-day period.

These findings provide evidence for the effect of massage in reducing anxiety and improving depression. However, this study suffers from self-stated problems in examining a "mixed bag" of conditions under the name of "adjustment disorder" and from being a small, single-site study. Even with these limitations, the study provides support and direction for continued investigation of massage therapy.

Ferrell-Torry and Glick[53] examined the effects of 2 days of 30-minute massage on cancer pain and anxiety. They used a convenience sample of nine patients, examining pain and anxiety with visual analog scales and anxiety using the State-Trait Anxiety Inventory (STAI-Y-1). Pulse and respiratory rates and blood pressure were also obtained before and after each session of massage. The findings were significant for reduction of pain and anxiety, increased relaxation, and changes in many of the physiologic measures obtained, which suggests that massage modified both anxiety and pain. By the authors' admission the study is exploratory, and the sample selection and size do not allow for generalization. Further, the nature of anxiety associated with pain and chronic illness such as cancer may be distinct from the psychiatric anxiety disorders discussed here.

ACUPUNCTURE

Tao[168] examined the use of acupuncture to reduce depression and anxiety in patients with chronic physical diseases. The 68 subjects (11 with anxiety, 8 with depression, 49 with both) were assigned in a single-blind, pre/postmeasure, noncontrolled study design. Changes in depression and anxiety were assessed using the Hospital Anxiety and Depression scale. The study reported that 70% of the patients with anxiety and 90% of patients with depression returned to normal levels.

The use of this work in treating anxiety and depression in patients with physical disease is a significant confounding variable in considering the pure anxiolytic effect of this treatment. Although the strength of these findings is limited by the lack of a control group, this study supports the need for further work in this area.

YOGA AND MEDITATION

Shannahoff-Khalsa and Beckett[158] examined the effect of Kundalini yoga versus a combination of relaxation response techniques and mindfulness meditation as a control group. A total of 25 subjects were randomly assigned to the groups after matching for age, gender, and "meditation status." Five measures were obtained, including the Yale-Brown Obsessive Compulsive Scale, Symptoms Checklist-90-Revised (SCL-90-R), Profile of Mood States, perceived stress scales, and Purpose in Life test. Brain imaging using 37-channel magnetometers was used in nonmeditating patients before and after treatment. Significant differences were reported at 3 months on all scales for those using Kundalini yoga and none for those receiving relaxation response techniques and mindfulness meditation.

This study's findings suggest significant impact for a specific form of yoga and little response to other forms of meditation. The small study size indicates that the negative finding for the control treatment should be viewed with caution because the risk of a type 2 error (accept null hypothesis when false) is high. The study builds on the common use of yoga techniques in stress reduction and points to treatments that may be more effective in a severe anxiety disorder. This area merits further exploration with larger sample size and more sophisticated design.

Another study compared the effect of meditation-based stress reduction programs with a relaxation program in addressing anxiety disorders.[92] The program was based on mindfulness meditation and involved 22 subjects prescreened with the SCL-90-R and Medical Symptom Checklist and then screened with a structured clinical interview meeting the *DSM* criteria for GAD or panic disorder (with or without agoraphobia).[2] Anxiety was measured using self-ratings, therapist ratings, HAMD scales, and Beck anxiety and depression scales before treatment and weekly throughout the treatment protocol, then after treatment monthly for 3 months. Patients taking medication were not excluded from the study because of small sample size. Subjects were assigned to one of two treatment groups, meditation or relaxation, without a control group. The report does not state whether subjects were randomly assigned to these groups. The descriptive data reported use of the patients as their own control. Statistics reported for each group did not show statistical significance on the SCL-90-R anxiety scales. Both the relaxation group and mindfulness meditation groups demonstrated a significant ($p > 0.001$) level on the HAMD rating, Beck anxiety and depression scales, and fear survey scheduled between their pretreatment and post-treatment results.

This study is consistent with the earlier findings of Lehrer et al.[99] in detecting only limited differences between similar treatment methods in 16 anxious subjects, as determined by the anxiety scale developed by the Institute of Personality and Ability Testing (IPAT). The study attempted to isolate the effects of these treatments in patients with anxiety disorders and identify longer-term effectiveness of these treatments. The study's small size and lack of control group limit the use of the findings to encouraging future research. The current understanding of panic disorder's etiology suggests a biologic connection, and its relationship to GAD is arguable, which weakens the findings by further limiting the sample for diagnosis.

DeBerry, Davis, and Reinhard[41] studied 32 geriatric subjects randomly assigned to one of three conditions: meditation-relaxation (MR), cognitive restructuring, and pseudotreatment control. The subjects were measured using the STAI and Beck depression inventory. The authors reported that MR was an effective modality for reducing state anxiety in anxious elderly individuals, and that constant practice of MR was required to maintain a reduction in anxiety. These findings are consistent with earlier findings from these authors.[39-41] The small cell size for each of the treatment conditions makes full endorsement of the findings risky because it is difficult to eliminate significant type 2 error in the treatment conditions for which no significant difference was found.

HERBAL TREATMENTS

Suanzaoretang

Suanzaoretang, an ancient Chinese remedy used for weakness, irritability, and insomnia, has been tested in double-blind controlled conditions against diazepam.[29] Ninety patients with Morbid Anxiety Inventory (MAI) scores between 14 and 30 were recruited from an anxiety clinic. The patients were divided into three conditions: suanzaoretang, 250 mg three times daily; diazepam, 2 mg three times daily; and placebo. The subjects were all given a 1-week placebo washout. Treatments were evaluated using the MAI, Hamilton Anxiety Scale, Digital Symbol Substitution Test, and self-rating of functioning (five-point Likert). Patients were also monitored for a variety of blood chemistry values. The patients were treated for 3 weeks on a regimen of active compounds. The findings indicated that suanzaoretang is an effective anxiolytic lacking the muscular tension–relieving and insomnia-relieving qualities of diazepam, which is consistent with the reports that suanzaoretang improved "psychomotor performance."

This study is also consistent with the current standard expected of a drug trial. Only the single site and the trial's size keep it from meeting the standards required of studies examining medications for clinical use. The authors recommended further investigation of suanzaoretang.[29] No follow-up work has been found in the literature search of MEDLARS.

Kava

Kava (kava-kava), the rhizome of the pepper plant *Piper methysticum*, has been widely used in the South Pacific as a narcotic drink. *Lactones*, the major constituents of kava, are considered to be pharmacologically active and are sold in Europe and the United States as standardized extracts for anxiety and tension. One of the best-selling herbal supplements in the United States, kava's recommended dose is 100 mg of extract with 70% lactones taken two or three times daily. Because kava is marketed as an herbal supplement, it is not required to undergo the strict quality and safety evaluations moderated by the FDA.[177]

Despite the supposed benefits, many researchers are skeptical about the safety of kava. Meseguer et al.[118] reported that a patient developed severe and persistent parkinsonism after being treated with kava extract for anxiety, leading to the proposal that kava derivatives could produce severe parkinsonism in individuals with genetic susceptibility.[118] Although using kava appears to have benefits on vagal cardiac control,[179] other side effects have been reported with kava in the treatment of anxiety.[77] Therefore all U.S. and European clinical trials were suspended in early 2002 pending a thorough investigation by the FDA on the safety of kava's components.

ELECTROSLEEP

Moore et al.[121] have reported a double-blind study with a crossover structure design in which they recruited 17 subjects with persistent anxiety and insomnia; the method of diagnosis was not discussed. Using a crossover design exposed the patient to electrosleep or a sham version of the treatment. There were 5 nights of treatment in each condition. Patients were assessed using the Likert self-rating scale for anxiety, insomnia, and depression; Taylor's Manifest Anxiety scale; Beck depression inventory; and Eysenck's personality inventory. No significant results were demonstrated between groups. The study's failure of diagnostic accuracy for inclusion and small sample size place it at risk for type 2 error, and thus it should be viewed with caution.

Flemenbaum[55] reported significantly positive results in a less rigorous, open-label clinical study with a 6-month follow-up. His study was uncontrolled and also was weakened by the use of patients from a number of outdated diagnostic categories.

HOMEOPATHY

The effectiveness of homeopathic treatment in patients with depression and anxiety was studied in 12 adults using individually selected homeopathic remedies.[63] Subjects had major depression, social phobia, or panic disorder. The patients either self-selected or were referred to this treatment after poor response to other treatments. Treatment length varied from 7 to 80 weeks. Outcomes were measured by a clinical global scale ($n = 12$), the self-rated SCL-90 scale ($n = 8$), and the Brief Social Phobia Scale ($n = 4$). The research reports that response rates were 58% on the clinical global improvement scale and 50% on the SCL-90 or the Brief Social Phobia Scale. Despite noble attempts, the study is examining different patient populations over differing time spans using different compounds. This study does not build a strong base for recommending homeopathic treatment.

McCutcheon[115] examined 72 adults with above-average anxiety scores who were randomly assigned to either antianxiety homeopathic treatment or a placebo for 15 days. A "four-measures," double-blind format was used, and determinations of pulse rate, sleep quality, and state and trait anxiety were obtained. Posttest comparisons were not significant except for a small reduction in amount of sleep loss for those receiving homeopathic treatment. In further analyses noted, subjects were unable to successfully predict their group assignment. The researcher noted that a homeopathic remedy aids in reducing the sleep loss often associated with anxiety.

▨ Schizophrenia and Psychotic Disorders

The illness now called *schizophrenia* has been recognized in most cultures and described throughout much of recorded history. The process of diagnosis in the West has evolved from descriptive and theoretic to criteria based, as in the *DSM*.[3] Characteristic symptoms of schizophrenia involve severe disturbance in several areas, including language and communication, content of thought, perception, affect, sense of self, volition, relationships to the outside world, and motor behavior.

Disturbances in *language and communication* include looseness of association, derailment, circumstantiality, tangentiality, neologisms, and "word salad." Disturbances of *thought content* are characterized by delusions or false fixed beliefs and ideas of reference. Disturbances of *perception* include auditory, visual, tactile, and olfactory hallucinations. Disturbances of *affect* may take a variety of forms, including lability and oddity, but most often the patient has a blunting or flattening of affect with little intensity or range. Disturbances in *sense of self* may include losing touch with one's self-identity or an overwhelming perplexity, doubt, or confusion about the meaning of one's life and illness. Disturbances in *volition* involve a decrease in self-initiated and goal-directed activity and invariably affect work performance and functioning in other roles. Disturbances in *outside relationships* are demonstrated by withdrawal from involvement with other people and attention directed inward toward self-absorbed, illogical ideas and fantasies. Disturbances in *motor behavior* range from greatly decreased reaction to the environment (e.g., catatonic stupor) to repetitive, ritualistic, or aggressive agitation.[70]

The disorder of schizophrenia is conceptualized as a syndrome that is heterogeneous in its cause, presenting picture, course, response to treatment, and outcome. Nevertheless, the syndrome is assumed to be an illness rather than merely a socially unacceptable or odd and eccentric set of behaviors.[87] Subtypes of schizophrenia include paranoid, disorganized, catatonic, undifferentiated, and residual.

In terms of both personal and societal costs, schizophrenia is one of the most devastating illnesses. An estimated 0.5% to 1% of the population suffers from schizophrenia. The incidence and prevalence rates of any psychiatric disorder, however, are a function of diagnostic criteria, and not all methods or studies reviewed here have similar diagnostic definitions. Schizophrenia usually strikes at an early age, so unlike patients with heart disease or cancer, schizophrenic patients usually live long after onset and continue to suffer from the typical stepwise deterioration of cognitive and emotional functioning.[171] Schizophrenia also creates an enormous financial burden on individuals, families, and society. Recent estimates of the direct and indirect costs of schizophrenia to society were between $10 and $20 billion, with approximately two thirds of costs resulting from the relative lack of productive employment. However, human suffering and the social and psychologic costs for patients and families cannot be measured monetarily.[87]

Currently, no established scientific cure exists for schizophrenia, but treatments have been identified that affect symptoms and level of functioning in patients. Antipsychotic medications have been rigorously studied but are not reviewed here. Some treatment approaches complement psychopharmacology or address the "living environment" stressors that can exacerbate psychotic symptoms. For example, inpatient "milieu therapy" has a long history as a treatment plan component,[88] and family "expressed emotion" has been identified as a factor in the severity and course of schizophrenic symptoms.[49] CAM therapy studies are reviewed by method where studies were identified. At times it is difficult to define what is "alternative."

Other psychotic disorders include schizoaffective disorder and mania. *Schizoaffective disorder* is essentially a diagnosis of both schizophrenia and an affective disorder, usually MDD or bipolar (formerly manic-depressive) disorder. *Mania* is characterized by a distinct period of abnormally or persistently elevated, expansive, or irritable mood for more than 1 week. Other symptoms common but not required for a diagnosis of mania include the following[3]:

- Inflated self-esteem or feelings of grandiosity
- Decreased need for sleep
- Rambling or pressured speech
- Racing thoughts
- Distractibility
- Increased risk-taking behavior
- Increased goal-directed behavior

HYPNOSIS

Hypnosis as a treatment method has historically been accepted as useful and safe for neurotic disorders and personality disorders since the early work done by Freud and his contemporaries. Hypnosis is not generally considered an alternative or complementary treatment, however, and hypnotherapy used with schizophrenic and psychotic patients has been doubted and debated for more than 100 years. The controversy surrounding the use of hypnosis with psychotic individuals centers on four main concerns: (1) psychotic patients were incapable of being hypnotized; (2) hypnosis might worsen psychotic symptoms; (3) the patient might enter and prefer the fantasy of hypnotic imagery; and (4) hypnosis might induce excessive dependency in the psychotic individual.

A review of the literature revealed evidence for and against these hypotheses. Scagnelli-Jobsis[152] reviewed a variety of clinical studies and case reports that question all four tenets. Baker[9] also identified potential benefits and focused on techniques that increase relaxation and improve ego strengths and self-image. Both authors emphasized that hypnotherapy is *not* a substitute for chemotherapy or other treatment modalities. Debate continues among hypnotherapists, however, with Spiegel[164] questioning the validity of Scagnelli-Jobsis'[152] hypothesis of lowered hypnotic responsivity in psychotic patients.[9,78]

The nature of hypnosis makes it difficult to complete controlled, blinded studies. The therapeutic relationship, induction techniques, and interventions in hypnotherapy are highly dependent on the style of the practitioner. Psychotherapy research and many CAM therapies wrestle with similar problems.

COGNITIVE-BEHAVIORAL THERAPY

Although medication is often used in the treatment of schizophrenia, a recent Cochrane review was done to evaluate the efficacy of cognitive-behavioral therapy

(CBT). A total of 22 papers that included 13 trials were evaluated. CBT did not reduce the rate of relapse and readmission to the hospital compared with other therapies, including medication. Interestingly, CBT did appear to influence patient discharge rate and compliance with therapy.[34]

MOVEMENT THERAPY

Inpatient psychiatric units regularly use recreational, art, music, occupational, relaxation, dance, and movement therapies in the milieu treatment of schizophrenic and psychotic patients. To evaluate the effect of movement therapies, the Volwiler Body Movement Analysis (VBMA) scale was developed. The scale provides a quantitative measure of 19 aspects of body movement. Data indicate that psychotic children were significantly different from control children in most categories of body movement.[177] This scale has been used by others in an attempt to confirm the effectiveness of movement and dance therapies, but rigorous controlled studies were not found in the literature.[6]

ACUPUNCTURE

Few clinical studies using acupuncture in psychotic disorders were identified. Keys[89] suggested that one reason is the diagnostic system differences between traditional Chinese medicine (TCM) and the Western approach.[5] Chronic pain, migraine, headache, anxiety, and other physical conditions may have an impact on the severity and course of psychotic disorders. For example, stress, physical pain, and irritability can exacerbate psychotic symptoms. Reducing these aggravating factors using acupuncture may improve the overall clinical picture.[35]

Shi and Tan[161] investigated the therapeutic effects of acupuncture treatment in 500 patients with schizophrenia. This study clearly exemplifies diagnostic criteria translation difficulties. According to TCM differentiation, patients were grouped by several types. "Manic-type" schizophrenic patients (181) had an excited state of mania based on the theory that the etiologic factor was "double yang." "Depressive-type" schizophrenic patients (140) were characterized by melancholy and tension and were thought to have "double yin." "Paranoid-type" schizophrenic patients (179) were exemplified by terror and worry thought to be related to the spleen. The specific subtype of schizophrenia directed the point locations of the acupuncture performed. The results cited were that 55% of schizophrenic patients were cured, 16.8% had remarkable improvement, and 16.6% showed no effect. These results appear impressive, but the broad range of the diagnosis of schizophrenia and the variety of different acupuncture interventions performed render these results questionable.[181]

HERBAL AND CHINESE MEDICINE

Minimal research has been identified on the use of botanic extracts, homeopathic agents, or TCM in the treatment of psychotic disorders. However, the use of these methods may be more widespread than this paucity of studies implies. Despite rigorous efforts, articles were not identified in the literature.

Ma, Ju, and Zhang[110] reported on 30 patients with chronic schizophrenia who received treatment with a variety of neuroleptic medications and were considered nonresponders. Seven immunologic functioning markers were measured, with six significantly different compared with a control group. In an attempt to regulate proportion and function of immune cells, 30 patients were given the immunomodulating herb *xin shen ling*. The Brief Psychosis Rating Scale (BPRS) and Nurses' Observation Scale for Inpatient Evaluation (NOSIE) were used to assess changes in clinical symptoms before and after treatment. The results showed that BPRS and NOSIE ratings before treatment were significantly higher than after treatment ($p < .05$). The clinical efficacy rate was 67%. The authors reported up to 3 years of follow-up, in some cases with better than expected relapse rates. This study, although using standard rating tools, testing for result significance, and presenting interesting possibilities, lacked a control group and clear diagnostic and dosing details.

Ma, Ju, and Zhang[110] also reported on the use of acupuncture combined with a medicinal concoction of several herbs called *Ding Jing Hong Pill*, a secret recipe handed down from an author's father. Fifty-three schizophrenic patients were given treatment (21 males, 32 females; 17 to 50 years of age), and length of treatment varied from 1 week to 30 days. The authors claimed that all patients were cured but provided few details of treatment or research methodology, making these results seem highly questionable.

Carod and Vazquez-Cabrera[23] presented a case report of a 34-year-old female schizophrenic patient who experienced significant reduction in presenting symptoms using herbal therapy in combination with neuroleptic medication. They suggested a possible complementary nature of the treatment.

DIETARY THERAPY

A review of the literature found a number of studies suggesting that dietary control or supplementation may have a complementary role in the current treatment of psychosis. Ascheim[8] proposed dietary interventions derived from established animal studies. He proposed diets in which essential amino acid composition has been modified to produce a defined imbalance of dopamine and norepinephrine precursors. Decreasing the amount of available dopamine complements the dopamine blockade by neuroleptic drugs and potentiates antipsychotic effects. This effect in turn might allow for lower neuroleptic doses and diminish drug-related side effects and risk of tardive dyskinesia. However, this report is primarily hypothetic and suggests further animal and human studies.

Bruinvels and Pepplinkhuizen[16] studied a group of schizoaffective patients with episodic psychosis and speculated that a disturbance in *serine* metabolism may be related to their psychotic symptoms. This group of patients was characterized by the occurrence of generalized sensory perceptual distortions of light, sound, shapes, and distances, especially at the onset of the psychosis. It was postulated that in this group, an increased demand for glycine, as in porphyria, may be the trigger for an increased production of 1-carbon units. The result would then be a greater endogenous production of beta-carotenes and isoquinolines, which may act as "psychotic" substances.[17]

After the patients recovered, serine, glycine, or glucose was administered orally to determine whether an enhancement of serine conversion would reintroduce psychotic symptoms. The authors suggested the results imply that a subgroup of schizoaffective patients may have a metabolic disturbance in the 1-carbon transfer system, and they reported evidence that psychotic symptoms may improve on a carbohydrate-rich, low-protein diet.[17,132] However, only 25 subjects were studied, and many other variables were not identified. Metabolic differences in psychotic patients merit further study.

Older studies examined the use of L-tryptophan in mania. Van Praag et al.[173] studied five manic patients in a double-blind, placebo-controlled crossover study using chlorpromazine and tryptophan and found that tryptophan was slightly superior in all parameters studied. Chambers and Naylor[26] completed a similar study with 10 female patients and found L-tryptophan no better than placebo. These conflicting conclusions illustrate the limitations of small numbers even in well-designed and controlled studies and the need to replicate results.

Rubin[146] discussed the possible clinical and etiologic overlap of psychotic disorders and *pellagra* (characterized by the "three Ds"—dementia, diarrhea, and dermatitis—and caused by a niacin deficiency). He discussed a newly discovered trace-3 essential fatty acid that provides the substrate on which niacin and other B vitamins act to form prostaglandins, and he postulated a common deficit in both disorders. Rubin reported on symptom improvement in 12 psychiatric patients with a variety of diagnoses, including schizophrenia, who were treated with linseed oil, a substance rich in the identified fatty acid. The study raises some interesting metabolic questions about diet and illness, but a clear limitation of the study method is that patients continued receiving their standard regimen of antipsychotic or antianxiety medication.[81-83,147]

Vlissides, Venulet, and Jenner[176] completed a double-blind controlled trial of gluten-free versus gluten-containing diet on an inpatient ward with 24 patients, most of whom suffered from psychotic disorders, especially schizophrenia, for 14 weeks using the Psychotic In-Patient profile (PIP). There were beneficial changes in the study patients between pretrial and gluten-free periods in five dimensions of the PIP. This improvement continued during the gluten-challenge period, but the authors attributed these changes to the increased attention the subjects received (Hawthorne effect). Two patients improved during the gluten-free period and relapsed when the gluten diet was reintroduced. The study concluded that the majority of psychotic patients are not affected by the elimination of gluten from the diet, but the authors readily acknowledged the difficulties and limitations in the study design. Freed et al.[58] and Harper et al.[73] explored the possibility that gluten impedes absorption of haloperidol. Diet-related absorption effects of medication are an area worthy of additional study.

CULTURE AND RELIGION

Cultural and religious beliefs have been shown to have a significant effect on an individual's mental and physical health. A large and growing body of ethnographic research and literature has been reviewed elsewhere.[95] Many medical and mental health practitioners, however, increasingly view illness from a perspective that considers the patient's cultural or religious beliefs.[109] Although these beliefs are not typically thought of as "alternative," a few case examples of treatment interventions for psychotic disorders are reviewed in which the cultural context was crucial to clinical improvement.[56,74,95]

Farmer and Falkowski[50] described psychotic illness in a Nigerian woman born in London who grew up in a family and community highly influenced by traditional Nigerian culture. She developed a brief postpartum psychotic episode and partially responded to chlorpromazine but worsened over the next few weeks. The quality of her psychosis became dominated by "delusional" beliefs about her ancestors, feeling she had spells placed on her, and hearing voices of people she knew in Africa. She believed that her illness was the result of "bewitchment," that psychiatric medication could only calm and not cure her, and that "strong medicine men from home" were needed to deal with "ju-ju" and break the spell on her. Her continued disturbed behavior remained resistant to both neuroleptic medication and ECT. Her husband was able to return with her to Nigeria for intervention by native healers, and soon a complete recovery occurred. A letter received from her husband 2 years later confirmed that she remained well.

Insomnia

Insomnia is difficulty initiating or maintaining sleep or nonrestorative sleep that lasts at least 1 month.[3] This lack of sleep results in clinically significant distress, which impairs social and occupational functioning. Insomnia is one of the *dyssomnias*, a group of disorders characterized by difficulty in initiating or maintaining sleep or by excessive sleepiness.

A hallmark of the dyssomnias is a core disturbance in the quality, amount, or timing of sleep with a marked preoccupation with the inability to attain restful sleep. Chronic insomnia can have a marked negative impact on mood, motivation, attention, energy levels, and concentration.[3] Chronically disturbed sleep can also be a symptom of mood disorders (MDD, mania), anxiety disorders, substance abuse, or chronic pain. Occasionally, sleep problems may result from situational anxiety, excessive physiologic stimulation (e.g., caffeine, strenuous exercise before retiring), or environmental factors (e.g., noise, temperature, lack of comfort with the bed).

Complaints of sleep disturbance increase with age and among women. This finding may be related to the decreased need for sleep and lack of exercise in elderly individuals and the perimenopausal symptoms (e.g., hot flashes) that affect some middle-aged women. The actual prevalence of primary insomnia is unknown, although U.S. population surveys report a 1-year prevalence rate of insomnia complaints of 30% to 40% in adults.[3]

Secondary insomnia, or sleep disorders resulting from a known underlying cause, is treated by attending to the primary etiologic factor, that is, treating the depressive or anxiety disorder or relieving the physical pain. The sleep disorder associated with drug abuse, particularly of heroin and cocaine, will often last for months after stopping abuse.

A National Institutes of Health (NIH) conference concluded that behavioral interventions such as relaxation training and biofeedback may produce improvement in some aspects of sleep.[127] However, some questions regarding whether the magnitude of improvement in sleep onset and total sleep time were clinically significant were raised. The CAM literature is replete with reports on the treatment of insomnia, but extremely limited with conclusive evidence of therapeutic effectiveness.

ACUPUNCTURE

Practitioners of TCM have used acupuncture for thousands of years to treat insomnia. Yi[189] reported on 86 cases of insomnia treated by double-point needle insertion. He reported "fairly satisfactory results in the treatment of insomnia" in all 86 patients. Clinical data were limited primarily to a discussion of the needle insertion technique. Any large trial that reports an improvement in 100% of the study subjects must be viewed with some level of skepticism.

Changlxin,[27] reporting in a published lecture on acupuncture treatment of insomnia, offers a poetic and philosophical description of insomnia from the Chinese perspective; however, no data or clinical cases are reported. Cangliang[20] published a synopsis of 62 patients with insomnia treated by *auricular point embedding therapy*. This form of acupuncture uses the embedding of *compositus semen vaccariae* (a traditional Chinese medicine) at specific auricular points. Of the 62 cases in the therapeutic group, 39 were rated as markedly improved, 30 as improved, and 3 as with no effect. A few cases were listed as both markedly improved and improved. This study is virtually impossible to assess from a Western perspective. Patient classification was based on (1) liver and kidney yin deficiency, (2) heart and spleen deficiency, (3) disturbance of the heart by phlegm-fire, and (4) yin deficiency leading to hyperactivity of fire. Although meaningful to the practitioner trained in these concepts, these classifications might be uninterpretable to Western scientists. This study also offered no references.

Leye et al.[102] reported a large series of 124 patients with dyssomnia treated with acupuncture at Sishencong points. Results were 73 cases (59%) cured, 26 cases (21%) markedly improved, 10 cases (8%) improved, and 15 cases (12%) unimproved. Only one case was presented, and no references were listed.

Nan and Qingming[126] compared auricular pressing (AP) therapy to a Western medicine control group, with both groups consisting of 80 subjects. Western control subjects were administered 10 mg of diazepam orally before sleep for 30 days. Of the AP group, 30 were cured, 35 improved, and 15 were considered ineffective. Of the Western (diazepam) group, 11 improved, and 69 were designated "ineffective." The authors concluded the AP group was "better than the Western medicine group." However, they did report that diazepam was more effective initially but lost effectiveness over time, whereas AP improved with time. The study sample included 80 patients with neurosis, 31 with neurasthenia, and 7 with cerebral trauma. This study offered no references and an inadequate description of methodology.

In 1992, Yukang[190] published a "short paper" on the therapeutic effect of acupuncture in treating 50 patients with insomnia, with results showing that all but 2 patients reported improvement. One case was presented as being representative of the entire sample. This report had no references, and content was very limited. All the reviewed reports on the use of acupuncture followed the same pattern of no references, scant description of methodology, and remarkably high response rates. Montakab and Langel,[120] in a 1994 review of acupuncture treatment of insomnia, concluded that polysomnographic studies are needed to verify the effectiveness of acupuncture. In 2001, Phillips and Skelton[133] reported that using a pre/posttest design, sleep quality in HIV-infected men and women could be modified through the use of acupuncture. Both sleep activity and sleep quality were found to "significantly be improved following 5 weeks of individualized acupuncture delivered in a group setting" to the 21 participants. The need for replication and a larger number of subjects with a strong sham control must be emphasized.

HERBAL TREATMENT: SUANZAORETANG

Chen and Hsich[30] reported on the use of suanzaoretang in the treatment of insomnia. Sixty patients with poorly defined sleep disorders were treated with 1 g of suanzaoretang 30 minutes before bedtime for 2 weeks. A 1-week placebo washout preceded active treatment. Results were that during active treatment, all sleep measures were significantly improved with no side effects observed. Having reported these remarkable although unbelievable results, the authors concluded that the compound merits further extensive investigation.

CRANIAL ELECTROSTIMULATION

Cranial electrostimulation (CES) is a therapeutic technique that uses low-level electrical signals applied to the eyelids and mastoid process to induce calming and ultimately sleep. In 1953, Gilyarovski et al.[67] coined the term "electrosleep" and applied the technique for the treatment of insomnia. The procedure was used almost exclusively in eastern Europe until the first International Symposium for Electrosleep was held in 1966.[124] Despite numerous reports of clinical effectiveness,[10,31] inadequacies in research design have resulted in skepticism in the West.[169]

Klawansky et al.[90] conducted a meta-analysis of randomized, controlled trials of CES and identified 18 trials of CES versus sham treatment. They uncovered significant methodologic flaws in the study designs and a failure to report the data needed to conduct a meta-analysis in reviewed studies. Although improvement was noted in treating anxious mood, no definitive data were available on efficacy for insomnia.

Four studies examining electrosleep have resulted in differing conclusions. Frankel, Buchbinder, and Synger[57] reviewed the effectiveness of electrosleep in treating chronic primary insomnia. This study identified many of the flaws in the clinical trials that reported efficacy and concluded that electrosleep is not an effective treatment for insomnia. Cartwright and Weiss[24] reported on a 2-year follow-up of 10 subjects with primary insomnia treated in a double-blind study of electrosleep. Results showed a modest improvement in the active treatment group and no residual therapeutic effects in the sham control group. The authors concluded that clear-cut improvements resulting from active treatment with electrosleep remained in doubt. Levitt and James[101] conducted a double-blind, placebo-controlled clinical trial of 13 subjects to assess the effectiveness of electrosleep. Their results showed that electrosleep was no better than placebo in improving sleep. Nagata et al.,[124] reporting on electrosleep in normal adults, insomniacs, and hypertensive patients, concluded that the procedure produced significant improvement in sleep latency, soundness of sleep, and mood at morning awakening.

The four prominent U.S. studies cited all concluded that electrosleep improved sleep and anxiety.[52,76,144,180] Despite the apparent controversy concerning effectiveness, no recent articles were identified in the literature.

LOW-ENERGY EMISSION THERAPY

Low-energy emission therapy (LEET), developed as a treatment for chronic insomnia, consists of low-amplitude-modulated electromagnetic fields delivered by means of a mouthpiece in direct contact with the oral mucosa. LEET was reported as safe, well tolerated, and effective in improving sleep in patients with chronic insomnia.[129] This large, well-designed study clearly demonstrated a reduction of insomnia.

Reite et al.[137] demonstrated that LEET was effective in inducing sleep in healthy volunteers in a scientifically sound clinical trial. The literature reviewed suggests the clinical efficacy of LEET in the treatment of insomnia.

HERBAL TREATMENT: VALERIAN

Valerian is an ancient herbal remedy used to treat anxiety and insomnia. Lindahl and Lindwall[104] reported that valerian was safe and effective in treating insomnia in 21 of 27 study subjects. The authors noted that their results could not be extrapolated to long-term use but believe long-term follow-up trials are indicated. Follow-up seems warranted based on the positive pilot data presented.

TRYPTOPHAN

Tryptophan, the metabolic precursor of serotonin, is one of the eight essential amino acids. Tryptophan has been reported to have therapeutic effectiveness in the treatment of insomnia.[14] In a comprehensive review of the literature, Schneider-Helmert and Spinweber[156] reported that L-tryptophan may be effective in alleviating *disorders of initiating and maintaining sleep* (DIMS) but concluded that, despite some sedative properties, the clinical utility, optimal dose, and mechanism of action remain to be determined. Demisch et al.[42] conducted the first reported double-blind placebo-controlled crossover study, but all the study findings were based on subjective ratings only. The results suggested a positive effect in select patient groups. The authors concluded that successful treatment with L-tryptophan is possible only if patients are carefully selected.

Despite its reported safety, a batch of contaminated tryptophan from Japan was discovered in the United States. A number of serious adverse events were reported to the FDA, which resulted in tryptophan being banned from sale in America.

MELATONIN

Melatonin is one of the most intensely advertised sleep aid "health" products sold in the United States. Melatonin's physiologic functions include regulation of sleep and synchronization of circadian rhythms. The significance of melatonin secretion in patients who complain of insomnia is unknown.[85] Butler[18] warned that no studies have determined the recommended dose, timing, duration of use, side effects, long-term effects, or interactions with other medications: "If melatonin does reset the body's clock, it may reset it wrong."[18] Insomnia might then worsen.

▧ Stress

Stress is a common experience and reaction to the world around us. Its purpose is presumed to be rooted in our primary survival instincts.[38] Stress allows us to attend to potentially threatening situations and muster mental and physical resources to cope with them. Many researchers have examined the effects of long-term arousal on both the psychologic and physical systems of the body. A simple review of a typical stress reduction handbook or medical or nursing textbook will reveal references on hypnosis, dietary modification, exercise, components of yoga (breathing and stretching), relaxation, meditation, herbal and homeopathic remedies, and encouragement to lead a more spiritual life as potential treatments.[38,157] These practices might now be considered more mainstream than alternative.

Stress is an inherently difficult area to study. Quantifying stress levels is problematic; if it is situational and thus changes with the passage of time, evaluating the effects of a treatment is difficult. Evaluating potent treatments that work quickly, such as a drug, is much easier than evaluation of subtle interventions. For the employee under stress at work, the full benefit of exercise efforts may not be effective for weeks, and the work stress and coping methods may not remain constant. Failure to address these issues allows skeptics to reject treatments as ineffective and others to endorse natural remedies that are largely unproved; this is clearly the case with stress. Inconsistent operational definitions and measurement tools result in problematic analysis. The studies reviewed here suffer from methodologic problems but indicate areas for future research.

EYE MOVEMENT DESENSITIZATION AND REPROCESSING

Eye movement desensitization and reprocessing (EMDR) was developed by Francine Shapiro in 1987 and promoted as a treatment for victims of trauma in 1989. The technique, as described by Shapiro, is a "comprehensive methodology for the treatment of the disturbing experiences that underlie many pathologies."[47] It is an integrated treatment model that incorporates aspects of cognitive, behavioral, psychodynamic, body-based, and systems therapies. The treatment consists of an eight-phase intervention that includes the use of eye movements or other left-right brain stimulation. Shapiro claims EMDR can rapidly relieve distress caused by a single trauma or a series of traumatic events.

To become an EMDR therapist, specific training is required. There are more than 17,000 trained EMDR therapists worldwide. In addition to the treatment of *post-traumatic stress disorder* (PTSD), other clinical applications are being explored. Although current neuroscience research is unable to provide a mechanism of action, EMDR practitioners have suggested a link to modulation of rapid eye movement (REM) sleep, dual attention, and bihemispheric involvement. Although admitting that well-controlled clinical outcomes research is currently scarce, Shapiro notes that a number of widely accepted psychotherapeutic techniques, such as systematic desensitization and flooding, were in use years before they were ultimately proven to be effective in methodologically sound research trials.

In a meta-analysis of 34 studies that examined EMDR's effectiveness in PTSD and other conditions, Davidson and Parker[37] concluded that EMDR showed an effect when compared with no treatment, but no significant effect was observed when EMDR was compared with other exposure techniques. "EMDR appears to be no more effective than other exposure techniques, and evidence suggests that the eye movements integral to the treatment, and to its name, are unnecessary."[37] In a separate analysis of the technique, Shepherd, Stein, and Milne[160] critically reviewed 16 published randomized controlled clinical trials comparing EMDR to other psychotherapy treatments for PTSD. Unfortunately, only five of the studies reported a blind assessment of outcome measures. Despite this methodologic limitation, EMDR did consistently demonstrate effectiveness in reducing symptoms. They concluded that the evidence supporting EMDR was of limited quality but that preliminary results were encouraging and warranted additional study, which seems appropriate. As an interesting addendum, Sack, Lempa, and Lamprecht[148] reported that when EMDR studies employ strong methodologic designs, calculate effect sizes, and provide treatment by "well-trained therapists" with an appropriate number of treatment sessions, the outcome results are "better" compared with studies that have weaker designs.

YOGA AND MEDITATION

Dostalek[43] explored the effectiveness of yoga in disease prevention and the reduction of stress. The study included 40 yoga practitioners and 40 nonyoga practitioners, each group divided equally based on gender. Participants were measured using the Perceived Guilt Index (PGI) Attitude Scale, PGI Health Questionnaire N-2, STAI, Presumptive Stressful Life Events Scale, and Jenkins Activity Survey. The findings indicated significant differences between male yoga and nonyoga practitioners in attitude toward yoga, neuroticism, state and trait anxiety, and stressful life events during the past year. Significant differences for females were found for attitude toward yoga, social desirability, and stressful life event scores during the past year. Yoga practitioners had significantly higher mean scores on yoga attitude and social desirability than did nonyoga practitioners.[43]

Schell, Allolio, and Schonecke[154] examined the effects of hatha yoga exercise in 25 healthy women. The authors examined a number of physiologic and psychologic measures in a nonrandomly assigned study comparing those experienced in yoga to a similar nonpracticing group. The endocrine measures proved not to be significant between the groups, but significant findings were reported in pulse, life satisfaction, excitability, aggressiveness, emotionality, and somatic complaints. The authors suggested that yoga groups have improved coping. The study's nonrandom assignment and small sample size again make it difficult to agree with the author's claims but provide suggestive evidence for the impact of yoga on stress. These studies suggest that yoga has a positive effect on stress as measured; however, they suffer from methodologic flaws, including nonrandom selection and assignment to treatment, which limit the scientific credibility of their findings.

Qi Gong

Ryu et al.[147] studied Qi Gong training and meditation to determine effects on stress hormone levels. Twenty subjects who were engaged in qi training for at least 4 months were enrolled in the study. Blood was drawn before, during, and after training to examine beta-endorphin, ACTH, and dehydroepiandrosterone sulfate (DHEA-S). The findings indicate significantly ($p < 0.05$) increased levels of beta-endorphin at both midtraining and posttraining draws. There were no significant differences for ACTH and DHEA-S.

The study points to hormonal changes that are related to stress reduction, but the sample suffers from a lack of a control group within the design and random selection. The findings are suggestive of and consistent with many studies on meditation (transcendental, Buddhist) and t'ai chi that point to the stress-relieving benefits of these activities.[107] However, most of these studies suffer from similar problems when examined in aggregate.

DANCE THERAPY

Lest'e and Rust[100] examined the effects of dance on anxiety in a "2 × 2" design, the two factors being *physical exercise* and *aesthetic appreciation*. College students ($n = 114$) were divided into four conditions: dance class, sports class, music class, and mathematics. The subjects did not have any psychopathologic conditions; stress or anxiety was measured using the STAI, and Likert self-reports assessed previous experience and level of interest. The results demonstrated significant decrease in anxiety for the students in the dance classes. This effect was more pronounced than for those in sports classes. The other classes showed no effect. The data indicated an effect beyond that of exercise in the reduction of state anxiety scores.

The authors have provided appropriate cautions about the use of their findings and their lack of generalizablity.[100] The findings provide an interesting variation on the use of dance to expand stress reduction or anxiolytic qualities of general exercise. This area seems to warrant further study.

HERBAL TREATMENTS

A number of herbal treatments have been anecdotally recommended for the treatment of anxiety or stress, including kava, valerian, hops, *Gingko biloba*, peppermint, and chamomile. Many of these herbal compounds have been extensively studied from a biochemical perspective.[79]

When reviewing the evidence for valerian root as an example for herbal treatments, the clinical trials were limited to two studies. Further searches failed to identify additional reports.[91,98] The extensive basic scientific work reflects the continuing search for effective herbal medicine treatments. Despite the broad use of these compounds by the public, limited research exists to support or deny their efficacy in stress reduction. This is especially true when evaluating duration of treatment effects or long-term safety.

STUDY RECOMMENDATIONS

Many of the areas reviewed in this section offer significant scientific support for their use as stress therapies, which is consistent with the experience in clinical practice. CAM methods are common interventions in the treatment of stress in a primary care practice. Despite the strength of the work that has been reviewed, several general issues merit discussion. The description of what defines stress, or being stressed, remains elusive. The lack of a discrete clinical entity weakens the research in this area. Comparison of the effectiveness of treatment between studies cannot be made with objectivity. Studies could be improved by employing double-blind, placebo-controlled designs where feasible.

SUMMARY

Exploration of research material in CAM medicine and psychiatric illness leads to several conclusions. A common flaw in all the studies reviewed is the relative lack of diagnostic rigor employed in the study design. Failure to identify a homogeneous patient population when studying an illness with a variety of clinical presentations is problematic.

Although this review identifies areas for potential future research in CAM and mental illness, the research literature remains sparse and weak in scientific validation for many, if not most, of the treatments reviewed. Except for *Hypericum* (St. John's wort) for mild depression, there are few valid replication studies of work with positive findings and few challenges of the studies with design weaknesses by CAM researchers. Spinella's text, *The Psychopharmacology of Herbal Medicine*, offers the most comprehensive review of this topic (see Suggested Readings).

Table 8-5 presents a summary and meta-analysis of several CAM therapies in psychiatry. Cognitive-behavioral therapies (CBTs) with components of relaxation, visual imagery, flooding, and other conditioning parameters, although not explicitly discussed in the text, demonstrate that positive research evidence exists regarding its

TABLE 8–5. **SELECT CAM THERAPIES USED IN PSYCHIATRY**

Diagnosis	Study/Results	Reference
HERBAL THERAPY: *HYPERICUM* (ST. JOHN'S WORT)		
Depression	Meta-analysis (*n* = 1757); superior to placebo	Linde et al.[105]
	8 of 14 studies; positive effect	Gelenberg[64]
	Patient surveys (*n* = 3250); positive effects	Woelk et al.[187]
	8 studies found response rate 23%-55% higher than with placebo, 6%-18% lower than with tricyclic antidepressants; few side effects	Gaster, Holroyd[62]
	Review, 107 articles; data revealed major action in neurochemical systems possibly involved with depression; little information on toxicity	Greeson et al.[71]
	Meta-analysis, 22 randomized controlled trials; more effective than placebo but not antidepressants; few adverse events reported	Whiskey et al.[184]
COGNITIVE-BEHAVIORAL THERAPY (CBT)		
Depression	Meta-analysis, multiple studies; positive effect	Wexler, Cicchetti[183]
	More than 65 studies; positive effects with pharmacotherapy	Gaffan et al.[60]
	48 controlled trials (*n* = 2765), versus wait list/antidepressant groups; more efficacious, better relapse rate on follow-up	Gloaguen et al.[68]
	6 studies (*n* = 217), pre/postdesign reports, significant effect sizes; useful for short-/long-term treatment of depression	Reinecke et al.[136]
Insomnia	Sleep improvement (?clinically significant)	NIH[127]
	Meta-analysis, 66 studies; greater magnitude and enhancement of sleep	Murtagh, Greenwood[123]
	Meta-analysis; decreased sleep latency, increased sleep maintenance	Morin et al.[122]
Anxiety, panic disorder, PTSD	Multiple studies; positive effects	Barlow, Cassandra[11]
Panic disorder	Meta-analysis, more than 20 studies; positive effect	Clum et al.[32]
Anxiety, panic, depression	Many patients improved/remained improved (panic); others with short-term improvement but did not remain improved (depression/GAD)	Westen, Morrison[182]
CRANIAL ELECTROSTIMULATION (CES)		
Anxiety	Meta-analysis, 8 studies; positive effects	Klawansky et al.[90]

NIH, National Institutes of Health; *PTSD*, posttraumatic stress disorder; *GAD*, generalized anxiety disorder.

solo or combined use (with medication), especially in the depressed and anxious patient. CBT and other forms of talk therapy are accepted, conventional treatments for depression, insomnia, and anxiety. Along with herbal treatment, these therapies represent alternatives to antidepressant drug treatments, for which there are strong meta-analysis reports for efficacy. (To integrate research information more completely, in 1996 the *Journal of Consulting and Clinical Psychology* published studies dealing with antidepressant drug therapies, and the *Archives of General Psychiatry* published reports on behavioral therapies.) One interesting area that needs to be "tracked" and continuously developed is the integration of medication with particular behavioral techniques so as to both maximize treatment benefit and reduce side effects of the drug(s). Another aspect would include a design evaluating the appropriateness of implementing CBT in the treatment protocol as certain psychotropic medications are being discontinued.[185]

Areas such as herbal medicine, bioelectric magnetic treatments, and EMDR offer promise. These treatments demonstrate effectiveness and are well studied. Improving the methodology of clinical trials may lead to more proven effective and efficient treatments. Indeed, some of yesterday's natural or alternative cures are today's mainstream insurance-reimbursable medicine. It is important for health care providers to maintain an open mind concerning nontraditional treatments while critically questioning unproven claims of effectiveness. Consumers of these products need to be educated about the existing state of knowledge and not left to assume the unproven advertising claims (largely testimonials) often reported. The rapidly growing number of patients seeking CAM treatments underscores this point.

REFERENCES

1. Adler N, Cave L: NIMH launches anxiety disorders education program. In NIH web page www.nih.gov//news/pr/oct96/nimh-22.htm, Washington, DC, 1996, National Institutes of Health.
2. American Psychological Association: *Diagnostic and statistical manual of mental disorders*, ed 3, revised (*DSM-III-R*), Washington, DC, 1987, American Psychiatric Press.
3. American Psychological Association: *Diagnostic and statistical manual of mental disorders*, ed 4, (*DSM-IV, TR*), Washington, DC, 2000, American Psychiatric Press.
4. Angoli A, Angreoli V, Cassacchia M: Effect of S-adenosyl-L-methionine (SAM) upon depressive symptoms, *J Psychiatr Res* 13:43, 1976.
5. Angst J, Woggond FJ, Schoefi KR: Treatment of depression: L-5HT vs. imipramine—results of two open and one double-blind clinical trial, *Arch Psychiatr Nerve Kr* 224:775, 1997.
6. Apter A et al: Movement therapy with psychotic adolescents, *Br J Med Psychol* 51:155, 1978.
7. Arnold LE: Screening and evaluating alternative and innovative psychiatric treatments: a contextual framework, *Psychopharmacol Bull* 30:61, 1994.
8. Ascheim E: Dietary control of psychosis, *Med Hypn* 41:327, 1993.
9. Baker L: The use of hypnotic techniques with psychotics, *Am J Clin Hypn* 25:283, 1983.
10. Banshchikov VM et al: Current status of the problem of electric sleep, *Vopr Kurortol Fizioter Lech Fiz Kult* 31:215, 1966.
11. Barlow DH, Cassandra LL: Advances in the psychosocial treatment of anxiety disorders: implications for national health care, *Arch Gen Psychiatry* 53:727, 1996.
12. Bell I et al: Brief communication: vitamin B1, B2, and B6 augmentation of tricyclic antidepressant treatment in geriatric depression with cognitive dysfunction, *J Am Coll Nutr* 11:159, 1992.
13. Bisset NG et al: *Herbal drugs and phytopharmaceuticals: a handbook for practice on a scientific basis*, Stuttgart, 1994, Medpharm Scientific.
14. Boman B: L-Tryptophan: a rational anti-depressant and a natural hypnotic? *Aust NZ J Psychiatry* 22:83, 1988.
15. Bradford HF: *Chemical neurobiology: an introduction to neurochemistry*, New York, 1986, Freeman.
16. Bruinvels J, Pepplinkhuizen L: Serine, glycine and carbohydrates in schizoaffective disorders, *Bibl Nutr Dicta* 38:168, 1986.
17. Bruinvels J et al: *Role of serine, glycine, and tetrahydrofolic P acid cycle in schizo-affective psychosis*, Chicester, NY, 1980, Wiley.
18. Butler R: Warnings about melatonin, *Geriatrics* 51(2):16, 1996.
19. Byerley W et al: 5-Hydroxytryptophan: a review of its antidepressant efficacy and adverse effects, *J Clin Psychopharmacol* 7:127, 1987.
20. Cangliang Y: Clinical observations of 62 cases of insomnia treated by auricular point imbedding therapy, *J Tradit Chin Med* 8:190, 1988.
21. Cantoni GL: S-adenosylmethionine: a new intermediate formed enzymatically from L-methionine and adenosine triphosphate, *J Biol Chem* 204:403, 1953.

22. Carney MWP, Chary TNK, Bottiglieri T: Switch mechanisms in affective illness and oral S-adenosylmethionine (SAM), *Br J Psychiatry* 150:43, 1987.

23. Carod FJ, Vazquez-Cabrera C: [A transcultural view of neurological and mental pathology in a Tzeltal Maya community of the Altos Chiapas], *Rev Neurol* 24:848, 1996.

24. Cartwright RD, Weiss M: The effects of electrosleep on insomnia revisited, *J Nerv Ment Dis* 161:134, 1975.

25. Cauffild JS: The psychosocial aspects of CAM, *Pharmacotherapy* 20:1289, 2000.

26. Chambers CA, Naylor GJ: L-Tryptophan in mania, *Br J Psychiatry* 132:555, 1978.

27. Changlxin X: Lectures on formulating acupuncture prescriptions: selection and matching of acupoints—acupuncture treatment of insomnia, *J Tradit Chin Med* 7:151, 1987.

28. Chen A: An introduction to sequential electric acupuncture (SEA) in the treatment of stress related physical and mental disorders, *Acupunct Electrother Res* 17:273, 1992.

29. Chen H, Hsiem MT, Shibuya TK: Suanzaoretang versus diazepam: a controlled double-blind study in anxiety, *Int J Clin Pharmacol Ther Toxicol* 24:646, 1986.

30. Chen HC, Hsich MT: Clinical trial of suanzaoretang in the treatment of insomnia, *Clin Ther* 7:334, 1985.

31. Chumakova LT, Kirllova ZA: Effectiveness of electrosleep, *Excerp Med* 128:20, 1966.

32. Clum GA et al: A meta-analysis of treatments for panic disorder, *J Consult Clin Psychol* 61:317, 1993.

33. Coppen A, Chaudhry S, Swade C: Folic acid enhances lithium prophylaxis, *J Affect Disord* 10:9, 1986.

34. Cormac I, Jones C, Campbell C: Cognitive behavior therapy for schizophrenia, Cochrane Library 1, 2002, Oxford (online: *update software*).

35. Das A: Schizophrenia and complementary treatments including acupuncture, *Towsen Lett* 105:250, 1992.

36. Davidson J et al: Homeopathic treatment of depression and anxiety, *Altern Ther* 3(1):46, 1997.

37. Davidson PR, Parker KC: Eye movement desensitization and reprocessing (EMDR): a meta-analysis, *J Consult Clin Psychol* 69:305, 2001.

38. Davis M, Eshelman R, McKay M: *The relaxation and stress reduction workbook*, ed 4, Oakland, Calif, 1995, New Harbinger.

39. DeBerry S: An evaluation of progressive muscle relaxation on stress related symptoms in a geriatric population, *Int J Aging Hum Dev* 14:255, 1981.

40. DeBerry S: The effects of meditation-relaxation on anxiety and depression in a geriatric population, *Psychother Theory Res Pract* 19:512, 1982.

41. DeBerry S, Davis S, Reinhard KE: A comparison of meditation-relaxation and cognitive/behavioral techniques for reducing anxiety and depression in a geriatric population, *J Geriatr Psychiatry* 22:231, 1989.

42. Demisch K et al: Treatment of severe chronic insomnia with L-tryptophan: results of double-blind cross-over study, *Pharmacopsychiatry* 20:242, 1987.

43. Dostalek C: Physiologic bases of yoga techniques in the prevention of diseases: CIANS-ISBM Satellite Conference Symposium—lifestyle changes in the prevention and treatment of disease, Hannover, Germany, 1992, *Homeost Health Dis* 35:205, 1994.

44. Dube KC: Nosology and therapy of mental illness in Ayurveda, *Comp Med East West* 4:209, 1978.

45. Dube KC, Kumar A, Dube S: Psychiatric training and therapies in Ayurveda, *Am J Chin Med* 13:13, 1985.

46. Eisenberg DM et al: Trends in CAM use in the U.S., 1990-1997, *JAMA* 280:1569, 1998.

47. *EMDR: basic principles, protocols, and procedures*, New York, 1995, Guilford.

48. Ernst E: [St. John's wort as antidepressive therapy], *Fortschr Med* 113:354, 1995.

49. Falloon IRH et al: Family management in the prevention of exacerbation of schizophrenia, *N Engl J Med* 306:1447, 1982.

50. Farmer AE, Falkowski WF: Maggot in the salt, snake factor and the treatment of atypical psychosis in West African women, *Br J Psychiatry* 146:446, 1985.

51. Fazio C et al: Effetti terapeutici e meccanismo d'azlone della S-adenosil-metionina (SAMe) nelle sindrml depressive, *Minerva Med* 64:1515, 1973.

52. Feighner JP, Braun SL, Oliver JE: Electrosleep treatment: double-blind study, *J Nerv Ment Dis* 157:121, 1973.

53. Ferrell-Torry A, Glick O: The use of therapeutic massage as a nursing intervention to modify anxiety and the perception of cancer pain, *Cancer Nurs* 16:93, 1993.

54. Field T et al: Massage reduces anxiety in child and adolescent psychiatric patients, *J Am Acad Child Adolesc Psychiatry* 31:125, 1992.

55. Flemenbaum A: Cerebral electrotherapy (electrosleep): an open-clinical study with a six-month follow-up, *Psychosomatics* 15:20, 1974.

56. Forsheim P: Cross-cultural views of self in the treatment of mental illness: disentangling the curative aspects of myth from the mythic aspects of cure, *Psychiatry* 53:304, 1990.

57. Frankel BL, Buchbinder R, Synger F: Ineffectiveness of electrosleep in chronic primary insomnia, *Arch Gen Psychiatry* 29:563, 1973.

58. Freed WJ et al: Wheat gluten impedes absorption of haloperidol, *Biol Psychiatry* 13:769, 1978.

59. Fujiwara J, Otsuki S: Subtype of affective psychosis classified by response on amine precursors and monoamine metabolism, *Folia Psychiatr Neurol* 28:94, 1974.

60. Gaffan EA et al: Research allegiance and meta-analysis: the case of cognitive therapy for depression, *J Consult Clin Psychol* 63:966, 1995.

61. Galanter M, Larson D, Rubenstone E: Christian psychiatry: the impact of evangelical belief on clinical practice, *Am J Psychiatry* 148:90, 1991.

62. Gaster B, Holroyd J: St. John's wort for depression: a systematic review, *Arch Intern Med* 160:152, 2000.

63. Gaus W, Hogel J: Studies on the efficacy of unconventional therapies: problems and designs, *Arzneimittelforschung* 45:88, 1995.

64. Gelenberg AJ: St. John's wort: nostrum for depression, *Biol Ther Psychiatry Newslett* 8:15, 1997.

65. George M et al: Daily repetitive transcranial magnetic stimulation (rTMS) improves mood in depression, *Neuroreport* 6:1853, 1995.

66. George MS, Keller TA, Post RM: Activation studies in mood disorders, *Psychiatr Ann* 24:648, 1994.

67. Gilyarovski VA et al: A's Electroson, *Medguaz* 6:10, 1953.

68. Gloaguen V et al: A meta-analysis of the effects of cognitive therapy in depressed patients, *J Affect Dis* 49:59, 1998.

69. Godfrey PSA et al: Enhancement of recovery from psychiatric illness by methylfolate, *Lancet* 336:392, 1990.

70. Goldman HH: *Review of general psychiatry*, ed 2, New York, 1988, Appleton & Lange.

71. Greeson JM, Sanford B, Monti DA: St. John's wort (*Hypericum perforatum*): a review of the current pharmacological, toxicological, and clinical literature, *Psychopharmacology (Berl)* 153:402, 2001.

72. Hansgen KD, Vesper J: Antidepressive Wirksamkeit eines hochdosierten *Hypericum*-extracktes, *Munch Med Wschr* 138:35, 1996.

73. Harper EH et al: Is schizophrenia rare if grain is rare? *Biol Psychiatry* 19:385, 1984.

74. Harrell S: Pluralism, performance and meaning in Taiwanese healing: a case study, *Culture Med Psychiatry* 15:45, 1991.

75. Harvard School of Public Health: Global health statistics. In Murray CJL, Lopez AD, editors: *Global burden of disease and injury series*, 1996, Cambridge, Mass, Harvard University.

76. Hearst ED et al: Electrosleep therapy: a double-blind trial, *Arch Gen Psychiatry* 30:463, 1974.

77. Hirsch M: What are the uses and dangers of kava? *Harv Ment Health Lett* 17:8, 2000.

78. Hodge JR: Can hypnosis help psychosis? *Am J Clin Hypn* 30:248, 1988.

79. Hoffman D: *The herbalist*, Hopkins, Minn, 1994, Hopkins Technology.

80. Holzl J: Zeitschrift fur Phytotherapie, *Inhalt Wirkmech Johannish* 14:255, 1993.

81. Horrobin DF: Prostaglandin deficiency and endorphin excess in schizophrenia: the case for treatment with penicillin, zinc and evening primrose oil, *J Orthomol Psychiatry* 8:13, 1979.

82. Horrobin DF: Niacin flushing, prostaglandin E and evening primrose oil: a possible objective test for schizophrenia, *J Orthomol Psychiatry* 9:33, 1980.

83. Horton EW: Prostaglandin E and schizophrenia, *Lancet* 1:313, 1980.

84. Hubner WD, Lande S, Podzuweit H: *Hypericum* treatment of mild depressions with somatic symptoms, *J Geriatr Psychiatr Neurol* 7(suppl 1):12, 1994.

84a. Hypericum Depression Study Group: Effect of *Hypericum perforatum* (St. John's Wort) in major depressive disorder; a randomized controlled trial, *JAMA* 287:1807, 2002.

85. James S et al: Melatonin administration in insomnia, *Neuropsychopharmacology* 3:19, 1990.
86. Kaneko M et al: L-5-HTP treatment and serum 5-HT level after L-5-HTP loading on depressed patients, *Neuropsychobiology* 5:232, 1979.
87. Kaplan HI, Sadock BJ: *Textbook of psychiatry*, New York, 1985, Williams & Wilkins.
88. Keith SJ, Matthew SM: Group, family, and milieu therapies and psychosocial rehabilitation in the treatment of the schizophrenic disorders. In Grinspoon L, editor: *Psychiatry 1982 annual review*, Washington, DC, 1982, American Psychiatric Press.
89. Keys S: Attitudes towards the use of acupuncture in the treatment of the elderly mentally ill, *Complement Ther Med* 3:242, 1995.
90. Klawansky S et al: Meta-analysis of randomized controlled trials of cranial electrostimulation, *J Nerv Ment Dis* 183:478, 1995.
91. Klich R: Verhaltenstorungen im Kindesaler und deren Therapie, *Med Welt* 26:1251, 1975.
92. Kobat-Zinn J et al: Effectiveness of meditation-based stress reduction programs in the treatment of anxiety disorders, *Am J Psychiatry* 149:936, 1992.
93. Koh TC: T'ai chi chuan, *Am J Chin Med* IX(1):15, 1981.
94. Komori T et al: Effects of citrus fragrance on immune function and depressive states, *Neuroimmunomodulation* 2:174, 1995.
95. Krieger MJ, Zussman M: The importance of cultural factors in a brief reactive psychosis, *J Clin Psychiatry* 42:248, 1981.
96. Kurland HD: ECT and Acu-EST in the treatment of depression, *Am J Chin Med* 4:289, 1976.
97. Larson D: Role of prayer in mental health, *Altern Complement Ther*, March/April 1996, p 91.
98. Leathwood PD, Chauffard F: Quantifying the effect of mild sedatives, *J Psychiatr Res* 17:115, 1982.
99. Lehrer PM et al: Progressive relaxation and medication: a study of the psychophysiological and therapeutic differences between the two techniques, *Behav Res Ther* 21:651, 1983.
100. Lest'e A, Rust J: Effects of dance on anxiety, *Percept Mot Skills* 58:767, 1984.
101. Levitt E, James N: A clinical trial of electrosleep therapy with a psychiatric inpatient sample, *Aust NZ J Psychiatry* 9:287, 1975.
102. Leye X, Leqing X, Xiufeng Y: 124 cases of dyssomnia treated with acupuncture at sishencong points, *J Tradit Chin Med* 14:171, 1994.
103. MICB: AMED: allied and alternative medicine, 1985 to date, Knight-Ridder Information (DataStar), Yorkshire, UK, Boston Spa West.
104. Lindahl O, Lindwall L: Double blind study of a valerian preparation, *Pharmacol Biochem Behav* 32:1065, 1988.
105. Linde K et al: St John's wort for depression: an overview and meta-analysis of randomized clinical trials, *Br J Med* 313:253, 1996.
106. Lipinski JF et al: An open trial of *S*-adenosylmethionine for the treatment of depression, *Am J Psychiatry* 141:448, 1984.
107. Liu G et al: Changes in brain stem and cortical auditory potentials during Qi-gong meditation, *Am J Chin Med* XVIII:95, 1990.
108. Lopez-Ibor JJ: Depressive AquaValenta Undaraskiete Depressionen, *Psychiatry* 152:35, 1976.
109. Lukoff D, Lu FG, Turner R: Cultural considerations in the assessment and treatment of religious and spiritual problems, *Psychiatr Clin North Am* 18:467, 1995.
110. Ma QH, Ju YL, Zhang ZL: [Immunological study of inefficiency schizophrenics with deficiency syndrome treated with xin shen ling], *Chung Hsi I Chieh Ho Tsa Chih* 11:215, 197, 1991.
111. Marcolongo R et al: Double-blind multicentre study of the activity of *S*-adenosyl-methionine in hip and knee osteoarthritis, *Curr Ther Res* 37:82, 1985.
112. Martinez B et al: *Hypericum* in the treatment of seasonal affective disorder, *J Geriatr Psychiatr Neurol* 7(suppl 1):29, 1994.
113. Martinsen EW, Hoffart A, Solberg O: Comparing aerobic with nonaerobic forms of exercise in the treatment of clinical depression: a randomized trial, *Compr Psychiatry* 30:324, 1989.
114. Matussek N et al: The effect of L-5-hydroxytryptophan alone and in combination with a decarboxylase inhibitor in depressive patients, *Adv Biochem Psychopharmacol* 11:399, 1974.
115. McCutcheon LE: Treatment of anxiety with a homeopathic remedy, *J Appl Nutr* 48:2, 1996.

116. Mendlewicz J, Youdin MBH: Antidepressant potentiation of 5-hydroxytryptophan by L-deprenyl in affective illness, *J Affect Dis* 2:137, 1980.

117. *Mental health: a report of the surgeon general*, Rockville, Md, 1999, National Institutes of Mental Health.

118. Meseguer E et al: Life-threatening parkinsonism induced by kava-kava, *Mov Dis* 17:195, 2002.

119. Micali M, Chiti D, Balestra V: Double blind controlled clinical trial of SAMe administered orally in chronic liver disease, *Curr Ther Res* 33:1004, 1983.

120. Montakab H, Langel G: The effect of acupuncture in the treatment of insomnia: clinical study of subjective and objective evaluation, *Schweiz Med Wochenschr Suppl* 62:49, 1994.

121. Moore JA et al: A double-blind study of electrosleep for anxiety and insomnia, *Biol Psychiatry* 10:59, 1975.

122. Morin CM et al: Nonpharmacological interventions for insomnia: a meta-analysis of treatment efficacy, *Am J Psychiatry* 151:1172, 1994.

123. Murtagh DR, Greenwood KM: Identifying effective psychological treatments for insomnia: a meta-analysis, *J Consult Clin Psychol* 63:79, 1995.

124. Nagata K et al: Studies of electrosleep on normal adults, insomniacs, and hypertensive patients, *Tok J Exp Med* 28:69, 1981.

125. Nakajima T, Kudo Y, Kaneko Z: Clinical evaluation of 5-hydroxytryptophan as an antidepressant drug, *Folia Psychiatr Neurol* 32:223, 1978.

126. Nan L, Qingming Y: Insomnia treated by auricular pressing therapy, *J Tradit Chin Med* 10:174, 1990.

127. National Institutes of Health: Integration of behavioral and relaxation approaches into the treatment of chronic pain and insomnia, *JAMA* 276:313, 1996.

128. Obeyesekere G: The theory and practice of psychological medicine in the ayurvedic tradition, *Culture Med Psychiatry* 1:155, 1977.

129. Pasche B et al: Effects of low energy emission therapy in chronic psychophysiological insomnia, *Sleep* 19:327, 1996.

130. Pauling L: On the orthomolecular environment of the mind: orthomolecular therapy, *Am J Psychiatry* 131:1251, 1974.

131. Pauling L: Orthomolecular psychiatry, *Science* 19:265, 1986.

132. Pepplinhwaizen L et al: Schizophrenia-like psychosis caused by a metabolic disorder, *Lancet* 1(8166):454, 1980.

133. Phillips KD, Skelton WD: Effects of individualized acupuncture on sleep quality in HIV disease, *J Assoc Nurses AIDS Care* 12:27, 2001.

134. Post RM, Weiss RB, Ketter TA: The temporal lobes and affective disorders: basic and clinical perspective. In Bolwig T, editor: *The temporal lobes and the limbic system*, London, 1992, Wrightson Biomedical.

135. Reilly D et al: Is evidence for homeopathic treatment reproducible? *Lancet* 344:1601, 1994.

136. Reinecke MA, Ryan NE, DuBois DL: Cognitive-behavioral therapy of depression and depressive symptoms during adolescence: a review and meta-analysis, *J Am Acad Child Adolesc Psychiatry* 37:26, 1998.

137. Reite M et al: Sleep inducing effect of low energy emission therapy, *Bioelectromagnetics* 15:67, 1994.

138. Researchers, Agency for Health Care Policy and Research: Depression in primary care, Clinical practice guideline no 5, Rockville, Md, 1993, US Department of Health and Human Services.

139. Reynolds EH, Stramentinoli G: Folic acid S-adenosyl-L-methionine and affective disorders, *Psychol Med* 13:705, 1983.

140. Rief W, Hermanutz M: Responses to activation and rest in patients with panic disorder and major depression, *Br J Clin Psychol* 35:605, 1996.

141. Roberge AC, Missala K, Sourkes TL: Alpha-methyltryptophan: effects on synthesis and degradation of serotonin in the brain, *Neuropharmacology* 11:197, 1972.

142. Romoli A: Ear acupuncture in psychosomatic medicine, *Acupunct Electrother Res* 18:185, 1993.

143. Rosenbaum JF et al: An open-label pilot study of oral S-adenosyl-L-methionine in major depression: interim results, *Psychopharmacol Bull* 1:189, 1988.

144. Rosenthal SH, Masserman JH: *Current psychiatric therapies*, vol 12, New York, 1972, Grune & Stratton.

145. Rovesti P, Colombo E: Aromatherapy and aerosol, *SPC* 19:475, 1973.

146. Rubin DO: The major psychoses and neuroses as omega-3 essential fatty acid deficiency syndrome: substrate pellagra, *Biol Psychiatry* 16:837, 1981.

147. Ryu H et al: Acute effect of Qigong training on stress hormonal levels in man, *Am J Chin Med* XXIV:193, 1996.

148. Sack M, Lempa W, Lamprecht F: Study quality and effect-sizes: a meta-analysis of EMDR treatment for posttraumatic stress disorder, *Psychother Psychosom Med Psychol* 51:350, 2001.

149. Saki M, Pogady J: [Newest advances in clinical phytotherapy in Chinese psychiatry], *Cesk Psychiatr* 90:48, 1994.

150. Sano I: L-5-Hydroxytryptophan (L-5HTP) therapie, *Folia Psychiatr Neurol* 26:7, 1972.

151. Sarai K: Oriental medicine as therapy for resistant depression: use of some herbal drugs in the Far East (Japan), *Prog Neuropsychopharmacol Biol Psychiatry* 16:171, 1992.

152. Scagnelli-Jobsis J: Hypnosis with psychotic patients: a review of the literature and presentation of the-oretical framework, *Am J Clin Hypn* 25:22, 1983.

153. Scavone JM: *Essentials of clinical research*, Boston, 1991, Healthways Communications.

154. Schell EJ, Allolio B, Schonecke W: Physiological and psychological effects of hatha-yoga exercise in healthy women, *Int J Psychosom* 41:46, 1994.

155. Schmidt U, Sommer H: St. John's wort extract in the ambulatory therapy of depression: attention and reaction ability are preserved, *Fortschr Med* 11:339, 1993.

156. Schnieder-Helmert D, Spinweber C: Evaluation of L-tryptophan for treatment of insomnia: a review, *Psychopharmacology* 89:1, 1986.

157. Schoen Johnson B: *Psychiatric–mental health nursing*, ed 4, New York, 1997, Lippincott.

158. Shannahoff-Khalsa DS, Beckett LR: Clinical case report: efficacy of yogic techniques in the treatment of obsessive compulsive disorders, *Int J Neurosci* 85:1, 1996.

159. Shelton RC et al: Effectiveness of St. John's wort in major depression: a randomized controlled trial, *JAMA* 285:1978, 2001.

160. Shepherd J, Stein K, Milne R: Eye movement desensitization and reprocessing in the treatment of post-traumatic stress disorder: a review of an emerging therapy, *Psychol Med* 30:863, 2000.

161. Shi Z, Tan M: An analysis of the therapeutic effect of acupuncture treatment in 500 cases of schizo-phrenia, *J Tradit Chin Med* 6:99, 1986.

162. Simon GE, Von Korff M, Barlow W: Healthcare costs of patients with recognized depression, *Arch Gen Psychiatry* 52:850, 1995.

163. Sourkes T: Alpha-methyltryptophan as a therapeutic agent, *Neuropsychopharmacol Biol Psychiatry* 15:935, 1991.

164. Spiegel D: Hypnosis with psychotic patients: comment on Scagnelli-Jobsis, *Am J Clin Hypn* 25:289, 1983.

165. Springe R: Some neuroendocrinologic effects of so-called anxiolytic music, *Int J Neurol* 19/20:186, 1986.

166. Takahashi S, Kondo H, Kato N: Effects of 5-hydroxytryptophan on brain monoamine metabolism and evaluation of its clinical effect in depressive patients, *J Psychiatr Res* 12:177, 1975.

167. Tanra AJ et al: TJS-010: a new prescription of kampo medicine with putative antidepressive and anxi-olytic properties: a behavioral study using experimental models for depression and anxiety, *Hiroshima J Med Sci* 43:145, 1995.

168. Tao DJ: Research on the reduction of anxiety and depression with acupuncture, *Am J Acupunct* 21:327, 1993.

169. Templer DI: The efficacy of electrosleep therapy, *Can Psychiatr Assoc J* 20:607, 1975.

170. Thomson J et al: The treatment of depression in general practice: a comparison of L-tryptophan, amitriptyline, and a combination of L-tryptophan and amitriptyline with placebo, *Psychol Med* 12:741, 1982.

171. Tolbott JA, Hales RE, Yudofsky SC: *Textbook of psychiatry*, Washington, DC, 1988, American Psychiatric Press.

172. Unutzer J et al: Mental disorders and the use of alternative medicine: results from a national survey, *Am J Psychiatry* 157:1851, 2000.

173. Van Hiele LJ: 5-Hydroxytryptophan in depression: the first substitution therapy in psychiatry, *Neuropsychobiology* 6:230, 1980.

174. Van Praag AJ et al: Tryphophan in mania, *Arch Gen Psychiatry* 30:56, 1974.

175. Van Praag HM: Management of depression with serotonin precursors, *Biol Psychiatry* 16:291, 1981.

176. Vlissides DN, Venulet A, Jenner FA: Gluten free/gluten load controlled trial in a secure ward population, *Br J Psychiatry* 148:447, 1986.

177. Volwiler-Gunning S, Holmes TH: Dance therapy with psychotic children: definition and quantitative evaluation, *Arch Gen Psychiatry* 28:707, 1973.

178. Wagner H, Bladt S: Inhibition of MAO by fractions and constituents of *Hypericum* extract, *J Geriatr Psychiatr Neurol* 7(suppl 1):65, 1994.

179. Watkins LL, Connor KM, Davidson JR: Effect of kava extract on vagal cardiac control in generalized anxiety disorder: preliminary findings, *J Psychopharmacol* 15:283, 2001.

180. Weiss MF: The treatment of insomnia through the use of electrosleep: an EEG study, *J Ment Dis* 157:108, 1973.

181. Wen ST: The development of psychiatric concepts in traditional Chinese medicine, *Arch Gen Psychiatry* 29:569, 1973.

182. Westen D, Morrison K: A multidimensional meta-analysis of treatments for depression, panic, and generalized anxiety disorder: an empirical examination of the status of empirically supported therapies, *J Consult Clin Psychol* 69:875, 2001.

183. Wexler BE, Cicchetti DV: The outpatient treatment of depression: implications of outcome research for clinical practice, *J Nerv Ment Dis* 180:277, 1991.

184. Whiskey E, Werneke U, Taylor D: A systematic review and meta-analysis of *Hypericum perforatum* in depression: a comprehensive review, *Int Clin Psychopharmacol* 16:239, 2001.

185. Whittal ML, Otto MW, Hong JJ: Cognitive-behavior therapy for discontinuation of SSRI treatment of panic disorder: a case series, *Behav Res Ther* 39:939, 2001.

186. Witte B et al: Treatment of depressive symptoms with a high concentration *Hypericum* preparation: a multicenter placebo-controlled double-bind study, *Fortschr Med* 113(28):404, 1995.

187. Woelk H, Burkard G, Grunwald J: Benefits and risks of the *Hypericum* extract LI: drug monitoring study with 3250 patients, *J Geriatr Psychiatr Neurol* 7(suppl 1):34, 1994.

188. Xiujuan Y: Clinical observation on needling extrachannel points in treating mental depression, *J Tradit Chin Med* 14:14, 1994.

189. Yi R: Eighty-six cases of insomnia treated by double point needling: dailing through to waiguan, *J Tradit Chin Med* 5:22, 1985.

190. Yukang W: An observation on the therapeutic effect of acupuncture in treating 50 cases of insomnia, *Int J Clin Acupunct* 3:91, 1992.

191. Zimilacher K, Battegay R, Gastpar M: L-5-Hydroxytryptophan alone and in combination with a peripheral decarboxylase inhibitor in the treatment of depression, *Neuropsychobiology* 20:28, 1988.

SUGGESTED READINGS

Brodie HK, Brodie SM: An overview of trends in psychiatry research, *Am J Psychiatry* 130:1309, 1973.

Daniel W: *Biostatistics: A foundation for analysis in the health sciences*, New York, 1995, Wiley.

Goleman D, Gurin J: *Mind body medicine: how to use your mind for better health*, Yonkers, 1993, Consumer Reports Books.

Lebot V, Merlin M, Lidstrom L: Kava: the pacific elixir, New Haven, Conn, 1997, Yale University Press.

Maxmen JS, Ward NG: *Essential psychopathology and its treatment*, ed 2 (revised for *DSM*-IV), New York, 1995, Norton.

Spinella M: *The psychopharmacology of herbal medicine*, Cambridge, 2001, MIT Press.

CHAPTER 9

Alcohol and Chemical Dependency

TACEY ANN BOUCHER, PATRICIA D. CULLITON,
and MILTON L. BULLOCK

Complementary and alternative medicine (CAM) has an extensive past in the field of substance abuse treatment. The use of herbs to treat the effects of alcohol consumption dates back hundreds of years. Sanitariums for people with drug and alcohol disorders used saline and electric baths in treatment in the late 1800s, and early in the twentieth century, street peddlers sold remedies for substance abuse even though the remedies themselves frequently contained morphine or cocaine in substantial doses.[151] Spirituality and prayer were introduced into mainstream addiction medicine in the 1900s and provide the foundation for the most common intervention for alcoholism in the United States.[32,146] Other methods such as acupuncture and nutrition are now widely used for the treatment of substance use disorders.

The progressive integration of CAM methods into addiction medicine has been bolstered by popular sentiment toward CAM and the desire of treatment counselors and physicians to broaden their treatment arsenals. The development of drug courts in numerous states, which often mandate offenders to acupuncture treatment programs, also has contributed to the merger of these treatment fields. Although research lags behind integration efforts, scientists and clinicians have generated useful preliminary data during the last three decades regarding treatment efficacy.

This chapter first presents information on the various forms of CAM therapies used to treat addictions. Second, an overview provides empiric findings relevant to the efficacy of CAM for the treatment of substance abuse. Third, we propose potential models for the integration of CAM with conventional or biomedicine and offer predictions concerning the future of CAM for the treatment of substance abuse.

◥ Epidemiology of Substance Abuse

The extraordinary prevalence of substance abuse in the United States and the attendant human and economic costs of this disease have been amply documented in the academic and popular literature.[88,145,210] The consequences of misuse and abuse vary widely, depending on the user's social environment, substance of choice, and pattern of use, but may result in hundreds of physiologic ailments and include any number of social costs. Each year, tobacco smoking is estimated to cause 400,000 deaths, alcohol use can be linked to approximately 100,000, and illicit drug use is associated with an additional 20,000 deaths. The consequences of alcohol and drug abuse cost U.S. taxpayers up to $276 billion annually, and 55% of this total is paid by people not abusing these substances.[4] Substance abuse is one of the most prevalent and costly diseases in the United States and a leading preventable cause of death.

◥ Theories on Dependence

Researchers agree that the causes of addiction are complex and probably varied.[143] Although many people use drugs such as nicotine and alcohol, the majority rarely misuse these substances.[93] Whereas some individuals with addiction move in and out of treatment programs for years or even throughout their lifetime, others may have spontaneous remission.[106,229] Genetics provides one method of explaining the etiology or epidemiology of addictive behaviors, but exceptions abound. However, no one theory has been able to explain the phenomenon known as addiction, or *dependence.*

Sociologists have typically focused on social interactions or cultural norms.[93,143] Social change, cultural expectations, inequalities in the social system, and the impact of labeling have all been cited as causal factors.[11,70] *Psychologic traditions* differ because their models of substance abuse typically implicate mental or behavioral disorders that arise out of physical and environmental factors. Substance abuse may provide relief from suffering or provide a stimulating distraction.[11,248] Recently, psychiatry has branched toward *physiologic approaches* and turned its attention to the role of genetics and neuroscience in the etiology and maintenance of addiction.[93,143]

PHYSIOLOGIC EXPLANATIONS: GENETICS AND NEUROSCIENCE

Despite cultural differences in the behavior manifestations of substance use, recent neurochemical and molecular findings provide strong evidence for physiologic models of dependence.[84] Research has shown that genetic influences are related to characteristics of alcohol and drug abuse, such as alcohol-metabolizing enzymes, personality traits, and related neurochemical receptors.[57,72,98,108] Although alcoholism has been the focus of research efforts, evidence suggests that genetic explanations may be applicable to other substances.[253]

Numerous advances have been made in neurochemistry and molecular biology, with profound implications for addictions research.* Knowledge of the molecular pharmacology of most drugs of abuse has led researchers to examine the roles of neurotransmitters in addiction. Findings have implicated serotonin, dopamine, and endogenous opioid activity in the brain in many aspects of drug use and abuse.[158,191] Explicating details about the neurotransmitter system, including the functions of dopamine, gamma-aminobutyric acid (GABA), and the neuropeptide corticotropin-releasing factor (CRF), is believed to be key in understanding the neurobiology of ethanol dependence.[116]

◤ Overview of Standard Treatments

Alcoholism is a heterogeneous disorder; numerous combinations of factors satisfy the diagnostic criteria, and it has been acknowledged that no single model or standardized package of care will suffice.[2,46,90,184] The same is true for a number of other drugs, including cocaine, opiates, and nicotine.[12,67] Dreams of finding a "magic bullet" to prevent or treat drug misuse are fading, leading researchers and treatment professionals to suggest increasing the frequency and intensity of treatment services and combining multiple therapies.[220]

CAM approaches offer treatment providers the opportunity to improve overall treatment outcomes by expanding and enhancing the treatment continuum. Treatment programs increasingly combine methods from both CAM and conventional frameworks to such an extent that in some areas therapies such as acupuncture and hypnosis are almost commonplace.

BEHAVIORAL THERAPIES

"Standard treatment" is somewhat of a misnomer when used to describe the behavioral and social approaches of contemporary chemical dependency treatment programs. Treatment has become highly specialized, with a variety of approaches and options available, including inpatient, residential, day care, and outpatient programs. The most frequently encountered behavioral techniques and components include comprehensive assessment, medical services, sociotherapies, psychosocial education, 12-step work, relapse prevention, cognitive therapies, psychotherapies, behavioral therapies, family therapy, occupational therapy, and brief interventions. Variations in the interpretation and application of each of these components contribute to program diversity. In recent years a wide variety of procedures, both psychologic and somatic, have been tried in the treatment of alcoholism. No one therapy has been definitively proved superior to another.[5,73,148,149,178,179]

---

*References 7, 63, 69, 124, 125, 158, 202, 231.

PHARMACOLOGIC THERAPIES

Alcohol

A variety of drug treatments are used in the treatment of alcohol dependence, including aversive drugs, opioid antagonists, selective serotonin reuptake inhibitors (SSRIs), and antidepressants.[220] *Disulfiram* is a common aversive agent. Despite some positive clinical trial data, however, dropout rates of patients using disulfiram have been prohibitively high,[59] and the use of disulfiram is generally discouraged.[220]

Two medications, *naltrexone* and *acamprosate* (calcium acetylhomotaurinate), have demonstrated the greatest efficacy in the treatment of alcohol dependence.[61,109,110] Although acamprosate is not approved for clinical use in the United States, both acamprosate and naltrexone appear to have a modest impact on abstinence. Clearly, however, neither functions as a magic bullet.[110,112] Current drug therapies appear to help reduce alcohol consumption and extend periods of abstinence rather than eliminate alcohol dependence. Questions about optimal treatments, dosages, and duration remain.[220]

Opiates

Three drug groups have been used in the pharmacologic treatment of opiate dependence: (1) opiate agonists, such as methadone and L-alpha-acetylmethadol (LAAM); (2) partial opiate agonists, such as buprenorphine; and (3) opiate antagonists, such as naltrexone.[90]

Cocaine

No pharmaceutical for the treatment of cocaine dependence has demonstrated wide-spread efficacy, although pharmacotherapy is considered a promising avenue for research.[121] Several therapies have shown a subjective impact on craving, but none has directly impacted dependence or use. The dopaminergic system has been the target of the majority of agents (dopamine agonists) because of its relationship to reinforcement. Serotonergic systems have been targeted with agents such as fluoxetine, ritanserin, and sertraline. Classic tricyclic antidepressants have also been used in treatment.[68,69]

Marijuana

Although the cause and effect are difficult to determine, dependence on marijuana appears to be driven by psychopathology rather than psychopharmacology. At this time, psychosocial interventions rather than medication are used to treat *Cannabis* dependence.[76]

Stimulants

Other dopamine agonists (e.g., bromocriptine) and tricyclic antidepressants (e.g., desipramine) have been used, but controlled research regarding treatment of amphetamine abuse is scarce.[105]

Sedative-Hypnotics (Benzodiazepines)

The pharmacologic treatment of benzodiazepine withdrawal typically involves the substitution of a less addictive barbiturate, such as phenobarbital. Anticonvulsants such as carbamazepine or valproate may also be substituted, although studies do not fully evaluate subsequent issues of craving.[247]

Hallucinogens

Despite their abuse potential, benzodiazepines may be used to treat negative reactions to hallucinogens. Medication is *not* used for the treatment of chronic abuse of hallucinogens; if treatment is necessary, psychotherapy or a 12-step program is recommended.[169]

Nicotine

Ironically, nicotine is one of the primary pharmacologic agent approved by the U.S. Food and Drug Administration (FDA) for the treatment of smoking cessation. Rather than being smoked, nicotine replacement therapy is administered using transdermal systems (patch), gum, spray, or inhaler. Sustained-release *bupropion* (e.g., Zyban) is also approved as a treatment for nicotine dependence. Bupropion is recommended as a first-line pharmacotherapy for smoking cessation and is often used in conjunction with nicotine replacement therapies.[227]

Two other therapies, *clonidine* and *nortriptyline*, are also often used as smoking cessation medications but are not currently FDA approved. Both should be used only under a physician's direction when first-line medications are contraindicated. Anxiolytics, benzodiazepines, beta-blockers, silver acetate, mecamylamine, and antidepressants other than bupropion and nortriptyline have not shown beneficial effects for smoking cessation and therefore are not recommended.[227]

◼ CAM Therapies for Chemical Dependency

This section reviews several substances based on the prevalence and severity of misuse/abuse and the extent of the CAM literature, including heroin and opiates, alcohol, cocaine, nicotine, and hallucinogens. Amphetamine and benzodiazepine abuse are also briefly discussed. The CAM methods selected for discussion are determined by the extent and quality of available literature and research; acupuncture is a focal point because of the large volume of literature.

ACUPUNCTURE

Acupuncture is highlighted in this chapter for two principal reasons. First, literature on the use of acupuncture for the overall treatment of substance abuse is more prevalent than for any other CAM method. In particular, a greater number of descriptive and controlled studies have been published regarding the efficacy of acupuncture. Second, acupuncture is the most widely used CAM method for the treatment of substance abuse, excluding spirituality and prayer in conventional 12-step programs. Acupuncture is even mandated for the treatment of offenders by many drug courts.

In the 1980s, crack cocaine, high rates of recidivism, and the lack of a magic bullet to treat substance use disorders provided the opportunity for acupuncture to enter the mainstream. Acupuncture had been growing in popularity for treating alcoholism, and data had been published indicating that acupuncture increases treatment retention.[29] The National Acupuncture Detoxification Association (NADA) was formed in 1985 as a membership and training organization with references to "barrier-free treatment."[41] The sudden influx of a new treatment population of young crack-smoking men and women who either were not receiving successful treatment or were in urban areas that could not serve the dramatic increase in treatment requests opened the way for acupuncture. It was believed that acupuncture would provide inexpensive and effective treatment for large numbers of individuals.

In the United States, NADA trainers have taught more than 4000 acupuncturists, counselors, nurses, and physicians how to perform acupuncture for substance abuse. Almost as many people have been trained in Europe, testament to the proliferation of NADA chapters throughout the world. An estimated 700 to 1000 chemical dependency programs in the United States are offering acupuncture for the treatment of addictions, and new programs are implemented regularly.[205]

Table 9-1 summarizes studies conducted on the use of acupuncture in alcohol and chemical dependency, and Table 9-2 presents major review articles on this CAM therapy. Articles were identified using a number of databases, including MEDLINE, *Excerpta Medica* (EMBASE), Cochrane Database of Systematic Reviews (COCH), Database of Abstracts of Reviews of Effectiveness (DARE), and *Cumulative Index to Nursing and Allied Health* (CINHAL). The bibliographies of selected articles then were reviewed to identify additional references. Despite the large number of studies, treatment protocols are often poorly designed or implemented; they lack methodologic rigor. Poorly designed studies may be characterized by insufficient sample size/power, inadequately defined hypotheses, inappropriate outcome measures, and/or substandard analyses. Furthermore, discrepancies in design and implementation or lack of standardization make it difficult to compare the outcomes of studies and impair our ability to draw conclusions. Some of these studies are reviewed in more detail later in this section.

Therapeutic Approach to Patient

NADA regards acupuncture as an adjunctive treatment for addictions. However, depending on location and the local policy of treatment admissions, entry into acupuncture for addictive disorders may occur by several different methods. Individuals may walk into a freestanding acupuncture clinic or program, can be mandated by a "drug court" to a particular acupuncture program, can be incarcerated in a jail or prison that offers acupuncture, or may be a client of a hospital-based, outpatient, or residential facility that offers acupuncture as part of its treatment regimen.

Once admission criteria have been met, however, the process for NADA-style acupuncture is relatively uniform. Patients receive treatment in a group setting, seated in large chairs with arms and high backs to provide support if they fall asleep during

TABLE 9–1. **STUDIES OF ACUPUNCTURE IN ALCOHOL AND CHEMICAL DEPENDENCY**

Study	Number	Design†	Methods‡	Journal
ALCOHOL				
*Bullock et al.[27] (2002)	503	s,b,r,l,p,c,f	Z,H,O,I	J Subst Abuse Treat
Bullock et al.[26] (1989)	80	s,b,l,p,c,f	Z,H,O,I	Lancet
Bullock et al.[29] (1987)	54	s,b,l,c	Z,H,O,I	Alcohol Clin Exp Res
Facchinetti et al.[53] (1985)	14	m,s,c	—,H,O,i	Subst Alcohol Actions Misuse
Lao[115] (1995)	30	l,c	—,H,O,I	Am J Acupunct
Lewenberg[119] (1985)	50/76	l,f	—,—,o,—	Clin Ther
Milanov, Toteva[144] (1993)	25	w,s,l	—,H,—,I	Am J Acupunct
Olms[160] (1984)	34 cases	w,l	—,—,—,—	Am J Acupunct
Sapir-Weise et al.[188] (1999)	72	s,b,r,l,p	—,H,O,I	Alcohol Alcoholism
Thorer, Volf[224] (1996)	35	s,b,r,c	—,H,O,—	Presented at conference
Timofeev[225] (1994)	48	s,l,f	—,—,—,—	Bull Exp Biol Med
Toteva, Milanov[226] (1996)	118	w,s,r,l,c,f	—,H,O,I	Am J Acupunct
Worner et al.[254] (1992)	56	s,r,l,c	—,H,O,I	Drug Alcohol Depend
COCAINE				
Avants et al.[8] (2000)	82	s,b,r,l,p,c	Z,H,O,I	Arch Intern Med
Avants et al.[9] (1995)	40	s,b,r,p	Z,H,O,i	J Subst Abuse Treat
*Bullock et al.[28] (1999)	438	s,b,r,l,p,c,f	Z,H,O,I	J Subst Abuse Treat
Gurevich et al.[78] (1996)	77	l,c,f	—,h,o,—	J Subst Abuse Treat
*Lipton et al.[122] (1994)	192	s,b,r,l,p,f	Z,H,O,I	J Subst Abuse Treat
*Margolin et al.[130] (2002)	620	s,b,r,l,p,c,f	Z,H,O,I	JAMA
Margolin et al.[133] (1993)	48	s,b,l,p	—,H,O,—	Am J Chin Med
Margolin et al.[132] (1993)	32	s,l,f	—,H,O,I	NIDA Res Monogr (abstract)
Otto et al.[163] (1998)	36	s,b,r,l,p, f +24	—,h,o,I Retro control	Am J Addict
Richard et al.[183] (1995)	228	s,r,l,c,f	—,H,O,i	J Sub Abuse Treat
Smith[204] (1988)	1500	l	—,—,—,I	Am J Acupunct
SMOKING CESSATION				
Choy et al.[33] (1983)	514	l,f	—,—,—,—	Am J Med
*Clavel-Chapelon[35] (1997)	996	s,b,r,l,p,c,f	Z,H,O,I	Prev Med
Clavel, Benhamou[36] (1985)	651	s,r,l,c,f	Z,H,o,I	Br Med J
Cottraux et al.[40] (1983)	558	s,r,l,c,f	Z,H,O,I	Behav Res Ther
Fuller[58] (1982)	194	s,l,f	—,—,—,—	Med J Aust
Gillams et al.[66] (1984)	81	s,b,r,l,p,c,f	—,—,O,I	Practitioner
Hackett et al.[79] (1984)	72	s,l,c,f	—,—,o,—	Practitioner
He et al.[81] (2001)	46	s,b,r,l,p,f	—,H,O,I	Prev Med
He et al.[82] (1997)	46	s,b,r,l,p	—,H,O,I	Prev Med
Lamontagne et al.[114] (1980)	75	s,r,l,c	—,H,O,I	Can Med Assoc J
Low[126] (1977)	150+	w,l,f	—,—,—,—	Med J Aust (letter)
Machovec, Man[128] (1978)	58	s,b,l,c,p,f	—,—,—,I	Am J Clin Hypn
Martin, Waite[135] (1981)	405	s,b,r,l,p,c	—,H,O,I	NZ Med J
Parker, Mok[165] (1977)	41	w,b,l,p,c,f	—,—,—,—	Am J Acupunct
Steiner et al.[212] (1982)	32	s,b,r,l,p	—,H,O,I	Am J Chin Med
Tan et al.[221] (1987)	418	s,b,l,p,c	—,—,o,—	Am J Acupunct
Waite, Clough[233] (1998)	79	s,b,r,l,p,f	Z,H,O,I	Br J Gen Pract
White et al.[251] (1998)	76	w,s,b,r,l,p	Z,H,O,I	Arch Intern Med
Yiming et al.[258] (2000)	336	s,d,r,l,p,f	Z,H,o,i	Am J Chinese Med
Zalessky et al.[259] (1983)	85	s,l,f	—,—,O,—	Acupunct Electrother Res
OPIATES				
ANIMAL STUDIES				
Choy et al.[34] (1978) Morphine	84	w,m,s,c	—,H,O,na	Biochem Biophys Res Commun

Ho et al.[85] (1979) Morphine	74/121	w,s,c	—,H,O,na	Neuropharmacology
Malin et al.[129] (1988) Opiates	56	w,s,c	—,H,O,na	Biol Psychiatry
Ng et al.[157] (1975) Morphine	36	w,s,c	—,H,O,N/A	Biol Psychiatry
Wen et al.[243] (1979) Morphine	14	m,s,c	—,H,O,N/A	Am J Chin Med
Yang and Kwok[257] (1986) Morphine	119	w,s,c	—,H,O,N/A	Am J Chin Med

HUMAN STUDIES

Clement-Jones[37] (1979) Heroin	12 + 50	w,m,s,c control	—,H,O,—	Lancet
Kroenig, Oleson[111] (1985) Narcotic/methadone	14	w,l	—,—,O,—	Int J Addict
Leung[118] (1977) Opiates	17	w,l,p	—,—,—,—	Am J Acupunct
Newmeyer et al.[155] (1984) Opiates	460/297	s,l,c,f	—,—,O,—	J Psychoactive Drugs
Sainsbury[187] (1974) Heroin	1	w, case	—,—,—,—	Med J Aust
Severson et al.[193] (1977) Heroin	8	s,l,f	—,—,—,l	Int J Addict
Shuaib[200] (1976) Opium+	19	w, case	—,—,—,—	Am J Chin Med
Washburn et al.[235] (1993) Opiates/heroin	100	s,b,r,l,p	—,H,O,i	J Subst Abuse Treat
Washburn et al.[234] (1990) Opiates (3 studies)	100	w,s,b,r,l,p	—,h,O,—	Multicultural Inquiry Res AIDS
	123	Demographic	—,—,O,—	
	63	w,s,l,c,f	—,—,O,—	
Wells et al.[237] (1995) Heroin/ cocaine	60	w,s,b,r,l,p,f	—,H,O,l	Am J Addict
Wen, Cheung[241] (1973) Opiates	40	w,l,f	—,—,o,—	Asian J Med
Wen, Teo[242] (1975) Opiates	70 (f)	w,s,l,c,f	—,—,O,—	Mod Med Asia
Wen[238] (1977) Opiates	6	w,s,l	—,—,o,—	Mod Med Asia
Wen et al.[245] (1978) Opiates	8 (f)	m,s,l	—,H,O,—	Bull Narc
Wen[240] (1980) Opiates	300	w,s,l,c,f	—,—,o,—	Am J Chin Med
Wen et al.[244] (1980) Heroin	37	m,s,l,c	—,H,O,—	Am J Chin Med

OTHER ADDICTIONS

Gurevich et al.[78] (1996) Dual diagnosis	77	l,c,f	—,—, o,—	J Subst Abuse Treat
Kao and Lu[94] (1974) Multiple	23	w,l,p	—,—,—,—	Am J Acupunct
Karrell[96] (1990) Polydrug	60	w,s,l,c,f	—,—,—,—	Addict Recov
Konefal et al.[107] (1994) Multiple	568	s,r,l,c	—,H,O,—	J Addict Dis
Margolin et al.[131] (1999) Cocaine/buprenorphine	34	m,s,l,c	—,H,O,—	J Altern Complement Ther
Margolin et al.[134] (1995) Cocaine/opiate	12	s,b,l, p	—,H,O,—	Am J Chin Med
Patterson[166] (1974) Multiple	40	w,l,f	—,—,—,—	Clin Med
Russell et al.[185] (2000) Multiple	86	s,l,c	—,H,O,—	J Subst Abuse Treat
Sacks[186] (1975) Multiple	187/ 642/ 15	Multiple case	—,—,—,—	Am J Acupunct
Shakur and Smith[195] (1979) Multiple	6	w, case	—,—,—,—	Am J Acupunct
Shwartz et al.[201] (1999) Multiple	8011	l,c,f	—,H,O,—	J Subst Abuse Treat
Sween et al.[219] (1996) Multiple	106	s,l,c	—,H,O,—	Presented at conference

*Best evidence.

†s, Prospective; b, single blind; r, randomized; l, clinical; p, placebo control; c, control group (other than placebo); f, follow-up; m, mechanism; w, addresses active withdrawal.

‡Z, Sample size appropriate (power calculated); H, same type of statistic used with H,o; O, outcome measurements valid; I, inclusion/exclusion criteria addressed; N/A, not applicable; lowercase z, h, o, and i indicate same criteria but incomplete or inadequate.

TABLE 9-2. **REVIEWS OF ACUPUNCTURE/CHEMICAL DEPENDENCY STUDIES**

Study*	Topic	Substance
Anonymous (1997)	General review; efficacy	General addiction; smoking
Blum et al.[17] (1978)	Neurochemical mechanism	Opiates
Brewington et al.[21] (1994)	Review of efficacy	Multiple drugs
Brumbaugh[24] (1993)	History and protocol	Multiple drugs
Brumbaugh[25] (1994)	Summary of practice	Multiple drugs
Center/Reviews[30] (2002)[a]	Acupuncture	Smoking cessation
Center/Reviews[31] (2002)[b]	Acupuncture	General addiction
Culliton, Kiresuk[41] (1996)	General review; efficacy	Multiple drugs
Lipton, Maranda[123] (1982)	Review of finding	Heroin
Mayer[138] (2000)	Acupuncture	Section on addictions
McLellan et al.[141] (1993)[c]	Research methodology	Multiple drugs
Mendelson[142] (1978)	Hypothesis of mechanism	Alcohol and heroin
Ng[156] (1996)	Review of 5 studies	Opiate
Omura[161] (1975)	Presentation	Multiple drugs
Schwartz[190] (1988)	Review of studies	Smoking
Sharps[198] (1977)	Overview of history	Multiple drugs
Smith et al.[207] (1982)	Acupuncture program	Addiction therapy
Smith, Khan[206] (1988)	General review	Multiple drugs
Ter Riet et al.[225] (1990)[b]	Review of efficacy	Multiple drugs
White et al.[249] (2002)[b]	Acupuncture	Smoking cessation
White et al.[250] (1999)[a]	Acupuncture	Smoking cessation
Whitehead[252] (1978)	Review of efficacy	Multiple drugs

*All studies are nonsystematic except a, meta-analysis; b, systematic review; and c, meeting summary.

the treatment. Subdued lighting, soft music, and caffeine-free herbal tea usually accompany the process. Both ears are swabbed with alcohol, then five $\frac{1}{2}$-inch, presterilized, disposable needles are placed in each ear. The NADA protocol uses the points Shen Men, sympathetic, kidney, liver, and lung (Figure 9-1). For 40 minutes the participants sit back and relax while the treatment takes place. Eating, talking, and walking around are discouraged, and the acupuncturist monitors the room to promote safety and comfort.

At the end of the session, the needles are removed and placed in a biohazard container for proper disposal, and the ears are wiped with a dry cotton ball to protect against the rare occurrence of a drop or two of blood. Again, varying from program to program, patient data collection may include an extensive history, various research instruments, and objective physiologic measures, but the standard requirement consists of a consent-to-treatment form and a precise record of date and number of treatments, symptoms, points used, and the response to the treatment. An acupuncturist or acupuncture detoxification specialist can treat several people within a short time, thereby creating a cost-efficient delivery system.

Key Concepts and Debates

The administration of acupuncture for the treatment of substance abuse has been standardized in the United States through the efforts of Michael Smith at Lincoln Hospital in New York City and eventually NADA. Acupuncture typically refers to *five-point bilateral acupuncture*, in which five tiny needles are placed in the cartilage ridge

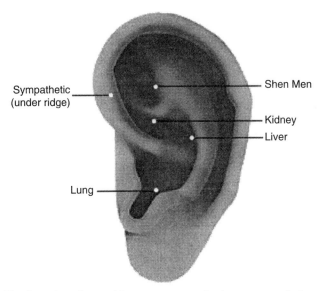

Sympathetic (under ridge)

Shen Men

Kidney

Liver

Lung

FIGURE 9–1. The five points often used in ear acupuncture for the treatment of substance abuse. The points are bilateral, and variations can exist in either number or placement.

and concha of each ear at the five points (Figure 9-1). However, variations exist within practice and research and are discussed below.

POINTS USED. Although the number of points used in addiction treatment has been standardized in clinical practice, this has not always been the case in the research setting. Although popular among practitioners, the five-point bilateral auricular protocol has typically been modified for research. The most widely recognized studies by Bullock[26-29] and Margolin[130] have traditionally used three-point or four-point protocols. Ulett has advocated one-point protocols, claiming that multiple points complicate interpretation.[141] Although body points are often used in clinical practice, they are rarely used in research. The appropriate points to insert the needle may be located using a *galvanometer*, a machine that measures skin conductivity, but these devices have been criticized as inaccurate.[141] Practitioners typically locate points visually or by patient reaction, such as sensitivity to pressure.

STAGES OF INTERVENTION. In biomedicine, substance abuse intervention occurs in stages. The medications offered to help patients through the primary stages of withdrawal are not necessarily the same ones offered during rehabilitation or for relapse prevention. Acupuncture was initially applied during the detoxification stage to help patients through withdrawal. In the United States during the 1980s, its use was extended to rehabilitation and relapse prevention. However, research has not clearly demonstrated the effectiveness of acupuncture as defined by these stages of treatment.

TREATMENT GOALS. Goals for acupuncture intervention may include decreased symptoms of withdrawal, relief from somatic symptoms, prevention of craving, increased treatment retention, hastened treatment readiness, improved quality of life, decreased substance use, and abstinence. These concepts may be measured using a variety of standardized instruments and laboratory testing.

Key Research Issues

A number of weaknesses frequently arise in substance abuse research,[41] particularly in studies employing acupuncture or other CAM methods. When designing a study, researchers often fail to differentiate between acceptable use and misuse of various substances. Although several standardized measurement tools exist, they are used infrequently or erratically in CAM research. In addition, the failure to recognize degrees of misuse often results in the inability to control for the "severity" of the addiction.

Comparison and control groups have often been inappropriate or absent from substance abuse and CAM research.[41] In acupuncture research there has been considerable debate over the use of sham or placebo treatments as controls. The five-point auricular acupuncture protocol generally has not been used in research because of the controversy over identifying an inactive placebo. Most acupuncturists believe that the puncturing of the ears by 10 or more needles could cause a generalized treatment effect by virtue of neurotransmitter mediation, regardless of their specific location. As stated earlier, the Minneapolis group has typically used three points, whereas the Yale group has settled on four in their acupuncture controlled studies. Whether auricular sham points constitute an adequate placebo is unknown, although preliminary research has been conducted.[9] As an alternative to using acupuncture needles at sham points, devices that deliver the sensation of a needle prick without puncturing the skin also are being developed.[56,95,214] These sham needling techniques are not yet being used in substance abuse research.

Success for the treatment of substance abuse has been evaluated using a variety of measures, including abstinence, decreased use, decreased cravings, diminished withdrawal symptoms, improved outlook, and increased productivity. These variations often make studies difficult to evaluate or compare. One research group may report intervention as successful because consumption was significantly reduced even though the majority of subjects relapsed, whereas another group may evaluate similar findings as a treatment failure. Data may actually be misleading if subjects who dropped out of treatment prematurely were excluded from the analysis.

Acupuncture research, in particular, has been criticized for its lack of clinical relevancy. The number and placement of needles used in research may differ from those used in a clinical setting, as may the environment and the therapist's interaction with the subject. Critics suggest that findings from this type of research cannot be generalized to the clinical setting.

HEROIN AND OPIATES

Acupuncture

Early research applying acupuncture for the treatment of substance use disorders was conducted in China on patients experiencing opiate withdrawal. In 1973, Wen and

Cheung[241] noticed that opium-addicted patients receiving *ear acupuncture* (EA) as a presurgical analgesic reported reduced withdrawal symptoms. Wen and others conducted a number of studies on humans and animals (see Table 9-1) and, despite debatable methods, made important distinctions between craving and abstinence and between detoxification and subsequent rehabilitation.[239,242]

Animal studies have generally reported positive findings for the treatment of opiate withdrawal, usually morphine.[34,85,129,157] Treatment of animals has focused on EA. The administration of EA in female WHT mice and Sprauge-Dawley rats has been reported to reduce opiate withdrawal symptoms such as wet dog shakes, teeth chattering, diarrhea, and abnormal posturing. Furthermore, preliminary animal research indicates that increases in plasma adrenocorticotropic hormone (ACTH) during withdrawal may be reduced during EA. The majority of human studies regarding EA and opiate withdrawal suffer from inadequate methodology. Despite clinical reports and preliminary trials that suggest EA decreases the symptoms and duration of withdrawal,[240-242] the efficacy of EA for the treatment of opiate withdrawal remains unknown.

Studies focused on opiate addictions that claim stronger research designs have used standardized auricular acupuncture rather than EA and have focused on relapse prevention rather than withdrawal.[235,237] One study suggests that standardized acupuncture may reduce 6-month detoxification readmission rates in some patients who list heroin as their drug of choice.[201] Still, however, no evidence at this time indicates that acupuncture is effective in the prevention of relapse in opiate dependency treatment.[21]

Other CAM Therapies

Other CAM therapies have been used for the treatment of opiate addiction, although efficacy has not been consistently shown (Table 9-3). Therapies include biofeedback,[5,22] yoga,[194] neuroelectric transcranial stimulation (NET),* transcendental meditation (TM),[64,159,162] nutrition,[14,150] and hallucinogens.[80,140,177,199] Table 9-3 reviews the outcomes of these studies as stated by the investigators/authors. The terms *positive*, *negative*, and *inconclusive* correspond to the authors' interpretation of the study results. For example, if the outcomes indicate that an intervention (e.g., yoga) was not effective for a particular condition (e.g., opiate dependence), the study would be considered "negative."

As discussed earlier, the methodologic rigor of research studies varies widely; studies frequently lack adequate sample size and appropriate outcome measures. Thus, the reader should be careful not to interpret a positive research finding as evidence of clinical efficacy; though outcomes might suggest that an intervention is effective, one or more poorly designed studies should not be considered persuasive evidence.

---

*References 3, 50, 51, 62, 71, 74, 91, 167, 168.

TABLE 9–3. **CAM THERAPIES FOR OPIATE DEPENDENCY AND WITHDRAWAL**

Study	Conclusion
BIOFEEDBACK	
Brinkman[22] (1978)	Positive
Fahrion[54] (1995)	Positive
YOGA	
Shaffer, Lasalvia[194] (1997)	Negative
NEUROLOGIC THERAPY	
Alling et al.[3] (1990)	Inconclusive
Ellison et al.[50] (1987)	Positive
Elmoghazy et al.[51] (1989)	Positive
Gariti et al.[62] (1992)	Negative
Gomez, Mikhail[71] (1978)	Positive
Gossop et al.[74] (1984)	Negative
Jarzembski[91] (1985)	Inconclusive
Patterson et al.[167] (1993)	Positive
Patterson et al.[168] (1994)	Positive
TRANSCENDENTAL MEDITATION	
Genderloos et al.[64] (1991)	Positive
O'Connell, Alexander[159] (1995)	Positive
Orme-Johnson, Farrow[162] (1977)	Positive
NUTRITION	
Beckley-Barrett, Mutch[14] (1990)	Positive
Mohs et al.[150] (1990)	Not applicable
HALLUCINOGENS	
Halpern[80] (1996)	Inconclusive
McKenna[140] (1996)	Inconclusive
Popik et al.[177] (1995)	Inconclusive
Sheppard[199] (1994)	Positive

ALCOHOL

Alcohol addiction has been treated by means of a wide variety of CAM therapies. However, two therapies have received significant attention in both popular and academic literature: acupuncture and nutrition therapy. Nutrition programs have not attained the same level of standardization as acupuncture programs, and no governing body for nutrition therapy is comparable to NADA. In 1990, however, the American Dietetic Association (ADA) issued a position statement that nutritional supplements, modified diets, and nutrition education can improve the efficacy of chemical dependency treatment, and to date this statement has not been revised.[14]

Acupuncture

Alcohol addiction was first treated with EA at Lincoln Hospital in New York. However, EA was replaced by auricular acupuncture when clinicians observed no difference between the two methods. Treatment standardization was motivated by early clinical findings,[195,203,206,207] resulting in the three-point to five-point protocols discussed earlier. Research has predominantly focused on human populations.

Several controlled studies have been published with generally positive outcomes, but few meet the standards of methodologic rigor. To date, the classic studies of Bullock et al.[26,29] have been the most rigorous and most frequently cited. In addition, the first and only large-scale, randomized, controlled trial of acupuncture for the treatment of alcoholism was recently completed by Bullock et al.[27] In the earlier studies, persons with chronic alcoholism were assigned to either true or sham acupuncture. In both studies the true-acupuncture group showed significantly decreased drinking episodes and desire to drink and fewer treatment readmissions than placebo control subjects. In the second study, significant effects were maintained through the 6-month follow-up; the placebo control group had more than twice the number of drinking episodes and readmissions to detoxification centers (Tables 9-4 and 9-5).

However, the recent large-scale study does not support previous findings.[27] The 503 subjects were recruited from a residential inpatient program and, in addition to conventional treatment, were randomized to one of the following four treatment conditions: (1) no acupuncture, (2) specific acupuncture (four-point ear), (3) nonspecific acupuncture (standardized sham), or (4) symptom-based acupuncture (individualized). This study was also concerned with clinically relevant models of delivery. The addition of a symptom-based acupuncture study arm allowed other therapeutic elements to be evaluated, including therapist-selected body points based on individual symptoms, music, dim lighting, and conversation.

TABLE 9–4. **COMPLETION RATES FOR TREATMENT PHASES AFTER ACUPUNCTURE AND PLACEBO TREATMENT FOR ALCOHOL ADDICTION***

Phase	Treatment (N = 40)	Control (N = 40)
I	37 (92.5%)	21 (52.5%)
II	26 (65%)	3 (7.5%)
III	21 (52.5%)	1 (2.5%)

From Bullock ML, Culliton PD, Olander RT: *Lancet* 1(8652):1436, 1989.
*Completion rates by treatment group for each phase, $p < 0.001$.

TABLE 9–5. **DETOXIFICATION CENTER ADMISSIONS AFTER ACUPUNCTURE AND PLACEBO TREATMENT FOR ALCOHOL ADDICTION**

Follow-Up Interval	ADMISSIONS (N)		MEAN (SEM) NO. OF ADMISSIONS	
	Treatment (75)	Control (186)	Treatment	Control
1 month*	25	59	0.62 (0.20)	1.54 (0.32)
3 months†	24	65	0.59 (0.17)	1.67 (0.42)
6 months†	26	62	0.69 (0.41)	1.56 (0.20)

From Bullock ML, Culliton PD, Oleander RT: *Lancet* 1(8652):1436, 1989.
*$p < .01$
†$p < .05$

Follow-up was done at 3, 6, and 12 months after treatment. With regard to alcohol consumption and desire for alcohol, Bullock et al.[27] found no significant differences between treatment groups. They concluded that, despite staff and patient perceptions of benefit, no support was found for the addition of acupuncture to conventional therapy for the treatment of alcoholism.

NUTRITION THERAPY

More than 20 studies have been published on the efficacy of nutrition therapies for the treatment of alcoholism.[13,77,137,246] Poor methodology and the lack of a standardized treatment protocol make evaluation of these studies difficult. Some therapies have involved the use of dietary supplements, whereas others studied complete diet changes. Despite difficulties in reporting, follow-up, or statistical power, a few studies have been identified as models for future inquiry.

The majority of animal studies have concentrated on dietary supplementation, particularly glutamine, thiamin, and zinc. In general these studies indicate that thiamin and zinc deficiencies can lead to increases in alcohol intake, whereas glutamine supplementation may decrease consumption. An early study conducted by Rogers, Pelton, and Williams[184] divided 50 Wistar rats into six groups. Each rat in five of the groups received 100 mg a day of either glutamine, glutamic acid, sodium glutamate, asparagine, or glycine. A sixth group received no supplements and served as controls. The glutamine group significantly decreased their alcohol consumption. The other five groups increased their consumption, but when the supplemented groups were compared with controls, the increases were not significant.

A link between *thiamin deficiency* and alcohol intake and metabolism was identified.[52,170] In a controlled trial, Eriksson, Pekkanen, and Rusi[52] noted that thiamin deficiency increased free-choice consumption in a mixed strain of rat derived from Wistar, Sprague-Dawley, and Long-Evans rats. High-thiamin, thiamin-deficient, and optimal-nutrition groups were given either water or ethanol during the first 4 weeks of research. During the last 3 weeks the alcohol-only group was given the choice between alcohol or water. Throughout the study the high-thiamin group drank significantly less alcohol than appropriate controls. However, the thiamin-deficient group did not clearly drink more alcohol unless consumption was related to the total energy or fluid intake during the free-choice period.

Pekkanen[170] induced thiamin deficiency in three ways: by means of diet or by the injection of one of two thiamin antagonists. Results of this controlled study indicated that the increase in ethanol intake is related to the roles of thiamin in the brain rather than to a reduction in food intake.

Collipp et al.[38] reported on three experiments on pair-fed Sprague-Dawley rats with *zinc deficiency*. Zinc deficiency did increase the voluntary intake of ethanol, which was statistically significant in the first (body weight, 58 to 81 g) and third (body weight, 120 to 199 g) experiments. After 6 weeks of the deficient diet, the percentage of alcohol consumed declined when a normal diet was administered.

Register et al.[181] attempted to look at the effects of *overall nutrition* rather than at the effects of specific supplements. One study compared the free-choice consumption of Sprague-Dawley rats fed six different diets designed to mimic human diets. A "teen-age" type of diet—with poor nutritional content—was administered to five groups. Some of the groups also received a spice mixture, a regular coffee mixture, decaffeinated coffee, a vitamin and mineral supplement, or a combination of these. The sixth group received an optimal diet. The rats fed the teen-age diet showed a progressive preference for drinking the alcohol solution. Caffeine also appeared to be a powerful inducer of free-choice consumption, whereas the spice mixture had no impact. Vitamin and mineral supplements did result in significantly reduced alcohol intake.

Although no large-scale clinical studies have been conducted, preliminary human trials have shown generally positive results using nutritional programs or supplements, including increased abstinence, reduced craving, and decreased depression.[16,18,23,43,137] For the most part, however, research has been piecemeal and methodologically unsound; results commonly lack an adequate sample size or sufficient controls.[150]

Blum, Trachtenberg, and Ransay[18] have conducted a series of trials on *amino acid supplements* for a variety of substance use disorders. Supplements are designed to restore brain neurotransmitter balance, increasing the availability of enkephalin in the brain, as well as levels of dopamine, norepinephine, serotonin, GABA, and aminergic neurotransmitters. Results of a trial ($n = 62$) showed significant improvement in retention, stress reduction, and ease of detoxification compared with placebos.

Gallimberti et al.[60] studied the impact of gamma-hydroxybutyric acid (GHB) on ethanol withdrawal. Despite a limited number of subjects in this double-blind trial ($n = 23$), GHB was superior to placebo in reducing symptoms of alcohol withdrawal, such as tremors, sweating, nausea, depression, anxiety, and restlessness.

DesMaisons[43] conducted a preliminary trial of a dietary protocol, recruiting 58 subjects with two drunk-driving offenses. She compared 29 subjects in the treatment group to 29 self-selected controls. Alcohol consumption and recidivism were significantly reduced in the treatment group.

Despite the positive outcomes of these preliminary trials, it is obvious that more rigorous studies must be conducted before claims of efficacy can be substantiated in regard to nutrition therapies. Further, the majority of human and animal studies have been restricted to alcohol abuse, neglecting the impact of nutrition therapies on other types of addiction. Strategic planning and some standardization of outcome measures are necessary if future research is to have a significant impact on the treatment of the addictions.

Other CAM Therapies

Numerous CAM methods have been used for the treatment of alcohol abuse and dependence (Table 9-6). As with Table 9-3, Table 9-6 reviews the outcomes of published studies as stated by the investigators/authors. The terms *positive, negative,* and *inconclusive* correspond to the authors' interpretation of the study results. Available literature reveals that the majority of studies conducted on the use of other CAM therapies are preliminary, often with inadequate sample size, follow-up, measures, or controls. Despite the bulk of research conducted on some methods, treatment protocols

TABLE 9–6. **CAM THERAPIES FOR ALCOHOL ABUSE AND DEPENDENCE**

Study	Conclusion
HYPNOSIS	
Edwards[49] (1966)	Negative
Jacobson, Silfverskiold[89] (1973)	Negative
Katz[97] (1980)	Inconclusive
Lenox, Bonny[117] (1976)	Not applicable
Smith-Moorhouse[209] (1969)	Positive
Stoil[213] (1989)	Inconclusive
Wadden, Penrod[232] (1981)	Inconclusive
BIOFEEDBACK	
DeGood, Vallee[42] (1978)	Not applicable
Denney et al.[44] (1991)	Positive
Fahrion[54] (1995)	Positive
Fahrion et al.[55] (1992)	Positive
Peniston[171] (1989)	Positive
Peniston, Kulkosky[172] (1990)	Positive
Peniston et al.[173] (1993)	Positive
Taub et al.[222] (1994)	Positive
Trudeau[228] (2000)	Not applicable
Weingarten et al.[236] (1980)	Not applicable
RESTRICTED ENVIRONMENTAL STIMULATION THERAPY (REST)	
Borrie[20] (1990)	Positive
Cooper et al.[39] (1988)	Positive
Rank, Suefeld[180] (1978)	Positive
PRAYER	
Miller[146] (1990)	Positive
Miller[147] (1997)	Positive
Muffler et al.[152] (1997)	Positive
Peteet[177] (1993)	Positive
YOGA	
Benson[15] (1969)	Positive
Nespor, Cs-Emy[154] (1994)	Positive
NEUROELECTRIC THERAPY (NET)	
Patterson[166] (1994)	Positive
Patterson et al.[167] (1993)	Positive
Smith, O'Neill[208] (1975)	Inconclusive
TRANSCENDENTAL MEDITATION (TM)	
Gelderloos et al.[64] (1991)	Positive
O'Connell, Alexander[159] (1995)	Positive
Orme-Johnson, Farrow[162] (1977)	Positive
HERBAL THERAPY	
Keung[99] (1993)	Positive
Keung, Vallee[101,102] (1993)	Positive
Keung, Vallee[104] (1994)	Positive
Keung et al.[103] (1995)	Positive
Li-Li et al.[120] (1985)	Positive
Overstreet et al.[164] (1996)	Positive
Petri, Takach[175] (1990)	Positive

Shanmugasundaram et al.[97] (1986)	Positive
Xie et al.[256] (1994)	Positive

EYE MOVEMENT DESENSITIZATION AND REPROCESSING (EMDR)

Shapiro et al.[197] (1994)	Positive

LIGHT THERAPY

Eastwood, Stiasny[48] (1978)	Inconclusive
Poikolainen[176] (1982)	Inconclusive
McGrath, Yahia[139] (1993)	Positive
Satel, Gawin[189] (1989)	Positive

HALLUCINOGENS

Halpern[80] (1996)	Positive
Ludwig et al.[127] (1970)	Negative
McKenna[140] (1996)	Inconclusive
Popik et al.[177] (1995)	Inconclusive
Rezvani et al.[182] (1995)	Positive
Sheppard[199] (1994)	Inconclusive

RELAXATION THERAPY

Taub et al.[222] (1994)	Negative

vary to such a degree that results are not comparable. As stated earlier, the reader should be careful not to interpret a positive research finding as evidence of clinical efficacy.

For example, more than 20 different protocols could be employed when treating addictive disorders with hypnosis, with therapists focusing on such features as reduced urge, symptom substitution, or cue sensitization.[97] Outcome measures may include abstinence, reduction in use, decreased cravings or symptoms of withdrawal, improved mood states or treatment retention, and increased productivity. Furthermore, the number of sessions and duration of treatment may vary, making it difficult to generalize findings even when the outcome measures are comparable. Therefore, whether the majority of studies report positive (biofeedback,[*] prayer,[146,147,152,174] light therapy,[48,139,176,189] herbs[†]), negative (hypnosis[‡]), or inconclusive (hallucinogens[§]) outcomes, little can be said about the efficacy of these methods.

Methodologic problems such as inadequate statistical analysis, inclusion/exclusion criteria, handling of dropouts, and reliability and validity of measurement tools reduce our confidence in other findings involving prayer,[146,147,152,174] yoga,[15,154] NET,[167,168,208] TM,[64,159,162] restricted environmental stimulation therapy (REST),[20,39,180] and relaxation.[222] Furthermore, despite clinical use, a few therapies either have been evaluated very little (e.g., eye movement desensitization and reprocessing,[197]) or not at all (e.g., homeopathy, aromatherapy) for the treatment of addictions.

---

[*]References 42, 44, 54, 55, 171-173, 222, 236.
[†]References 99-104, 120, 164, 175, 196, 256.
[‡]References 49, 89, 97, 117, 209, 213, 232.
[§]References 80, 127, 140, 177, 182, 199.

COCAINE

Acupuncture

Cocaine is included here because of its widespread use and abuse potential. At present, no known, effective treatment exists for cocaine dependence. Although the crack cocaine epidemic helped open doorways to acupuncture as a treatment method, little has been done to study the application of acupuncture or other CAM methods to this disorder. While clinical and case reports have shown promise for the treatment of craving and depression and for promoting abstinence,[10,132,133] randomized controlled trials have failed to replicate these positive findings.

Lipton, Brewington, and Smith[122] randomly assigned 192 patients to true or sham four-point auricular treatment. Forty-two patients were excluded from analysis. Only 30 patients completed two or more weeks of treatment. Of these 30 subjects, the true acupuncture treatment group showed greater mean decreases in the levels of cocaine metabolites in their urine. However, no differences were found in treatment retention or self-report.

Bullock et al.[28] conducted two linked but concurrent studies of three-point auricular acupuncture in the treatment of cocaine addiction. The first study randomly assigned 236 residential clients to true, sham, or conventional treatment. True acupuncture in this study involved the use of three auricular points. In the second study, true five-point acupuncture was administered to 202 randomly selected day-treatment clients at three dose levels (8, 16, or 28 treatments). In both studies, acupuncture was administered in conjunction with standardized treatment. The studies failed to confirm the efficacy of acupuncture for the treatment of cocaine addiction. Overall, no significant differences were found between the true, sham, psychosocial, and dose-response groups on any outcomes, including retention, abstinence, and mood states.

Margolin et al.[130] recently completed a multisite randomized controlled trial. The 620 subjects were randomized into three treatment groups: (1) standardized four-point auricular acupuncture, (2) needle insertion control (sham, or nonspecific acupuncture), and (3) relaxation control. Treatment was administered for 8 weeks, with a 3-month and a 6-month follow-up. Subjects received minimal concurrent psychosocial treatment in the form of weekly individual counseling sessions. Avants et al.[8] published initial findings from one of the sites ($n = 82$) and concluded that the findings supported the use of acupuncture for the treatment of cocaine addiction. When the data were pooled, however, Margolin et al.[100] found no differences by treatment condition on any outcome measure.

In their conclusion, Bullock et al.[28] suggest that the lack of a no-treatment control may have masked treatment effects, whereas Margolin and Avants[131] conclude that they found no evidence to support acupuncture as a stand-alone treatment. Together, these studies[28,122,130] do not support the use of acupuncture for the treatment of cocaine addiction.

Other CAM Therapies

A few other CAM methods have been used in clinical settings for the treatment of cocaine abuse and addiction (Table 9-7). With the exception of hallucinogens, for

TABLE 9–7. **CAM THERAPIES FOR COCAINE ABUSE AND ADDICTION**

Study	Conclusion
TRANSCENDENTAL MEDITATION	
Gelderloos et al.[64] (1991)	Positive
O'Connell, Alexander[159] (1995)	Positive
Orme-Johnson, Farrow[162] (1977)	Positive
NUTRITION THERAPY	
Beckley-Barrett, Mutch[14] (1990)	Positive
Blum et al.[19] (1988)	Positive
Horne[87] (1988)	Positive
Mohs et al.[150] (1990)	Not applicable
HERBAL THERAPY	
Upton[230] (1994)	Positive
HALLUCINOGENS	
McKenna[140] (1996)	Inconclusive
Popik et al.[177] (1995)	Inconclusive
Sershen et al.[192] (1994)	Positive
NEUROELECTRIC THERAPY (NET)	
Gariti et al.[62] (1992)	Negative
Patterson et al.[167] (1993)	Positive
Patterson et al.[168] (1994)	Positive

which the literature is mostly inconclusive,[140,177,192] the findings of preliminary studies have been positive. As with Table 9-3, Table 9-7 reviews the outcomes of published studies as stated by the investigators/authors. The terms *positive, negative,* and *inconclusive* correspond to the authors' interpretation of the study results. Methodologic problems, however, including inadequate controls, a lack of statistical analysis, absence of follow-up data, and failure to use standardized measurement tools, along with variations in treatment protocol, reduce our confidence in the validity of these findings (TM,[64,159,162] NET,[62,167,168] nutrition,[14,19,87,150] herbs[230]). As stated earlier, the reader should be careful not to interpret a positive research finding as evidence of clinical efficacy.

NICOTINE

Hypnosis

The American Medical Association (AMA) has approved hypnosis as a valid medical treatment; thus clinicians have applied hypnosis for the treatment of numerous symptoms, including the treatment of nicotine addiction. As with nutrition therapies, hypnotic procedures have not been standardized for the treatment of addictions, and patients may be exposed to any of 20 or more strategies.[97]

Although the mechanism is unknown, a number of physiologic changes occur during hypnosis. Memory, cognition, perception, and physiology may be altered in susceptible subjects. Hypnosis may reduce sympathetic nervous system activity, oxygen consumption, and carbon dioxide elimination; lower blood pressure and heart rate; and increase activity in certain types of brain waves.[211]

Although preliminary findings with hypnosis have been promising, studies have been repeatedly criticized for lack of commonality, insufficient data reporting, lack of proper control groups, and inadequate follow-up procedures.[75,86,92,97] Results of controlled trials vary significantly, with rates of abstinence ranging from 0% to 88%.[75] For example, Lambe, Osier, and Franks[113] conducted a randomized controlled trial ($n = 180$) and reported a 21% abstinence rate for the treatment group compared with 6% of controls. At 6 months the rates were 21% and 22%, respectively. These statistics were inflated, however, because 50% of the hypnosis group dropped out of the study after randomization and were apparently excluded from the analysis rather than included as treatment failures. Generally, higher success rates seem linked to a number of factors, such as longer sessions, more sessions, presence of adjunctive treatment, and suggestions tailored to patient goals and fears rather than standardized suggestions.[86]

In a recent systematic review of the literature, Abbot et al.[1] evaluated nine randomized controlled studies with a 6-month follow-up and could find no evidence that hypnotherapy was more effective than control therapies. They concluded that evidence is insufficient for the recommendation of hypnotherapy as a specific treatment for smoking cessation. Still, the reviewers suggest that additional large-scale trials, with clearly defined interventions and appropriate comparison groups, are needed to determine efficacy.

Other CAM Therapies

Several other therapies have been used to treat addiction to nicotine (Table 9-8). The efficacy of acupuncture has been assessed in a number of trials;* however, reviews of this literature have evaluated findings as either negative or inconclusive.[21,225] Furthermore, an acupuncture consensus conference held by the NIH concluded that acupuncture was not useful in the treatment of smoking cessation.[6] As with Table 9-3, Table 9-8 reviews the outcomes of published studies as stated by the investigators/authors. The terms *positive, negative,* and *inconclusive* correspond to the authors' interpretation of the study results.

Restricted environmental stimulation therapy (REST) also deserves mention. Numerous studies have reported reduction in use and improvements in mode states for chamber REST, although the methods used have not been ideal.[12,215-217] For cocaine, overall the findings of preliminary studies have been positive.

In general, however, small sample size, inadequate data handling and analysis, lack of follow-up, inadequate controls, failure to select subjects randomly or to report inclusion/exclusion criteria, and variations in treatment protocol reduce our confidence in the validity of these findings (nutrition,[14,47,150] massage,[83] light therapy,[45] TM,[64,159,162] biofeedback,[42,54] relaxation,[225,254] electrical stimulation[65]). As stated earlier, the reader should be careful not to interpret a positive research finding as evidence of clinical efficacy.

---

*References 30, 33, 35, 36, 40, 66, 114, 126, 128, 135, 212, 249, 250.

TABLE 9–8. **CAM THERAPIES FOR NICOTINE ADDICTION**

Study	Conclusion
ACUPUNCTURE	
Brewington et al.[21] (1994)	Negative
Choy et al.[33] (1983)	Positive
Clavel, Benhamou[36] (1985)	Negative
Cottraux et al.[40] (1983)	Negative
Gillams et al.[66] (1984)	Negative
Lamontagne et al.[114] (1980)	Negative
Low[126] (1977)	Positive
Machovec, Man[128] (1978)	Negative
Martin, Waite[135] (1981)	Negative
Steiner et al.[212] (1982)	Negative
Ter Reit et al.[225] (1990)	Negative
RESTRICTED ENVIRONMENTAL STIMULATION THERAPY (REST)	
Barabasz et al.[12] (1986)	Positive
Suedfeld[215] (1990)	Positive
Suedfeld, Ikard[216] (1974)	Positive
Suedfeld et al.[217] (1972)	Positive
NUTRITION THERAPY	
Beckley-Barrett, Mutch[14] (1990)	Positive
Douglass et al.[47] (1985)	Positive
Mohs et al.[150] (1990)	Not applicable
MASSAGE THERAPY	
Hernandez-Reif et al.[83] (1999)	Positive
LIGHT THERAPY	
Dilsaver, Majchrzak[45] (1988)	Positive
TRANSCENDENTAL MEDITATION	
Gelderloos et al.[64] (1991)	Positive
O'Connell, Alexander[159] (1995)	Positive
Orme-Johnson, Farrow[162] (1977)	Positive
BIOFEEDBACK	
DeGood, Ballee[42] (1978)	Not applicable
Fahrion[54] (1995)	Positive
RELAXATION THERAPY	
Surawy, Cox[218] (1986)	Not applicable
Wynd[255] (1992)	Positive

HALLUCINOGENS

As stated earlier, chronic abuse of hallucinogens is not typically treated by addiction medicine programs. Treatment for the abuse of hallucinogens has focused primarily on withdrawal. Overall, abuse of hallucinogens has not been a focal point for CAM treatments. However, limited evidence indicates that flotation REST may help alleviate the symptoms of withdrawal and diminish the psychotic-like symptoms of people who have taken phencyclidine (PCP) or lysergic acid diethylamide (LSD).[20]

Hallucinogens present a special case in the field of CAM, since attention has focused on these drugs as potential treatments for alcohol and drug disorders rather than as agents of abuse. The two drugs that have received the most attention are LSD and ibogaine. *LSD* affects serotonin receptors, and advocates believe it to be an effective anticraving agent. However, despite the positive findings of case studies, a review of controlled studies suggests that LSD is not an effective treatment for alcoholism.[127]

Ibogaine, a stimulant with hallucinogenic properties at high doses, is an *N* methyl-D-aspartate (NMDA) antagonist. Preliminary data indicate efficacy in attenuating the development of tolerance and in decreasing the symptoms of dependence.[138] Ibogaine is available at treatment centers in several European countries; however, no controlled clinical data are available on the use of ibogaine for the treatment of addictions. Ibogaine is listed as a Schedule I substance in the United States and therefore is not available for uses other than research.[177,182,199]

BENZODIAZEPINES AND AMPHETAMINES

The only controlled trial that has been conducted using CAM for the treatment of benzodiazepine withdrawal studied relaxation and electromyogram biofeedback.[153] Although the trial was controlled, the sample size was seven. Findings were reportedly negative, although follow-up was only conducted for the relaxation group.

Acupuncture has been used for the treatment of both benzodiazepine and methamphetamine addictions. Although several clinical studies are under way, no solid data are available.

N Future of CAM in Substance Misuse and Abuse

CAM seems destined to lose its distinct identity within the realm of behavioral interventions for the treatment of addictions. Although considered CAM in other fields of medicine, spirituality and prayer have become mainstream in the treatment of addictions as the foundation for the majority of 12-step programs. With the rise of drug courts and walk-in detoxification programs throughout the United States, acupuncture seems destined to take a similar path. Furthermore, consumer interest in CAM appears to be increasing the popularity of a number of methods, such as nutrition.

Despite the increasing integration of CAM with behavioral treatments, the divide between *pharmacologically based* addiction medicine programs and *psychosocial* chemical dependency treatment programs is expanding. Researchers and clinicians have begun to encourage patients to use pharmacologic and behavioral treatments in conjunction with each other. However, methadone maintenance and other addiction medicine programs often provide limited psychosocial support, and psychosocial programs may not offer pharmacologic therapies. Insurance and consumer dollars have been targeted at psychosocial treatment, whereas research dollars have been filtered into drug trials, reinforcing the division between addiction medicine programs and chemical dependency treatment programs.

SUMMARY

The lack of sound research hinders our ability to make clinical recommendations regarding CAM and substance misuse. At present, however, it seems reasonable to state that acupuncture is safe and cost-effective and may be helpful in the treatment of addictions. Several nutritional therapies, such as zinc supplements, glutamine, and healthful diets, have shown positive trends in preliminary laboratory tests, as have a number of other methods (Tables 9-3 and 9-6 to 9-8). High-quality research is needed to further our understanding both of CAM and of the physiology of addictions.

Because chemical dependency treatment centers and addiction medicine clinics have been unable to find reliable "magic bullet" treatments, new methods to help clients with detoxification, relapse prevention, symptom relief, treatment readiness, and retention are needed. The integration of CAM may increase the treatment arsenal, but quality research must first be conducted. Federal funding for CAM research has been increasingly available, and the National Center for Complementary and Alternative Medicine (NCCAM) provides a central location for information and assistance. Thus opportunities for addiction researchers interested in CAM have increased. With the proper research and guidance, some CAM therapies for the treatment of addiction offer promise.

REFERENCES

1. Abbot NC, Stead LF, White AR, Barnes J: Hypnotherapy for smoking cessation, Cochrane Library 1, 2002 (online: *update software*).
2. Allen J: Overview of alcoholism treatment: settings and approaches, *J Ment Health Admin* 16(2):5562, 1989.
3. Alling FA, Johnson BD, Elmoghazy E: Cranial electrostimulation (CES) use in the detoxification of opiate-dependent patients, *J Subst Abuse Treat* 7:173, 1990.
4. Amaro H: An expensive policy: the impact of inadequate funding for substance abuse treatment, *Am J Public Health* 89(5):657, 1999.
5. Annis HM: Is inpatient rehabilitation of the alcoholic cost effective? Con position, *Adv Alcohol Subst Abuse* 1/2:175, 1985.
6. Anonymous: Acupuncture, *NIH Consensus Statement* 15(5):1, 1997.
7. Anton RF, Kranzler HR, Meyer RE: Neurobehavioral aspects of the pharmacotherapy of alcohol dependence, *Clin Neurosci* 3:145, 1995.
8. Avants SK, Margolin A, Holford TR, Kosten TR: A randomized controlled trial of auricular acupuncture for cocaine dependence, *Arch Intern Med* 160(15):2305, 2000.
9. Avants SK, Margolin A, Chang P, et al: Acupuncture for the treatment of cocaine addiction, *J Subst Abuse Treatm* 12(3):195, 1995.
10. Avants SK, Margolin A, Kosten TR: Cocaine abuse in methadone maintenance programs: integrating pharmacotherapy with psychosocial interventions, *J Psychoactive Drugs* 26(2):137, 1994.
11. Babor T: Social, scientific and medical issues in the definition of alcohol and drug dependence. In Edwards G, Lader M, editors: *The nature of drug dependence*, Monograph, Society for the Study of Addictions, New York, 1990, Oxford University Press.
12. Barabasz AF, Baer L, Sheehan DV, Barabasz M: A three-year follow-up of hypnosis and restricted environmental stimulation therapy for smoking, *Int J Clin Exp Hypn* 34(3):169, 1986.
13. Beasley JD, Grimson RC, Bicker AA, et al: Follow-up of a cohort of alcoholic patients through 12 months of comprehensive biobehavioral treatment, *J Subst Abuse Treat* 8(3):133, 1991.
14. Beckley-Barrett LM, Mutch PB: nutrition intervention in treatment and recovery from chemical dependency, Position paper, American Dietetic Association, *ADA Rep* 90(9):1274, 1990.

15. Benson H: Yoga for drug abuse, *N Engl J Med* 281(20):1133, 1969.
16. Biery JR, Williford JH, McMullen EA: Alcohol craving in rehabilitation: assessment of nutrition therapy, *J Am Diet Assoc* 91(4):463, 1991.
17. Blum K, Newmeyer JA, Whitehead C: Acupuncture as a common mode of treatment for drug dependence: possible neurochemical mechanisms, *J Psychedelic Drugs* 10(2):105, 1978.
18. Blum K, Trachtenberg MC, Ramsay JC: Improvement of inpatient treatment of the alcoholic as a function of neurotransmitter restoration: a pilot study, *Int J Addict* 23(9):991, 1988.
19. Blum K et al: Enkephalinase inhibition and precursor amino acid loading improves inpatient treatment of alcohol and polydrug abusers: double-blind placebo-controlled study of the nutritional adjunct SAAVE, *Alcohol* 5(6):481, 1988.
20. Borrie RA: The use of restricted environmental stimulation therapy in treating addictive behaviors, *Int J Addict* 25(7A/8A):995, 1990.
21. Brewington V, Smith M, Lipton D: Acupuncture as a detoxification treatment: an analysis of controlled research, *J Subst Abuse Treat* 11(4):289, 1994.
22. Brinkman DN: Biofeedback application to drug addiction in the University of Colorado drug rehabilitation program, *Int J Addict* 13(5):817, 1978.
23. Brown RJ, Blum K, Trachtenberg MC: Neurodynamics of relapse prevention: a neuronutrient approach to outpatient DUI offenders, *J Psychoactive Drugs* 22(2):173, 1990.
24. Brumbaugh AG: Acupuncture: new perspectives in chemical dependency treatment, *J Subst Abuse Treat* 10(1):35, 1993.
25. Brumbaugh AG: Acupuncture. In Miller NS, editor: *Principles of addiction medicine*, Chevy Chase, Md, 1994, American Society of Addiction Medicine.
26. Bullock ML, Culliton PD, Olander RT: Controlled trial of acupuncture for severe recidivist alcoholism, *Lancet* 1(8652):1435, 1989.
27. Bullock ML, Kiresuk TJ, Sherman RM, et al: A large randomized placebo-controlled study of auricular acupuncture for alcohol dependence, *J Subst Abuse Treat* 22(2):71, 2002.
28. Bullock ML, Kiresuk TJ, Pheley AM, et al: Auricular acupuncture in the treatment of cocaine abuse: a study of efficacy and dosing, *J Subst Abuse Treat* 16(1):31, 1999.
29. Bullock ML, Umen AJ, Culliton PD, Olander RT: Acupuncture treatment of alcoholic recidivism: a pilot study, *Alcohol Clin Exp Res* 11(3):292, 1987.
30. Center for Reviews and Dissemination Reviewers: A meta-analysis of the effectiveness of acupuncture in smoking cessation, *Database of Abstracts of Reviews of Effectiveness* 1, 2002.
31. Center for Reviews and Dissemination Reviewers: Acupuncture and addiction treatment, *Database of Abstracts of Reviews of Effectiveness* 1, 2002.
32. Chappel J: Long-term recovery from alcoholism, *Rec Adv Addict Dis* 16(1):177, 1993.
33. Choy DS, Lutzker L, Meltzer L: Effective treatment for smoking cessation, *Am J Med* 75(6):1033, 1983.
34. Choy YM, Tso WW, Fung KP, et al: Suppression of narcotic withdrawals and plasma ACTH by auricular electroacupuncture, *Biochem Biophys Res Commun* 82(1):305, 1978.
35. Clavel-Chapelon F, Paoletti C, Benhamou S: Smoking cessation rates 4 years after treatment by nicotine gum and acupuncture, *Prev Med* 26(1):25, 1997.
36. Clavel F, Benhamou S: Helping people to stop smoking: randomised comparison of groups being treated with acupuncture and nicotine gum with control group, *Br Med J* 291:1538, 1985.
37. Clement-Jones V, McLoughlin L, Lowry PJ, et al: Acupuncture in heroin addicts: changes in met-enkephalin and β-endorphin in blood and cerebrospinal fluid, *Lancet* 2(8139):380, 1979.
38. Collipp PJ, Kris VK, Castro-Magana M, et al: The effects of dietary zinc deficiency on voluntary alcohol drinking in rats, *Alcoholism* 8(6):556, 1984.
39. Cooper GD, Adams HB, Scott JC: Studies in reduced environmental stimulation therapy (REST) and reduced alcohol consumption, *J Subst Abuse Treat* 5(2):61, 1988.
40. Cottraux JA, Harf R, Boissel JP, et al: Smoking cessation with behaviour therapy or acupuncture: a controlled study, *Behav Res Ther* 21(4):417, 1983.
41. Culliton P, Kiresuk T: Overview of substance abuse acupuncture treatment research, *J Altern Complement Med* 2(1):149, 1996.
42. DeGood DE, Valle RS: Self-reported alcohol and nicotine use and the ability to control occipital EEG in a biofeedback situation, *Addict Behav* 3:13, 1978.

43. DesMaisons KB: Addictive nutrition as a treatment intervention for multiple offense drunk drivers, Dissertation, 1996, Union Institute.

44. Denney MR, Baugh JL, Hardt HD: Sobriety outcome after alcoholism treatment with biofeedback participation: a pilot inpatient study, *Int J Addict* 26(3):335, 1991.

45. Dilsaver SC, Majchrzak MJ: Bright artificial light produces subsensitivity to nicotine, *Life Sci* 42:225, 1988.

46. Donovan DM, Marlatt GA: Behavioral treatment. In Galanter M, editor: *Recent developments in alcoholism*, vol 11, Ten years of progress, New York, 1993, Plenum, p 397.

47. Douglass JM, Rasgon IM, Fleiss PM, et al: Effects of a raw food diet on hypertension and obesity, *South Med J* 78(7):841, 1985.

48. Eastwood MR, Stiasny LS: Psychiatric disorder, hospital admission and season, *Arch Gen Psychiatr* 35:769, 1978.

49. Edwards G: Hypnosis in treatment of alcohol addiction: controlled trial, with analysis of factors affecting outcome, *Q J Stud Alcohol* 27(2):221, 1966.

50. Ellison F, Ellison W, Daulonded JP, Daubech JF: Opiate withdrawal and electrostimulation: double blind experiment, *L'Encephale* 13:225, 1987.

51. Elmoghazy EE, Johnson BD, Alling FA: A pilot study of a neurostimulator device vs. methadone in alleviating opiate withdrawal symptoms: problems of drug dependence, NIDA Research Monograph No 95, Rockville, Md, 1989, National Institute of Drug Abuse.

52. Eriksson K, Pekkanen L, Rusi M: The effects of dietary thiamin on voluntary ethanol drinking and ethanol metabolism in the rat, *Br J Nutr* 43(1):1, 1980.

53. Facchinetti F, Petraglia F, Nappi G, et al: Functional opioid activity varies according to the different fashion of alcohol abuse, *Subst Alcohol Actions Misuse* 5:6, 1985.

54. Fahrion SL: Human potential and personal transformation, *Subtle Energies* 6(1):55, 1995.

55. Fahrion SL, Walters ED, Coyne L, Allen T: Alterations in EEG amplitude, personality factors and brain electrical mapping after alpha-theta brainwave training: a controlled case study of an alcoholic in recovery, *Alcohol Clin Exp Res* 16(3):547, 1992.

56. Fink M, Gutenbrunner C, Rollnik J, Karst M: Credibility of a newly designed placebo needle for clinical trials in acupuncture research, *Forsch Komplement Klass Naturheilk* 8(6):368, 2001.

57. Froelich JC: Genetic factors in alcohol self-administration, *J Clin Psychiatry* 56(suppl 7):15, 1995.

58. Fuller JA: Smoking withdrawal and acupuncture, *Med J Aust* 1(1):28, 1982.

59. Fuller RK, Branchey L, Brightwell DR, et al: Disulfiram treatment of alcoholism: a VA cooperative study, *JAMA* 11:1449, 1986.

60. Gallimberti L, Canton G, Gentile N, et al: Gamma-hydroxybutyric acid for treatment of alcohol withdrawal syndrome, *Lancet* 2(8666):787, 1989.

61. Garbutt JC, West SL, Carey TS, et al: Pharmacological treatment of alcohol dependence: a review of the evidence, *JAMA* 281(14):1318, 1999.

62. Gariti P, Auriacombe M, Incmikoski R, et al: A randomized double-blind study of neuroelectric therapy in opiate and cocaine detoxification, *J Subst Abuse* 4(3):299, 1992.

63. Gawin FH: Chronic neuropharmacology of cocaine: progress in pharmacotherapy, *J Clin Psychiatry* 49(suppl):11, 1988.

64. Gelderloos P, Walton KG, Orme-Johnson D, Alexander CN: Effectiveness of the transcendental meditation program in preventing and treating substance misuse: a review, *Int J Addict* 26(3):293, 1991.

65. Georgiou AJ, Spencer CP, Davies GK, Stamp J: Electrical stimulation therapy in the treatment of cigarette smoking, *J Subst Abuse* 10(3):265, 1998.

66. Gillams J, Lewith GT, Machin D: Acupuncture and group therapy in stopping smoking, *Practitioner* 228:341, 1984.

67. Glynn TJ, Greenwald P, Mills SM, Manley MW: Youth tobacco use in the United States: problem, progress, goals and potential solutions, *Prev Med* 22(4):568, 1993.

68. Gold MS: Cocaine (and crack): clinical aspects. In Lowinson JH, Ruiz P, Millman RB, Langrod JG, editors: *Substance abuse: a comprehensive textbook*, ed 3, Baltimore, 1997, Williams & Wilkins, p 181.

69. Gold MS, Miller NS: Cocaine (and crack): neurobiology. In Lowinson JH, Ruiz P, Millman RB, Langrod JG, editors: *Substance abuse: a comprehensive textbook*, ed 3, Baltimore, 1997, Williams & Wilkins, p 166.

70. Goldstein A: Introduction. In Goldstein A, editor: *Molecular and cellular aspects of the drug addictions*, New York, 1989, Springer-Verlag, p xiii.

71. Gomez E, Mikhail AR: Treatment of methadone withdrawal with cerebral electrotherapy (electrosleep), *Br J Psychiatry* 134:111, 1978.

72. Goodwin DW: *Genetic influences in alcoholism*, Chicago, 1987, Year Book.

73. Goodwin DW, Gabrielli WF: Alcohol: clinical aspects. In Lowinson JH, Ruiz P, Millman RB, Langrod JG, editors: *Substance abuse: a comprehensive textbook*, ed 3, Baltimore, 1997, Williams & Wilkins, p 142.

74. Gossop M, Bradley B, Strang J, Connell P: The clinical effectiveness of electrostimulation vs. oral methadone in managing opiate withdrawal, *Br J Psychiatry* 144:203, 1984.

75. Green JP, Lynn SJ: Hypnosis and suggestion-based approaches to smoking cessation: an examination of the evidence, *Int J Clin Exp Hypn* 48(2):195, 2000.

76. Grinspoon L, Bakalar JB: Marihuana. In Lowinson JH, Ruiz P, Millman RB, Langrod JG, editors: *Substance abuse: a comprehensive textbook*, ed 3, Baltimore, 1997, Williams & Wilkins, p 199.

77. Guenther RM: Nutrition and alcoholism, *J Appl Nutr* 35:44, 1983.

78. Gurevich MI, Duckworth D, Imhof JE, Katz JL: Is auricular acupuncture beneficial in the inpatient treatment of substance abusing patients? A pilot study, *J Subst Abuse Treat* 13(2):165, 1996.

79. Hackett GI, Burke P, Harris I: An anti-smoking clinic in general practice, *Practitioner* 228:1079, 1984.

80. Halpern JH: The use of hallucinogens in the treatment of addiction, *Addict Res* 4(2):177, 1996.

81. He D, Medbo JI, Hostmark AT: Effect of acupuncture on smoking cessation or reduction: an 8-month and 5-year follow-up study, *Prev Med* 33(5):364, 2001.

82. He D, Berg JE, Hostmark AT: Effects of acupuncture smoking cessation or reduction for motivated smokers, *Prev Med* 26(2):208, 1997.

83. Hernandez-Reif M, Field T, Hart S: Smoking cravings are reduced by self-massage, *Prev Med* 28(1):28, 1999.

84. Higgins ST: Comments. In Onken LS, Blaine JD, Boren JJ, editors: *Integrating behavioral therapies with medications in the treatment of drug dependence*, NIDA Research Monograph No 150, Rockville, Md, 1995, US Department of Health and Human Services, p 170.

85. Ho WK, Wong HK, Wen HL: The influence of electroacupuncture on naloxone-induced morphine withdrawal. III. The effect of cyclic-AMP, *Neuropharmacology* 18(11):865, 1979.

86. Holroyd J: Hypnosis treatment for smoking: an evaluative review, *Int J Clin Exp Hypn* 28(4):341, 1980.

87. Horne DE: Clinical impressions of SAAVE and tropamine, *J Psychoactive Drugs* 20(3):333, 1988.

88. Institute for Health Policy: *Substance abuse: the nation's number one health problem—key indicators for policy*, Princeton, NJ, 1993, Brandeis University for Robert Wood Johnson Foundation.

89. Jacobson NO, Silfverskiold NA: Controlled study of a hypnotic method in the treatment of alcoholism, with evaluation by objective criteria, *Br J Addict* 68:25, 1973.

90. Jaffe JH, Knapp CM: Opiates: clinical aspects. In Lowinson JH, Ruiz P, Millman RB, Langrod JG, editors: *Substance abuse: a comprehensive textbook*, ed 3, Baltimore, 1997, Williams & Wilkins, p 158.

91. Jarzembski WB: Electrical stimulation and substance abuse treatment, *Neurobehav Toxicol Teratol* 7:119, 1985.

92. Johnston EJ, Donoghue JR: Hypnosis and smoking: a review of the literature, *Am J Clin Hypn* 13(4):265, 1971.

93. Kalant H: The nature of addiction: an analysis of the problem. In Goldstein A, editor: *Molecular and cellular aspects of the drug addictions*, New York, 1989, Springer-Verlag.

94. Kao AH, Lu LYC: Acupuncture procedure for treating drug addiction, *Am J Acupunct* 2:201, 1974.

95. Kaptchuk TJ: Placebo needle for acupuncture, *Lancet* 352(9132):992, 1998.

96. Karrell R: Acupuncture in an adolescent treatment setting, *Addict Recov* 10:24, 1990.

97. Katz N: Hypnosis and the addictions: a critical review, *Addict Behav* 5:41, 1980.

98. Kendler KS, Kessler RC: A population-based twin study of alcoholism in women, *JAMA* 268(14):1877, 1992.

99. Keung WM: Biochemical studies of a new class of alcohol dehydrogenase inhibitors from Radix Puerariae, *Alcohol Clin Exp Res* 17(6):1254, 1993.

100. Keung WM, Vallee BL: Kudzu root: an ancient Chinese source of modern antidipsotropic agents, *Phytochemistry* 47(4):499, 1998.

101. Keung WM, Vallee BL: Daidzin and daidzein suppress free-choice ethanol intake by Syrian golden hamsters, *Proc Natl Acad Sci USA* 90(21):10008, 1993.

102. Keung WM, Vallee BL: Daidzin: a potent, selective inhibitor of human mitochondrial aldehyde dehydrogenase, *Proc Natl Acad Sci USA* 90(4):1247, 1993.

103. Keung WM, Vallee BL: Therapeutic lessons from traditional Oriental medicine to contemporary occidental pharmacology. In Jansson B, Jornvall H, Rydberg U, et al, editors: *Toward a molecular basis of alcohol use and abuse*, Boston, 1994, Birkhauser Verlag, p 371.

104. Keung WM, Lazo O, Kunze L, Vallee BL: Daidzin suppresses ethanol consumption by Syrian golden hamsters without blocking acetaldehyde metabolism, *Proc Natl Acad Sci USA* 92(19):8990, 1995.

105. King GR, Ellinwood EH: Amphetamines and other stimulants. In Lowinson JH, Ruiz P, Millman RB, Langrod JG, editors: *Substance abuse: a comprehensive textbook*, ed 3, Baltimore, 1997, Williams & Wilkins, p 207.

106. Klingemann HK: Coping and maintenance strategies of spontaneous remitters from problem use of alcohol and heroin in Switzerland, *Int J Addict* 27(12):1359, 1992.

107. Konefal J, Duncan R, Clemence C: The impact of the addition of an acupuncture treatment program to an existing Metro-Dade County outpatient substance abuse treatment facility, *J Addict Dis* 13(3):71, 1994.

108. Kosten TR, Kreck MJ, Ragunath J, Kleber HB: A preliminary study of beta endorphin during chronic naltrexone maintenance treatment in ex-opiate addicts, *Life Sci* 31(1):55, 1986.

109. Kranzler HR: Pharmacotherapy of alcoholism: gaps in knowledge and opportunities for research, *Alcohol Alcoholism* 35(6):537, 2000.

110. Kranzler HR, Van Kirk J: Efficacy of naltrexone and acamprosate for alcoholism treament: a meta-analysis, *Alcohol Clin Exp Res* 25(9):1335, 2001.

111. Kroenig RJ, Oleson TD: Rapid narcotic detoxification in chronic pain patients treated with auricular electroacupuncture and naloxone, *Int J Addict* 20:1347, 1985.

112. Krystal JH, Cramer JA, Krol WF, Kirk GF, Rosenheck RA: Naltrexone in the treatment of alcohol dependence, *N Engl J Med* 345(24):1734, 2001.

113. Lambe R, Osier C, Franks P: A randomized controlled trial of hypnotherapy for smoking cessation, *J Fam Pract* 22(1):61, 1986.

114. Lamontagne Y, Annable L, Gagnon MA: Acupuncture for smokers: lack of long-term therapeutic effect in a controlled study, *Can Med Assoc J* 122(7):787, 1980.

115. Lao HH: A retrospective study on the use of acupuncture for the prevention of alcoholic recidivism, *Am J Acupunct* 32(1):29, 1995.

116. Lê AD, Kiianmaa K, Cunningham CL, et al: Neurobiological processes in alcohol addiction: symposium, *Alcohol Clin Exp Res* 25(5):1448, 2001.

117. Lenox JR, Bonny H: The hypnotizability of chronic alcoholics, *Int J Clin Exp Hypn* 24(4):419, 1976.

118. Leung A: Acupuncture treatment of withdrawal symptoms, *Am J Acupunct* 5:43, 1977.

119. Lewenberg A: Electroacupuncture and antidepressant treatment of alcoholism in a private practice, *Clin Ther* 7(5):611, 1985.

120. Li-Li F, O'Keefe DD, Powell WJ: Pharmacologic studies on *Radix puerariae*: effect of puerarin on regional myocardial blood flow and cardiac hemodynamics in dogs with acute myocardial ischemia, *Chin Med J* 98(11):821, 1985.

121. Lima AR, Lima MS, Soares BGO, Farrell M: Carbamazepine for cocaine dependence, Cochrane Library 1, 2002 (online: *update software*).

122. Lipton DS, Brewington V, Smith M: Acupuncture for crack-cocaine detoxification: experimental evaluation of efficacy, *J Subst Abuse Treat* 11(3):205, 1994.

123. Lipton DS, Maranda MJ: Detoxification from heroin dependency: an overview of method and effectiveness: evaluation of drug treatment programs, *Adv Alcohol Subst Abuse* 2(1):31, 1982.

124. Litten RZ, Allen JL: Pharmacotherapies for alcoholism: promising agents and clincial issues, *Alcohol Clin Exp Res* 15(4):620, 1991.

125. Litten RZ, Allen J, Fertig J: Pharmacotherapies for alcohol problems: a review of research with focus on developments since 1991, *Alcohol Clin Exp Res* 20(5):859, 1996.

126. Low S: Acupuncture and nicotine withdrawal, *Med J Aust* 2:687, 1977 (letter).

127. Ludwig A, Levine J, Stark L: *LSD and alcoholism: a clinical study of treatment efficacy,* Springfield, Ill, 1970, Thomas.
128. Machovec FJ, Man SC: Acupuncture and hypnosis compared: 58 cases, *Am J Clin Hypn* 21(1):45, 1978.
129. Malin DH, Murray JB, Crucian GP, et al: Auricular microelectrostimulation: naloxone-reversible attenuation of opiate abstinence syndrome, *Biol Psychiatry* 24:886, 1988.
130. Margolin A, Kleber HD, Avants SK, et al: Acupuncture for the treatment of cocaine addiction: a randomized controlled trial, *JAMA* 287(1):55, 2002.
131. Margolin A, Avants SK: Should cocaine-abusing, buprenorphine-maintained patients receive auricular acupuncture? Findings from an acute effects study, *J Altern Complement Med* 5(6):567, 1999.
132. Margolin A, Avants SK, Kosten TR, Chang P: Acupuncture reduces cocaine abuse in methadone-maintained patients, NIDA Research Monograph No 32, Washington, DC, 1993, US Department of Health and Human Services.
133. Margolin A, Chang P, Avants SK, Kosten TR: Effects of sham and real auricular needling: implications for trials of acupuncture for cocaine addiction, *Am J Chin Med* 21(2):103, 1993.
134. Margolin A, Avants SK, Chang P, et al: A single-blind investigation of four auricular needle puncture configurations, *Am J Chin Med* 23(2):105, 1995.
135. Martin GP, Waite PM: The efficacy of acupuncture as an aid to stopping smoking, *NZ Med J* 93(686):421, 1981.
136. Mash DC, Kovera CA, Pablo J, et al: Ibogaine: complex pharmacokinetics, concerns for safety, and preliminary efficacy measures, *Ann NY Acad Sci* 914:394, 2000.
137. Mathews-Larson J, Parker RA: Alcoholism treatment with biochemical restoration as a major component, *Int J Biosocial Res* 9(1):92, 1987.
138. Mayer DJ: Acupuncture: an evidence-based review of the literature, *Annu Rev Med* 51:49, 2000.
139. McGrath RE, Yahia M: Preliminary data on seasonally related alcohol dependence, *J Clin Psychiatry* 54(7):260, 1993.
140. McKenna DJ: Plant hallucinogens: springboards for psychotherapeutic drug discovery, *Behav Brain Res* 73:109, 1996.
141. McLellan AT, Grossman DS, Blaine JD, Haverkos HW: Acupuncture treatment for drug abuse: a technical review, *J Subst Abuse Treat* 10(6):569, 1993.
142. Mendelson G: Acupuncture and cholinergic suppression of withdrawal symptoms: a hypothesis, *Br J Addict* 73:166, 1978.
143. Meyer RE: Finding paradigms for the future of alcoholism research: an interdisciplinary perspective, *Alcohol Clin Exp Res* 25(9):1393, 2001.
144. Milanov I, Toteva S: Acupuncture treatment of tremor in alcohol withdrawal syndrome, *Am J Acupunct* 21(4):319, 1993.
145. Miller NS: Mortality risks in alcoholism and effects of abstinence and addiction treatment, *Psychiatr Dis North Am* 22(2):371, 1999.
146. Miller WR: Spirituality: the silent dimension in addiction research, 1990 Leonard Ball Oration, *Drug Alcohol Rev* 9:259, 1990.
147. Miller WR: Spiritual aspects of addictions treatment and research, *Mind/Body Med* 2(1):37, 1997.
148. Miller WR, Hester RK: Inpatient alcoholism treatment: who benefits? *Am Psychologist* 41:794, 1986.
149. Miller WR, Rollnick S: *Motivational interviewing,* New York, 1991, Guilford.
150. Mohs ME, Watson RR, Leonard-Green T: Nutritional effects of marijuana, heroin, cocaine and nicotine, *J Am Diet Assoc* 90(9):1261, 1990.
151. Morgan HW, editor: *Drugs in America: a social history, 1800-1980,* Syracuse, NY, 1981, Syracuse University Press.
152. Muffler J, Langrod JG, Richardson JT, Ruiz P: Religion. In Lowinson JH, Ruiz P, Millman RB, Langrod JG, editors: *Substance abuse: a comprehensive textbook,* ed 3, Baltimore, 1997, Williams & Wilkins, p 492.
153. Nathan RG, Robinson D, Cherek DR: Alternative treatments for withdrawing the long-term benzodiazepine user: a pilot study, *Int J Addict* 21(2):195, 1986.
154. Nespor K, Cs-Emy L: [Alcohol and drugs in Central Europe: problems and possible solutions], *Casop Lekaru Ceskych* 133(16):483, 1994.

155. Newmeyer T, Johnson G, Klot S: Acupuncture as a detoxification modality, *J Psychoactive Drugs* 16:241, 1984.
156. Ng L: Auricular acupuncture in animals: effects of opiate withdrawal and involvement of endorphins, *J Altern Complement Med* 2(1):61, 1996.
157. Ng L et al: Modification of morphine withdrawal syndrome in rats following transauricular electro-stimulation: an experimental paradigm for auricular electroacupuncture, *Biol Psychiatry* 10:575, 1975.
158. Nutt DJ: Addiction: brain mechanisms and their treatment implications, *Lancet* 347:31, 1996.
159. O'Connell DF, Alexander CN: Introduction: recovery from addictions using transcendental meditation and Maharishi Ayur-Veda. In O'Connell DF, Alexander CN, editors: *Self recovery: treating addictions using transcendental meditation and Maharishi Ayur-Veda*, New York, 1995, Harrington Park Press.
160. Olms JS: New: an effective alcohol abstinence acupuncture treatment, *Am J Acupunct* 12(2):145, 1984.
161. Omura Y: Electro-acupuncture for drug addiction withdrawal, *Acupunct Electrother Res* 1:231, 1975.
162. Orme-Johnson DW, Farrow JJ, editors: *Scientific research on the transcendental meditation program: collected papers*, vol 1, Rheinweiler, West Germany, 1977, MERU Press.
163. Otto KC, Quinn C, Sung YF: Auricular acupuncture as an adjunctive treatment for cocaine addiction: a pilot study, *Am J Addict* 7(2):164, 1998.
164. Overstreet DH, Lee YW, Rezvani AH, et al: Suppression of alcohol intake after administration of the Chinese herbal medicine NPI-028 and its derivatives, *Alcohol Clin Exp Res* 20(2):221, 1996.
165. Parker L, Mok M: The use of acupuncture for smoking withdrawal, *Am J Acupunct* 5:363, 1977.
166. Patterson MA: Electro-acupuncture in alcohol and drug addictions, *Clin Med* 81:9, 1974.
167. Patterson MA, Patterson L, Flood NV, et al: Electrostimulation in drug and alcohol detoxification: significance of stimulation criteria in clinical success, *Addict Res* 1:130, 1993.
168. Patterson MA, Krupitsky E, Flood N, et al: Amelioration of stress in chemical dependency detoxification by transcranial electrostimulation, *Stress Med* 10:115, 1994.
169. Pechnick RN, Ungerleider JT: Hallucinogens. In Lowinson JH, Ruiz P, Millman RB, Langrod JG, editors: *Substance abuse: a comprehensive textbook*, ed 3, Baltimore, 1997, Williams & Wilkins, p 230.
170. Pekkanen L: Effects of thiamin deprivation and antagonism on voluntary ethanol intake in rats, *J Nutr* 110(5):937, 1980.
171. Peniston EG: Alpha-theta brainwave training and beta-endorphin levels in alcoholics, *Alcohol Clin Exp Res* 13(2):271, 1989.
172. Peniston EG, Kulkosky PJ: Alcoholic personality and alpha-theta brainwave training, *Med Psychother* 3:37, 1990.
173. Peniston EG et al: EEG alpha-theta brainwave synchronization in Vietnam theater veterans with combat-related post-traumatic stress disorder and alcohol abuse, *Adv Med Psychother* 6:37, 1993.
174. Peteet JR: A closer look at the role of a spiritual approach in addictions treatment, *J Subst Abuse Treat* 10(3):263, 1993.
175. Petri G, Takach G: Application of herbal mixtures in rehabilitation after alcoholism, *Plant Med* 56(6):692, 1990.
176. Poikolainen K: Seasonality of alcohol-related hospital admissions has implications for prevention, *Drug Alcohol Depend* 10:65, 1982.
177. Popik P, Layer RT, Skolnick P: 100 years of ibogaine: neurochemical and pharmacological actions of a putative anti-addictive drug, *Pharmacol Rev* 47(2):235, 1995.
178. Powell BJ, Penick EC, Read MR, Ludwig AM: Comparison of three outpatient treatment interventions: a twelve-month follow-up of men alcoholics, *J Stud Alcohol* 46(4):309, 1985.
179. Project MATCH Research Group: Matching alcoholism treatments to client heterogeneity: Project MATCH posttreatment drinking outcomes, *J Stud Alcohol* 58(1):7, 1997.
180. Rank D, Suedfeld P: Positive reactions of alcoholic men to sensory deprivation, *Int J Addict* 13(5):807, 1978.
181. Register UD, Marsh SR, Thurston DT, et al: Influence of nutrients on intake of alcohol, *J Am Diet Assoc* 61:159, 1972.
182. Rezvani AH, Overstreet DH, Lee Y: Attenuation of alcohol intake by ibogaine in three strains of alcohol-preferring rats, *Pharmacol Biochem Behav* 52(3):615, 1995.

183. Richard AJ, Montoya ID, Nelson R, Spence RT: Effectiveness of adjunct therapies in crack cocaine treatment, *J Subst Abuse Treat* 12(6):401, 1995.
184. Rogers LL, Pelton RB, Williams RJ: Amino acid supplementation and voluntary alcohol consumption by rats, *J Biol Chem* 220(1):321, 1956.
185. Russell LC, Sharp B, Gilbertson B: Acupuncture for addicted patients with chronic histories of arrest: A pilot study of the Consortium Treatment Center, *J Subst Abuse Treat* 19:199, 2000.
186. Sacks L: Drug addiction, alcoholism, smoking, obesity, treated by auricular staple puncture, *Am J Acupunct* 3:147, 1975.
187. Sainsbury MJ: Acupuncture in heroin withdrawal, *Med J Aust* 2(3):102, 1974.
188. Sapir-Weise R, Berglund M, Frank A, Kristenson H: Acupuncture in alcoholism treatment: a randomized out-patient study, *Alcohol Alcoholism* 34(4):629, 1999.
189. Satel SL, Gawin FH: Seasonal cocaine abuse, *Am J Psychiatry* 146:534, 1989.
190. Schwartz JL: Evaluation of acupuncture as a treatment for smoking, *Am J Acupunct* 16:135, 1988.
191. Sellers EM, Higgins GA, Sobell MB: 5-HT and alcohol abuse, *Trends Pharmacol Sci* 13(2):69, 1992.
192. Sershen H, Hashim A, Lajtha A: Ibogaine reduces preference for cocaine consumption in C57BL/6 by mice, *Pharmacol Biochem Behav* 47:13, 1994.
193. Severson L, Markoff RA, Chin-Hoon A: Heroin detoxification with acupuncture and electrical stimulation, *Int J Addict* 12(7):911, 1977.
194. Shaffer HJ, Lasalvia TA: Comparing Hatha yoga with dynamic group psychotherapy for enhancing methadone maintenance treatment: a randomized clinical trial, *Altern Ther Health Med* 3(4):57, 1997.
195. Shakur M, Smith MO: The use of acupuncture in the treatment of drug addiction, *Am J Acupunct* 7(3):223, 1979.
196. Shanmugasundaram E, Subramaniam U, Santhini R, Shanmugasundaram K: Studies on brain structure and neurological function in alcoholic rats controlled by an Indian medicinal formula (SKV), *J Ethnopharmacol* 17:225, 1986.
197. Shapiro F, Vogelmann-Sine S, Sine LF: Eye movement desensitization and reprocessing: treating trauma and substance abuse, *J Psychoactive Drugs* 26(4):379, 1994.
198. Sharps H: Acupuncture and the treatment of drug withdrawal symptoms, *Pharmchem Newslett* 1, 1977.
199. Sheppard SG: A preliminary investigation of ibogaine: case reports and recommendations for further study, *J Subst Abuse Treat* 11(4):379, 1994.
200. Shuaib BM: Acupuncture treatment of drug dependence in Pakistan, *Am J Chin Med* 4(4):403, 1976.
201. Shwartz M, Saitz R, Mulvey K, Brannigan P: The value of acupuncture detoxification programs in a substance abuse treatment system, *J Sub Abuse Treat* 17(4):305, 1999.
202. Simon EJ: Opiates: neurobiology. In Lowinson JH, Ruiz P, Millman RB, Langrod JG, editors: *Substance abuse: a comprehensive textbook*, ed 3, Baltimore, 1997, Williams & Wilkins.
203. Smith MO: Chinese theory of acupuncture detoxification, *Am J Acupunct* 12(4):386, 1985.
204. Smith MO: Acupuncture treatment for crack: clinical survey of 1500 patients treated, *Am J Acupunct* 16(3):241, 1988.
205. Smith MO: Lincoln Hospital acupuncture detoxification: the early days. Paper presented at National Acupuncture Detoxification Association annual meeting, Chicago, 1997.
206. Smith MO, Khan I: An acupuncture programme for the treatment of drug-addicted persons, *Bull Narc* 40(1):35, 1988.
207. Smith MO et al: Acupuncture treatment of drug addiction and alcohol abuse, *Am J Acupunct* 10(2):161, 1982.
208. Smith RB, O'Neill L: Electrosleep in the management of alcoholism, *Biol Psychiatry* 10(6):675, 1975.
209. Smith-Moorhouse PM: Hypnosis in the treatment of alcoholism, *Br J Addict* 64:47, 1969.
210. *Socioeconomic evaluations of addictions treatment: executive summary*, Washington, DC, 1993, Center of Alcohol Studies, Rutgers University.
211. Spiegel D, Bloom JR, Kraemer HC, Gottheil E: Effect of psychosocial treatment on survival of patients with metastatic breast cancer, *Lancet* 2(8668):888, 1989.
212. Steiner RP, Hay DL, Davis AW: Acupuncture therapy for the treatment of tobacco smoking addiction, *Am J Chin Med* 10:107, 1982.

213. Stoil M: Problems in the evaluation of hypnosis in the treatment of alcoholism, *J Subst Abuse Treat* 6:31, 1989.

214. Streitberger K, Kleinhenz J: Introducing a placebo needle into acupuncture research, *Lancet* 352(9125):364, 1998.

215. Suedfeld P: Restricted environmental stimulation and smoking cessation: a fifteen-year progress report, *Int J Addict* 25:861, 1990.

216. Suedfeld P, Ikard F: The use of sensory deprivation in facilitating the reduction of cigarette smoking, *J Consult Clin Psychol* 42:888, 1974.

217. Suedfeld P et al: An experimental attack on smoking: attitude manipulation in restricted environments. III, *Int J Addict* 7:721, 1972.

218. Surawy C, Cox T: Smoking behaviour under conditions of relaxation: a comparison between types of smokers, *Addict Behav* 11(2):187, 1986.

219. Sween JA, Shabazz CD, Carter D: The short-term symptom-relief effect of acupuncture on men and women in a residential drug and alcohol treatment program: results of a pilot study. Paper presented at the National Acupuncture Detoxification Association (NADA) conference, Portland, Ore, 1996.

220. Swift RM: Drug therapy: drug therapy for alcohol dependence, *N Engl J Med* 340(19):1482, 1999.

221. Tan C, Sin T, Huang X: The use of laser on acupuncture points for smoking cessation, *Am J Acupunct* 15:137, 1987.

222. Taub E, Steiner SS, Weingarten E, Walton KG: Effectiveness of broad-spectrum approaches to relapse prevention in severe alcoholism: a long-term, randomized, controlled trial of transcendental meditation, EMG biofeedback and electronic neurotherapy, *Alcohol Treat Q* 11:187, 1994.

223. Ter Riet G, Kleijnen J, Knipschild A: Meta-analysis of studies into the effect of acupuncture on addiction, *Br J Gen Pract* 40(338):379, 1990.

224. Thorer H, Volf N: Acupuncture after alcohol consumption: a sham controlled assessment. Paper presented to British Medical Acupuncture Society, London, 1996.

225. Timofeev MF: Internal inhibition: a form of nonconflict breaking mental alcohol dependence in narcology, *Bull Exp Biol Med* 117(2):149, 1994.

226. Toteva S, Milanov I: The use of body acupuncture for treatment of alcohol dependence and withdrawal syndrome: a controlled study, *Am J Acupunct* 24(1):19, 1996.

227. *Treating tobacco use and dependence: clinical practice guidelines,* US Department of Health and Human Services, Washington, DC, 2000, US Government Printing Office.

228. Trudeau D: The treatment of addictive disorders by brain wave biofeedback: a review and suggestions for future research, *Clin Electroenceph* 31(1):13, 2000.

229. Tuchfield BS: Spontaneous remission in alcoholics: empirical observations and theoretical implications, *J Stud Alcohol* 42(7):626, 1981.

230. Upton R: *Minimizing the effects of addiction and withdrawal through herbal and nutritional support (alcohol and cocaine),* Anaheim, Calif, 1994, Expo West.

231. Valenzuela CF, Harris RA: Alcohol: neurobiology. In Lowinson JH, Ruiz P, Millman RB, Langrod JG, editors: *Substance abuse: a comprehensive textbook,* ed 3, Baltimore, 1997, Williams & Wilkins.

232. Wadden TA, Penrod JH: Hypnosis in the treatment of alcoholism: a review and appraisal, *Am J Clin Hypn* 24(1):41, 1981.

233. Waite NR, Clough JB: A single-blind, placebo-controlled trial of a simple acupuncture treatment in the cessation of smoking, *Br J Gen Pract* 48(433):1487, 1998.

234. Washburn A, Keenan P, Nazareno J: Preliminary findings: study of acupuncture-assisted heroin detoxification, *Multicultural Inquiry Res AIDS* 4:3, 1990.

235. Washburn AM et al: Acupuncture heroin detoxification: a single-blind clinical trial, *J Subst Abuse Treat* 10(4):345, 1993.

236. Weingarten E, Hartman L, Holcomb Z: Frontalis EMG of dropouts from inpatients treatment for alcoholism, *Int J Addict* 15(7):1113, 1980.

237. Wells E, Jackson R, Diaz O, et al: Acupuncture as an adjunct to methadone treatment services, *Am J Addict* 4(3):198, 1995.

238. Wen HL: Fast detoxification of drug abuse by acupuncture and electrical stimulation (AES) in combination with naloxone, *Mod Med Asia* 13:13, 1977.

239. Wen HL: Acupuncuture and electrical stimulations (AES) outpatient detoxification, *Mod Med Asia* 15:39, 1979.

240. Wen HL: Clinical experience and mechanism of acupuncture and electrical stimulation (AES) in the treatment of drug abuse, *Am J Chin Med* 8(4):349, 1980.

241. Wen HL, Cheung SYC: Treatment of drug addiction by acupuncture and electrical stimulation, *Asian J Med* 9:138, 1973.

242. Wen HL, Teo SW: Experience in the treatment of drug addiction by electro-acupuncture, *Mod Med Asia* 11:23, 1975.

243. Wen HL, HO WKK, Ling N, et al: The influence of electro-acupuncture on naloxone-induced morphine withdrawal. II. Elevation of immunoassayable beta-endorphin activity in the brain but not the blood, *Am J Chin Med* VII(3):237, 1979.

244. Wen HL, Ho WK, Ling N, et al: Immunoassayable beta-endorphin level in the plasma and CSF of heroin addicted and normal subjects before and after electroacupuncture, *Am J Chin Med* 8:154, 1980.

245. Wen HL, Ng TH, Ho WKK, et al: Acupuncture in narcotic withdrawal: a preliminary report on biochemical changes in the blood and urine of heroin addicts, *Bull Narc* 30(2):31, 1978.

246. Werbach MR: *Nutritional influences on mental illness: a sourcebook of clinical research*, Tarzana, Calif, 1991, Third Line Press.

247. Wesson DR, Smith DE, Ling W, Seymour RB: Sedative-hypnotics and tricyclics. In Lowinson JH, Ruiz P, Millman RB, Langrod JG, editors: *Substance abuse: a comprehensive textbook*, ed 3, Baltimore, 1997, Williams & Wilkins.

248. Westermeyer J, Lyfoung T, Westermeyer M, Neider J: Opium addiction among Indochinese refugees in the U.S.: characteristics of addictions and their opium use, *Am J Drug Alcohol Abuse* 17(3):267, 1991.

249. White AR, Rampes H, Ernst E: Acupuncture for smoking cessation, Cochrane Library 1, 2002 (online: *update software*).

250. White AR, Resch KL, Ernst E: A meta-analysis of acupuncture techniques for smoking cessation, *Tobacco Control* 8(4):393, 1999.

251. White AR, Resch KL, Ernst E: Randomized trial of acupuncture for nicotine withdrawal symptoms, *Arch Intern Med* 158(20):2251, 1998.

252. Whitehead PC: Acupuncture in the treatment of addiction: a review and analysis, *Int J Addict* 13(1):1, 1978.

253. Winger G, Hofmann FG, Woods JH: *A handbook on drug and alcohol abuse: the biomedical aspects*, ed 3, New York, 1992, Oxford University Press.

254. Worner TM, Zeller B, Schwarz H, et al: Acupuncture fails to improve treatment outcome in alcoholics, *Drug Alcohol Depend* 30(2):169, 1992.

255. Wynd CA: Relaxation imagery used for stress reduction in the prevention of smoking relapse, *J Adv Nurs* 17(3):294, 1992.

256. Xie CI, Lin RC, Antony V, et al: Daidzin: an antioxidant isoflavonoid, decreases blood alcohol levels and shortens sleep time induced by ethanol intoxication, *Alcohol Clin Exp Res* 18(6):1443, 1994.

257. Yang MMP, Kwok JSL: Evaluation on the treatment of morphine addiction by acupuncture: Chinese herbs and opioid peptides, *Am J Chin Med* 14:46, 1986.

258. Yiming C, Changxin Z, Ung WS, Lei Z, Kean LS: Laser acupuncture for adolescent smokers: a randomized double-blind controlled trial, *Am J Chin Med* 28:443, 2000.

259. Zalesskiy V, Belousova I, Frolov G: Laser-acupuncture reduces cigarette smoking: a preliminary report, *Acupunct Electrother Res* 8:297, 1983.

SUGGESTED READINGS

Lowinson JH, Ruiz P, Millman RB, Langrod JG, editors: *Substance abuse: a comprehensive textbook*, ed 3, Baltimore, 1997, Williams & Wilkins.

Onken LS, Blaine JD, Boren JJ, editors: Integrating behavioral therapies with medications in the treatment of drug dependence, NIDA Research Monograph No 150, Rockville, Md, 1995, US Department of Health and Human Services.

CHAPTER 10

Pain

ANN GILL TAYLOR, DANIEL I. GALPER, KAREN
D'HUYVETTER, CHERYL BOURGUIGNON, and
DEBRA E. LYONS

The high incidence and prevalence of pain have led both health professionals and persons experiencing pain to explore the potential effectiveness of complementary and alternative medicine (CAM) to reduce their pain and enhance comfort. One national survey indicated that 42% of the U.S. population had used one or more CAM modalities during the previous year, including the following therapies used to treat pain: chiropractic, relaxation techniques, therapeutic massage, and acupuncture.[57] The philosophy underlying CAM is one that fosters a sense of well-being, human integrity, and healing the person rather than curing the disease. These factors have a potentially important role in relieving pain. Many CAM therapists operate from a partnership perspective in which the patient is viewed as an active participant in the therapy, enhancing a sense of control and self-efficacy, factors shown to be important in the effective management of pain.[1,198] The popularity of CAM therapies for pain may be sending the message that multiple factors have great importance for the patient.

This chapter reviews studies testing the effects of CAM modalities for pain relief when used either as a single therapy or as an adjunct to conventional pain management interventions. The most important findings for health care providers and patients are reviewed in this chapter and summarized in the accompanying tables. To uncover published articles, the authors searched major databases (MEDLINE, PRE-MEDLINE, PsychINFO, CINAHL, Cochran databases) from the date of origin through early 2002. Additional hand searching of reference lists from published articles and book chapters was conducted to obtain further published materials. Because the quality of CAM research has improved dramatically over the past several years, we emphasize studies published since 1997. The review includes primary randomized controlled trials and meta-analyses combining controlled clinical studies, which offer

This chapter was prepared with partial support from grant award T32 AT00052, funded by the National Center for Complementary and Alternative Medicine, National Institutes of Health.

the strongest evidence. For some CAM modalities and conditions with limited research, however, the authors reviewed the best available published investigations, including quasi-experimental and uncontrolled studies.

N Definition and Types of Pain

Pain is a ubiquitous feature of life and one of the primary reasons that individuals seek assistance within the health care system. Despite notable advances in the understanding of pain mechanisms and management, the cause of an individual's pain is frequently not understood. Moreover, even when a clear etiology can be established, the pain is often inadequately managed.[231] The inherent subjectivity of pain is an impediment to its understanding and treatment. Pain can persist without an identifiable injury or disorder; likewise, injury can occur without pain. Thus the relationship between tissue damage and pain is not isomorphic (one to one). In addition to biochemical and physiologic factors, a range of behavioral, affective, cognitive, and sociocultural factors influence an individual's experience of pain. These factors not only influence the perception of the pain experience, but also may have implications for the efficacy and selection of treatment methods.

Pain is defined as an unpleasant sensory and emotional experience associated with actual or potential tissue damage or described in terms of such damage.[117] Pain is typically classified as one of three types: acute, chronic, or cancer-related. *Acute pain* is associated with tissue damage that results from surgery, trauma, or painful medical procedures. Acute pain generally serves a biologically useful function by bringing attention to an underlying pathologic condition that, once identified, may be treated.[235] Acute pain is expected to diminish with healing and time. In contrast, pain associated with trauma that persists beyond the usual healing period, or pain that accompanies a disease process that persists for extended periods, can be considered *chronic pain*.[231]

Cancer-related pain may have characteristics of both acute and chronic pain because it can result from disease processes (e.g., bone metastases, nerve compression or infiltration) or treatment therapies (e.g., surgery, radiation). Cancer patients often report suffering that is not directly related to their pain but rather results from psychologic issues (e.g., fear, worry associated with financial ruin) associated with the diagnosis of cancer.[200] However, patients with cancer often report a high magnitude of pain-related suffering, because the pain can serve as a constant reminder of the cancer.

N Epidemiology of Pain

Pain is a high-priority symptom related to the problems of cancer, heart disease and stroke, diabetes, acquired immunodeficiency syndrome (AIDS), trauma, and chronic disabling conditions for more than 120 million persons in the United States. Pain costs the U.S. economy at least $100 billion in lost productivity and health care each year.[60,231] A Louis Harris & Associates poll found that pain resulted in 50 million lost work days and $3 billion in lost wages per year.[137] The combined expense associated with the treatment of back pain, migraine headaches, and arthritis alone amounts to an estimated $40 billion annually.

The prevalence of pain in the United States has been evaluated in a number of reports. A representative national survey of 1539 households found that back problems, arthritis, sprains or strains, and headache were among the 10 most frequently reported principal medical conditions.[58] Anxiety and depression, which often accompany painful conditions, were also cited among the top 10 conditions.

The National Center for Health Statistics (NCHS) reported the prevalence of painful conditions to be, from most frequent to least frequent, arthritis, back pain, lower extremity pain, migraine headache, ischemic heart disease, intervertebral disk disorders, upper extremity pain, gout and gouty arthritis, and neuralgia or neuritis.[6] Similarly, *The Nuprin Pain Report* indicated that headaches, backaches, muscle pains, joint pains, and (pre-) menstrual pains are the most common painful problems for adults, and respondents reported having three to four physical pain problems every year.[228] In addition, back symptoms, stomach pain, cramps, spasms, headache, chest pain, and knee pain were among the principal reasons for medical visits.[206]

About 8 million U.S. citizens have cancer or a history of cancer. The incidence of cancer-related pain depends on the type and stage of the cancer. Persons with cancer may have acute pain associated with diagnostic procedures and therapy, chronic pain associated with the disease or therapy, and pain associated with conditions other than cancer.[73] An estimated 30% to 45% of patients with cancer have moderate to severe pain, and almost 75% of patients with advanced cancer report less-than-adequate pain control.[22,152] *Breakthrough pain,* rated from severe to excruciating, is a problem for an estimated 64% of persons with cancer.[186] Cancer patients receiving home-based care report higher levels of pain than hospitalized patients.[68]

Prevalence of moderate to severe pain is also high among hospitalized individuals in general. Some reports have suggested that 58% to 75% of hospitalized adults have excruciating pain.[42,52,156] Indeed, as many as three quarters of postoperative patients have moderate to unbearable pain 24 hours after surgery, and 65% have moderate to unbearable pain 72 hours after surgery.[5]

Researchers are learning more about the neuroanatomic pathways and neurophysical and neurochemical mechanisms involved in pain. However, the *subjective* nature of the pain experience in individuals with all types of pain specifically challenges those studying pain as well as clinicians. Although the basic physiology of pain transmission may be similar in all humans, there are pronounced individual differences related to a number of factors, including genetic makeup, endocrine activity, central and autonomic nervous system activity, immune system function, stress, age, gender, environment, and sociocultural background. These factors are thought to account for a significant amount of variability in both the experience of pain and the response to conventional and CAM therapies.

Despite advances in pharmacology, improvements in modes of delivery of analgesia, development of guidelines for pain management for a number of different populations, and education of physicians and nurses about pain management, the incidence of pain remains high. Optimal patient care involves knowledge of the phenomenon of pain, technical skills to implement pain management guidelines, and an ethical obligation to manage pain. The present review of the literature suggests that CAM therapies with demonstrated efficacy can be considered an integral part of pain management.

⬛ Acute Postoperative and Procedural Pain

More than 23 million surgical procedures are performed each year in the United States alone. No matter how skillfully conducted, operations produce tissue damage and pain. Pain triggers a metabolic stress response that increases tissue breakdown, metabolic rate, blood clotting, and water retention. Pain in postoperative patients leads to shallow breathing and cough suppression in an effort to "splint" the traumatized site, causing increased pulmonary secretions and pneumonia. Unrelieved pain also may delay the return of normal gastric and bowel function in the postoperative patient.[5]

Patients differ in their response to postoperative pain and conventional analgesics. The Acute Pain Management Guideline Panel[5] recommended an aggressive and flexible approach to postoperative pain management, incorporating both pharmacologic and nonpharmacologic therapies to control pain and reduce procedure-related anxiety and stress. Effective pain management not only increases patient comfort and satisfaction but also may provide additional benefits, including earlier mobilization, more rapid healing, shortened hospital stays, and reduced costs.

CAM research has increasingly focused on developing and testing interventions to assist with procedural and postoperative pain. Because opioids remain the gold standard for the management of acute postoperative pain, CAM interventions have been used adjunctively in an effort to decrease pain and analgesic use. Thus, to the extent that adjunctive CAM modalities may reduce the need for excessive pain medication, they also reduce medication side effects.[5] In contrast, analgesic medications may be ineffective or contraindicated for pain associated with many medical procedures, including diagnostic and treatment procedures that require conscious sedation. In these instances, adjunctive CAM modalities may decrease procedure-related pain and distress.

Building on earlier studies that contained many methodologic problems, recent randomized controlled trials (RCTs) have been conducted on hypnosis, imagery, positive suggestions, relaxation, music, acupuncture, acupressure, massage, magnets, and transcutaneous electrical nerve stimulation (TENS) for procedural and postoperative pain management (Table 10-1).

These studies reflect a number of high-quality RCTs that have found several mind-body techniques to benefit patients undergoing surgery (and invasive medical procedures) compared with usual care and with various control conditions. Specifically, evidence suggests that hypnosis, imagery, positive suggestion, and relaxation instructions, delivered by either trained investigators or audiotapes, often reduce medication needs.[66,136,154,159,162] To a lesser extent, these studies reported reduced pain and anxiety, as well as enhanced physical recovery and physiologic stability. A few studies have also demonstrated that preoperative, intraoperative, and postoperative *music* can reduce surgical patients' reported pain intensity and distress, as well as anxiety and

Text continued on p. 331.

TABLE 10-1. **STUDIES OF CAM THERAPIES FOR PROCEDURAL AND POSTOPERATIVE PAIN**

Study	Sample	Intervention	Design	Measurement	Major Findings
ACUPUNCTURE					
Felhendler, Lisander[67] (1996)	Knee arthroscopy 40 subjects (15 F, 25 M); mean age 36 (range 15-66) Group 1 (n = 20): *acupressure stimulation (AS)*; mean age 32 (range 24-44) Group 2 (n = 20): placebo/ sham stimulation (PS); mean age 35 (range 29-45)	Both groups: postoperative analgesics AS group: stimulation with dental tool at 15 traditional acupoints on contralateral side PS group: stimulation with dental tool at 15 nonacupoints 2 cm from true acupoints	Randomized controlled trial (RCT) Repeated measures Patient blinded	Pain visual analog score (VAS) Analgesic use Laser Doppler blood flow Skin temperature Heart rate Blood pressure	AS group had significantly decreased pain at 60 minutes (p <.05) and 24 hours after treatment (p <.0001) vs. PS group. No significant differences between groups on physiologic variables
Gupta et al.[101] (1999)	Knee arthroscopy 42 subjects Group 1 (n = 21; 11 F, 10 M): *acupuncture*; mean age 40.1 (SD 19.4) Group 2 (n = 21; 7 F, 14 M): control; mean age 47.4 (SD 19.6)	Both groups: usual pre/ postoperative care Acupuncture group: preemptive analgesia (after induction but before surgery) with needle stimulation for 5 minutes at 5 acupoints on same side of body as surgery Control group: no adjunctive treatment	RCT Repeated measures Anesthetist blinded	Pain VAS Pain: verbal score Analgesic requirements	No significant differences between groups on any outcomes
Stener-Victorin et al.[220] (1999)	Oocyte aspiration, in vitro fertilization 150 women Group 1 (n = 75): *electroacupuncture (EA)*; mean age 33.3 (range 25-42) Group 2 (n = 75): conventional anesthetic; mean age 34.4 (range 25-46)	All patients: local anesthetic (paracervical block) EA group: high-intensity stimulation at 5 acupoints 30 minutes before aspiration; "de qi" sensation attained for each session Conventional treatment group: alfentanil	RCT Prospective Repeated measures	Abdominal pain VAS Pain related to oocyte aspiration VAS Adequacy of anesthesia VAS Stress VAS Duration of discomfort VAS Nausea VAS	No significant differences between EA and conventional anesthetic

(Continued)

TABLE 10–1. **STUDIES OF CAM THERAPIES FOR PROCEDURAL AND POSTOPERATIVE PAIN—cont'd**

Study	Sample	Intervention	Design	Measurement	Major Findings

Kotani et al.[133] (2001)	Elective abdominal surgery
	Upper abdominal ($n = 98$)
	• Group 1 ($n = 50$; 21 F,
	  29 M): acupuncture; mean
	  age 52 (15)
	• Group 2 ($n = 48$; 18 F,
	  30 M): control; mean
	  age 55 (14)
	Lower abdominal ($n = 77$)
	• Group 1 ($n = 39$; 12 F,
	  27 M): acupuncture; mean
	  age 55 (10)
	• Group 2 ($n = 38$; 13 F,
	  25 M): control; mean
	  age 55 (11)
		All patients: standardized
		preoperative medication
		and anesthesia
		Acupuncture group (Acu):
		insertion of needles at
		14 sites for 4 postoperative
		days
		Control group (Con):
		needles positioned at
		acupoints but not inserted
			RCT
			Repeated measures
			Double blinded (except
			acupuncturist)
				Numeric rating scale
				(NRS): 0-3
				• Incisional pain
				• Deep visceral pain
				• Overall pain relief
				• Drowsiness
				• Pruritus
				• Nausea
				• Vomiting
				Daily morphine consumption
				Cortisol
				Epinephrine (E)
				Norepinephrine (NE)
				Dopamine
				Vital signs
					Upper abdominal surgery
					patients
					• Both groups: significantly
					  decreased incisional and
					  deep visceral pain
					• Acu: significantly decreased
					  pain on postoperative day 2
					  ($p < .05$) vs. Con
					Lower abdominal surgery patients
					• Acu: significantly decreased
					  pain on postoperative days 1
					  and 2 ($p < .05$) vs. Con
					Upper and lower abdominal
					surgery patients
					• Acu: significantly (50%)
					  decreased morphine consumption
					  ($p < .01$) vs. Con
					• Acu: significantly decreased
					  postoperative nausea/vomiting
					  ($p < .05$) vs. Con
					• Acu: significantly decreased E
					  and cortisol elevation 1 hour into
					  surgery ($p < .01$) vs. Con
					• No significant differences
					  between Acu and Con on other
					  measures
					• Acu: no complications

ELECTRICAL STIMULATION

Benedetti et al.[16] (1997)	Thoracic surgery 324 subjects Group 1 (n = 103): active *transcutaneous electrical nerve stimulation* [TENS] (AT) Group 2 (n = 106): placebo TENS (PT) Group 3 (n = 115): usual-care control	All patients: standard postoperative care AT group: 2 hours of adjunctive postoperative high-frequency stimulation (100 Hz) around incision site PT group: same procedures but with inactive TENS unit	RCT Prospective Patient blinded	Time to request for further analgesia Analgesic use: patient-controlled analgesia (PCA) Pain intensity: NRS 0-10	AT was not effective for decreased pain and medication use in patients who underwent posterolateral thoracotomy (patients with high pain level). AT resulted in significantly increased time to request for analgesia (p <.001) for patients who underwent muscle-sparing thoracotomy, costotomy, and sternotomy (patients with mild to moderate pain level). AT was effective as sole anesthetic for more than 9 hours postsurgery in patients who underwent video-assisted thoracoscopy (patients with minimal to mild pain level).
Wang et al.[243] (1997)	Elective lower abdominal surgery 100 women (25 each group) Group 1: *high-intensity acupoint TENS* (High); mean age 43 (8) Group 2: *low-intensity acupoint TENS* (Low); mean age 45 (9) Group 3: sham TENS at acupoints (*Sham*); mean age 44 (9)	All patients: usual postoperative pain control through PCA All active TENS patients: 30 minutes of stimulation every 2-3 hours, given with alternating frequencies (2 Hz/100 Hz) every 3 seconds; all TENS at Hegu acupoint on nondominant hand and	RCT Prospective Patient and data collector blinded	Pain VAS Morphine: PCA intake PCA duration Sedation VAS Fatigue VAS Discomfort VAS Nausea VAS Dizziness VAS Length of hospitalization	*High:* 65% decreased morphine intake (p <.05) vs. all other groups *High:* decreased duration of PCA (p <.01) vs. all other groups *High:* decreased nausea (p <.05) vs. Sham and UC *High:* decreased dizziness (p <.05) vs. all other groups

(Continued)

Study	Sample	Intervention	Design	Measurement	Major Findings
	Group 4: usual care with PCA only (UC); mean age 44 (10)	on both sides of incision High: 9-12 mA Low: 4-5 mA			*High:* decreased pruritus (p <.05) vs. UC *Low:* significantly decreased pain (p <.05) vs. Sham (but not UC) No significant differences between groups in length of hospitalization or other outcomes
Chen et al.[35] (1998)	Elective total abdominal hysterectomy or myomectomy 100 women (25 each group) Group 1: *acupoint TENS* (Acu); mean age 43 (13) Group 2: *incisional TENS* (Inc); mean age 44 (13) Group 3: *shoulder TENS* (Sho); mean age 44 (13) Group 4: *sham acupoint TENS* (Sham); mean age 45 (12)	All patients: usual pre/postoperative analgesia (PCA) All TENS groups: 30 minutes of stimulation (or sham) given every 2-3 hours, given with alternating frequencies (2 Hz/100 Hz) every 3 seconds; high-intensity stimulation: 9-12 mA *Acu:* bilaterally at classic Chinese acupoints (Zusanli; ST36) *Inc:* at dermatomes next to incision *Sho:* bilaterally at deltoid *Sham:* placebo at same acupoints as Acu	RCT Prospective Patient and data collector blinded	Pain VAS PCA (morphine) intake PCA duration Sedation VAS Fatigue VAS Discomfort VAS Nausea VAS Length of hospitalization	*Acu* and *Inc* TENS groups had significantly decreased postoperative PCA intake (p <.05) vs. Sho and Sham groups *Acu* and *Inc:* significantly decreased duration of postoperative PCA (p <.05) vs. Sho and Sham *Acu* and *Inc:* significantly increased pain relief (p <.05) vs. Sho and Sham *Acu* and *Inc:* significantly decreased nausea and dizziness (p <.05) vs. Sho and Sham No significant differences between groups on other outcomes
Hamza et al.[104,105] (1999)	Elective total abdominal hysterectomy or myomectomy 100 women (25 each group)	All patients: usual pre/postoperative analgesia (PCA) All TENS groups: 30 minutes of stimulation (or sham) every 2-3 hours	RCT Prospective Patients and data collectors blinded	Pain VAS PCA (morphine) intake PCA duration Sedation VAS Fatigue VAS Discomfort VAS	No significant differences in pain were found among groups *Mix:* significantly decreased morphine intake (p <.05) vs. all other groups (53% less than Sham)

Reference	Sample	Design/Intervention	Outcome Measures	Results
	Group 1: *high-frequency TENS* (100 Hz); mean age 44 (11) Group 2: *low-frequency TENS* (2 Hz); mean age 43 (11) Group 3: *mixed-frequency TENS* (2 Hz/100 Hz) (Mix); mean age 45 (10) Group 4: *sham TENS control*; mean age 43 (9)	All TENS administered to both sides of incision at high intensity (9-15 mA) with bidirectional current and changing pulse width	Nausea VAS Dizziness VAS Length of hospitalization	*Mix:* significantly decreased 24-hour sedation and 48-hour discomfort ($p < .05$) vs. Sham All active TENS groups: significantly decreased morphine intake, duration of PCA, and PCA demands ($p < .05$); significantly decreased 24-hour nausea and pruritus ($p < .05$); and significantly decreased 24-hour sedation ($p < .05$) vs. Sham *Mix:* significantly decreased 24-hour dizziness and 48-hour discomfort ($p < .05$) vs. Sham No significant differences between groups in length of hospitalization
Robinson et al.[195] (2001)	Diagnostic colonoscopy 33 subjects Group 1 ($n = 10$): medication only; mean age 56.40 (12.53) Group 2 ($n = 10$): *active TENS;* mean age = 47.80 (18.86) Group 3 ($n = 13$): sham TENS; mean age 53.23 (16.45)	All patients: usual preoperative medication (midazolam) Active TENS group: adjunctive stimulation for 5 minutes before procedure Sham TENS group: nonfunctioning TENS unit for 5 minutes before procedure	RCT Prospective Investigator blinded	Pain: NRS 1-100 (physician rated) Procedure discomfort Procedure distress Procedure satisfaction
				No significant differences were found among groups

(Continued)

TABLE 10–1. STUDIES OF CAM THERAPIES FOR PROCEDURAL AND POSTOPERATIVE PAIN—cont'd

Study	Sample	Intervention	Design	Measurement	Major Findings
HYPNOSIS, IMAGERY, AND SUGGESTION					
McLintock et al.[159] (1990)	Elective abdominal hysterectomy 60 women Group 1 (n = 30): *positive suggestions*; mean age 40.5 (range 37-44) Group 2 (n = 14): control; mean age 40.8 (range 39-43)	Both groups: preoperative temazepam/anesthesia and postoperative PCA Positive-suggestion group listened to an audiotape during surgery with suggestions for successful outcomes Control group was played a blank tape	RCT Prospective Repeated measures Double blind	Pain VAS 24-hour pain medication use (PCA) Nausea/vomiting	Positive-suggestion group had significantly decreased (23%) pain medication (p <.028) vs. control No significant differences between groups in postoperative pain No significant differences between groups in nausea/vomiting
Weinstein, Au[245] (1991)	Angioplasty for coronary artery disease 32 subjects Group 1 (n = 16): hypnosis (Hyp); mean age 60 (8) Group 2 (n = 16): standard care (SC); mean age 59 (11)	Both groups: usual preoperative medication Hyp: adjunctive presurgical hypnosis with posthypnotic suggestions (about 30 minutes), as well as support/prompting during surgery SC: no adjunctive treatment	RCT Prospective Unblinded Convenience sample	Heart rate Blood pressure Pain medication use Catecholamines: epinephrine (E), norepinephrine (NE)	Hypnosis group had significantly decreased pain medication use (p = .05) vs. SC group Hyp: significantly increased NE at start of procedure (p <.01) vs. SC Hyp: significantly greater drop in total catecholamines at end of procedure (p <.025) vs. SC No significant difference between groups in procedure time
Faymonville et al.[65] (1995)	Plastic surgery under local anesthesia and conscious sedation 337 subjects	All patients: usual care with IV sedation Some patients: adjunctive preoperative	Retrospective Group comparison Unblinded Convenience sample	Anxiety VAS Postoperative pain VAS	Hypnosis and relaxation groups: significantly decreased intraoperative anxiety (p <.01) vs. IV group

Study	Sample	Design	Intervention	Outcomes	Results
	Group 1 (n =137; 25.4% F, 74.6% M): intravenous (IV) sedation only; mean age 38.7 (15) Group 2 (n =172; 70.8% F, 29.2% M): *hypnosis*; mean age 36.3 (18) Group 3 (n = 28; 85.7% F, 14.3% M): *relaxation*; mean age 41.0 (15)		induction of hypnosis (successful hypnosis) or relaxation (unsuccessful hypnosis)		Hypnosis and relaxation groups: significantly decreased postoperative anxiety (p <.01) vs. IV group Hypnosis group: 70% decrease in intraoperative pain (p <.001) vs. IV group Hypnosis group: significantly decreased postoperative pain (p <.001) vs. IV group Relaxation group: 60% decrease in intraoperative pain (p <.01) vs. IV group Hypnosis and relaxation groups: significantly decreased sedative use (p <.01) vs. IV group Patients preferred hypnosis and relaxation to IV sedation alone.
Manyande et al.[154] (1995)	Abdominal surgery 51 subjects (21 F, 30 M); mean age 45 (range 22-76) Group 1 (n = 26): *imagery*; mean age 47 (13.8) Group 2 (n = 25): control; mean age 44 (15.4)	RCT	All patients: usual preoperative medication, anesthesia, and postoperative analgesia Imagery group listened to an audiotape preoperatively with imagery and relaxation instructions to assist with coping Control group listened to an audiotape preoperatively with information about the hospital	Pain intensity VAS Pain distress VAS Pain coping VAS State anxiety: Spielberger State-Trait Anxiety Inventory (STAI) Cortisol Epinephrine (E) Norepinephrine (NE) Heart rate (HR) Blood pressure Postoperative analgesic use	Imagery group had significantly decreased pain intensity (p <.05) and pain distress (p <.01) vs. control group Imagery: significantly increased pain coping (p <.01) Imagery: significantly decreased postoperative analgesic use (p <.05) Imagery: significantly decreased cortisol at induction and during recovery (p <.01)

(Continued)

Study	Sample	Intervention	Design	Measurement	Major Findings
					Imagery: significantly increased NE at induction and during recovery ($p < .001$) Imagery: decreased maximum HR during surgery and recovery ($p < .01$) Both groups had equal reductions in state anxiety ($p < .001$), indicating that imagery was not effective in reducing state anxiety.
Ashton et al.[15] (1997)	Elective coronary artery bypass surgery 32 subjects Group 1 (n = 20): *self-hypnosis* Group 2 (n = 12): routine care (RC)	Self-hypnosis group: preoperative adjunctive training in self-hypnosis for relaxation and symptom management before and after surgery RC control group: no adjunctive treatment	RCT with stratification by age, gender, and hypnotizability (HIP) Prospective Surgeon and data collector blinded	HIP Profile of Mood States (POMS) Analgesic requirements	Self-hypnosis patients who complied with treatment had significantly decreased pain medication requirements ($p = .046$) vs. RC, but self-hypnosis group used significantly more pain medication ($p = .022$) vs. RC Self-hypnosis group: significantly decreased postoperative POMS tension ($p = .0317$) Compliance with self-hypnosis: 100% (preoperative) and 65% (postoperative)

| Faymonville et al.[66] (1997) | Elective plastic surgery under local anesthesia and conscious sedation 56 subjects Group 1 (n = 31; 89% F, 11% M): hypnosis (Hyp); mean age = 36 (14) Group 2 (n = 25; 84% F, 16% M): support control (SC); mean age 34 (10) | Both groups: local anesthesia and postoperative analgesia Hyp: hypnotic induction and pleasant imagery during surgery (word "hypnosis" not used) SC: emotional support with continuous stress management strategies and reassurance No direct suggestions for analgesia given to either group | RCT Prospective Patient blinded | Pain VAS Anxiety VAS Perceived control VAS Medication use Vital signs Postoperative nausea/vomiting (N/V) | Hypnosis group had significantly decreased intraoperative and postoperative pain (p <.02) vs. support group Hyp: significantly decreased intraoperative sedative use (p <.001) vs. SC Hyp: significantly decreased postoperative anxiety (p <.04) vs. SC Hyp: significantly greater perceived intraoperative control (p <.01) vs. SC Hyp: significantly more stable vital signs (p <.002) vs. SC Hyp: significantly decreased postoperative N/V (p <.001) vs. SC |
| Tusek et al.[233] (1997) | First elective abdominal surgery for colorectal disorders 130 subjects; mean age 40 Group 1 (n = 65): guided imagery (GI); mean age 40 (14) Group 2 (n = 65): standard-care control (SC); median age 39 | Both groups: routine care with postoperative pain medication and support GI: multimodal imagery and music (twice daily) adjunctive therapy before and after surgery, as well as music during surgery SC: no adjunctive treatment | RCT Prospective Repeated measures Unblinded | Pain: NRS 0-100 Anxiety: NRS 0-100 Narcotic (PCA) requirement Time to first bowel movement (BM) Postoperative side effects Sleep quality Length of hospitalization | Guided imagery group had significantly decreased total analgesic requirement (p <.001) vs. support group GI: significantly decreased worst and lowest pain (p <.001) vs. SC GI: significantly attenuated anxiety (p <.001) vs. SC GI: significantly decreased time to first BM (p <.003) vs. SC No significant difference between groups for median length of stay or other outcomes |

(Continued)

TABLE 10–1. STUDIES OF CAM THERAPIES FOR PROCEDURAL AND POSTOPERATIVE PAIN—cont'd

Study	Sample	Intervention	Design	Measurement	Major Findings
					Imagery patients reported benefits for postoperative sleep, recovery, and anxiety
Mauer et al.[158] (1999)	Orthopedic and surgery 60 subjects (11 F, 49 M) Group 1 (n = 30): hypnosis (Hyp) Group 2 (n = 30): usual-treatment control (UC)	*Hyp*: standardized 20-minute hypnotic intervention with instructions for relaxation and suggestions for positive outcomes *UC*: no adjunctive treatment	Quasi-experimental Groups run in separate cohorts Repeated measures Consecutive patients	Pain intensity: NRS 0-10 Pain effect: NRS 0-10 State anxiety (STAI) Trait anxiety (STAI) Postsurgical recovery (surgeon rated) Postsurgical complications	Hypnosis group had significantly decreased pain intensity and pain effect (p <.002) on first 3 postoperative days vs. UC group *Hyp*: significantly decreased state anxiety on postoperative day 4 (p <.001) vs. UC *Hyp*: significantly increased postsurgical recovery (p = .004) vs. UC *Hyp*: significantly decreased complications (p = .016) vs. UC
Lang et al.[136] (2000)	Percutaneous vascular and renal procedures 241 subjects (127 F, 114 M); median age 56 (18-92) 55% inpatients 45% day patients Group 1 (n = 82; 44 F, 38 M): hypnosis; median age 54 Group 2 (n = 80; 40 F, 40 M): attention control; median age 57 Group 3 (n = 79; 43 F, 36 M): standard-care	Hypnosis group had intraoperative attention and adjunctive self-hypnotic relaxation training Attention control group received only structured attention SC group received typical care at the university hospital	RCT Prospective Repeated measures Unblinded	Pain: NRS 0-10 Anxiety: NRS 0-10 Standard drug units	Hypnosis significantly attenuated pain vs. SC (p <.0001) and attention (p = .0259) Hypnosis significantly attenuated anxiety (p = .0022) vs. SC Hypnosis group had significantly decreased average procedure duration (p = .0016) vs. SC group Hypnosis and attention groups had significantly

Author	Subjects	Design	Intervention	Outcomes	Results
	control (SC); median age 57				decreased drug use (p <.0001) vs. SC group Hypnosis group had significantly increased hemodynamic stability vs. attention (p <.0041) and SC (p <.0009) groups.
Renzi et al.[192] (2000)	Surgery for benign anorectal diseases 86 subjects Group 1 (n = 43; 22 F, 21 M): *imagery*; mean age 48 (range 25-72) Group 2 (n = 43; 15 F, 28 M): standard care (SC); mean age 44 (range 18-70)	RCT Prospective Unblinded Consecutive patients	All patients: pre/ postoperative anesthesia Imagery group listened to recorded guided imagery and music to increase relaxation before, during, and after surgery (30-minute audiotape) SC group: no adjunctive treatment	Postoperative pain VAS Sleep quality VAS First micturition (normal or difficult) Medication use	No significant difference between groups in postoperative pain (p = .07) Imagery group had significantly increased sleep (p = .01) vs. SC group No significant differences between groups in medication use (hypnotics, analgesics) No significant difference between groups in difficulty of micturition
Cupal, Brewer,[46] (2001)	Anterior cruciate ligament (ACL) reconstructive surgery 30 subjects (10 each group; 14 F, 16 M) Mean age 28.2 (SD 8.2) Group 1: *imagery* Group 2: *placebo* Group 3: usual care, physical therapy (PT)	RCT Prospective Only physical therapists were blinded Consecutive patients	All patients: postsurgical PT Imagery treatment: 10 individualized, standardized sessions of relaxation and guided imagery over 6 months, as well as daily audiotaped sessions Placebo treatment: attention, support, and encouragement Usual care: only PT	Reinjury anxiety: NRS 0-10 Pain: NRS 0-10 Knee strength: Cybex 6000 isokinetic dynamometer	Imagery group had significantly decreased pain at 24 weeks postsurgery vs. placebo and PT (p <.05) groups Imagery group had significantly increased knee strength at 24 weeks postsurgery vs. placebo (p <.003) and PT (p <.02) groups Imagery group had significantly decreased reinjury anxiety at 24 weeks postsurgery vs. placebo and PT (p <.05) groups

(Continued)

TABLE 10–1. **STUDIES OF CAM THERAPIES FOR PROCEDURAL AND POSTOPERATIVE PAIN** —cont'd

Study	Sample	Intervention	Design	Measurement	Major Findings
					Patients reported moderate compliance with use of tape (4.4 uses/wk)
Montgomery et al.[165] (2002)	Excisional breast biopsy surgery 20 patients; mean age 50.11 (10.94) Group 1 ($n = 10$): *hypnosis* Group 2 ($n = 10$): usual-treatment control (UC)	Hypnosis group received adjunctive hypnosis with a standardized (10-minute) preoperative hypnotic induction and intervention tool (suggestions for relaxation/recovery). Trained clinical psychologist provided hypnosis. UC group: no adjunctive treatment	RCT Unblinded Consecutive patients	Pain VAS Distress VAS Pain expectations VAS Distress expectations VAS Medical care satisfaction VAS	Hypnosis group had significantly decreased postsurgery pain ($p < .001$) and decreased distress ($p < .025$) vs. UC group Postintervention (preoperative) pain expectations were significantly correlated with postoperative pain ($r = .69$, $p < .001$), indicating that pain expectations were important predictors of treatment outcome Postintervention (preoperative) distress was significantly correlated with postoperative distress ($r = .53$, $p < .015$) Postintervention (preoperative) distress expectations were significantly correlated with postoperative distress ($r = .71$, $p < .001$) No significant difference between group in treatment satisfaction

MAGNET THERAPY

Study	Sample/Groups	Intervention	Design	Outcome Measures	Results
Man et al.[151] (1999)	Suction lipectomy 20 subjects; age range 18-75 Group 1 (n = 10): *magnets* Group 2 (n = 10): sham	Magnetic treatment group wore magnetic patches for 14 days (with ceramic magnets oriented in one direction; 150 to 400 gauss) over suctioned areas of skin. Sham group wore unmagnetized patches	RCT Double blind Repeated measures	Pain VAS Daily pain log Skin discoloration: 0-10 (observer rated) Edema: 0-10 (observer rated)	Magnet group had significantly decreased (37%-65%) pain (p <.05) vs. sham group Magnet group had significantly decreased discoloration (p <.05) vs. sham group Magnet group had significantly decreased edema (p <.05) vs. sham group No significant differences were found between groups in regard to side effects

MASSAGE THERAPY

Study	Sample/Groups	Intervention	Design	Outcome Measures	Results
Hulme et al.[114] (1999)	Laparoscopic sterilization 59 women Group 1 (n = 30): *massage* Group 2 (n = 29): standard care (SC)	Both groups: standard postoperative analgesia as needed at discharge Massage group: adjunctive 5-minute foot massage preoperatively SC group: no adjunctive treatment	RCT Prospective Unblinded Repeated measures	Pain: NRS 0-10 Analgesic use Perceived treatment efficacy	Both massage and UC groups had significantly decreased pain (p <.008) No significant differences between groups were found on any measured outcome
Hattan et al.[108] (2002)	Coronary artery bypass graft surgery 25 patients (5 F, 20 M); mean age 63.12 (9.35) Group 1 (n = 9): *massage* Group 2 (n = 9): *relaxation* Group 3 (n = 7): usual-care control (UC)	All patients: standard care Adjunctive massage and relaxation on postoperative day 2 Massage group: one 20-minute foot massage from trained massage therapist Relaxation group: 20 minutes of progressive muscle relaxation through audiotape	RCT Pretest/posttest Unblinded Consecutive patients	Pain VAS Anxiety VAS Tension VAS Calm VAS Relaxation VAS Blood pressure Heart rate Respiratory rate	Massage group had significantly increased "calm" scores (p = .014) vs. relaxation and UC groups No significant difference among groups on pain and other VAS scores No significant differences among groups on physiologic outcomes

(Continued)

TABLE 10–1. **STUDIES OF CAM THERAPIES FOR PROCEDURAL AND POSTOPERATIVE PAIN—cont'd**

Study	Sample	Intervention	Design	Measurement	Major Findings
Taylor et al.[227] (2002)	Abdominal laparotomy for removal of suspected cancer 146 subjects (105 completed study) Group 1 (n = 34): *massage;* mean age 53.8 (11.7) Group 2 (n = 35): *vibration;* mean age = 56.3 (13.3) Group 3 (n = 36): standard care (SC); mean age 58.4 (10.0)	UC group: no adjunctive treatment All patients: standard postoperative care Massage group: adjunctive massages (45 minutes) from licensed massage therapist on 3 consecutive evenings after surgery Vibration group: adjunctive vibration therapy (20-minute sessions) using physioacoustics on 3 consecutive evenings after surgery (and additional sessions as desired)	RCT Prospective Investigator blinded Repeated measures	Pain: NRS 0-10 Anxiety: NRS 0-10 Distress: NRS 0-10 24 hour pain medication use (PCA) Blood pressure Cortisol Length of hospitalization Postoperative complications	Trend for decreased pain and distress in massage group, but not significant when statistically controlling for multiple outcomes and comparisons No significant difference between groups on other outcomes
MUSIC THERAPY Koch et al.[130] (1998)	Urologic procedures using spinal anesthesia (study 1) or lithotripsy treatment (study 2) Study 1 (n = 34) • Group 1 (n = 15; 13% F, 87% M): *music;* mean age 53 (12) • Group 2 (n = 19; 15% F, 85% M): control; mean age 54 (15) Study 2 (n = 44) • Group 1 (n = 22; 56% F, 44% M): *music;* mean age 53 (12)	All patients: patient-controlled sedation (study 1) or patient-controlled anesthesia (study 2) Patients in music groups listened to self-selected intraoperative music through a headset	RCT	*Study 1* • Heart rate • Blood pressure • Perceived level of sedation score (patient report) • Sedative use • Duration of stay in postanesthesia care • Pulse oximetry *Study 2* • PCA use • Pain VAS • Sedation VAS	*Study 1* • Music group had significantly decreased sedative use (p <.001) vs. control group • No other significant difference between groups *Study 2* • Music group had significantly decreased PCA (analgesic) use • No significant difference between groups for pain or other measures

Study	Sample	Design	Intervention	Outcome measures	Results
	• Group 2 (n = 21; 20% F, 80% M): control; mean age 54 (15)			• Perceived level of sedation • Score (patient report) • Heart rate • Blood pressure • STAI • Adverse events (n)	No significant differences were found between groups Low to moderate pain levels may have limited potential treatment effects
Broscious et al.[29] (1999)	Open heart surgery requiring chest tube removal (acute pain) 156 subjects; mean age 66.35 (9.7) Group 1 (n = 70; 17 F, 53 M): music Group 2 (n = 36; 14 F, 22 M): white noise Group 3 (n = 50; 18 F, 32 M): standard-care control (SC)	RCT Prospective	Interventions provided during chest tube removal (about 10 minutes) Music group listened to a tape with self-selected music White noise group listened to tape with only white noise (to control for distraction)	Pain: NRS 0-10 Narcotic intake Heart rate Blood pressure	
Good et al.[91,92] (1999, 2001)	Major abdominal surgery 617 patients (500 completed study; 413 F, 87 M); mean age 45.37 (11.03) Group 1 (n = 111): usual-care control (UC) Group 2 (n = 116): relaxation only Group 3 (n = 122): music only Group 4 (n = 109): relaxation and music (Combo)	RCT Prospective Multisite Pre/posttest Repeated measures Patient blinded Convenience sample	All patients: usual analgesia Audiotaped interventions given pre/postoperatively Relaxation-only group: tape-recorded training on jaw muscular relaxation Music-only group: self-selected soothing music from investigator choices Combo group: tape with both relaxation and self-selected music	Pain sensation VAS Pain distress VAS Opioid intake	All treatment groups had significantly decreased pain (p <.05) vs. UC group Combo: significantly decreased pain sensation and distress (p <.027) vs. relaxation and significantly decreased pain distress (p = .023) vs. music No significant differences between relaxation and music on any outcomes. 84%-95% of patients achieved mastery of techniques by day 1

(Continued)

TABLE 10-1. STUDIES OF CAM THERAPIES FOR PROCEDURAL AND POSTOPERATIVE PAIN—cont'd

Study	Sample	Intervention	Design	Measurement	Major Findings
					Treatment effects were similar on postoperative days 1 and 2 for ambulatory and resting pain ($p < .001$)
Jacobson[118] (1999)	Intravenous (IV) insertion 110 subjects Group 1 ($n = 36$): *music* Group 2 ($n = 38$): *saline* Group 3 ($n = 36$): *control*	Music group listened to preferred music Saline group: 0.1 ml 0.9% intradermal saline infiltrated over IV site Control group: usual IV insertion	RCT Prospective	Pain intensity VAS Pain distress VAS IV Catheter Insertion Rating Scale	No differences were found among groups
RELAXATION THERAPY					
Miró, Raich[162] (1999)	Hysterectomy 92 women; mean age 55 (29-59) Group 1 ($n = 46$): *relaxation* Group 2 ($n = 46$): *attention control*	Relaxation group received brief preoperative relaxation training (30 minutes) and 1 week of home practice Control group received attention, support, and information	RCT Participant blinded	Pain: NRS 0-10 (standing, walking, bed positioning) Analgesic use Activity level: 0-100 Coping style (Miller Behavioral Style Scale): patients divided into low ($n = 43$) and high ($n = 49$) monitors	Relaxation group had significantly decreased pain ($p = .06-.001$) vs. attention group Relaxation group had significantly decreased interference with activities ($p < .001$) vs. attention group No significant difference between groups in analgesic use ($p < .06$) Coping style (high or low monitor) did not moderate treatment effects

medication use.[92,130] Other trials have not replicated these findings.[29] However, many studies have found that music can reduce anxiety in hospitalized patients.[63] Therefore, if music has an effect on the pain experience, it is likely indirect (i.e., mediated by anxiety/distress reduction).

In contrast to earlier research, more recent RCTs have found TENS to be an effective complementary therapy for pain control among patients undergoing various types of elective surgery. In particular, a series of studies demonstrated lower postoperative pain ratings, less medication use, and fewer treatment side effects among patients receiving several hours of TENS therapy.[35,105,243] However, brief TENS did not benefit a small sample of patients during diagnostic colonoscopy.[195] The literature suggests that TENS is most useful for low to moderate pain, and the degree of benefit appears to depend on the location, intensity, and frequency of the stimulation.[251] Also, these TENS studies have included mostly women, and demonstrated benefits may not generalize to men.

Another study within the CAM program area of *bioelectromagnetics* found that 2 weeks of exposure to static magnets reduced pain, edema, and wound discoloration in patients undergoing suction lipectomy.[151] However, further studies are needed to investigate fully the potential benefits of magnetic therapies in the surgical setting.

Within the CAM program area of body-based therapies, studies have found acupuncture and acupressure to reduce postoperative pain and pain medication consumption compared with usual care and placebo/sham conditions,[67,133] although other studies have not found an effect.[220] Likewise, a few studies have examined the effects of massage on postoperative pain, anxiety, recovery, and analgesic use. Although these studies have not found *massage* significantly more effective than usual postoperative care due to limited sample sizes and high intersubject variability, the results suggest that massage therapy may enhance postoperative outcomes among some patients.[108,114,227] Massage appears to reduce anxiety among acute and critical care patients,[194] but the available literature does not currently support massage for postoperative pain management.

N Pain Associated with Traumatic Injuries

Trauma produced by accidents ranks third as the cause of death in industrialized societies. Those who survive the initial trauma experience both immediate and delayed onset of pain that requires management.[242] The most widely studied and validated CAM modalities used in the treatment of pain associated with traumatic injuries have included herbs and natural products, hypnosis, and massage (Table 10-2).

Herbs and other natural products have been found to reduce itching and antihistamine use associated with burn healing[157] and pain associated with ear infections.[202] Two recent RCTs using homeopathic preparations did not demonstrate reduced muscle pain or analgesic use among long distance runners with muscle soreness.[237,238] Additional research is needed before any conclusion can be drawn about all these products.

Text continued on p. 339.

TABLE 10–2. **STUDIES OF CAM THERAPIES FOR PAIN ASSOCIATED WITH TRAUMATIC INJURIES**

Study	Sample	Intervention	Design	Measurement	Major Findings
BIOFEEDBACK					
Schoenberger et al.[208] (2001)	Traumatic brain injury 12 subjects (10 F, 2 M) Group 1: immediate treatment Group 2: wait-list control	Treatment group: Flexyx neurotherapy—electroencephalographic (EEG) biofeedback, 25 sessions over 5-8 weeks Control group: wait list	Randomized controlled trial (RCT)	Symptom Rating Scale (SRS) Beck Depression Inventory (BDI) Multidimensional Fatigue Inventory (MFI) Symptom Checklist (SCL-90-R) Auditory Verbal Learning Test (AVLT) Paced Auditory Serial Addition Test (PASAT) Digit Span Backwards (DSB)	SRS improved with treatment ($p < .01$) BDI improved with treatment ($p < .02$) SCL-90 general fatigue and mental fatigue subscales improved with treatment ($p < .02$) AVLT interference and delayed recall subscales improved with treatment ($p < .05$) PASAT improved with treatment ($p < .02$) Adverse events: headache (3), dizziness (4), nausea (1), tingling (1) DSB improved with treatment ($p < .05$) Other tests: Rey-Osterrieth Complex Figure, Trail Making Test, Controlled Oral Word Association, Digit Symbol
Greco et al.[96] (1997)	Temporomandibular disorder (TMD) 361 subjects (321 F, 40 M; 90% white, 7% black, 3% other) Group 1 ($n = 103$): traumatic onset Group 2 ($n = 258$): nontraumatic onset	Intraoral appliance Biofeedback: six weekly 75-minute sessions	Prospective treatment outcome study	McGill Pain Questionnaire (MPQ) Multidimensional Pain Inventory (MPI) Beck Depression Inventory (BDI) Coping Strategies Questionnaire (CSQ) TMD pain	Clinical outcomes improved regardless of group

HERBAL THERAPY AND SUPPLEMENTS

Matheson et al.[157] (2001)	Itch during burn healing 34 subjects Group 1 (n = 17; 2 F, 15 M): paraffin and oatmeal; age 32 ±6 Group 2: paraffin only (n = 17 3 F, 14 M; age 28 ±6	Oatmeal group: liquid paraffin and 5% colloidal oatmeal; bath oil Control group: liquid paraffin alone	RCT Double blind	Pain rating Itch rating Antihistamine use	Oatmeal group reported half the itch complaints as control group Oatmeal group requested half as many antihistamines as control group
Sarrell et al.[202] (2001)	Ear pain associated with otitis media 103 subjects; ages 6-18 Group 1 (n = 61; 32 F, 29 M): Otikon Group 2 (n = 42; 22 F, 20 M): anesthetic	Treatment group: Otikon (herbal ear drop formulation) Control group: ametocaine/ phenazone anesthetic	RCT	Pain-o-meter	Pain scores 30 minutes after administration of ear drops were lower for herbal group (p = .007) than control group No adverse events were noted
Thompson et al.[230] (2001)	Muscle soreness in shuttle runners 9 men; age 28.4 ±1.3 Group 1 (n = 4): vitamin C first Group 2 (n = 5): placebo first	Treatment group: 1 g vitamin C 2 hours before 90-minute intermittent shuttle running test Control group: placebo before exercise	RCT Double blind Repeated measures	Blood lactate Blood glucose Plasma volume Plasma vitamin C Creatine kinase (CK) Aspartate transaminase Methylenedioxy-amphetamine Uric acid Serum cortisol Vitamin E Total iron Heart rate	Plasma vitamin C concentrations were higher in treatment group and increased over course of exercise (p <.01) Decline in muscle function in vitamin C group (p <.05) No difference in muscle soreness between groups Other tests: perceived exertion, sweat loss, sprint times, food consumption
Van Wieringen et al,[234] (2001)	Chronic whiplash 81 subjects (59 F, 22 M); age 33.4 ± 10.7 Group 1 (n = 41): melatonin Group 2 (n = 40): placebo	Treatment group: melatonin, 5 mg daily, 5 hours before dim-light melatonin onset (DLMO) Control group: placebo 5 hours before DLMO	RCT Randomized in blocks of 10	Sleep diary Medical Outcomes Study–Short Form-36 (MOS SF-36) Pain score Concentration Polysomnography Actigraphy DLMO	Melatonin group advanced their melatonin onset (p = .02) Melatonin group advanced their wake-up time (p = .02) No difference in pain score was found between groups

(Continued)

TABLE 10–2. **STUDIES OF CAM THERAPIES FOR PAIN ASSOCIATED WITH TRAUMATIC INJURIES—cont'd**

Study	Sample	Intervention	Design	Measurement	Major Findings
Freund, Schwartz[78] (2000)	Whiplash 26 subjects (15 F, 11 M); ages 29-75 Group 1 (n = 14): botulinum toxin Group 2 (n = 12): saline	Treatment group: 100 U botulinum toxin-A (Botox) in 1 ml saline injected in 5 tender cervical trigger points Control group: 1 ml saline injected in trigger points	RCT Double blind	Neck pain visual analog scale (VAS) Shoulder pain VAS Head pain VAS Range of motion (ROM) Vernon-Mior functional index	Botox group increased ROM (p <.01) vs. placebo group Botox group decreased pain (p <.01) vs. placebo group
Stjernberg, Berglund[222] (2000)	Tick bites 100 subjects Group 1 (n = 50): garlic first Group 2 (n = 50): placebo first	Treatment group: garlic, 1200 mg/day in capsule for 8 weeks followed by 2-week washout Placebo group: 8 weeks	RCT with crossover Prospective Double blind	Tick bite frequency	Significant reduction in tick bites with garlic consumed (p = .04); relative risk 0.70 (95% confidence interval 0.54-0.90)
Buchman et al.[30] (1999)	Gastrointestinal (GI) injury in marathon runners 23 subjects Group 1 (n = 13; 5 F, 8 M): arginine Group 2 (n = 10; 2 F, 8 M): glycine	Treatment group: L-arginine 10 g three times daily for 14 days before marathon Control group: glycine (placebo) 10 g three times daily for 14 days before marathon	RCT Double blind	CK Amylase Lipase Salicylate concentration Serum amino acid concentration Occult blood GI distress Intestinal permeability	No clear benefit of arginine or glycine supplementation on GI injury
Starley et al.[219] (1999)	Full-thickness and infected burns 32 patients	Flesh of papaya mashed into paste and applied to wound	Single group	Observation of wound cleanliness	Wounds treated with papaya needed less debridement.
HOMEOPATHY					
Vickers et al.[238] (1998)	Muscle soreness in long distance runners 400 subjects Group 1 (n = 200, 44 F, 156 M): homeopathy; age 42.5 (11.1)	Treatment group: homeopathic Arnica 30x, 5 pills twice a day beginning evening before race and continued for 9 doses	RCT Double blind Placebo controlled	Visual analog scale (VAS)	No difference between groups

Study	Sample	Intervention	Design	Outcome Measures	Results
	Group 2 (n = 200; 62 F, 138 M): placebo; age:42.4 (10.0)	Control group: placebo on same dosing schedule			No difference between groups Three individuals in placebo group and four in homeopathy group experienced adverse events
Vickers et al.[237] (1997)	Exercise-induced muscle soreness 56 subjects Group 1 (n = 29; 18 F, 11 M): homeopathy; median age 30.9 (1.01) Group 2 (n = 27; 15 F, 12 M): placebo; median age 30.4 (1.11)	Treatment group: Homeopathic Arnica 30c plus Rhus Tox 30c plus sarcolactic acid 30c Control group: placebo	RCT Randomized in blocks of 4	Muscle soreness Analgesic use	

HYPNOSIS, IMAGERY, AND SUGGESTION

Study	Sample	Intervention	Design	Outcome Measures	Results
Frenay et al.[77] (2001)	Burns 26 subjects Group 1 (n = 11; 3 F, 8 M): hypnosis; median age 47.9 (13.5) Group 2 (n = 15; 10 F, 5 M): stress reduction; median age: 35.9 (10.7)	Hypnosis group: eye fixation, muscle relaxation, permissive and indirect suggestion Stress reduction group: deep breathing, relaxation, and positive evocation	Prospective RCT	VAS	Hypnosis decreased anxiety over stress reduction (p <.05)
Wright, Drummond[253] (2000)	Burns 30 patients; ages 4-48 (8 F, 22 M) Group 1 (n = 15): hypnosis Group 2 (n = 15): standard care	Hypnosis group: modified rapid induction analgesia (RIA) script (relaxation and suggestion) Control: standard dressing change	RCT	Pain rating Tellegen Absorption Scale	Pain intensity and distress decreased in RIA group (p <.001) vs. control group Medication use decreased in RIA group (p <.01) vs. control group The greater the capacity for absorption, the larger the pain decrease
Ginandes, Rosenthal[88] (1999)	Bone fractures 23 subjects; ages 21-49 Group 1 (n = 11; 9 F, 2 M): hypnosis Group 2 (n =12; 9 F, 3 M): control	Hypnosis group: six individual office visits addressing normative stages in fracture healing in accelerated time frame, plus tapes Control: usual care	RCT	Radiologic assessment Orthopedic assessment Pain assessment	No significant difference between groups

(Continued)

TABLE 10-2. **STUDIES OF CAM THERAPIES FOR PAIN ASSOCIATED WITH TRAUMATIC INJURIES—cont'd**

Study	Sample	Intervention	Design	Measurement	Major Findings
Patterson, Pracek[181] (1997)	Burns 61 subjects (10 F, 51 M) Group 1: *hypnosis*; median age 36.86 (12.10) Group 2: control	Hypnosis group: rapid induction analgesia (RIA) Control group: usual care	RCT	VAS Effectiveness of hypnosis	Patients with high initial pain ratings experienced decreased pain with hypnosis (p <.05) vs. control group
MANIPULATION Pellow, Brantingham[182] (2001)	Ankle inversion sprain 30 subjects Group 1 (n = 15; 9 F, 6 M): *adjustment*; median age 23.7 Group 2 (n = 15; 2 F, 13 M): placebo; median age 26.1	Treatment group: manual adjustment of ankle Placebo group: sham ultrasound for 5 minutes	RCT	MPQ Pain numeric rating scale (NRS) Ankle dorsiflexion Ligament tenderness Functional evaluation	Adjustment group had significantly decreased pain over placebo group Adjustment group had significantly increased ankle dorsiflexion range of motion over placebo group Adjustment group had significantly increased ankle functioning over placebo group
MASSAGE THERAPY Field et al.[69] (2000)	Burns 20 subjects Group 1 (n = 10; 70% M, 10% white, 60% Hispanic, 30% black): *massage*; age 37 ±14 Group 2 (n = 10; 70% M, 10% white, 70% Hispanic, 20% black): control; age 39 ±13	Treatment group: massage 30 minutes twice weekly for 5 weeks on localized nongrafted wound area Control group: standard care	RCT	Itch rating VAS McGill Pain Questionnaire (MPQ) State-Trait Anxiety Inventory (STAI) Profile of Mood States (POMS)	Massage decreased itching (p <.001), pain (p <.05), and depressed mood (p <.005) vs. standard care

Study	Population/Groups	Design	Outcomes Measured	Results
Field et al.[70] (1998)	Burns 28 subjects; 86% M, 41% Hispanic, 30% black, 29% white Group 1 (n = 14): *massage* Group 2 (n = 14): *control*	Treatment group: massage 20 minutes daily for 1 week Control group: standard treatment	RCT	VAS MPQ STAI Present Pain Inventory POMS Behavioral observation Heart rate Cortisol levels	Massage decreased STAI score (p <.001) vs. standard care Massage increased positive behaviors (p <.01) vs. standard care Massage decreased salivary cortisol levels (p <.05) vs. standard care No difference in pain between groups

MUSIC THERAPY

Study	Population/Groups	Design	Outcomes Measured	Results
Fratianne et al.[76] (2001)	Burn debridement 25 subjects (9 F, 16 M); ages 7-83 Group 1: *music first* Group 2: *control first*	Treatment: music therapist improvised song lyrics referencing patient's imagery and deep breathing Control: standard care	RCT with crossover	Heart rate Pain Anxiety Behavioral observation	Music decreased pain (p = .008) vs. standard care
Tanabe et al.[226] (2001)	Musculoskeletal trauma 77 subjects; median age 41 (17.54) Group 1 (n = 24): *distraction* Group 2 (n = 24): *ibuprofen* Group 3 (n = 28): *control*	Distraction group: music plus standard care Ibuprofen group: ibuprofen plus standard care Control group: standard care alone (ice, elevation, immobilization)	Controlled trial	Pain ratings Satisfaction with pain management	No differences were found among groups

THERAPEUTIC TOUCH

Study	Population/Groups	Design	Outcomes Measured	Results
Turner et al.[232] (1998)	Burns 99 subjects Group 1 (n = 62; 76% M, 74% white, 26% black): *therapeutic touch;*	Treatment group: therapeutic touch (TT) practitioner centers, then clears, directs, or balances patient's energy flow for	RCT	MPQ VAS pain VAS anxiety VAS satisfaction Credibility of therapy form	TT decreased pain (p <.005) vs. sham TT decreased anxiety (p = .031) vs. sham TT decreased CD8+ cells by

(Continued)

TABLE 10–2. **STUDIES OF CAM THERAPIES FOR PAIN ASSOCIATED WITH TRAUMATIC INJURIES—cont'd**

Study	Sample	Intervention	Design	Measurement	Major Findings
	Ages 15-68 Group 2 (n = 37; 78% M, 76% white, 24% black): sham; ages 20-64	5-20 minutes Sham group: random, mimicked TT movements while counting 7s backward		Effectiveness with therapy form CD4+ cells CD8+ cells	13%; sham increased by 46.5% TT increased CD4+ cells by 15.2%; sham increased by 48.3% TT increased total lymphocyte count by 1.1%; sham increased by 38.6%
VIRTUAL REALITY					
Hoffman et al.[109] (2001)	Burn physical therapy 7 patients; ages 9-32 (1 F, 6 M) Group 1 Group 2: control	Virtual reality group: "Cyberworlds": patients could manipulate environment during physical therapy Control: standard physical therapy	Single group Repeated measures	VAS	Virtual reality decreased pain (p <.01) vs. standard therapy

In the CAM program area of mind-body therapies, several recent studies have found hypnosis to reduce pain, anxiety, and/or analgesic use among persons undergoing burn wound debridement.[77,181,253] These studies support earlier research demonstrating efficacy of hypnosis in the treatment of burn pain[164] and indicate that hypnosis may be more effective for patients who report high levels of pain.[181] Other researchers found that music used to reinforce imagery and deep breathing was effective in reducing pain associated with burn treatment.[76] The literature also revealed evidence that massage therapy,[69,70] as well as therapeutic touch,[232] may be useful adjunctive modalities in the management of burn pain and related symptoms. Because most of the studies reviewed included small sample sizes, further studies are needed to replicate and extend these findings.

◤ Musculoskeletal Pain

Musculoskeletal disorders are a worldwide cause of pain and suffering. This discussion addresses acute and chronic pain associated with the muscles and joints in the back, neck, shoulders, and extremities. On a national scale, back, neck, shoulder, and extremity pain are the most common, debilitating, and expensive pain problems in terms of lost productivity.[110,228] For example, national statistics indicate a yearly prevalence of *low back problems* in the U.S. population of 15% to 20%.[12] Low back problems are the main reason for office visits to primary care physicians and rank third among reasons for surgical procedures.[47] Estimates of total annual societal costs of back pain range from $20 to $50 billion.[170]

According to a recent report, musculoskeletal problems are also the most common health problems associated with CAM use.[179] Therefore, CAM therapies with proven effectiveness for musculoskeletal pain have potential cost-saving implications, not only in terms of reducing time lost from work, but also in avoiding more costly and invasive medical procedures. Many clinical trials have been conducted to examine the efficacy of CAM modalities on musculoskeletal pain. In recent years, larger and more rigorous studies have revealed that acupuncture and manipulation have been the most studied CAM treatments (Table 10-3).

In recent RCTs, *acupuncture* has been found beneficial for relieving chronic neck pain,[116] chronic low back pain,[37,142] and shoulder pain.[54,129] These studies provide further evidence that acupuncture may be useful as an adjunctive therapy for musculoskeletal pain.[174]

The clinical guidelines for acute lower back problems in adults recommend that after serious spinal conditions (e.g., fracture, tumor, infection, cauda equina) and nonspinal pathologic conditions (vascular, abdominal, urinary tract, or pelvic disease that can cause referred back pain) are ruled out, *spinal manipulation* can be used to provide symptomatic relief and improve function.[4] A meta-analysis of the chiropractic literature showed that chiropractic treatment hastened recovery from back strains and sprains.[135]

Systematic reviews[61,131] and meta-analyses[2,11] of early studies on spinal manipulation were inconclusive because of design flaws. More recent studies of spinal manipulation

Text continued on p. 354.

TABLE 10–3. **STUDIES OF CAM THERAPIES FOR MUSCULOSKELETAL PAIN**

Study	Sample	Intervention	Design	Measurement	Major Findings
ACUPUNCTURE					
Green et al.[97] (2002)	Lateral elbow pain 4 studies	Acupuncture	Systematic review	Pain Function Disability Quality of life Strength Satisfaction with treatment	Acupuncture provided pain relief longer than placebo Acupuncture was more likely to reduce pain after one treatment Acupuncture was more likely to result in participant report of improvement No difference in pain was found with laser acupuncture vs. placebo
Ter Riet et al.[229] (1990)	Chronic pain, including back 51 clinical trials	Acupuncture	Meta-analysis	Quality measure of studies	Results suggest efficacy of acupuncture remains doubtful based on quality of studies
Patel et al.[180] (1989)	Regional pain in lower back and other sites 14 clinical trials	Acupuncture	Meta-analysis	Number of patients showing improvement	Pooled results suggest effectiveness of acupuncture in low back pain
Lu et al.[147] (2001)	Head and neck pain syndromes 25 subjects (14 F, 11 M); ages 32-80 (mean 55.3) Group 1: acupuncture Group 2: acupuncture and hypnosis	Acupuncture once a week for 3 weeks, followed by washout period, followed by hypnosis for 3 sessions	Single group, crossover design with washout	Visual analog scale (VAS) pain	Acupuncture decreased acute and chronic pain, but not psychogenic pain ($p < .0001, .0002, .42$) compared with baseline Hypnosis decreased all types of pain ($p < .005, .0004, .003$)

Study	Population	Design	Treatment	Outcome Measures	Results
Inrich et al.[116] (2001)	Chronic neck pain 177 subjects (117 F, 60 M): ages 39-65, 165 subjects completed study Group 1 (n = 49): *acupuncture* Group 2 (n = 59): *massage* Group 3 (n = 57): sham laser acupuncture	RCT Placebo and alternative treatment Multisite	All treatments: 30 minutes 5 times over 3 weeks	VAS pain with motion Range of motion (ROM) Short Form Health Survey (SF-36)	Decreased pain related to ROM in acupuncture vs. massage, but not acupuncture vs. sham (p <.005) Decreased pain on motion by 50% in acupuncture group, 32% in sham group, and 25% in massage group (p <.008) *Adverse effects:* 33% had pain or vegetative response to acupuncture, 7% had adverse effects to massage, 21% to sham acupuncture
Birch, Jamison[18] (1998)	Chronic myofascial neck pain 46 subjects Group 1 (n = 15; 85.7% F): relevant *acupuncture;* median age 40.9 Group 2 (n = 16; 76.9% F): irrelevant acupuncture; median age 38.0 Group 3 (n = 15; 85.7% F): no acupuncture; median age 38.6	RCT	Relevant acupuncture: 30 minutes twice weekly for 4 weeks, then once weekly for 4 weeks, then once every other week for 2 weeks Irrelevant acupuncture: following same schedule as relevant	Comprehensive Pain Evaluation Questionnaire (CPEQ) McGill Pain Questionnaire (MPQ) Pain intensity rating SF-36 Symptom checklist (SCL-90-R) Medication diary Belief and helpfulness Blood pressure Heart rate	Relevant acupuncture decreased pain and intensity ratings after treatment more than other groups (p <.05) Previous acupuncture experience was correlated with confidence that acupuncture would relieve pain (p <.05)
David et al.[48] (1998)	Chronic neck pain 70 subjects Group 1 (n = 33; 23 F, 10 M): *acupuncture;* median age 48 Group 2 (n = 28; 18 F, 10 M): physiotherapy; median age 44	Randomized convenience sample	Acupuncture vs. standard mobilization techniques	Pain VAS Northwick Park Neck Pain Questionnaire (NPQ) ROM General Health Questionnaire (GHQ)	No significant differences were found between groups

(Continued)

TABLE 10–3. **STUDIES OF CAM THERAPIES FOR MUSCULOSKELETAL PAIN**—cont'd

Study	Sample	Intervention	Design	Measurement	Major Findings
Cherkin et al.[37] (2001)	Chronic low back pain 262 subjects Group 1 (n = 94; 52% F, 82% white): *acupuncture;* median age 45.3 (11.5) Group 2 (n = 78; 69% F, 82% white): *massage;* median age 45.7 (11.4) Group 3 (n = 90; 56% F, 89% white): self-care; median age 44.9 (11.5)	Acupuncture: TCM needling, electrical stimulation, manual manipulation of needles, indirect "moxibustion," infrared heat, cupping, exercise Massage: Swedish, deep tissue, neuromuscular, trigger and pressure point work) Self-education: high-quality book, two professionally demonstrated videotapes	RCT without stratification	Modified Roland Disability Scale (RDS) National Health Interview Survey (NHIS) Medication use Satisfaction with care SF-12 Exercise	74% rated massage very helpful vs. 46% for acupuncture ($p < .001$) Significant treatment effects favoring massage emerged after 10 weeks ($p < .02$) Massage and acupuncture groups reported more satisfaction with care vs. self-care group (50% vs. 37% vs. 13%; adjusted $p < .001$) Medication use decreased in acupuncture and massage groups but not in self-care group ($p < .05$) At 1-year follow-up, massage was superior to acupuncture on symptoms ($p < .002$) Adverse events: 11% of acupuncture group and 13% of massage group reported significant discomfort or pain during or shortly after treatment
Leibing et al.[142] (2002)	Chronic low back pain 131 subjects; median age 48.1 (9.7) Group 1 (n = 40; 22 F, 18 M): *acupuncture;* age 47.9 (11.1)	All treatments: 20- to 30-minute sessions over 12 weeks Treatment group: fixed traditional body and ear acupuncture	Randomized Placebo controlled Prospective	Pain VAS Pain Disability Index (PDI) Psychologic distress Spinal flexion	Acupuncture decreased pain intensity over control ($p < .001$) Acupuncture decreased pain disability over control ($p < .001$)

Study	Subjects	Intervention	Design	Outcome measures	Results
	Group 2 (n = 45; 27 F, 18 M): sham acupuncture; age 49.0 (9.4) Group 3 (n = 46): control; median age 47.5 (8.9)	Sham group: minimal needle penetration distant from verum Control group: active physiotherapy			Acupuncture decreased psychologic distress over sham acupuncture (p <.04) and control (p.02) At 9-month follow-up, both acupuncture and sham acupuncture decreased pain disability over control (p <.01)
Wedenberg et al.[244] (2000)	Low back and pelvic pain in pregnancy 48 women; ages 21-36 Group 1 (n = 28): *acupuncture* Group 2 (n = 18): *physiotherapy*	Acupuncture: 30 minutes 3 times/wk for 2 weeks, then twice/wk for 2 weeks, totaling 10 sessions in 1 month Physiotherapy: 50 minutes once or twice a week, totaling 10 sessions in 6-8 weeks	RCT	Pain VAS Disability rating index	Acupuncture decreased pain after treatment in morning and evening vs. physiotherapy (p <.02) Acupuncture significantly decreased disability scores after treatment vs. physiotherapy
Yi-Kai et al.[254] (2000)	Intractable low back pain; lumbar diskectomy 24 patients (7 F, 17 M); ages 26-67	Traditional silver needle acupuncture centered about a tender spot, with moxa burned on each needle	Single group pre/posttest	Total Tenderness Score System	Acupuncture decreased pain after treatment (p = .000 to .004 depending on site)
Giles, Muller[87] (1999)	Chronic spinal pain syndromes 77 subjects; ages 34-49 Group 1 (n = 20: 13 F, 7 M): *acupuncture* Group 2: (n = 36; 17 F, 19 M): *manipulation* Group 3 (n =21; 17 F, 4 M): *drugs*	Acupuncture: with low-volt electrical stimulation Manipulation: high velocity, low amplitude Medication: Tenoxicam with ranitidine	RCT	Oswestry Disability Index (ODI) Neck Disability Index Pain VAS Pain frequency	Manipulation decreased disability scores for back and neck pain (p <.004; p <.001) Manipulation decreased pain frequency (p <.007). 43% of subjects crossed over to another treatment because of inefficacy or side effects

(Continued)

TABLE 10-3. **STUDIES OF CAM THERAPIES FOR MUSCULOSKELETAL PAIN—cont'd**

Study	Sample	Intervention	Design	Measurement	Major Findings
Grant et al.[94] (1999)	Chronic back pain in elderly patients 60 subjects Group 1: (n = 30; 30 F, 2 M; 20 home, 12 hospitalized): acupuncture; ages 60-90 Group 2: (n = 27; 24 F, 4 M; 13 home, 15 hospitalized): TENS; ages 60-83	Acupuncture: twice weekly for 4 weeks Transcutaneous electrical nerve stimulation (TENS): 50 Hz 30minutes to 6 hours daily	RCT	VAS Pain numeric rating scale (NRS) Number of analgesics Spinal flexion	Analgesic use decreased 50% with acupuncture and 33% with TENS (p <.05) Acupuncture increased spinal flexion (p <.05), but improvement not maintained at 3-month follow-up
Branco, Naeser[25] (1999)	Carpal tunnel syndrome 36 hands, 31 subjects (22 F, 9 M); ages 24-84 Laser acupuncture and TENS	Laser acupuncture: 670 nm continuous wave, 5 mW, 1-7 J/point for 21 minutes TENS <900 µA, 282 Hz for 2 minutes, then 9.25 Hz for 18 minutes	Open treatment protocol Repeated measures	McGill Pain Questionnaire (MPQ)	Pain was significantly reduced after treatment (p <.0001)
Dyson-Hudson et al.[54] (2001)	Shoulder pain in wheelchair users 18 subjects Group 1 (n = 9; 2 F, 7 M): acupuncture; median age 49.6 (11.3) Group 2: (n = 9; 2 F, 7 M): Trager; age 40.6 (10.1)	Acupuncture: 20 to 30 min for 10 sessions Trager tablework and mental gymnastics: 45 min for 10 sessions	RCT	Performance-Corrected Wheelchair User's Shoulder Pain Index (PC-WUSPI)	Acupuncture decreased? pain after treatment (p <.001) Trager decreased pain after treatment (p <.05)
Kleinhenz et al.[129] (1999)	Rotator cuff tendinitis 53 subjects Group 1 (n = 26; 12 F, 14 M): acupuncture; median age 33.72(7.91) Group 2 (n = 27; 9 F, 18 M): placebo needling; median age: 37.37 (10.08)	Acupuncture: needle insertion into deep tissues Placebo needle: blunt tip does not penetrate skin; produces tingling sensation Both groups received 4 sessions (20 min each)	RCT	Modified Constant Murley Score	Acupuncture decreased pain over placebo needling (p <.01)

Study	Condition/Subjects	Intervention	Design	Outcome Measures	Results
Jensen et al.[120] (1999)	Patellofemoral pain syndrome 70 subjects Group 1 (n = 36; 20 F, 16 M): *acupuncture*; median age 29 Group 2 (n = 34; 21 F, 13 M; control; median age 33.4	If no improvement, 4 additional sessions at alternate sites Acupuncture: 20-25 min, repeated twice weekly for 4 weeks Control	RCT with block randomization	Cincinnati Rating Scale (CRS) VAS pain Analgesic use Stairs-Hopple test Atrophy	Acupuncture decreased symptoms, function, and pain at 12 months after treatment over control (p <.02)
BIOFEEDBACK					
Deepak, Behari[50] (1999)	Hand dystonia (writer's cramp) 13 women; ages 19-62 Group 1 (n = 10): *biofeedback*	Electromyographic (EMG) biofeedback once every 2 weeks	Single group Convenience sample	Visual analog scale (VAS) Handwriting improvement	9 of 10 in biofeedback group improved from 37% to 93% in handwriting
Dursun et al.[53] (2001)	Patellofemoral pain syndrome 60 subjects Group 1 (n = 30; 24 F, 6 M): *biofeedback*; median age 36.9 (9.2) Group 2 (n = 30; 24 F, 6 M; control; age 36.6 (10.6)	EMG biofeedback: 30-minute sessions 3 days a week for 4 weeks Control: usual exercise program	RCT	VAS pain Functional Index Questionnaire (FIQ)	Mean contraction values of vastus lateralis muscle increased in biofeedback group over control group (p <.007) No difference between groups on VAS or FIQ
ELECTRICAL STIMULATION					
Milne et al.[161] (2002)	Chronic low back pain 5 studies: *transcutaneous electrical nerve stimulation*	TENS Acupuncture-like TENS Sham TENS	Meta-analysis	Standardized mean differences between conditions	No statistically significant differences between active TENS group and other groups
Price, Pandyan[188] (2002)	Poststroke shoulder pain 4 studies: *surface electrical stimulation (ES)*	Any form of surface electrical stimulation (ES) technique including functional electrical stimulation (FES), TENS, and other	Meta-analysis	Prevention or treatment of shoulder pain	No significant change in pain incidence No significant change in pain intensity ES improved pain-free ROM

(Continued)

TABLE 10-3. **STUDIES OF CAM THERAPIES FOR MUSCULOSKELETAL PAIN—cont'd**

Study	Sample	Intervention	Design	Measurement	Major Findings
White et al.[249] (2000)	Chronic nonradiating neck pain 68 subjects (37 F, 31 M); ages 27-80	Acupuncture Local dermatomal stimulation (DS) Remote DS	Randomized Sham controlled Investigator blinded Crossover	VAS pain Short Form Health Survey (SF-36) Analgesic use	Local DS decreased pain scores vs. remote DS and acupuncture ($p < .01$) Local DS decreased analgesic use over remote DS and acupuncture ($p < .05$) All conditions provided improvement from baseline, but significantly greater with local DS ($p < .05$)
Ghoname et al.[85] (1999)	Low back pain 60 subjects (31 F, 29 M); median age 42 (1.9) Group 1: PENS Group 2: Sham PENS Group 3: TENS Group 4: Exercise	Percutaneous electrical nerve stimulation (PENS): 4 Hz width, 0.5 millisecond Sham PENS TENS Flexion/extension exercise	Randomized Single blind Sham controlled Crossover	SF-36 VAS pain Analgesic use Effectiveness scale	PENS, TENS, and sham PENS all showed improved SF-36 scores over baseline ($p = .007$, $p < .02$, $p < .02$) PENS and TENS decreased VAS pain scores ($p < .007$, $p < .03$) PENS decreased oral analgesic use by 50% ($p < .009$) 91% of patients preferred PENS
Hamza et al.[104] (1999)	Low back pain 75 subjects (41 F, 34 M); ages 21-76	PENS: 0, 15, 30, 45 minutes; alternating frequency of 15 and 30 Hz for 60 minutes 3 times weekly for 2 weeks, with 1 week off between 2 series	Randomized Sham controlled Crossover	SF-36 VAS Analgesic use	All PENS treatments improved SF-36 scores over baseline ($p < .01$, $p < .001$, $p < .001$) All PENS decreased pain scores over baseline ($p < .05$, $p < .01$, $p < .01$) All PENS improved degree of pain, physical activity, and sleep quality scores over baseline ($p < .05$, $p < .01$, $p < .01$).

Study	Condition/Subjects	Intervention	Design	Outcome Measures	Results
Rompe et al.[197] (2001)	Chronic lateral epicondylitis of elbow; 60 subjects; Group 1 (n = 30; 16 F, 14 M): shock waves plus cervical adjustment; ages 35-65; Group 2 (n = 30; 16 F, 14 M): previous shock waves; ages 37-68	Shock wave therapy: 1000 impulses of 0.16 mJ/mm² at lateral elbow plus manual adjustment of cervical spine; Monotherapy with shock waves in past 3 years	Prospective, Matched, Single blind, Controlled	Pain rating, VAS, Grip strength	All PENS decreased analgesic use ($p < .05$, $p < .01$, $p < .01$). No difference between groups
Werners et al.[248] (1999)	Low back pain; 152 subjects; Group 1 (n = 74; 57% M): *interferential*; median age 38.3 (9.4); Group 2 (n = 73; 51% M): *traction*; age 38.2 (9.5)	Interferential therapy: (electrotherapy at frequencies between 30 and 60 Hz); Standard motorized lumbar traction with simultaneous massage	RCT stratified by age, gender, work, and sick leave status	Oswestry Disability Index (ODI), VAS	No difference between groups

HERBAL THERAPY AND SUPPLEMENTS

Study	Condition/Subjects	Intervention	Design	Outcome Measures	Results
Chrubasik et al.,[40] 2001	Low back pain; 228 subjects; Group 1 (n = 114; 72 F, 42 M): *willow bark*; median age 63; Group 2 (n = 114; 74 F, 40 M): NSAID; age 59	Willow bark: 240 mg salicin for 4 weeks; Nonsteroidal antiinflammatory drug: Rofecoxib (COX-2 inhibitor), 12.5 mg for 4 weeks	Open randomized study	VAS, Modified Arhus index, Total Pain Index (TPI), Treatment success	No significant difference between groups; Willow bark about 40% less expensive than NSAID

HYPNOSIS, IMAGERY, AND SUGGESTION

Study	Condition/Subjects	Intervention	Design	Outcome Measures	Results
Malone et al.[150] (1988)	Chronic pain conditions, including back; 109 studies	Nonpharmacologic treatment	Meta-analysis	Effect size, Proportion of improved patients	Positive effect size suggests short-term efficacy of relaxation and behavioral techniques
Hasenbring et al.[107] (1999)	Acute sciatic pain; 59 subjects (24 F, 35 M); ages 25-78; 24 subjects dropped out or	Risk factor–based cognitive-behavioral therapy (CB) 1 hour/wk	RCT	Pain intensity, Physical dysfunction, Immobility in everyday life	BF group decreased pain over CB and control groups ($p < .05$)

(Continued)

TABLE 10-3. **STUDIES OF CAM THERAPIES FOR MUSCULOSKELETAL PAIN** —cont'd

Study	Sample	Intervention	Design	Measurement	Major Findings
	were excluded before baseline measurements Group 1 (n = 12): *cognitive behavioral* Group 2 (n = 11): *biofeedback* (BF) Group 3 (n = 12): usual care	Standardized electromyographic (EMG) BF: 20 minutes/wk for 12 weeks Control: usual medical care		Beck Depression Inventory (BDI) Analgesic use	CB treatment decreased pain over BF at discharge and 6-month follow-up (p <.05) Immobility decreased 85.7% in CB group and 30% in BF group Depression decreased in CB and BF groups over control group (p <.01 and p <.05)
MAGNET THERAPY Collacott et al.[43] (2000)	Chronic low back pain 20 subjects (1 F, 19 M); median age 60 (12); 2 groups	Magnet: 282-300 gauss at surface Demagnetized sham magnet: 6 h/d, 3d/w 1 week per treatment with 1-week washout	Randomized Double blind Placebo controlled Crossover	VAS Pain Rating Index (PRI) Range of motion (ROM)	No difference between groups
MANIPULATION Ernst, Harkness[61] (2001)	Chronic low back pain and other conditions 8 studies	*Spinal manipulation*	Systematic review	Difference between sham and active treatment	Most rigorous studies indicated that spinal manipulation is not associated with clinically relevant therapeutic effects
Koes et al.[131] (1996)	Chronic low back pain Acute low back pain 36 RCTs	*Spinal manipulation*	Systematic review	Pain intensity Patient report of improvement	53% of trials showed better results for manipulation group vs. reference treatment Five trials showed improvement in subgroups. Ten trials showed no difference Six studies demonstrated long-term effects

Study	Sample	Intervention	Design	Outcomes	Results
Shekelle et al.[211] (1992)	Chronic low back pain 5 controlled studies	Spinal manipulation	Meta-analysis	Pain Functional outcomes	Insufficient data to support or refute efficacy of spinal manipulation Study designs varied, and results from studies were contradictory
Anderson et al.[11] (1992)	Acute and chronic back pain 23 RCTs	Spinal manipulation	Meta-analysis	Pain Functional outcomes	Consistent trend for spinal manipulation to produce better results than other therapies Most studies assessed outcomes within first month of treatment; few assessed outcomes beyond 3 months
Abenhaim, Bergeron[2] (1992)	Acute and chronic back pain 21 RCTs	Spinal manipulation	Meta-analysis	Pain Functional outcomes	Some indication of short-term effectiveness in relieving acute and chronic back pain Long-term effect not adequately evaluated
Bronfort et al.[27] (2001)	Chronic neck pain 191 subjects Group 1 ($n = 64$; 59.4% F): *manipulation* plus exercise; median age 45 (10.5) Group 2 ($n = 63$; 60.3% F): *exercise*; age 43.6 (10.5) Group 3 ($n = 64$; 57.8% F): *manipulation*; age 44.3 (11.0)	1. Manipulation: 15 minutes, short lever, low amplitude, high velocity *plus* 45 minutes strengthening exercise, aerobics, and light stretching 2. Exercise: 15-20 minutes, aerobics and progressive resistance 3. Manipulation: 15 minutes *plus* 45-minute sham microcurrent	Randomized Parallel group Single blind	Pain scale Neck Disability Index (NDI) SF-36 Satisfaction with care Neck performance	Satisfaction with care increased with manipulation plus exercise over manipulation alone ($p < .05$) Manipulation plus exercise and exercise alone increased strength, endurance, and range of motion over manipulation alone ($p < .05$) Long-term follow-up showed manipulation plus exercise and exercise alone decreased pain over manipulation alone ($p = .04$).

(Continued)

TABLE 10-3. **STUDIES OF CAM THERAPIES FOR MUSCULOSKELETAL PAIN—cont'd**

Study	Sample	Intervention	Design	Measurement	Major Findings
Schiller[207] (2001)	Thoracic spine syndromes 30 subjects Group 1 (n = 15; 8 F, 7 M): manipulation; ages 16-55 Group 2 (n = 15; 8 F, 7 M): placebo; ages 16-55	Spinal manipulation Nonfunctional ultrasound	RCT Single blind Comparative	Range of motion (ROM) Oswestry Disability Index (ODI) McGill Pain Questionnaire (MPQ) Numerical Pain Rating Scale (NPR)	Manipulation decreased pain score (p <.025) Manipulation increased flexibility (p <.025)
Wood et al.[252] (2001)	Cervical spine dysfunction 30 subjects Group 1 (n = 15; 10 F, 5 M): mechanical manipulation; ages 20-59 Group 2 (n = 15; 9 F, 6 M): manipulation; ages 20-59	Activator-assisted mechanical manipulation Standard manipulation	RCT	NPR MPQ Neck Disability Index (NDI) ROM	Both groups had significantly decreased pain No difference was noted between groups
Jordon et al.[121] (1998)	Chronic neck pain 119 subjects (88 F, 31 M) Group 1 (n = 40; 30 F, 10 M): training; ages 23-50 Group 2 (n = 39; 29 F, 10 M): physiotherapy; ages 20-58 Group 3 (n = 40; 29 F, 11 M): chiropractic; ages 28-53	1. Aerobics, stretching, isometrics 2. Hot packs, massage, ultrasound, traction, exercise 3. High-velocity, low-amplitude adjustment, and trigger point work	RCT	Self report disability scale Physician's global assessment ROM	All groups had decreased pain All groups had increased endurance No difference was noted among groups
Burton et al.[34] (2000)	Symptomatic lumbar disk herniation 40 subjects (21 F, 19 M); median age 41.9 (10.6) Group 1 (n = 20): manipulation Group 2 (n = 20): chemonucleolysis	Manipulation: stretching, low amplitude, high velocity Chemonucleolysis: single injection of chymopapain under general anesthesia	RCT Single blind	Pain VAS Roland Disability Questionnaire (RDQ) Distress and risk assessment	Decreased pain in both groups No difference between groups

Study	Condition/Subjects/Groups	Intervention	Design	Outcome Measures	Results
Andersson et al.[13] (1999)	Low back pain 178 subjects Group 1 (n=83; 49 F, 34 M): *osteopathic care*; age 28.5 (10.6) Group 2 (n=72; 40 F, 32 M): *allopathic care*; age 37.0 (11.0)	Osteopathic manual therapy Standard medical therapy	RCT	VAS RDQ ODI ROM Medication use	Osteopathic group used less medication (p <.001) than allopathic group Osteopathic group used less physical therapy (p <.05) than allopathic group
Cherkin et al.[36] (1998)	Low back pain 321 subjects Group 1 (n=66; 42% F): booklet; age 40.1 (11.2) Group 2 (n=122; 53% F): *chiropractic*; age 39.7 (9.4) Group 3 (=133; 48% F): *physiotherapy*; age 40.7 (10.7)	1. Educational booklet 2. Exercise, book, and lumbar support 3. Short-lever, high-velocity thrust	RCT without stratification Multisite	VAS RDQ National Health Interview Survey (NHIS) Care rating	Bothersome nature of low back pain differed at baseline, 4 weeks, and 12 weeks (p <.04) Physiotherapy group decreased symptoms at 4 weeks vs. booklet group (p <.02)
Kivimaki, Pohjolainen[128] (2001)	Frozen shoulder 24 subjects (12 F, 12 M) Group 1 (n=13): *steroid plus manipulation* Group 2 (n=11): *anesthesia plus manipulation*	Steroid: betamethasone, 1 ml, *plus manipulation* Anesthetic: lidocaine, 4 ml, *plus manipulation*	RCT	ROM Pain medication	Both groups improved No difference was found between groups
Bronfort et al.[26] (2000)	Sciatica 20 subjects Group 1 (n=6; 3 F, 3 M): *medical*; age 48.5 (9.8) Group 2 (n=7; 3 F, 4 M): *chiropractic*; age 46.2 (10.1) Group 3 (n=7; 2 F, 5 M): *steroid*; age 39.4 (11.3)	1. Medication 2. Spinal manipulation, massage, traction 3. Epidural steroid injection	Randomized Three-group parallel Single blind	Modified Roland Scale Pain rating Improvement rating Bothersomeness Frequency Satisfaction Medication use ROM	All groups improved No difference was found among groups

(Continued)

TABLE 10-3. STUDIES OF CAM THERAPIES FOR MUSCULOSKELETAL PAIN—cont'd

Study	Sample	Intervention	Design	Measurement	Major Findings
MASSAGE					
Furlan et al.[80] (2002)	Low back pain 4 studies	Massage Manipulation TENS Corsets	Meta-analysis	Change in low back pain	Limited evidence that massage less effective than manipulation Moderate evidence that massage less effective than TENS
Preyde[187] (2000)	Low back pain 98 subjects Group 1 (n = 25; 56% F): comprehensive *massage;* median age 47.9 (16.2) Group 2 (n = 25; 56% F): soft tissue *manipulation;* age 46.5 (18.4) Group 3 (n = 22; 41% F): exercise; age 48.4 (12.9) Group 4 (n = 26; 54% F): placebo; age 41.9 (16.6)	1. Soft tissue manipulation, remedial exercise, posture education 2. Soft tissue manipulation only 3. Exercise only 4. Sham laser treatment	RCT	Roland Disability Questionnaire (RDQ) McGill Pain Questionnaire (MPQ) State Anxiety Index (SAI) ROM	Comprehensive massage decreased RDQ score (p <.006) vs. all other groups Comprehensive massage decreased MPQ score (p <.006) Comprehensive massage decreased SAI score (p <.006)
THERAPEUTIC TOUCH					
Blankenfield et al.[19] (2001)	Carpal tunnel syndrome 21 subjects Group 1 (n = 11; 5 F, 6 M): *therapeutic touch* (TT) first; age 57.4 (14.9) Group 2 (n = 10; 5 F, 5 M): sham TT first; median age 55.2 (13.1)	Therapy: energy exchange to facilitate healing Sham: mimicked TT motion while counting backward	RCT Single blind Partial crossover	Electroneurometer Pain scores	No difference between groups
Lin et al.[145] (1998)	Chronic musculoskeletal pain and anxiety 90 subjects Group 1 (n = 31; 27 F, 4 M): *TT;* age 77.8 (8.21)	TT: 20-minute energy exchange to facilitate healing MT: 20-minute mimicked TT motion	RCT Multisite	Pain NRS STAI Salivary cortisol	Pain significantly decreased in TT group (p <.001; effect size 0.92) vs. MT and UC groups

Study	Sample	Treatment	Design	Outcomes measured	Results
	Group 2 (n = 29; 22 F, 7 M); mimic touch (MT); age 75.65 (9.68) Group 3 (n = 30; 17 F, 3 M): usual care (UC); median age 80 (7.77)	UC: standard care			Anxiety significantly decreased in TT group (p <.01; effect size 0.35). Salivary cortisol showed no change
YOGA Garfinkel et al.[83] (1998)	Carpal tunnel syndrome (CTS) 42 subjects (28 F, 13 M) Group 1 (n = 22): yoga; mean age 48.9 (range 17-68) Group 2 (n = 20): control; mean age 48.7 (range 18-70)	Yoga: 8 weekly sessions (60-90 minutes/session) of instruction in structural alignment, upper body postures, and stretching to improve flexibility (Iyengar approach to hatha yoga); all sessions ended with relaxation technique Control: wrist splint to supplement treatment	RCT Repeated measures Data collector blinded	Pain intensity VAS Grip strength Change in Phalen sign (measure of CTS) Hours of disturbed sleep/night Median nerve sensory conduction Median nerve motor conduction	Yoga group had significantly decreased pain (p = .02) vs. control group Yoga group had significantly increased Phalen sign (p = 0.008) vs. control group Yoga group had significantly increased grip strength (p = .009) vs. control group No significant differences were found between groups on nerve conduction tests and other outcomes

have reported positive results for chronic neck pain,[27,121] low back pain,[13] and thoracic spine syndrome,[207] often with prolonged pain relief. However, other studies on spinal manipulation showed no direct benefit of manipulation over medication.[26] Spinal manipulation can be beneficial for some patients, and reasons for patient failure with this modality need to be explored.

Two recent studies reported positive effects of massage on low back pain and related symptoms,[37,187] although a systematic review of four other studies concluded that massage was less effective than other conservative therapies for low back pain.[80] Finally, two studies reviewed on carpal tunnel syndrome reported contrasting outcomes. One study found that real therapeutic touch was not significantly better than sham therapeutic touch,[19] whereas another study found yoga to improve pain reports as well as other subjective and objective measures of carpal tunnel syndrome.[83] However, in an elderly population experiencing chronic musculoskeletal pain, researchers found that real therapeutic touch significantly reduced the report of pain and anxiety compared with sham therapeutic touch and a usual-care group.[145] This study suggests that therapeutic touch can be a beneficial therapy when administered for a sufficient length of time and duration.

Research on electrical stimulation also reported mixed results; however, the studies with more rigorous methodology had the most favorable outcomes.[85,104,250] Few studies have tested the effects of other CAM modalities such as herbal and magnetic products. In one study on low back pain, willow bark was found to be as effective as the antiinflammatory drug rofecoxib, a COX-2 inhibitor.[40]

◼ Rheumatoid Arthritis

Surveys indicate that 28% to 67% of persons diagnosed with rheumatoid arthritis (RA) report use of CAM therapies.[122,190] These therapies include acupuncture, herbs and other natural products, vibration, relaxation, hypnosis, and imagery (Table 10-4).

The frequent use of herbal products by those suffering pain and related symptoms of RA has led researchers to give emphasis to research testing the efficacy of these products. Patients with RA who were given *gamma-linoleic acid* (GLA) (found in borage seed oil, black currant oil, and evening primrose oil) for its antiinflammatory properties reported moderately decreased pain and joint tenderness and swelling, and reduced disease activity compared with placebo.[144,256] A review of 7 RCTs of GLA reported improvements in some measures, but due to the variation in methodology and quality of the studies, the authors were unable to make recommendations regarding the use of GLA.[146] RCTs provide some evidence of the beneficial effects of fish oil in RA. Specifically, these studies have found decreased pain ratings, tender joint counts, and morning stiffness,[240] although negative findings have also been reported.[75,119]

A placebo-controlled study evaluating the effects of vitamin E (an antioxidant) suggested that it may reduce pain ratings in patients with RA.[55] In another RCT, patients who consumed a diet high in monounsaturated and polyunsaturated fatty acids and low in saturated fatty acids were found to have a reduced number of swollen

Text continued on p. 363.

TABLE 10–4. STUDIES OF CAM THERAPIES FOR RHEUMATOID ARTHRITIS

Study	Sample	Intervention	Design	Measurement	Major Findings
ACUPUNCTURE					
David et al.[49] (1999)	Rheumatoid arthritis (RA) 56 patients; ages 46-66 Group 1 (n = 29): acupuncture first Group 2 (n = 27): placebo first	Acupuncture: single point Placebo: sham acupuncture	Randomized controlled trial (RCT) with crossover Randomized order of interventions	Erythrocyte sedimentation rate (ESR) C-reactive protein (CRP) Visual analog scale (VAS) Swollen joints (n) Analgesics (n) General Health Questionnaire Disease Activity Score	No differences between groups Adverse effects: none
HERBAL THERAPY AND SUPPLEMENTS					
Andjelkovic et al.[14] (1999)	RA 19 patients (12 F, 7 M); ages 23-72 (mean 55)	Activated form of vitamin D	Open-label trial	Ritchie Articular Index (RAI) Pain ESR CRP Rheumatoid factor (RF)	89% had positive effect (45% remission, 44% satisfactory effect) Decreased number of painful swollen joints Decreased RAI Decreased ESR and CRP
Chopra et al.[39] (2000)	RA 182 patients (F/M=5:1); mean age 45 Group 1 (n = 89): ayurvedic plant Group 2 (n = 93): placebo	Ayurvedic plant–derived formula RA-1	RCT Double blind	ESR Interleukin-6 (IL-6) CRP RF Joint count: pain and tenderness Joint swelling Grip strength Walking time Physician and patient global assessments Morning stiffness	Large placebo response Active group showed improvement in the primary measures, but not significantly different from placebo Increased proportion with 50% reduction in swollen joint count in active group

(Continued)

TABLE 10-4. **STUDIES OF CAM THERAPIES FOR RHEUMATOID ARTHRITIS—cont'd**

Study	Sample	Intervention	Design	Measurement	Major Findings
Edmonds et al.[55] (1997)	RA 42 patients Group 1 (n = 20; 16 F, 4 M): *vitamin E*; mean age 55.4 (15.1) (range 24-75) Group 2 (n = 22; 15 F, 7 M): placebo; mean age 52.0 (10.3) (range 32-66)	Vitamin E: 1200 mg daily	Multicenter RCT Double blind Placebo controlled	Pain VAS Modified Health Assessment Questionnaire (MHAQ) RAI Morning stiffness Pain VAS ESR CRP RF Complete blood count (CBC) Lipids	Pain decreased in vitamin E group Patient global assessment of efficacy was 60% in vitamin E group vs. 31.8% for placebo No significant differences in RAI, morning stiffness, or number of swollen joints After removal of vitamin E for 8 weeks, groups again showed no differences
Leventhal et al.[144] (1993)	RA 37 patients Group 1 (n = 19): GLA Group 2 (n = 18): placebo	GLA: gamma-linolenic acid	RCT Double blind Placebo controlled	Pain VAS Physician and patient global assessment of disease activity Tender/painful joints Swollen joints (n) Morning stiffness Grip strength ESR, RF, CBC	GLA group had the following: • Decreased pain • Decreased tender or painful joint counts • Decreased swollen joint counts • Decreased physician-rated disease activity • Moderate overall improvement Placebo group did not improve on any measure
Little, Parsons[146] (2001)	RA 11 studies	Herbs and supplements (GLA: gamma-linolenic acid)	Systematic review (NSAID: nonsteroidal anti-inflammatory drug)	Pain Mobility Grip strength NSAID use Lipids	GLA: 7 studies found some improvement, but methodology and quality varied, difficult to draw conclusions

Study	Population/Groups and Intervention	Design	Outcomes measured	Results
			Fatty acids Quality of life	Possible pain decrease, decrease in morning stiffness, and decrease in joint tenderness
Sarzi-Puttini et al.[203] (2000)	RA 50 patients Group 1 (n = 25; 19 F, 6 M; 22 finished): *diet therapy*; mean age 49.6 Group 2 (n = 25; 20 F, 5 M; 21 finished): *control*; mean age 50.3 Diet therapy: high in mono/polyunsaturated fatty acids and low in saturated fatty acids with restriction of certain dietary items Control: typical well-balanced diet	RCT Double blind	Pain VAS RAI Tender swollen joints Morning stiffness Physician and patient global assessments Health Assessment Questionnaire (HAQ) Body Mass Index (BMI) CBC, RF CRP, ESR High-density lipoprotein (HDL) Paulus index for global response to treatment	Diet therapy group had the following: • Decreased RAI • Decreased tender and swollen joint counts • Trend toward decreased pain • Decreased ESR When adjusted for BMI and baseline values, only number of tender joints and ESR remained significantly decreased
Volker et al.[240] (2000)	RA 26 patients Group 1 (n = 13): *fish oil*; age 54 (4) Group 2 (n = 13): *placebo*; age 60 (3) Fish oil: (60% omega-3 fatty acids) 40 mg/kg of body weight given daily over 15 weeks Placebo: [50% corn oil, 50% olive oil)	RCT Double blind	Tender and swollen joint count Morning stiffness Pain VAS Global assessment of arthritis activity HAQ Lipid analysis	Fish oil group had significant within-group differences in pain, HAQ, and morning stiffness from baseline to 15 weeks Fish oil group had significant decreases in morning stiffness and HAQ vs. placebo No signs of improvement were seen at 4-week and 8-week follow-up in either group
Zurier et al.[256] (1996)	RA 56 patients Group 1 (n = 28; 26 F, 2 M; 22 finished): *GLA*; mean age 57.4 (9.98) GLA: gamma-linolenic acid Placebo: sunflower seed oil	RCT Double blind Placebo controlled	Pain VAS Tender or painful joint count Swollen joint count HAQ Grip strength	Within-group differences from baseline to 6 months for the GLA group involved decreases in (1) tender and swollen joint counts,

(Continued)

TABLE 10-4. STUDIES OF CAM THERAPIES FOR RHEUMATOID ARTHRITIS—cont'd

Study	Sample	Intervention	Design	Measurement	Major Findings
	Group 2 (n = 28; 23 F, 5 M; 19 finished); placebo; mean age 54.6 (13.58)			Global assessment of disease activity Morning stiffness ESR, RF, CBC Fatty acid analysis	(2) morning stiffness, (3) pain, (4) HAQ score, and (5) global assessment of disease activity GLA group had decreased pain, decreased joint counts, and decreased HAQ vs. placebo GLA group was 6.5 times more likely to experience meaningful improvement than placebo group When GLA discontinued for 3 months, GLA group experienced exacerbation of disease and symptoms
HOMEOPATHY Fisher, Scott[71] (2001)	RA 58 patients (46 F, 12 M); mean age 54	180 active homeopathic remedies vs. 180 placebo remedies Disease-modifying antirheumatic drugs (DMARDs)	RCT with crossover Convenience sampling Stratified by NSAIDs and DMARDs	Pain VAS RAI Morning stiffness ESR	Active treatment did not improve RA symptoms Pain was lower at 6 months in placebo group than active group RAI, ESR, and morning stiffness were similar for active and placebo arms Overall, the 58 subjects (combined active and placebo groups) at 6 months had pain decreased by 18%, ESR decreased by 11%, and morning stiffness increased by 43%

HYDROTHERAPY

Verhagen et al.[236] (2000)	RA and osteoarthritis (OA) 10 studies	Balneotherapy: hydrotherapy or spa therapy	Systematic review World Health Organization/ International League Against Rheumatism (WHO/ILAR)	WHO/ILAR core set of end points; at least one had to be among the main outcome measures Pain measures Patient and physician global assessments Physical disability Swollen/tender joints Acute-phase reactants Radiographs of joints	Positive findings reported in most studies, but methodology flawed Overall, poor methodologic quality of studies Only 3 studies had between-group analyses Data were scarce in papers No answer on effectiveness can be given
Welch et al.[247] (2001)	RA 4 studies	Thermotherapy: heat and cold applied superficially	Systematic review Tender joints (n) Swollen joints (n) Physician and patient global assessments Functional status CRP Radiologic damage	Ice: not significant on inflammation Heat: not significant on joint tenderness, stiffness, or destruction Subjects liked heat therapy, but only 41% thought long-lasting benefit and 47% that heat decreased morning stiffness Ice/heat massage: not significant in pain threshold No significant differences in pain, stiffness, or preference between ice or heat therapy

HYPNOSIS, IMAGERY, AND SUGGESTION

Horton-Hausknecht et al.[113] (2000)	RA 66 patients Group 1 (n = 26): *hypnosis* Group 2 (n = 20): relaxation Group 3 (n = 20): control	1. Hypnosis and imagery group: imagery specific to reducing immune reactivity and symptom severity 2. Relaxation group	Quasi-experimental design Pain VAS Joint pain and swelling Morning stiffness Arthritis Impact Measurement Scale (AIMS) ESR, CRP	Hypnosis/imagery group had the following: • Decreased pain • Decreased joint swelling • Decreased stiffness • Decreased ESR

(Continued)

TABLE 10–4. **STUDIES OF CAM THERAPIES FOR RHEUMATOID ARTHRITIS—cont'd**

Study	Sample	Intervention	Design	Measurement	Major Findings
		3. Wait-list control group		Leukocyte number Beck Depression Inventory (BDI) Daily Hassles Questionnaire (DHQ) Tellegen Absorption Scale (TAS) Health locus of control (HLOC) Number of practices	• Moderate effect sizes in improvement of pain, joint swelling, and stiffness Dose effect of imagery practices: those who practiced more had greater clinical improvements Wait-list control group had increased leukocyte count
Sharpe et al.[210] (2001)	RA 45 patients Group 1 (n = 23; 16 F, 7 M): *cognitive-behavioral training* (CBT); mean age 54.1 (14.3) Group 2 (n = 22; 16 F, 6 M): control; mean age 56.9 (12.8)	CBT: with relaxation, pain management, and self-help strategies Control: standard care	RCT	Pain (10-point scale) Pain index (pain intensity × duration) HAQ RAI ESR, CRP Hospital Anxiety and Depression Scales (HADS) Coping Strategy Questionnaire (CSQ)	CBT group had decreased depression after therapy and at 6 months vs. control group CBT group had decreased CRP after therapy but not at 6 months vs. control group RAI: CBT group had greater improvement in joint tenderness and pain vs. control group Decreased pain in both groups over study No significant differences in ESR and HAQ
RELAXATION Leibing et al.[143] (1999)	RA 39 patients Group 1 (n = 19; 13 F, 6 M): *cognitive-behavioral therapy* (CBT); mean	CBT: with relaxation, imagery, and pain management strategies	RCT	Pain VAS MPQ Pain diary Hannover Functional Ability Questionnaire (HFAQ)	Within-group analyses: CBT group had the following: • Increased CRP • Decreased depression

			Measures	Results
	age 55.3 (10.9) Group 2 (n = 20; 16 F, 4 M): control; mean age 48.5 (11.6)		ESR, CRP Grip strength Swollen joints (n) Medication use State-Trait Anxiety Inventory (STAI) Depression scale Arthritis Helplessness Index (AHI) Bernese Coping Modes	• Decreased AHI • Decreased affective pain ratings Between-group analyses: CBT group had the following: • Decreased depression • Decreased anxiety • Decreased AHI • Decreased affective pain ratings
Lundgren, Stenstrom[149] (1999)	RA 68 patients; ages 28-70; mean 57 Group 1 (n = 37; 30 F, 7 M): relaxation training (RT) Group 2 (n = 31; 22 F, 9 M): control	RCT RTG: relaxation training group Control group	Arthritis impact measurement scales (AIMS) Nottingham Health Profile (NHP) Sickness Impact Profile-RA (SIP-RA) Arthritis Self-Efficacy Scale (ASES) Index of muscle function (IMF) Pain VAS ESR	From baseline to after treatment, within-group analyses: RTG group had the following: • Increase in some quality of life indicators (self-care, recreation, pastime abilities) • No differences in pain or disease activity Between groups, RTG had the following: • Increased muscle endurance and arm function • No differences in pain or disease activity • No differences at 12-month follow-up

(Continued)

TABLE 10-4. STUDIES OF CAM THERAPIES FOR RHEUMATOID ARTHRITIS—cont'd

Study	Sample	Intervention	Design	Measurement	Major Findings
SPIRITUAL HEALING					
Le Gallez et al.[140] (2000)	RA 29 patients; ages 40-74; mean 50 Group 1 (no M): physician and *spiritual healer* Group 2 (only 2 M): physician only	MD and spiritual healer MD only	Assessed by blind observer	Personality Grip strength RAI Summated change score Pain score (1-5) Morning stiffness HAQ ESR, CRP, CBC	No changes in either group comparing baseline to 24 weeks Healer group had improvement in change score at 16 weeks, but not maintained at 24 weeks vs. MD-only group
VIBRATION THERAPY					
Nader et al.[171] (2001)	RA 176 patients; *n* for RA = 4	1. Maharishi Vedic vibration technology (sound and conscious mind) 2. Sham vibration control	RCT Double blind	Rated change in pain from 0% to 100% relief of pain	Pain decreased in vibration group vs. control group Effect size = 1.79, even though sample size was very small

and painful joints and decreased erythrocyte sedimentation rate (ESR), although there was only a trend toward decreased pain ratings.[203]

Several modalities used by with persons diagnosed with RA have limited support in the literature. Studies on acupuncture have yielded mixed results.[49,64] Relaxation as a single modality has not led to reduced pain ratings, although more favorable outcomes have been reported when relaxation is combined with imagery and hypnosis.[113,143,149] Additional RCTs are needed to provide evidence of the effectiveness of CAM modalities in the treatment of pain and related symptoms of RA.

◤ Headache

Headache is one of the most common pain problems among individuals of all ages, and effective treatment remains a challenge for health care professionals.[177] Although headaches are often treated pharmacologically, many persons also use various forms of physical and behavioral treatments.[28,57,189] CAM modalities used by those with migraine and tension headaches include acupuncture, herbs and natural products, homeopathy, biofeedback, relaxation and imagery, and manipulation (Table 10-5).

A large body of research has investigated the effectiveness of relaxation, imagery, biofeedback, and cognitive-behavioral therapy (CBT) in the treatment of migraine and tension headaches. A 1995 National Institutes of Health (NIH) technology assessment panel concluded that a number of behavioral and relaxation interventions may be useful adjunctive modalities for the management of headache pain in adults.[174] Based on study designs and consistency of findings, moderate evidence supported the conclusion that biofeedback was more effective than relaxation and no treatment in relieving migraine headache. However, the evidence was less clear when biofeedback was compared with psychologic placebo. Several meta-analyses supported the effectiveness of electromyographic (EMG) biofeedback, hypnosis, relaxation and imagery, and CBT for the reduction of headache activity.[21,111,112,115] More recently, one large-scale clinical trial found that the addition of imagery to individualized headache therapy significantly decreased headache activity.[153] Finally, treatment combining thermal biofeedback with progressive muscle relaxation and breathing exercises was significantly more effective than physical therapy in relieving migraine headache pain.[155]

Herbal and other natural therapies have yielded mixed results in the treatment of chronic headaches. One RCT found high-dose riboflavin (vitamin B_2) significantly more effective than placebo in reducing headache frequency.[209] A meta-analysis of four studies testing the effects of the herb feverfew (*Tanacetum parthenium*) in the prevention of migraine headaches was inconclusive. Although the results of three studies suggested beneficial effects, the largest and highest quality study found no significant effect compared with placebo.[185] Likewise, a multicenter RCT on the use of magnesium demonstrated no significant differences in headache activity compared with placebo.[183]

Most studies investigating the effects of acupuncture on migraine and tension headaches demonstrated beneficial outcomes, with decreased headache duration and

Text continued on p. 372.

TABLE 10–5. STUDIES OF CAM THERAPIES FOR HEADACHE

Study	Sample	Intervention	Design	Measurement	Major Findings
ACUPUNCTURE					
Karst et al.[124] (2000)	Tension headache 39 subjects Group 1 (n = 21; 11 F, 7 M): acupuncture; mean age 50.4 (13.5) Group 2 (n = 18; 8 F, 13 M): placebo; mean age 47.3 (16.5)	Treatment group: acupuncture Control group: placebo	Randomized controlled trial (RCT) Double blind	Visual analog scale (VAS) Pressure pain thresholds (PPTs) Clinical global improvement Nottingham Health Profile Everyday-Life-Questionnaire Freiburg Questionnaire	PPTs increased after acupuncture VAS scores decreased in both groups
Melchart et al.[160] (2001)	Headache (HA) 26 studies	Acupuncture (Acu) Sham acupuncture	Systematic review	Studies had to measure at least one clinical outcome related to HA: • HA frequency • HA intensity • Global assessment of HA	Majority of trials had methodologic or reporting shortcomings In 8 studies (migraine, tension HA), Acu was significantly superior to sham In 4 studies, trend was in favor of Acu Two studies showed no intergroup difference Ten studies yielded contradictory results when Acu was compared to other treatments Two studies were uninterpretable
Gao et al.[213] (1999)	Migraine headache 64 subjects (46 F, 18 M); ages 15-58 Group 1 (n = 32): acupuncture Group 2 (n = 32): drug treatment	Acupuncture prescriptions combined distant and local acupoints (selected by differential diagnosis) Drug treatment: ergot plus caffeine in acute phase, with Zhentianwan (Chinese herb) during remission	RCT	Headache status after 1 year: • Cured: no symptoms or recurrence • Improved: symptoms disappeared completely but recurred in 1 year • No effect: recurrence of symptoms	Acupuncture group: 75.0% cured; 18.8% improved; 6.2% no effect Drug treatment group: 34.4% cured; 28.1% improved; 37.5% no effect

Study	Condition/Subjects	Design	Intervention	Outcome Measures	Results
Vincent et al.[239] (1989)	Migraine headache 32 subjects Group 1: *acupuncture* Group 2: Control	RCT	Treatment group: true acupuncture Control group: placebo acupuncture	Headache diary Medication use	Overall effectiveness rates differed significantly, as follows: • Acupuncture: 93.8% • Drug treatment: 62.5% True acupuncture significantly more effective in relieving pain than sham acupuncture 43% decrease in pain scores in true acupuncture group 38% decrease in medication use in true acupuncture group Results maintained at 4-month and 1-year follow up
White et al.[249] (2000)	Tension headache 50 subjects Group 1 (n = 25; 18 F, 7 M; 15 completed): *acupuncture*; mean age 49.8 (2.9) Group 2 (n = 25; 20 F, 5 M; 19 completed): control; mean age 48.2 (2.9)	RCT Multisite	Treatment group: true acupuncture Control group: sham acupuncture	Daily HA diary: number, duration, severity of HAs; number of analgesics HA intensity VAS General Health Questionnaire (GHQ) Global assessment of change	No difference between acupuncture and sham groups on any outcome variable Both groups reported significant decrease in symptoms
BIOFEEDBACK					
Rokicki et al.[196] (1997)	Tension headache 43 subjects Group 1 (n = 29; 25 F, 4 M): *biofeedback*; mean age 19 Group 2 (n = 14; 12 F, 2 M: control; mean age 18.6	RCT	Electromyographic (EMG) biofeedback with progressive muscle relaxation	Masseter EMG recorded while electrically stimulating EMG activity: frontalis, trapezius (right, left) Daily HA diary: HA pain 4 times/day Headache activity score Number of HA-free days/week	Biofeedback group had the following: • Decreased EMG activity in all muscles tested across study • Improvement in HA activity • Increased number of HA-free days • Trend toward decreased analgesic use

(Continued)

TABLE 10–5. **STUDIES OF CAM THERAPIES FOR HEADACHE—cont'd**

Study	Sample	Intervention	Design	Measurement	Major Findings
ELECTRICAL STIMULATION					
Solomon et al.[215] (1989)	Headache 100 subjects; ages 20-70 (mean 41.5) Group 1 (n = 50): electrotherapy Group 2 (n = 50): placebo	Active transcranial electrotherapy stimulator with high-frequency, extremely low-level current Placebo: electrotherapy stimulator	RCT Multicenter Double blind	Medication intake HA locus of control scale (HSLC) HA self-efficacy scale (HSES)	• Decrease in external locus of control scores • increase in HSES across study Biofeedback group: 51.7% had at least 50% reduction in headache activity vs. 15% in control group
			RCT Multicenter Double blind	HA severity Patient and physician global assessments	36% of active group rated unit as highly or moderately effective vs. 16% of placebo group Active group had 35% decrease in pain vs. 18% decrease in placebo group
HERBAL THERAPY AND SUPPLEMENTS					
Pfaffenrath et al.[183] (1996)	Migraine headache 69 subjects (64 F, 5 M); ages 18-64 Group 1 (n = 35): magnesium Group 2 (n = 34): control	Treatment: magnesium, aspartate hydrochloride trihydrate Control: placebo	RCT Multinational Multicenter Double blind Placebo controlled	Headache diary: intensity, duration, symptoms, triggers, medications Patient and physician global assessments Complete blood count Aspartate transaminase (AST, SGOT) Alanine transaminase (ALT, SGPT) Bilirubin Magnesium Ca, Na, K, and Cr	Number of responders (at least 50% reduction in HA intensity or duration) was 10 in each group No benefit with magnesium vs. placebo 33% of magnesium group rated magnesium superior to previously used medications vs. 11% of placebo group 45.7% of magnesium group reported primarily mild

Study	Subjects	Intervention	Design	Outcomes measured	Results
Pitler et al.[185] (2001)	4 trials 194 subjects	Feverfew vs. placebo	Systematic review	Trial measured clinical outcomes related to headache (HA): • HA frequency • Nausea/vomiting • Lost work days	adverse events (e.g., soft stool, diarrhea) 23.5% in placebo group had mild adverse events Trial was discontinued. Three trials suggested beneficial effects of feverfew compared with placebo. Trial with highest methodologic quality found no significant difference between feverfew and placebo. Overall, results favored feverfew, but efficacy not established beyond reasonable doubt
Schoenen et al.[209] (1998)	Migraine headache 55 subjects (43 F, 12 M); ages 18-62 Group 1 (n = 28): *riboflavin* Group 2 (n = 27): *placebo*	Treatment group: riboflavin, 400 mg daily for 3 months Control group: placebo	RCT Double blind	HA diary HA severity Presence of nausea or vomiting HA medications used HA duration in hours	Riboflavin group had the following: • Decreased HA frequency, severity, and duration • Decreased number of days with migraine • Higher 50% responder rate Effect of riboflavin begins after 1 month and is maximal after 3 months
HOMEOPATHY Walach et al.[241] (2000)	Migraine, tension, and cluster headaches 87 subjects 94 in original study (54: previous homeopathy) Half carried on with homeopathic treatment	1-year follow-up after homeopathic intervention	Follow-up study to double-blind, placebo-controlled RCT	6-week HA diary with frequency, duration, and intensity of HA Follow-up questionnaire	During original RCT, both homeopathic and placebo groups had reduction in HAs, with no indication that homeopathic treatment was better

(Continued)

TABLE 10–5. **STUDIES OF CAM THERAPIES FOR HEADACHE—cont'd**

Study	Sample	Intervention	Design	Measurement	Major Findings
					At 1-year follow-up, both groups had slight further reduction in Has, but again, no group differences
HYPNOSIS, IMAGERY, AND SUGGESTION					
Mannix et al.[153] (1999)	Tension headache 260 subjects; mean age 40.5 Group 1 (n = 129; 84.5% F): *imagery* Group 2 (n = 131; 74.1% F): control	Guided imagery with individualized headache therapy Control with individualized headache therapy but no guided imagery	RCT	Headache diary, with HA frequency, severity Patient global assessment HA disability inventory Short Form Medical Outcomes Study (SF-36)	Guided imagery and control groups both improved in HA frequency, HA severity, and disability caused by HA 21.7% of imagery group reported HAs were much better vs. only 7.6% of control group Imagery group had significantly more improvement in some SF-36 domains (pain, vitality, mental health)
MANIPULATION					
Bove, Nilsson[24] (1998)	Tension headache 75 subjects (49 F, 26 M); ages 20-59 Group 1 (n = 38): *manipulation* Group 2 (n = 37): placebo	Spinal manipulation and deep friction massage Placebo with deep friction massage and low-power laser light	RCT	Daily hours of HA Pain intensity per episode Daily analgesic use recorded in diaries	No significant differences between groups Both groups had significant decrease in mean daily HA hours and mean number of analgesics used per day HA pain intensity was unchanged in either group
Launso et al.[139] (1999)	Migraine and tension headaches 220 subjects (81% F): ages 25-54	Reflexology	Quasi-experimental	HA diary Medication use Patient evaluation	78% reported they were cured or had relief at completion of study

Source	Population/Intervention	Design	Outcome Measures	Results
Marcus et al.[155] (1998)	Migraine headache *Study 1* 88 women; ages 20-58; mean 37 (10.9) Group 1 (n = 30): physical therapy Group 2 (n = 39): relaxation with biofeedback *Study 2* Study 1 subjects without significant decrease in HA score Group 1 (n = 11): physical therapy (previous relaxation with biofeedback) Group 2 (n = 19): relaxation with biofeedback (previous therapy)	RCT *Study 1* Physical therapy (PT) Relaxation with thermal biofeedback (RTB) *Study 2* RTB if failed PT PT if failed RTB	Qualitative patient interviews 3 months after treatment Multidimensional Pain Inventory (MPI) Center for Epidemiological Studies–Depression (CESD) Daily HA diaries HA index (HI)	At 3-month follow-up, 81% were helped (16% reported as cured and 65% had relief) 19% of those who had formerly taken drugs to control HA were able to stop medication *Study 1* 13% of PT group had at least a 50% decrease in HI score 51% of RTB group had at least a 50% decrease in HI score RTB group had greater clinical improvement with decreased MPI and CESD vs. PT group *Study 2* Both groups improved with treatment: 47% of PT group, 50% of RTB group Overall, PT alone did not help migraine, but if failed RTB initially, adding PT was helpful
Nelson et al.[176] (1998)	Migraine headache 218 subjects Group 1 (n = 77; 79.2% F): *manipulation;* mean age 36.1 (11.4) Group 2 (n = 70; 82.9% F): mean age 37.4 (10.9) Group 3 (n = 71; 74.6% F): manipulation and	RCT 1. Spinal manipulation therapy (SMT) 2. Amitriptyline drug treatment 3. Combined SMT and drug treatment	Daily HA diary HA pain: 0-10 score HI: weekly sum of HA activity Over-the-counter (OTC) medication use SF-36	Decrease in HI from baseline to end of treatment • SMT: 40% • Amitriptyline: 49% • Combined: 41% Decrease in HI from baseline to follow-up: • SMT: 42% • Amitriptyline: 24% • Combined: 25%

(Continued)

TABLE 10-5. STUDIES OF CAM THERAPIES FOR HEADACHE—cont'd

Study	Sample	Intervention	Design	Measurement	Major Findings
	amitriptyline; mean age 40.2 (9.8)				No group differences in pain, OTC medication use, or SF-36 health status Age, gender, smoking, weight, duration of complaint, work interference, psychologic overlay, and level of depression were not significant predictors of HI score
RELAXATION					
Bogaards, ter Kuile[21] (1994)	Recurrent tension headache 78 studies	Relaxation, EMG biofeedback, and cognitive-behavioral interventions	Meta-analysis	Daily HA diary Global ratings	Significant decrease in HA activity with cognitive therapy alone or in combination with EMG biofeedback compared with placebo and no treatment
Holroyd, Penzien[112] (1990)	Migraine headaches 60 clinical trials	Propranolol, relaxation/biofeedback, progressive muscle relaxation, relaxation response training, autogenic training	Meta-analysis	Headache Index	43% decrease in HA in both propranolol and relaxation/biofeedback training groups Significant difference in improvement with two treatments vs. placebo group (14% reduction) and untreated patients (no improvement)

Author (Year)	Condition/Subjects	Intervention	Study Design	Outcome Measures	Results
Holroyd, Penzien[111] (1986)	Recurrent tension headache 37 studies	EMG biofeedback, progressive muscle relaxation, meditation, autogenic training, biofeedback and relaxation, false biofeedback (control)	Meta-analysis	Headache activity Proportion of improved patients	Significantly greater improvement in headache activity with EMG biofeedback, relaxation, and combined interventions than with control; No significant difference among interventions; Negative relationship between age and treatment outcomes, suggesting older persons are less likely to respond to relaxation and behavioral techniques
Hyman et al.[115] (1989)	Headache and variety of clinical symptoms 48 studies	Relaxation alone, or combined with imagery, progressive muscle relaxation, rhythmic breathing, Benson's Relaxation Technique	Meta-analysis	Effect sizes for varied outcomes including headache pain	Positive effect sizes suggest effectiveness of relaxation techniques in treating headache and other chronic symptoms; Number of studies for any one condition was small
Malone et al.[150] (1988)	Chronic pain conditions, including migraine and tension HAs 109 studies	Nonpharmacologic treatments for chronic pain conditions	Meta-analysis	Effect sizes and proportion of improved patients for a variety of outcomes	Positive effect size suggests short-term efficacy of relaxation and behavioral techniques for migraine/tension HAs

THERAPEUTIC TOUCH

Author (Year)	Condition/Subjects	Intervention	Study Design	Outcome Measures	Results
Keller, Bzdek[127] (1986)	Tension headache 60 subjects Group 1: therapeutic touch Group 2: placebo	Therapeutic touch (TT) Placebo TT	RCT	McGill-Melzack Pain Questionnaire	70% decrease in pain in TT group vs. 37% in placebo group

intensity.[124,160,213,239] However, one multisite RCT for episodic tension headaches found no difference in treatment response between true and sham acupuncture,[249] and several other studies yielded either contradictory or negative results.[160]

Mixed results also occurred with various types of manipulation. One RCT found spinal manipulation to be as effective as *amitriptyline* (Elavil, a tricyclic antidepressant) in reducing headache pain and activity.[176] In another RCT the combined effects of spinal manipulation and deep friction massage for tension headaches were not superior to placebo and deep friction massage, but both groups had significantly decreased hours of headache and daily analgesic use.[24]

Studies have failed to support other CAM modalities for reducing headache activity. A RCT found that classic homeopathy was no better than placebo after treatment and at 1-year follow-up.[241] A few studies have examined modalities such as transcranial electrotherapy[215] and therapeutic touch.[127] However, major methodologic flaws make it difficult to evaluate the treatment effects in these studies. Future RCTs are needed to clarify further the effectiveness of these CAM modalities in the treatment of chronic headaches.

◣ Neuropathic Pain

Neuropathic pain syndromes are difficult to treat. Several drugs are known to have limited efficacy, but complete pain relief is rarely achieved. Because of the limitations of conventional modalities in relieving neuropathic pain, the effectiveness of several complementary modalities has been tested, including acupuncture,[3,212] electrical stimulation,[8,106,134] and vibration therapy[178] (Table 10-6).

These studies provide preliminary evidence for use of acupuncture, electrical stimulation, and vibration therapy for relieving neuropathic pain. However, future RTCs are needed to discern the active treatment response versus the response caused by the high percentage of participants in the sham groups who also reported decreased pain.

◣ Dental Pain

Several alternatives to traditional dental anesthesia have been tested in adults, including acupuncture,[216] electrical stimulation,[168,205] hypnosis,[86] and music therapy[90] (Table 10-7).

These studies provide strong evidence that alternative forms of pain control in dentistry are well accepted by many patients. However, results of these studies were mixed in terms of satisfactory pain relief through CAM methods. Also, postoperative episodes of vomiting were increased in the hypnosis group in one study.[86] Given the small sample sizes of these studies, further investigations using larger samples are needed to make generalizations regarding the effectiveness of alternative methods of dental pain control and related symptom management.

Text continued on p. 378.

TABLE 10–6. **STUDIES OF CAM THERAPIES FOR NEUROPATHIC PAIN**

Study	Sample	Intervention	Design	Measurement	Major Findings
ACUPUNCTURE					
Abuaisha et al.[3] (1998)	Consecutive outpatients with peripheral diabetic neuropathy 44 patients (32 M, 12 F); mean age 57.2 (range 29-79) 29 patients were receiving standard medical treatment (pain medication)	Patients received six courses of classic acupuncture over 10 weeks to both lower limbs	Pre/posttest Prospective	Pain visual analog scale (VAS) Sleep VAS Neuropathy disability score (NDS) Vibration perception threshold (VPT) Hemoglobin (HbA$_{1c}$)	Significantly decreased pain (p <.01) after acupuncture No significantly change in sleep (p = .09) after acupuncture No significant changes in NDS, VPT, or HbA$_{1c}$ after acupuncture
Shlay et al.[212] (1998)	Human immunodeficiency virus (HIV) and lower extremity peripheral neuropathy 250 subjects Group 1 (n = 121; 88% M): true acupuncture (TA); mean age 40.9 (6.8) Group 2 (n = 118; 92% M): sham acupuncture (SA); age 41.7 (8.3) Group 3 (n = 71; 94% M): amitriptyline; age 40.1 (7.1) Group 4 (n = 88; 88% M): placebo; age 39.9 (5.9)	All patients: usual medical care Separate and combined effects of acupuncture (TA) and amitriptyline Interventions: 14 weeks 1. TA group: standard needle acupuncture at true acupoints 2. SA group: needle stimulation at false/control points 3. Amitriptyline group: 25-75 mg of active drug 4. Placebo amitriptyline group: inert capsules (identical in appearance to amitriptyline)	Randomized controlled trial (RCT) Prospective Repeated measures Double blind (not blinded to pharmacist or acupuncturist) Factorial design	Pain (Gracely scale) Global pain relief Quality of life (QOL) Physician evaluation: • Muscle strength • Sensory ability • Lower extremity reflex	All groups had decreased pain through study No significant differences between groups were found for any measured outcome Placebo effect or use of standardized protocol may explain lack of effect for acupuncture Amitriptyline dose may have been too low to have an effect

(Continued)

TABLE 10-6. **STUDIES OF CAM THERAPIES FOR NEUROPATHIC PAIN—cont'd**

Study	Sample	Intervention	Design	Measurement	Major Findings
ELECTRICAL STIMULATION					
Ahmed et al.[8] (1998)	Acute-onset (<72 hours) herpes zoster lesions 50 patients (23 M, 27 F) Group 1 (n = 25; 52% F, 48% M): *percutaneous electrical nerve stimulation* (PENS); mean age 56 (15) Group 2 (n = 25; 56% F, 44% M): medication only; mean age 53 (15)	PENS group: low-intensity (5 mA) variable-frequency (4-100 Hz) electrical stimulation from acupuncture-like needles around the lesions (three 30-minute sessions/wk for 2 weeks) Medication-only group: 150 mg famciclovir (1 week)	RCT Prospective Repeated measures Participant blinded	Pain VAS Activity VAS Sleep quality VAS Location/severity of cutaneous lesions (blind observer)	PENS group had significantly decreased pain (67% pain reduction; p <.05) vs. medication group (45% pain reduction) PENS group had significantly decreased postherpetic neuralgia pain at 3- and 6-month follow-up (p <.05) vs. medication group PENS group had more rapid resolution and healing of lesions (p <.05) vs. medication group No other significant differences were found between groups
Kumar et al.[134] (1998)	Type 2 diabetes and persistent painful lower extremity peripheral neuropathy 23 patients; ages 31-70 Group 1 (n = 14; 10 F, 4 M): adjunctive TENS; mean age 59 (2) Group 2 (n = 9; 3 F, 6 M): adjunctive sham TENS; mean age 58 (4)	All patients: usual care with amitriptyline Active TENS group: 12 weeks of adjunctive (in-home) H-wave stimulation of variable intensity and frequency (30 minutes daily) Sham control group: same procedure with inactive electrotherapy machine	RCT Prospective Repeated measures Participant and data collector blinded	Neuropathic pain and discomfort: graded 0-5 Neuropathy symptoms Current Perception Test (CPT)	Active TENS group had significantly decreased pain (55% pain relief; p <.03) vs. sham TENS groups (47% pain relief) Neuropathy symptoms recurred after discontinuing TENS
Hamza et al.[106] (2000)	Long-standing type 2 diabetes and persistent peripheral neuropathy (>6 months)	All patients: 3 weeks (three 30-minute sessions/wk) of either active or sham PENS, counterbalanced,	RCT Repeated measures Investigator blinded Crossover design	Pain VAS Physical activity VAS Sleep quality VAS Analgesic use QOL (SF-36)	Active PENS group had the following significant effects vs. sham PENS group:

	50 patients (28 F, 22 M); mean age 55 (9) Group 1 (n = 25): active PENS; mean age 56 (8) Group 2 (n = 25): sham PENS; mean age 54 (9)	with 1-week washout between treatments Active PENS group: high-intensity (maximum tolerable intensity without muscle contraction) bilateral electrical stimulation via 10 acupuncture-like needles stimulated at alternating frequencies of 15 and 30 Hz every 3 seconds Sham PENS group: same placement but no electrical stimulation		Beck Depression Inventory (BDI) Profile of Mood States (POMS)	• Decreased pain (p <.05) • Increased activity and sleep (p <.05) • Increased QOL (p <.05) • Decreased depression (p <.01) • Decreased POMS scores (p <.01) • Decreased analgesic use (p <.05) 92% of patients preferred active PENS for pain and numbness
RELAXATION					
Grunert et al.[100] (1990)	Persistent reflex sympathetic dystrophy (RSD) 20 patients (7 F, 13 M); ages 23-64	All patients had failed to benefit from usual medical care Therapy with autogenic suggestions, thermal biofeedback, and relaxation exercises to enhance thermal self-regulation and coping Total sessions:15-60 (mean 23.6)	Pre/posttest	Subjective pain rating Hand temperature	Patients had significantly decreased pain (p <.0001) after treatment Pain remained significantly decreased at 1-year follow-up Patients were able to increase hand temperature by 7° to 10° F (p <.0001) after treatment
VIBRATION THERAPY					
Paice et al.[178] (2000)	HIV with persistent (≥1 month) neuropathic pain 40 patients; mean age 41 (6) Group 1 (n = 20): active vibration Group 2 (n = 20): sham vibration	Active vibration group: 45-minute session of foot vibration therapy (58.3 Hz) using mechanical foot massager Sham vibration group: inactive foot massager	RCT Double blind	Pain intensity: numeric rating scale (NRS) 0-10 Brief Pain Inventory-Revised (BPI)	Both groups had significantly decreased pain (p <.005) Vibration group had 67.3% (±33.1%) decreased pain vs. 55.0% (±32.0%) for sham group No significant differences were found between groups for pain (p = .19)

TABLE 10–7. **STUDIES OF CAM THERAPIES FOR DENTAL PAIN**

Study	Sample	Intervention	Design	Measurement	Major Findings
ACUPUNCTURE					
Lao et al.[138] (1999)	Oral surgery (third molar extraction) 39 patients; ages 18-34 Group 1 (n = 19; 8 F, 11 M): acupuncture; mean age 23.4 (4.7) Group 2 (n = 20; 9 F, 11 M): placebo; age 24.0 (3.8)	Both groups: usual pre/postoperative care Acupuncture group: postoperative needle stimulation and manual needle manipulation at 4 acupoints on same side of body as the surgery; "De qi" sensation attained at each session Placebo control group: same procedure without needle insertion	Randomized controlled trial (RCT) Patient and surgeon blinded Repeated measures	Pain intensity: 0-3 Time pain free Time until moderate pain Time until analgesic use Expectations	Acupuncture group had following significant effects vs. control group: • Increased time pain free (p = .01) • Increased time until analgesic use (p = .01) • Increased time to moderate pain (p = .008) • Decreased analgesic use (p = .05) No significant differences between groups in positive expectations
ELECTRICAL STIMULATION					
Schafer et al.[205] (2000)	Healthy individuals subjected to stimulation with electric pulp tester 66 subjects	Three transcutaneous electrical nerve stimulation (TENS) devices with extraoral and intraoral electrodes	Double blind Placebo controlled	Pain perception threshold	No difference in pain thresholds
HYPNOSIS, IMAGERY, AND SUGGESTION					
Ghoneim et al.[86] (2000)	Dental surgery (extraction of third molar) 60 patients; age range = 18-35 Group 1 (n = 30): hypnosis; mean age 22.8 (2.3) Group 2 (n = 30): standard care (SC); 23.6 (5.1)	Hypnosis group: self-hypnosis audiotape daily for 1 week preoperatively and immediately presurgery SC control group: no adjunctive treatment	RCT Prospective Unblinded	Pain visual analog scale (VAS) Nausea VAS State-Trait Anxiety Inventory (STAI) Blood pressure Heart rate Postoperative analgesia tablets	Hypnosis group had significantly attenuated anxiety (p = .03) vs. SC group Hypnosis group had significantly increased vomiting (p <.02) vs. control group

Study	Sample/Procedure	Intervention	Design	Outcomes measured	Results
Enqvist, Fischer[59] (1997)	Removal of third mandibular molars 69 patients Group 1 (n = 33; 19 F, 14 M): *hypnosis*; mean age 27.7 (6.23) Group 2 (n = 36; 17 F, 19 M): control; mean age 28.5 (5.35)	Both groups: same pre/postoperative medical care Hypnosis group: mailed 20-minute hypnosis tape to use daily for 1 week before surgery Control group: no adjunctive treatment	RCT	Postoperative complications Vomiting Pain VAS Anxiety VAS Analgesic use	No significant differences were found between groups for analgesic use and other outcomes No significant differences in pain were found between groups Control group had significantly increased preoperative anxiety ($p = .002$) vs. hypnosis group Hypnosis group had significantly decreased postoperative analgesic use ($p = .005$) vs. control group Hypnosis group rated the tape as moderately effective
MUSIC THERAPY Goff et al.[90] (1997)	Crown preparation 80 patients Group 1: *music* Group 2: nitrous oxide (N_2O) Group 3: music plus N_2O Group 4: control	1. Music listening 2. N_2O administration 3. Music and N_2O administration 4. Usual care	RCT	Serum immunoglobulin A IgA (S-IgA) Anxiety and stress (scales not specified)	S-IgA levels were lower in female patients

N Cancer-Related Pain

Uncontrolled pain is prevalent among patients with cancer, often contributing to increased distress, reduced quality of life, and increased health care utilization.[89] Cancer patients may experience acute or chronic pain from the disease process, diagnostic procedures, treatment (surgery, chemotherapy, radiation), or preexisting conditions.[84,225] Cancer pain is dynamic and ever changing and therefore requires careful and frequent assessment to determine the specific etiology and optimal course of treatment.[41,152]

According to Rowlingson and Hamill,[199] "the diagnosis of cancer intensifies the emotional impact of pain, so attention must be given to the psychosocial aspects of the disease." Patients with cancer should have the expectation of pain control as an integral aspect of their care throughout the course of the disease.[172] Consequently, although drug therapies, often delivered by patient-controlled analgesia (PCA), remain the cornerstone of pain management for persons with cancer, nonpharmacologic CAM interventions that increase pain coping skills, as well as feelings of hope and control, can be useful adjunctive therapies.

Patients diagnosed with cancer are among the highest users of CAM modalities. Population-based surveys suggest that about 50% to 75% of cancer patients use CAM interventions to enhance health status and decrease treatment-related side effects such as pain and nausea.[141,166] In contrast to several other pain populations reviewed in this chapter, relatively few CAM modalities have been studied for cancer-related pain (Table 10-8).

The National Cancer Institute (NCI) and Management of Cancer Pain Guideline Panel[152] currently recommend massage as a nonpharmacologic method of pain management. Recent quasi-experimental studies have found immediate benefits for *massage* on pain and anxiety among individuals with cancer.[95,221] Few studies, however, have examined the longer-term effects of massage on pain and related outcomes (e.g., medication use) in cancer populations. One recent RCT, comparing massage therapy to a usual-care control group, found reduced nausea, anxiety, and distress, but no reductions in pain or medication use, in patients undergoing bone marrow transplants.[7] Further studies are necessary to examine the effects of longer-term massage on pain outcomes among men and women with cancer.

Because massage may have relatively small effects on cancer-related pain, some of which may be mediated by reductions in anxiety and distress,[89] massage may be most effective when combined with relaxation, imagery, or hypnosis. When used adjunctively with conventional cancer care, these interventions have reduced the report of pain in patients undergoing bone marrow transplants,[148,223,224] increased comfort after radiation therapy,[132] and reduced anxiety and nausea.[175,191] The clinical guidelines for cancer-related pain control recommend the incorporation of relaxation and behavioral techniques early in the course of the disease, while patients have the energy and strength to learn and practice these strategies.[152]

Text continued on p. 384.

TABLE 10–8. STUDIES OF CAM THERAPIES FOR CANCER-RELATED PAIN

Study	Sample	Intervention	Design	Measurement	Major Findings
ACUPUNCTURE					
Alimi et al.[10] (2000)	Cancer; analgesics for chronic pain 20 patients; mean age 54.3 (11.3)	Adjunctive auricular acupuncture at sites of electrodermal response	Descriptive Consecutive patients	Pain intensity visual analog scale (VAS; ≥30 mm)	Average pain intensity decreased by 33% at day 60 ($p < .00001$) vs. day 0
HYPNOSIS, IMAGERY, AND SUGGESTION					
Spiegel, Bloom[217] (1983)	Primary breast carcinoma and metastases 54 patients Group 1a (n = 11): support only; mean age = 54 Group 1b (n = 19): support with adjunctive self-hypnosis; mean age 54 Group 2 (n = 24): standard care (SC); mean age 55	Treatment groups met weekly for 90-minute sessions of supportive psychotherapy Self-hypnosis group: taught techniques to enhance coping with pain SC group: no-contact control	Randomized controlled trial (RCT) Prospective Repeated measures Physician blinded	Pain intensity: numeric rating scale (NRS) 0-10 Pain suffering: 0-10 Pain frequency Pain duration Affective response: Profile of Mood States (POMS)	Both support groups had significantly decreased pain intensity and suffering ($p < .03$) vs. SC group Support group receiving hypnosis had the lowest pain intensity and suffering No difference was found among groups in number or length of pain episodes Improved mood in treatment groups was significantly associated with change in pain sensation (Spearman $\rho = .36$, $p = .05$)
Syrjala et al.[224] (1992)	Hematologic malignancy or lymphoma; first bone marrow transplant 45 patients (19 F, 26 M); mean age 32.7 (19-49) Group 1 (n = 12; 6 F, 6 M): hypnosis; mean	Intervention groups: two 90-minute training sessions and home practice (preadmission) as well as two weekly 30-minute booster sessions (hospital)	RCT Repeated measures	Mucositis pain intensity VAS Nausea VAS Emesis: NRS 0-3 Opioid intake	Only hypnosis group had significantly decreased oral mucositis pain over 3 weeks ($p = .011$) CBT was not significantly more effective than control on any outcmes

(Continued)

TABLE 10–8. **STUDIES OF CAM THERAPIES FOR CANCER-RELATED PAIN—cont'd**

Study	Sample	Intervention	Design	Measurement	Major Findings
	age 32.3 (range 22-45) Group 2 (n = 11; 6 F, 5 M): *cognitive-behavioral training* (CBT); mean age 33.3 (23-44) Group 3 (n = 12; 5 F, 7 M): therapist contact; mean age 30.9 (19-49) Group 4 (n = 10; 2 F, 8 M): usual care; mean age 34.6 (19-49)	1. Hypnosis group: training and hypnosis audiotapes 2. CBT group: coping skills training (relaxation, but not hypnosis or imagery) 3. Therapist contact group: equal time and attention from therapist as hypnosis and CBT groups 4. Usual care group: no-contact control			No treatment had a significant effect on nausea, emesis, or opioid intake Women reported less pain than men (p = .001)
Syrjala et al.[225] (1995)	Leukemia, myelodysplasia, or lymphoma; first bone marrow transplant 94 patients (41 F, 53 M); mean age 36 (9.4) Group 1 (n = 23): *hypnosis* Group 2 (n = 24): *CBT* Group 3 (n = 24): *support* Group 4 (n = 23): usual care (*UC*)	Intervention groups: two 90-minute training sessions (preadmission) and home practice and two weekly 20- to 40-minute booster sessions (hospital) 1. Hypnosis group: structured training (labeled as "relaxation and imagery") 2. CBT group: coping skills training (relaxation, imagery) 3. Support group: supportive therapy with equal time/attention from therapist as hypnosis/CBT groups 4. UC group: no-contact control	RCT Stratified for total body radiation and gender Repeated measures	Oral pain VAS Nausea VAS Opioid intake: patient-controlled analgesia (PCA) Oral mucositis index Symptom Check List (SCL-90-R)	Both hypnosis and CBT groups had significantly decreased oral pain (p <.009) vs. UC group No significant differences were found between hypnosis and CBT groups on any outcomes, indicating additional CBT skills did not enhance benefits of hypnosis alone No differences between groups were found for opioid intake (p = .25) Oral mucositis index was significantly correlated with oral pain (r = .43; p <.001) and opioid intake (r = 45; p <.001)

Study	Sample	Design	Intervention	Measures	Results
Kolcaba, Fox[132] (1999)	Radiation treatment (RT) for early-stage breast cancer 53 women Group 1 (n = 26): guided imagery Group 2 (n = 27): no-treatment control	RCT	Guided imagery group listened to audiotape (soft jazz music) with imagery to increase comfort; patients instructed to use tape daily during and following RT	Radiation Therapy Comfort Questionnaire State-Trait Anxiety Inventory (STAI)	Guided imagery group had significantly increased comfort (p = .05) vs. control Greatest treatment effects 3 weeks after RT Pretreatment anxiety was positively correlated with comfort (r = .30 to .60; p = .05) Age was negatively correlated with anxiety (r = −.16; p = .05)
MASSAGE					
Ahles et al.[7] (1999)	Autologous bone marrow transplants 34 patients (26 F, 8 M); mean age 41 (9.3) Group 1 (n = 16; 14 F, 2 M): massage; mean age 41.3 (9.4) Group 2 (n = 18; 12 F, 6 M): control; mean age 42.3 (9.5)	RCT Repeated measures	Massage group: 20-minute upper body massages (2-3 times/wk) from trained massage therapist during hospitalization for treatment Control group: usual care (told to have quiet time for 20 min/day)	Pain: NRS 0-10 Distress: NRS 0-10 Fatigue: NRS 0-10 Nausea: NRS 0-10 Opioid intake Anxiolytic use Antiemetic use Blood pressure (BP) Heart rate Respiration rate Speilberger STAI Beck Depression Inventory (BDI) POMS	Across all measurement points, massage group had significantly decreased diastolic BP (p = .01), distress (p = .02), nausea (p = .01), and state anxiety (p < .0001) vs. control Massage group had significantly decreased fatigue (p = .02) at day 7 vs. control Massage group had significantly decreased state anxiety (STAI) at midtreatment (p = .02) vs. control Most robust treatment effects were seen after first week of treatment

(Continued)

TABLE 10-8. **STUDIES OF CAM THERAPIES FOR CANCER-RELATED PAIN—cont'd**

Study	Sample	Intervention	Design	Measurement	Major Findings
Grealish et al.[95] (2000)	Cancer (32 with metastatic disease) 87 patients (52 F, 35 M; mean age 58.2 (range 18-88)	10-minute foot massage on 2 of 3 evenings; patients served as own controls on third evening (control session)	Quasi-experimental Within-subject design Randomly assigned order of massage and control Repeated measures	Pain intensity VAS Nausea VAS Relaxation VAS Activity: NRS 0-4	No differences between groups were found for pain or medication intake Pain intensity was significantly decreased after both massage sessions ($p < .01$) vs. control session Nausea was significantly decreased after both massage sessions ($p < .01$) vs. control session Relaxation was significantly increased after both massage sessions ($p < .01$) vs. control No significant gender differences were found
Stephenson et al.[221] (2000)	23 hospitalized patients (15 F, 8 M) with breast (13) and lung (10) cancer reporting anxiety; mean age 68.7 (2.69)	30-minute reflexology session (with 15 minutes targeting pain areas and cancer site) one evening; patients served as own controls on another evening (control session)	Quasi-experimental Within-subject design Randomly assigned order of reflexology and control	McGill Pain Questionnaire Short Form (MPQ-SF) Anxiety VAS Analgesic intake	Significantly decreased anxiety after reflexology session ($p < .001$) vs. control Significantly decreased pain (MPQ-SF) after reflexology session ($p .05$) among patients with breast cancer vs. controls No significant difference was found between treatments in analgesic intake

RELAXATION

Luebbert et al.[148] (2001)

| Studies of patients with cancer receiving adjunctive *relaxation training and imagery* | Weighted effect sizes calculated for pain, other treatment-related symptoms, and emotional adjustment

Various relaxation techniques, some including imagery | Meta-analysis | Pain
Other treatment-related symptoms
Negative emotions | Relaxation training had significant positive effects on pain and related symptoms vs. control group

Relaxation training had significant positive improvements in depression, anxiety, and hostility vs. control group

Relaxation was equally effective for patients undergoing different medical procedures |

◼ Temporomandibular Joint Pain

Temporomandibular joint disorders (TMDs) are syndromes marked by jaw pain and dysfunction (e.g., limited range of motion). Because traditional medical interventions are often not effective for TMDs, patients often turn to CAM modalities in an effort to reduce pain and enhance quality of life. Although few CAM modalities have been rigorously investigated, support exists for several CAM modalities to reduce TMJ pain (Table 10-9).

EMG biofeedback, both with and without additional relaxation training, has been found more effective than no treatment and psychologic placebo controls for TMD pain and clinical outcomes.[45,72,163] Studies have also found relaxation to be similar in effect to EMG biofeedback[79] and more effective than hypnosis.[218] A number of studies have demonstrated reduced TMD pain and symptoms following treatment with acupuncture, but this research is preliminary. Further rigorous research is needed to replicate these findings.[62]

◼ Fibromyalgia

Fibromyalgia, which affects up to 20% of all patients seen in rheumatology practices, is a syndrome characterized by diffuse musculoskeletal pain, fatigue, stiffness, sleep disturbance, and resistance to treatment. Many persons with fibromyalgia seek CAM modalities as adjunctive therapy to conventional medical care in hope of finding more effective pain and symptom relief than that achieved through current conventional medical treatment (Table 10-10).

A review of seven studies (three RCTs, three prospective cohort studies, one retrospective cohort study) reported increased pain thresholds and decreased pain ratings and medication use with acupuncture treatment, though some persons experienced exacerbations of their pain after the acupuncture.[17]

Results from several studies suggest that imagery, relaxation, and hypnosis can be effective in the management of fibromyalgia by improving pain ratings and functional status and decreasing the number of positive tender points.[*] EMG biofeedback alone[201] and biofeedback combined with exercise[32] were effective in decreasing pain ratings and tender point counts. However, a later study comparing biofeedback, exercise, combined biofeedback and exercise, and an educational attention control found no difference among groups in pain ratings, disease activity, myalgic scores, or sleep.[31] Additional research is needed before conclusions can be drawn about the effectiveness of CAM modalities for persons diagnosed with fibromyalgia.

---

*References 44, 74, 102, 123, 125, 126.

Text continued on p. 396.

TABLE 10–9. **STUDIES OF CAM THERAPIES FOR TEMPOROMANDIBULAR JOINT (TMJ) PAIN AND TEMPOROMANDIBULAR DISORDER (TMD)**

Study	Sample	Intervention	Design	Measurement	Major Findings
BIOFEEDBACK Funch, Gale[79] (1984)	Chronic TMJ pain 57 subjects Group 1 (n = 30): electromyographic (EMG) *biofeedback*; mean age 43 (15) Group 2 (n = 27): *relaxation*; mean age 35.6 (12.7)	Biofeedback group: EMG biofeedback (bilateral electrodes over masseter area) for reduced EMG on painful side of jaw Relaxation group: three tape-recorded relaxation procedures (weekly in investigator's office) and tapes at home	Randomized controlled trial (RCT) Repeated measures	Pain: numeric rating scale (NRS) 0-5 (from pain diary) Taylor Manifest Anxiety Inventory	No significant difference was found between groups for average percentage of pain (p = .10) Response to relaxation was negatively associated with duration of TMJ symptoms (r = -.45; p <.01) and positively associated with number of comorbid disorders (r = .39 and .46; p <.05) Response to EMG biofeedback was positively associated with age (r = .43; p <.05), marriage (r = .49; p <.01), and time with TMJ symptoms (r = .35; p <.05) and negatively associated with history of equilibration treatment (r = -.38 and .36; p <.05) and family support (r = -.47; p <.01)

(Continued)

TABLE 10–9. **STUDIES OF CAM THERAPIES FOR TEMPOROMANDIBULAR JOINT (TMJ) PAIN AND TEMPOROMANDIBULAR DISORDER (TMD)**—cont'd

Study	Sample	Intervention	Design	Measurement	Major Findings
Flor, Birbaumer[22] (1993)	Chronic back pain (CBP) or TMJ pain and TMD 78 subjects; 21 TMD, 57 CBP; mean age 42.43 (9.68) Group 1 (n = 26; 16 F, 10 M): *electromyographic biofeedback* (EMG-BFB); mean age 40.88 (10.01) Group 2 (n = 26; 16 F, 10 M): *cognitive-behavioral therapy* (CBT); mean age 42.56 (9.42) Group 3 (n = 26; 18 F, 8 M): conservative medical treatment; mean age 43.85 (9.62)	EMG-BFB group: biofeedback at site of pain to reduce muscle tension, but no specific relaxation training CBT group: instruction in pain and stress management skills, including progressive muscle relaxation Medical group: best available conservative medical care (e.g., medication, physical therapy, chiropractic, massage, bite plates)	RCT Stratified by pain type	West Haven-Yale Multidimensional Pain Inventory (MPI) Medication intake Pain catastrophizing and coping: Pain-Related Self-Statements scale and Pain-Related Control Scale (PRCS) Pain-related doctor visits (n)	EMG-BFB group had significantly decreased MPI pain severity after treatment ($p < .05$) vs. medical group EMG-BFB group had significantly decreased MPI pain severity and pain interference at 6 months ($p < .05$) vs. CBT and medical groups EMG-BFB group had significantly decreased pain catastrophizing (posttreatment), affective distress (posttreatment, 6 months), and increased MPI active coping (posttreatment) ($p < .05$) vs. CBT and medical groups Both EMG-BFB and CBT groups had significantly increased MPI active coping at 6 months ($p < .001$) vs. medical group EMG-BFB group had decreased pain-related physician visits at 24 months ($p < .01$) Duration of pain problem was strongest predictor of response ($r = -.308$; $p < .01$)

| Mishra et al.[163] (2000)
Gardea et al.[81] (2001) | Chronic TMD
94 subjects (77 F, 17 M); mean age 35.76 (9.92)
Group 1 (n = 23; 18 F, 5 M): *biofeedback (BFB)*; mean age 38.13 (10.95)
Group 2 (n = 22; 18 F, 4 M): *cognitive-behavioral skills training (CBST)*; mean age 35.55 (9.14)
Group 3 (n = 24; 21 F, 3 M): BFB and CBST (Combo); mean age 34.13 (8.26)
Group 4 (n = 25; 20 F, 5 M); no treatment control (NTC); mean age 35.24 (11.16) | Diagnosed using research diagnostic criteria (RDC)
All treatment groups: 12 sessions (over 8 weeks)
1. BFB group: EMG and temperature biofeedback and relaxation training with electrodes placed over frontalis muscles
2. CBST group: instruction in pain and stress management skills, including progressive muscle relaxation
3. Combo group: components of both BFB and CBST | RCT
Repeated measures
Unblinded | RDC characteristic pain intensity: 0-100
Pain-related disability: RDC graded chronic pain status: 0-4
Profile of Mood States (POMS)
Limitations in mandibular functioning | No significant change in EMG or stress reactivity was seen after treatments
Physiologic reactivity was negatively associated with response to EMG-BFB ($r = -.42$; $p < .01$) and positively associated with practice of relaxation and distraction (for both: $r = .55$; $p < .01$)
Reported use of cognitive distortions was negatively associated with response to CBT ($r = -.48$; $p < .01$)
BFB, CBST, and Combo groups all had significantly decreased pain intensity ($p < .05$) vs. NTC group
BFB group had significantly decreased pain intensity ($p = .014$) vs. NTC group
BFB and Combo groups had significantly decreased pain intensity at 1-year follow-up ($p < .024$) vs. NTC group
CBST group had significantly decreased pain-related disability at 1-year follow-up ($p = .02$) vs. NTC group
BFB, CBST, and Combo groups all had significantly increased POMS ($p < .001$) |

(Continued)

TABLE 10-9. STUDIES OF CAM THERAPIES FOR TEMPOROMANDIBULAR JOINT (TMJ) PAIN AND TEMPOROMANDIBULAR DISORDER (TMD)—cont'd

Study	Sample	Intervention	Design	Measurement	Major Findings
Crider, Glaros[45] (1999)	TMD 12 studies, including 6 controlled trials	EMG biofeedback (EMG-BFB) training used alone or with other stress management techniques EMG-BFB directed at masseter/frontalis sites	Meta-analysis	Pain Clinical outcomes (from examination)	Significantly larger effect sizes were found for pain with EMG-BFB vs. control group 69% of EMG-BFB patients were rated "significantly improved" vs. 35% of control patients Significantly larger effect sizes were found for clinical outcomes with EMG-BFB vs. control group Conclusion: available research supports the use of EMG biofeedback for TMD

HYPNOSIS, IMAGERY, AND SUGGESTION

Study	Sample	Intervention	Design	Measurement	Major Findings
Stam et al.[218] (1984)	Persistent TMD 41 subjects; mean age 25.7 (range 15-41) Group 1 (n = 12): relaxation Group 2 (n = 15): hypnosis Group 3 (n = 14): wait-list control (WLC)	Relaxation group: four weekly sessions of progressive relaxation and instruction in pain coping skills Hypnosis group: same relaxation intervention labeled as "hypnosis" and preceded by hypnotic induction WLC: no intervention	RTC Stratified by hypnotic susceptibility Repeated measures	Pain intensity VAS Peak pain (derived from pain diary) Jaw sounds with jaw opening Jaw opening limitations (self-report) Hypnotic susceptibility	Relaxation group had significantly decreased peak pain ($p < .05$) vs. hypnosis and WLC Both hypnosis and relaxation groups had significantly increased jaw opening by week 4 ($p < .01$) vs. WLC All groups had significantly decreased pain intensity after treatment ($p < .05$), but no significant differences between groups

Study	Sample	Intervention	Design	Outcome Measures	Results
Simon, Lewis[214] (2000)	Chronic TMD with failure to respond to conservative treatment and no evidence of organic TMJ changes 23 subjects (20 F, 3 M); mean age 33 (range 20-52)	All patients: six sessions of adjunctive group hypnosis	Quasi-experimental Pre/posttest Treatment group vs. wait-list patient group	Pain frequency: NRS 1-7 Pain duration: 0-600 min/ episode Pain intensity: NRS 0-10 Outpatient medical visits Improvement (%)	Pain reduction was significantly correlated with hypnotic susceptibility ($r = .44$ to $.60$; $p < .01$) Patients had significantly decreased pain frequency, duration, and intensity after hypnosis ($p < .001$) vs. no significant change in wait-list patients Treatment gains with hypnosis were maintained at 6-month follow-up. 71% of patients reported improvement in pain after hypnosis Patients had significantly decreased outpatient visits after treatment ($p = .006$)

TABLE 10-10. STUDIES OF CAM THERAPIES FOR FIBROMYALGIA

Study	Sample	Intervention	Design	Measurement	Major Findings
ACUPUNCTURE					
Berman, Swyers[17] (1999)	Fibromyalgia 7 studies	Acupuncture	Evidence-based review	Pain intensity Pain thresholds Sleep Biochemical markers (serotonin, substance P) Medication use	High-quality RCTs found the following 1. Acupuncture group had decreased pain intensity and increased pain thresholds 2. Decreased medication use may be *clinically* significant even though not statistically significant 3. Exacerbations of fibromyalgia pain may occur, or some patients may feel worse after acupuncture Prospective studies demonstrated similar findings; one also found improvement in sleep quality and serotonin and substance P Retrospective study of efficacy of several CAM therapies found that patients rated acupuncture as providing the best and longest lasting pain reduction
Deluze et al.[51] (1992)	Fibromyalgia 70 subjects (54 F, 16 M) Group 1: *electroacupuncture* (EA) Group 2: placebo	EA group: 6 sessions over 2 weeks Placebo acupuncture group: same program but needling 2 mm from true sites	Randomized controlled trial (RCT) Double blind	Pain threshold Pain intensity rating Stiffness Analgesics: self-report Sleep quality Perceived general state	EA group had significant improvement in all outcomes except one measure EA group had 70% improvement in pain threshold vs. 4% in placebo group

BIOFEEDBACK

Study	Population	Design	Intervention	Outcome Measures	Results
Buckelew et al.[32] (1992)	Fibromyalgia 119 subjects Group 1: *biofeedback* Group 2: exercise Group 3: combo Group 4: control	RCT	1. Biofeedback only 2. Exercise only 3. Combined biofeedback/ exercise 4. Education and attention control	Self-efficacy for function Tender point pain	Significant improvement in tender points and self-efficacy for function maintained only by biofeedback/exercise group at follow-up
Buckelew et al.[31] (1998)	Fibromyalgia 119 subjects (108 F, 11 M); mean age 44.0 (9.6) Group 1 (n = 29): *biofeedback and relaxation* Group 2 (n = 28): exercise Group 3 (n = 30): combination Group 4 (n = 30): control	RCT	6-week individual training phase and 2-year maintenance regimen 1. Biofeedback and relaxation 2. Exercise only 3. Biofeedback and relaxation combined with exercise 4. Education and attention control	Tender point index (TPI) Myalgic scores Disease activity: physician rating Pain visual analog scale (VAS) Pain behavior observation Arthritis Impact Measurement Scale (AIMS) SCL-90 Center for Epidemiological Studies–Depression (CES-D) Arthritis Self-Efficacy Scale (ASES) Sleep problems	No significant differences were found among groups in disease severity, pain VAS, pain behavior, myalgia scores, and sleep at 6 weeks TPI decreased in all treatment groups at 6 weeks Pain VAS was decreased in all treatment groups at 6 weeks Pain behavior decreased in all treatment groups at 3-month and 1-year follow-up
Sarnoch et al.[201] (1997)	Fibromyalgia 18 subjects (16 F, 2 M); mean age 51 (5)	Quasi-experimental	Electromyographic (EMG) biofeedback	Pain EMG activity (trapezius) Muscular sensitivity Helplessness Belief of control (effect size[ES] = .55)	After EMG biofeedback training: • Decreased pain intensity • Decreased EMG activity (ES = 1.33) • Increased muscular discrimination or sensitivity (ES = .79)

(Continued)

TABLE 10-10. STUDIES OF CAM THERAPIES FOR FIBROMYALGIA—cont'd

Study	Sample	Intervention	Design	Measurement	Major Findings
ELECTRICAL STIMULATION					
Mueller et al.[167] (2001)	Fibromyalgia 30 subjects (27 F, 3 M); ages 27-69; mean 50.7 (12)	Brain wave intervention, EEG-driven stimulus (EDS) Massage and physical therapy (PT) added later in study	Quasi-experimental	Modified Fibromyalgia Impact Questionnaire (FIQ-M) Tender points (TP) SCL-90 R Pain VAS Sleep VAS Fatigue VAS Depression VAS Anxiety VAS Cognitive clouding VAS	Differences from baseline to immediately before start of massage and PT: • Decreased pain, TP, fatigue, depression, anxiety, and cognitive clouding • Increased sleep quality Differences from start of massage and PT to end of study: • Further decreases in pain • Maintenance of other treatment gains
HERBAL THERAPY AND SUPPLEMENTS					
Edwards et al.[56] (2000)	Fibromyalgia 12 women (9 completed study); mean age 45.6 (5.9) Groups 1, 2, and 3: *anthocyanidin* Group 4: Placebo	1. Anthocyanidins, 40 mg/day 2. Anthocyanidins, 80 mg/day 3. Anthocyanidins, 120 mg/day 4. Placebo control	RCT Double blind Crossover	Pain (5-point scale) Sleep (5-point scale) Investigator and patient global efficacy assessments General Health Questionnaire (GHQ)	All anthocyanidin groups had decreased sleep disturbances No significant group differences in pain, fatigue, or patient ratings of global efficacy Investigators' ratings showed significant decrease in fatigue in those taking 80 mg/day vs. placebo group
HYPNOSIS, IMAGERY, AND SUGGESTION					
Burckhardt et al.[33] (1994)	Fibromyalgia 99 women Group 1: education plus	1. Education and cognitive-behavioral training (CBT) 2. Education and physical	RCT	Fibromyalgia Impact Questionnaire (FIQ) Tender point pain	Significant improvement in both treatment groups in FIQ and QOL

Study	Subjects	Intervention	Design	Outcomes	Results
		cognitive-behavioral training Group 2: education plus physical training Group 3: control therapy (PT) 3. Wait-list control		Quality of life (QOL)	Significant reduction in number of tender points in both treatment groups Education plus PT group had significantly better outcomes at 3-month follow-up
Creamer et al.[44] (2000)	Fibromyalgia 28 subjects (20 completed study)	Relaxation, CBT, and Qi Gong	Quasi-experimental	FIQ TP Pain VAS Sleep VAS Patient and physician global assessments SF-36 Depression-BDI Coping Strategies Questionnaire (CSQ) HAQ	The following improved after treatment: • FIQ total scores • Sleep • HAQ • BDI • Patient global assessment All improvements remained at 4-month follow-up except depression
Fors, Gotestam[74] (2000)	Fibromyalgia 58 women; mean age 45.7 (10) Group 1 (n = 17): *guided imagery* Group 2 (n = 22): education with imagery Group 3 (n = 19): control	1. Guided imagery (pleasant nature scene) and relaxation 2. Education, with relaxation and imagery of natural pain-killing systems in body 3. Control: subjects talked about fibromyalgia problems	RCT	Pain VAS Anxiety VAS	Imagery and patient education (with imagery) groups had decreased pain and anxiety vs. control group Imagery and patient education with imagery groups did not differ from each other
Keel[126] (1998)	Fibromyalgia 32 subjects (27 completed study) Group 1 (n = 14; 12 F, 2 M):	1. Treatment group: relaxation, CBT, and education combined 2. Control group	RCT	Freiburg Personality Inventory (FPI) Locus of control (LOC) Pain diary	Experimental group had decreased pain over study vs. control group, who had increased pain

(Continued)

TABLE 10-10. **STUDIES OF CAM THERAPIES FOR FIBROMYALGIA**—cont'd

Study	Sample	Intervention	Design	Measurement	Major Findings
	relaxation plus CBT plus education; age 48 Group 2 (n = 13; 12 F, 1 M): control; age 50			Sleep disturbance Pain duration	7 patients from experimental group and 2 from control group showed significant clinical improvement in 3 of 6 parameters At follow-up, improvement was still present in 5 experimental cases but in none of controls
MAGNET THERAPY Alfano et al.[9] (2001)	Fybromyalgia 119 subjects (93% F; 94 completed all 6 months of study); mean age 45.4 (8.0) Group 1 (n = 37): functional A Group 2 (n = 33): functional B Group 3 (n = 17): sham A Group 4 (n = 15): sham B Group 5 (n = 17): control	1. Functional magnet pad A (MagnetiCo) 2. Functional magnet pad B (Nikken) 3. Sham pad A 4. Sham pad B 5. Control: usual care	RCT Subjects stratified based on FIQ scores, then randomly assigned to group	Pain: NRS 0-10 FIQ pain rating Tender points (TPs) Functional status (FIQ)	Functional pad A group had significantly decreased pain intensity vs. sham group No significant group differences in number of TPs or in FIQ scores, although functional pad groups showed improvement in proper direction
MANIPULATION Blunt et al.[20] (1997)	Fibromyalgia 21 subjects (19 completed study); ages 25-70 Group 1 (n = 10): *chiropractic* Group 2 (n = 9): control	Chiropractic group: soft tissue massage, stretching, spinal manipulation Control group: wait list	RCT Crossover design	Pain VAS TPs Range of motion (ROM): cervical and lumbar spine Strength testing Oswestry Disability Index (ODI) Neck Pain Disability Index (NDI)	Chiropractic group had improved pain, ROM, and straight-leg raising vs. control group

Haines, Haines[103] (2000)	Fibromyalgia 15 women; mean age 51.1 (10.4)	Chiropractic (30 treatments) with ischemic compression and spinal manipulation	Quasi-experimental	Pain VAS for 12 parts of body Fatigue: NRS 0-10 Sleep quality: 0-10	Nine patients (60%) responded with at least 50% improvement in pain Respondents (vs. nonrespondents) had the following: • Decreased pain intensity • Decreased fatigue • Increased sleep quality Improvements in pain and sleep (but not fatigue) were maintained at 1 month

VIBRATION AND MUSIC THERAPY

Chesky et al.[38] (1997)	Fibromyalgia 26 subjects Group 1 (n = 13; 11 F, 2 M): vibration; mean age 51 (9.1) Group 2 (n = 13; 13 F): placebo; age 46.7 (10.7)	Treatment group: musically fluctuating vibration (60-300 Hz) Placebo group: sinusoidal vibration (20 Hz)	RCT Double blind Placebo controlled	Tender Point Index (TPI) Pain VAS Dolorimeter Pain Threshold (TPA)	Vibration did not significantly alter pain VAS Vibration group had improved TPI and TPA from pretest to posttest vs. control group TPI did not differ between groups TPA was better in vibration group vs. placebo group

◼ Pain Associated with Vascular Insufficiency

Vascular insufficiency represents a major public health problem, contributing to ischemic pain (i.e., intermittent claudication, angina), vascular complications, neuropathy, disability, and death.[246] Current medical care includes treatment with dietary modification, exercise, medication, and bypass surgery.[82,169,255] Because these therapies are less effective than desired, CAM modalities may be of value in the treatment of pain associated with vascular insufficiency.

A few case studies and clinical trials suggest that *thermal biofeedback,* alone or in combination with relaxation strategies and hypnotic suggestions, may improve pain-free walking, blood flow, and blood pressure in individuals with intermittent claudication.[93,98,193,204] However, few recent studies have been conducted to extend these findings and test additional CAM modalities for vascular pain and related symptoms. Recent studies have examined the effects of electrical stimulation and the herb *Ginkgo biloba* (Table 10-11). According to a recent meta-analysis of eight randomized, placebo-controlled, double-blind trials, *G. biloba* is more effective than placebo for increasing pain-free walking.

SUMMARY

Evidence supports the use of a number of well-defined CAM modalities for reducing pain and promoting comfort in patients with acute, chronic, and cancer-related pain. This state-of-the-art review reveals that the most evidence available supports the use of behavioral interventions, including relaxation, imagery, and hypnosis, although there is need for replication of many of these studies using rigorous methodology and adequate sample size. In addition, this review supports the NIH Consensus Conference on Acupuncture[173] showing efficacy of acupuncture for postoperative dental pain, and evidence strongly suggests that acupuncture may also be beneficial for pain and related symptoms after other surgical procedures. Evidence is increasing to support the use of electrostimulation for decreasing pain in selected acute and chronic pain conditions. A wide range of herbal and natural products also have demonstrated positive effects in pain management. Rarely, however, have these studies been replicated using similar populations and treatment conditions.

Data are insufficient in some cases to conclude that one CAM method is better than another for a given pain condition. One approach may be more effective than another for a given *individual,* however, emphasizing the importance of individual differences in the treatment of acute, chronic, and cancer-related pain. In recommending CAM modalities in which evidence is inconclusive, patients are most likely to receive benefit from those for which they hold the most positive expectations. Future studies customizing CAM interventions to patient characteristics are needed.

Current and future research will reveal additional data to support the appropriateness and adequacy of CAM interventions in reducing pain and promoting comfort when used alone or in conjunction with conventional interventions. These investigations should include assessment of physiologic dimensions of pain and the impact of

TABLE 10–11. **STUDIES OF CAM THERAPIES FOR VASCULAR PAIN**

Study	Sample	Intervention	Design	Measurement	Major Findings
ELECTRICAL STIMULATION					
Borjesson et al.[23] (1997)	Angina 30 patients Group 1 (n = 14): *transcutaneous electrical nerve stimulation* (TENS) Group 2 (n = 16): placebo	TENS vs. placebo control	Single blind Placebo controlled	Continuous vector cardiography Cardiac enzyme leakage Analgesic use: 24 hour	TENS decreased number of silent ischemic ST change vector magnitude episodes (p = .02) TENS decreased duration of ST change (p = .01)
HERBAL THERAPY AND SUPPLEMENTS					
Pittler, Ernst[184] (2000)	Intermittent claudication 8 studies	Ginkgo biloba	Randomized controlled trials (RCTs) Double blind		Ginkgo biloba significantly improved pain-free walking (weighted mean difference: 34 m [95% confidence interval]; 26-43 m) In studies using similar methodologic features (ergometer speed 3 km/hr, inclination 12%), this difference was 33 m in favor of G. biloba (95% CI); 22-43 m) Adverse effects were rare, mild, and transient Studies suggest that G. biloba extract may be superior to placebo in symptomatic treatment of intermittent claudication
Gregory et al.[99] (2002)	Superficial second-degree burns	Propolis cream (made from a natural product) for treatment of minor burns (superficial second degree) in ambulatory care setting	Experimental	Wounds cultured for microbial growth Wounds photographed: • Inflammation • Cicatrization	Wounds treated with Propolis skin cream consistently showed less inflammation and more rapid cicatrization than those treated with silver sulfadiazine (Silvadene)

pain and pain reduction on body systems. The next decades will bring new discoveries that will enhance our knowledge and skills in promoting comfort and reducing pain in populations across the age span in all clinical settings. Challenges to clinicians are (1) to overcome perceived organizational, bureaucratic, financial, and attitudinal barriers to the integration of therapies for which there is demonstrated efficacy and (2) to work with patients who are seeking ways to be active and responsible partners in the treatment of their pain.

REFERENCES

1. Abeles RP: Schemas, sense of control, and aging. In Rodin J, Schaie KW, editors: *Self-directedness: causes and effects through the life course,* Mahwah, NJ, 1990, Lawrence Erlbaum Associates.
2. Abenhaim L, Bergeron AM: Twenty years of randomized clinical trials of manipulative therapy for back pain: a review, *Clin Invest Med* 15:527, 1992.
3. Abuaisha BB, Costanzi JB, Boulton AJ: Acupuncture for the treatment of chronic painful peripheral diabetic neuropathy: a long-term study, *Diabetes Res Clin Pract Suppl* 39:115, 1998.
4. Acute Low Back Problems Guideline Panel: Acute low back problems in adults. Clinical practice guideline no 14, AHCPR pub no 95-0642, Agency for Health Care Policy and Research, Public Health Service, Rockville, Md, 1994, US Department of Health and Human Services.
5. Acute Pain Management Guideline Panel: Acute pain management: operative or medical procedures and trauma. Clinical practice guideline no 1, AHCPR pub no 92-0032, Agency for Health Care Policy and Research, Public Health Service, Rockville, Md, 1992, US Department of Health and Human Services.
6. Adams PF, Benson V: Current estimates from the National Health Interview Survey, 1991, *Vital Health Stat* 10, 1992.
7. Ahles TA, Tope DM, Pinkson B, et al: Massage therapy for patients undergoing autologous bone marrow transplantation, *J Pain Sympt Manage* 18:157, 1999.
8. Ahmed HE, Craig WF, White PF, et al: Percutaneous electrical nerve stimulation: an alternative to antiviral drugs for acute herpes zoster, *Anesth Analg* 87:911, 1998.
9. Alfano AP, Taylor AG, Foresman PA, et al: Static magnetic fields for treatment of fibromyalgia: a randomized controlled trial, *J Altern Complement Med* 7:53, 2001.
10. Alimi D, Rubino C, Leandri EP, et al: Analgesic effects of auricular acupuncture for cancer pain, *J Pain Sympt Manage* 19:81, 2000.
11. Anderson R, Meeker WC, Wirick BE, et al: A meta-analysis of clinical trials of spinal manipulation, *J Manipulative Physiol Ther* 15:181, 1992.
12. Andersson GBJ: The epidemiology of spinal disorders. In Frymoyer W, editor: *The adult spine: principles and practice,* New York, 1991, Raven.
13. Andersson GBJ, Lucente T, Davis AM, et al: A comparison of osteopathic spinal manipulation with standard care for patients with low back pain, *N Engl J Med* 34:1426, 1999.
14. Andjelkovic Z, Vojinovic J, Pejnovic N, et al: Disease modifying and immunomodulatory effects of high dose 1 alpha (OH) D3 in rheumatoid arthritis patients, *Clin Exp Rheumatol* 17:453, 1999.
15. Ashton C, Whitworth GC, Seldomridge JA, et al: Self-hypnosis reduces anxiety following coronary artery bypass surgery: a prospective, randomized trial, *J Cardiovasc Surg* 38:69, 1997.
16. Benedetti F, Amanzio M, Casadio C, et al: Control of postoperative pain by transcutaneous electrical nerve stimulation after thoracic operations, *Ann Thorac Surg* 63:773, 1997.
17. Berman BM, Swyers JP: Complementary medicine treatments for fibromyalgia syndrome, *Baillieres Best Pract Res Clin Rheumatol* 13:487, 1999.
18. Birch S, Jamison RN: Controlled trial of Japanese acupuncture for chronic myofascial neck pain: assessment of specific and nonspecific effects of treatment, *Clin J Pain* 14:248, 1998.
19. Blankfield RP, Sulzmann C, Fradley LG, et al: Therapeutic touch in the treatment of carpal tunnel syndrome, *J Am Board Fam Pract* 14:335, 2001.
20. Blunt KL, Rajwani MH, Guerriero RC: The effectiveness of chiropractic management of fibromyalgia patients: a pilot study, *J Manipulative Physiol Ther* 20:389, 1997.

21. Bogaards MC, ter Kuile MM: Treatment of recurrent tension headache: a meta-analytic review, *Clin J Pain* 10:174, 1994.

22. Bonica JJ: Cancer pain. In Bonica JJ, editor: *The management of pain,* Malvern, Pa, 1990, Lea & Febiger.

23. Borjesson M, Eriksson P, Dellborg M, et al: Transcutaneous electrical nerve stimulation in unstable angina pectoris, *Coron Artery Dis* 8:530, 1997.

24. Bove G, Nilsson N: Spinal manipulation in the treatment of episodic tension-type headache: a randomized controlled trial, *JAMA* 280:1576, 1998.

25. Branco K, Naeser M: Carpal tunnel syndrome: clinical outcome after low-level laser acupuncture, microamps transcutaneous electrical nerve stimulation, and other alternative therapies—an open protocol study, *J Altern Complement Med* 5:5, 1999.

26. Bronfort G, Evans R, Anderson AV, et al: Nonoperative treatments for sciatica: a pilot study for a randomized clinical trial, *J Manipulative Physiol Ther* 23:536, 2000.

27. Bronfort G, Evans R, Nelson B, et al: A randomized clinical trial of exercise and spinal manipulation for patients with chronic neck pain, *Spine* 26:788, 2001.

28. Bronfort G, Nilsson N, Assendelft WJJ, et al: Noninvasive physical treatments for chronic headache, Cochrane Library 1, 2002.

29. Broscious SK: Music: an intervention for pain during chest tube removal after open heart surgery, *Am J Crit Care* 8:410, 1999.

30. Buchman AL, O'Brien W, Ou CN, et al: The effect of arginine or glycine supplementation on gastrointestinal function, muscle injury, serum amino acid concentrations and performance during a marathon run, *Int J Sports Med* 20:315, 1999.

31. Buckelew SP, Conway R, Parker J, et al: Biofeedback/relaxation training and exercise interventions for fibromyalgia: a prospective trial, *Arthritis Care Res* 11:196, 1998.

32. Buckelew SP, Parker JC, Conway R, et al: The effects of biofeedback and exercise on fibromyalgia: a controlled trial, *Arch Phys Med Rehabil* 73:980, 1992.

33. Burckhardt CS, Mannerkorpi K, Hedenberg L, et al: A randomized, controlled clinical trial of education and physical training for women with fibromyalgia, *J Rheumatol* 21:714, 1994

34. Burton AK, Tillotson KM, Cleary J: Single-blind randomised controlled trial of chemonucleolysis and manipulation in the treatment of symptomatic lumbar disc herniation, *Eur Spine J* 9:202, 2000.

35. Chen L, Tang J, White PF, et al: The effect of location of transcutaneous electrical nerve stimulation on postoperative opioid analgesic requirement: acupoint versus nonacupoint stimulation, *Anesth Analg* 87:1129, 1998.

36. Cherkin D, Deyo RA, Battie M, et al: A comparison of physical therapy, chiropractic manipulation, and provision of an educational booklet for the treatment of patients with low back pain, *N Engl J Med* 339:1021, 1998.

37. Cherkin D, Eisenberg D, Sherman KJ, et al: Randomized trial comparing traditional Chinese medical acupuncture, therapeutic massage, and self-care education for chronic low back pain, *Arch Intern Med* 161:1081, 2001.

38. Chesky KS, Russel IJ, Lopez Y, et al: Fibromyalgia tender point pain: a double-blind, placebo-controlled pilot study of music vibration using the music vibration table, *J Musculoskeletal Pain* 5:33, 1997.

39. Chopra A, Lavin P, Patwardhan B, et al: Randomized double blind trial of an ayurvedic plant derived formulation for treatment of rheumatoid arthritis, *J Rheumatol* 27:1365, 2000.

40. Chrubasik S, Kunzel O, Model A, et al: Treatment of low back pain with a herbal or synthetic anti-rheumatic: a randomized controlled study—willow bark extract for low back pain, *Rheumatology* 40:1388, 2001.

41. Cleeland CS, Syrjala KL: How to assess cancer pain. In Turk D, Melzack R, editors: *Pain assessment,* New York, 1992, Guilford Press.

42. Cohen FL: Postsurgical pain relief: patients' status and nurses' medication choices, *Pain* 9:265, 1980.

43. Collacott EA, Zimmerman JT, White DW, et al: Bipolar permanent magnets for the treatment of chronic low back pain, *JAMA* 283:1322, 2000.

44. Creamer P, Singh BB, Hochberg MC, et al: Sustained improvement produced by nonpharmacologic intervention in fibromyalgia: results of a pilot study, *Arthritis Care Res* 13:198, 2000.

45. Crider AB, Glaros AG: A meta-analysis of EMG biofeedback treatment of temporomandibular disorders, *J Orofac Pain* 13:29, 1999.

46. Cupal DD, Brewer BW: Effects of relaxation and guided imagery on knee strength, re-injury anxiety, and pain following anterior cruciate ligament reconstruction, *Rehabil Psych* 46:28, 2001.
47. Cypress BK: Characteristics of physician visits for back symptoms: a national perspective, *Am J Public Health* 73:389, 1983.
48. David J, Modi S, Aluko AA, et al: Chronic neck pain: a comparison of acupuncture treatment and physiotherapy, *Br J Rheumatol* 37:1118, 1998.
49. David J, Townsend S, Sathanathan R, et al: The effect of acupuncture on patients with rheumatoid arthritis: a randomized, placebo-controlled cross-over study, *Rheumatology* 38:864, 1999.
50. Deepak KK, Behari M: Specific muscle EMG biofeedback for hand dystonia, *Appl Psychophysiol Biofeedback* 24:267, 1999.
51. Deluze C, Bosia L, Zirbs A, et al: Electroacupuncture in fibromyalgia: results of a controlled trial, *BMJ* 305, 1992.
52. Donovan M, Dillon P, McGuire L: Incidence and characteristics of pain in a sample of medical surgical inpatients, *Pain* 30:69, 1987.
53. Dursun N, Dursun E, Kilic Z: Electromyographic biofeedback: controlled exercise versus conservative care for patellofemoral pain syndrome, *Arch Phys Med Rehabil* 82:1692, 2001.
54. Dyson-Hudson TA, Shiflett SC, Kirshblum SC, et al: Acupuncture and Trager psychophysical integration in the treatment of wheelchair user's shoulder pain in individuals with spinal cord injury, *Arch Phys Med Rehabil* 82:1038, 2001.
55. Edmonds SE, Winyard PG, Guo R, et al: Putative analgesic activity of repeated oral doses of vitamin E in the treatment of rheumatoid arthritis: results of a prospective placebo-controlled double-blind trial, *Ann Rheum Dis* 56:649, 1997.
56. Edwards AM, Blackburn L, Christie S, et al: Food supplements in the treatment of primary fibromyalgia: a double-blind, crossover trial of anthocyanidins and placebo, *J Nutr Environ Med* 10:189, 2000.
57. Eisenberg DM, Davis RB, Ettner SL, et al: Trends in alternative medicine use in the United States, 1990-1997: results of a follow-up national survey, *JAMA* 280:1569, 1998.
58. Eisenberg DM, Kessler RC, Foster C, et al: Unconventional medicine in the United States: Prevalence, costs, and patterns of use, *N Engl J Med* 328:246, 1993.
59. Enqvist B, Fischer K: Preoperative hypnotic techniques reduce consumption of analgesics after surgical removal of third mandibular molars: a brief communication, *Int J Clin Exp Hypn* 45:102, 1997.
60. Erickson P, Wilson R, Shannon I: Statistical notes. Years of healthy life. In *Healthy people 2000,* Report no 7, Centers for Disease Control and Prevention, National Center for Health Statistics, Washington, DC, 1995, US Department of Health and Human Services.
61. Ernst E, Harkness E: Spinal manipulation: a systematic review of sham-controlled, double-blind, randomized clinical trials, *J Pain Sympt Manage* 24:879, 2001.
62. Ernst E, White AR: Acupuncture as a treatment for temporomandibular joint dysfunction: a systematic review of randomized trials, *Arch Otolaryngol Head Neck Surg* 125:269, 1999.
63. Evans D: The effectiveness of music as an intervention for hospital patients: a systematic review, *J Adv Nurs* 37:8, 2002.
64. Ezzo J, Berman B, Hadhazy VA, et al: Is acupuncture effective for the treatment of chronic pain? A systematic review, *Pain* 86:217, 2000.
65. Faymonville ME, Fissette J, Mambourg PH, et al: Hypnosis as adjunct therapy in conscious sedation for plastic surgery, *Reg Anesth* 20:145, 1995.
66. Faymonville ME, Mambourg PH, Joris J, et al: Psychological approaches during conscious sedation. Hypnosis versus stress reducing strategies: a prospective randomized study, *Pain* 73:361, 1997.
67. Felhendler D, Lisander B: Pressure on acupoints decreases postoperative pain, *Clin J Pain* 12:326, 1996.
68. Ferrell BR, Schneider C: Experience and management of cancer pain at home, *Cancer Nurs* 11:84, 1988.
69. Field T, Peck M, Hernandez-Reif M, et al: Postburn itching, pain, and psychological symptoms are reduced with massage therapy, *J Burn Care Rehabil* 21:189, 2000.
70. Field T, Peck M, Krugman S, et al: Burn injuries benefit from massage therapy, *J Burn Care Rehabil* 19:241, 1998.
71. Fisher P, Scott DL: A randomized controlled trial of homeopathy in rheumatoid arthritis, *Rheumatology (Oxford)* 40:1052, 2001.

72. Flor H, Birbaumer N: Comparison of the efficacy of electromyographic biofeedback, cognitive-behavioral therapy, and conservative medical interventions in the treatment of chronic musculoskeletal pain, *J Consult Clin Psychol* 61:653, 1993.

73. Foley KM: The treatment of cancer pain, *N Engl J Med* 313:84, 1985.

74. Fors EA, Gotestam KG: Patient education, guided imagery and pain related talk in fibromyalgia coping, *Eur J Psychiatry* 14:233, 2000.

75. Fortin PR, Lew RA, Liang MH, et al: Validation of a meta-analysis: the effects of fish oil in rheumatoid arthritis, *J Clin Epidemiol* 48:1379, 1995.

76. Fratianne RB, Prensner JD, Huston MJ, et al: The effect of music-based imagery and musical alternate engagement on the burn debridement process, *J Burn Care Rehabil* 22:47, 2001.

77. Frenay MC, Faymonville ME, Devlieger S, et al: Psychological approaches during dressing changes of burned patients: a prospective randomised study comparing hypnosis against stress reducing strategy, *Burns* 27:793, 2001.

78. Freund BJ, Schwartz M: Treatment of whiplash associated with neck pain with botulinum toxin-A: a pilot study, *J Rheumatol* 27:481, 2000.

79. Funch DP, Gale EN: Biofeedback and relaxation therapy for chronic temporomandibular joint pain: predicting successful outcomes, *J Consult Clin Psychol* 52:928, 1984.

80. Furlan AD, Brosseau L, Welch V, et al: Massage for low back pain, Cochrane Library 1, 2002.

81. Gardea MA, Gatchel RJ, Mishra KD: Long-term efficacy of biobehavioral treatment of temporomandibular disorders, *J Behav Med* 24:341, 2001.

82. Gardner AW, Poehlman ET: Exercise rehabilitation programs for the treatment of claudication pain: a meta-analysis, *JAMA* 274:975, 1995.

83. Garfinkel MS, Singhal A, Katz WA, et al: Yoga-based intervention for carpal tunnel syndrome: a randomized trial, *JAMA* 280:1601, 1998.

84. Gaston-Johansonn F, Ohly KV, Fall-Dickson JM, et al: Pain, psychological distress, health status, and coping in patients with breast cancer scheduled for autotransplantation, *Oncol Nurs Forum* 26:1337, 1999.

85. Ghoname EA, Craig WF, White PF, et al: Percutaneous electrical nerve stimulation for low back pain, *JAMA* 281:818, 1999.

86. Ghoneim MM, Block RI, Sarasin DS, et al: Tape-recorded hypnosis instructions as adjuvant in the care of patients scheduled for third molar surgery, *Anesth Analg* 90:64, 2000.

87. Giles LGF, Muller R: Chronic spinal pain syndromes: a clinical pilot trial comparing acupuncture, a nonsteroidal anti-inflammatory drug, and spinal manipulation, *J Manipulative Physiol Ther* 22:376, 1999.

88. Ginandes CS, Rosenthal DI: Using hypnosis to accelerate the healing of bone fractures: a randomized controlled pilot study, *Altern Ther Health Med* 5:67, 1999.

89. Glover J, Dibble SL, Dodd MJ, et al: Mood states of oncology outpatients: does pain make a difference? *J Pain Sympt Manage* 10:120, 1995.

90. Goff LC, Pratt RR, Madrigal JL: Music listening and S-IgA levels in patients undergoing a dental procedure, *J Arts Med* 5:22, 1997.

91. Good M, Stanton-Hicks M, Grass JA, et al: Relaxation and music to reduce postsurgical pain, *J Adv Nurs* 33:208, 2001.

92. Good M, Stanton-Hicks M, Grass JA, et al: Relief of postoperative pain with jaw relaxation, music and their combination, *Pain* 81:163, 1999.

93. Grabowska MJ: The effect of hypnosis and hypnotic suggestion on blood flow in the extremities, *Polish Med J* 10:1044, 1971.

94. Grant DJ, Bishop-Miller J, Winchester DM, et al: A randomized comparative trial of acupuncture versus transcutaneous electrical nerve stimulation for chronic back pain in the elderly, *Pain* 82:9, 1999.

95. Grealish L, Lomasney A, Whiteman B: Foot massage: a nursing intervention to modify the distressing symptoms of pain and nausea in patients hospitalized with cancer, *Cancer Nurs* 23:237, 2000.

96. Greco CM, Rudy TE, Turk DC, et al: Traumatic onset of temporomandibular disorders: positive effects of a standardized conservative treatment program, *Clin J Pain* 13:337, 1997.

97. Green S, Buchbinder R, Barnsley L, et al: Acupuncture for lateral elbow pain, Cochrane Library 1, 2002.

98. Greenspan K, Lawrence PF, Esposito DB, et al: The role of biofeedback and relaxation therapy in arterial occlusive disease, *J Surg Res* 29:387, 1980.

99. Gregory SR, Piccolo N, Piccolo MT, et al: Comparison of propolis skin cream to silver sulfadiazine: a naturopathic alternative to antibiotics in treatment of minor burns, *J Altern Complement Med* 8:77, 2002.

100. Grunert BK, Devine CA, Sanger JR, et al: Thermal self-regulation for pain control in reflex sympathetic dystrophy syndrome, *J Hand Surg Am* 15:615, 1990.

101. Gupta S, Francis JD, Tillu AB, et al: The effect of pre-emptive acupuncture treatment on analgesic requirements after day-case knee arthroscopy, *Anaesthesia* 54:1204, 1999.

102. Haanen HCM, Hoenderdos HTW, vanRomunde LKJ, et al: Controlled trial of hypnotherapy in the treatment of refractory fibromyalgia, *J Rheumatol* 18:72, 1991.

103. Hains G, Hains F: A combined ischemic compression and spinal manipulation in the treatment of fibromyalgia: a preliminary estimate of dose and efficacy, *J Manipulative Physiol Ther* 23:225, 2000.

104. Hamza MA, Ghoname EA, White PF, et al: Effect of the duration of electrical stimulation on the analgesic response in patients with low back pain, *Anesthesiology* 91:1622, 1999.

105. Hamza MA, White PF, Ahmed HE, et al: Effect of the frequency of transcutaneous electrical nerve stimulation on the postoperative opioid analgesic requirement and recovery profile, *Anesthesiology* 91:1232, 1999.

106. Hamza MA, White PF, Craig WF, et al: Percutaneous electrical nerve stimulation: a novel analgesic therapy for diabetic neuropathic pain, *Diabetes Care* 23:365, 2000.

107. Hasenbring M, Ulrich HW, Hartmann M, et al: The efficacy of a risk factor-based cognitive behavioral intervention and electromyographic biofeedback in patients with acute sciatic pain: an attempt to prevent chronicity, *Spine* 24:2525, 1999.

108. Hattan J, King L, Griffiths P: The impact of foot massage and guided relaxation following cardiac surgery: a randomized controlled trial, *J Adv Nurs* 37:199, 2002.

109. Hoffman H, Patterson D, Carrougher G, Sharar S: Effectiveness of virtual reality pain control with multiple treatments, *Clin J Pain* 17:229, 2001.

110. Holbrook T: *The frequency of occurrence, impact, and cost of selected musculoskeletal conditions in the United States,* Chicago, 1984, American Academy of Orthopedic Surgeons.

111. Holroyd KA, Penzien DB: Client variables and the behavioral treatment of recurrent tension headache: a meta-analytic review, *J Behav Med* 9:515, 1986.

112. Holroyd KA, Penzien DB: Pharmacological versus non-pharmacological prophylaxis of recurrent migraine headache: a meta-analytic review of clinical trials, *Pain* 42:1, 1990.

113. Horton-Hausknecht JR, Mitzdorf U, Melchart D: The effect of hypnosis therapy on the symptoms and disease activity in rheumatoid arthritis, *Psychol Health* 14:1089, 2000.

114. Hulme J, Waterman H, Hillier VF: The effect of foot massage on patients' perception of care following laparoscopic sterilization as day case patients, *J Adv Nurs* 30:460, 1999.

115. Hyman RB, Feldman HR, Harris RB, et al: The effects of relaxation training on clinical symptoms: a meta-analysis, *Nurs Res* 38:216, 1989.

116. Inrich D, Behrens N, Molzen H, et al: Randomised trial of acupuncture compared with conventional massage and "sham" laser acupuncture for treatment of chronic neck pain, *BMJ* 322:1, 2001.

117. International Association for the Study of Pain, Subcommittee on Taxonomy: Pain terms: a list with definitions and notes on usage, *Pain* 8:249, 1979.

118. Jacobson AF: Intradermal normal saline solution, self-selected music, and insertion difficulty effects on intravenous insertion pain, *Heart Lung* 28:114, 1999.

119. James MJ, Cleland LG: Dietary n-3 fatty acids and therapy for rheumatoid arthritis, *Semin Arthritis Rheum* 27:85, 1997.

120. Jensen R, Gothesen O, Liseth K, et al: Acupuncture treatment of patellofemoral pain syndrome, *J Altern Complement Med* 5:521, 1999.

121. Jordon A, Bendix T, Nielsen H, et al: Intensive training, physiotherapy, or manipulation for patients with chronic neck pain: a prospective, single-blinded, randomized clinical trial, *Spine* 23:311, 1998.

122. Kaboli PJ, Doebbeling BN, Saag KG, et al: Use of complementary and alternative medicine by older patients with arthritis: a population-based study, *Arthritis Rheum* 45:398, 2001.

123. Kaplan KH, Goldenberg DL, Galvin-Nadeau M: The impact of meditation-based stress reduction on fibromyalgia, *Gen Hosp Psychiatry* 15:284, 1993.

124. Karst M, Rollnik JD, Fink M, et al: Pressure pain threshold and needle acupuncture in chronic tension-type headache: a double-blind placebo-controlled study, *Pain* 88:199, 2000.

125. Keefe FJ, Caldwell DS: Cognitive behavioral control of arthritis pain, *Med Clin North Am* 81:277, 1997.

126. Keel PJ, Bodoky C, Gerhard U, et al: Comparison of integrated group therapy and group relaxation training for fibromyalgia, *Clin J Pain* 14:232, 1998.

127. Keller E, Bzdek VM: Effects of therapeutic touch on tension headache pain, *Nurs Res* 35:101, 1986.

128. Kivimaki J, Pohjolainen T: Manipulation under anesthesia for frozen shoulder with and without steroid injection, *Arch Phys Med Rehabil* 82:1188, 2001.

129. Kleinhenz J, Streitberger K, Windeler J, et al: Randomised clinical trial comparing the effects of acupuncture and a newly designed placebo needle in rotator cuff tendinitis, *Pain* 83:235, 1999.

130. Koch ME, Kain ZN, Ayoub C, et al: The sedative and analgesic sparing effect of music, *Anesthesiology* 89:300, 1998.

131. Koes BW, Assendelft WJJ, Van der Heijden GJMG, et al: Spinal manipulation for low back pain: an updated systematic review of randomized clinical trials, *Spine* 21:2860, 1996.

132. Kolcaba K, Fox C: The effects of guided imagery on comfort of women with early stage breast cancer undergoing radiation therapy, *Oncol Nurs Forum* 26:67, 1999.

133. Kotani N, Hashimoto H, Sato Y, et al: Preoperative intradermal acupuncture reduces postoperative pain, nausea and vomiting, analgesic requirement, and sympathoadrenal responses, *Anesthesiology* 95:349, 2001.

134. Kumar D, Alvaro MS, Julka IS, et al: Diabetic peripheral neuropathy: effectiveness of electrotherapy and amitriptyline for symptomatic relief, *Diabetes Care* 21:1322, 1998.

135. LaBan MM, Taylor RS: Manipulation: an objective analysis of the literature, *Orthop Clin North Am* 23:451, 1992.

136. Lang EV, Benotsch EG, Fick LJ, et al: Adjunctive non-pharmacological analgesia for invasive medical procedures: a randomised trial, *Lancet* 355:1486, 2000.

137. Langreth R: Science yields powerful new therapies for pain, *Wall Street J* sectionB, p 1, Aug 20, 1996.

138. Lao L, Bergman S, Hamilton GR, et al: Evaluation of acupuncture for pain control after oral surgery: a placebo-controlled trial, *Arch Otolaryngol Head Neck Surg* 125:567, 1999.

139. Launso L, Brendstrup E, Arnberg S: An exploratory study of reflexological treatment for headache, *Aletrn Ther Health Med* 5:57, 1999.

140. Le Gallez P, Dimmock S, Bird HA: Spiritual healing as adjunct therapy for rheumatoid arthritis, *Br J Nurs* 9:695, 2000.

141. Lee MM, Lin SS, Wrensch MR, et al: Alternative therapies used by women with breast cancer in four ethnic populations, *J Natl Cancer Inst* 92:42, 2000.

142. Leibing E, Leonhardt U, Koster G, et al: Acupuncture treatment of chronic low-back pain: a randomized, blinded, placebo-controlled trial with 9-month follow-up, *Pain* 96:189, 2002.

143. Leibing E, Pfingsten M, Bartmann U, et al: Cognitive-behavioral treatment in unselected rheumatoid arthritis outpatients, *Clin J Pain* 15:58, 1999.

144. Leventhal LJ, Boyce EG, Zurier RB: Treatment of rheumatoid arthritis with gamma linolenic acid, *Ann Intern Med* 119:867, 1993.

145. Lin Y-S, Taylor AG: Effects of therapeutic touch in reducing pain and anxiety in an elderly population, *Int Med* 1:155, 1998.

146. Little C, Parsons T: Herbal therapy for treating rheumatoid arthritis, Cochrane Library 1, 2001.

147. Lu DP, Lu GP, Kleinman L: Acupuncture and clinical hypnosis for facial and head and neck pain: a single crossover comparison, *Am J Clin Hypn* 44:141, 2001.

148. Luebbert K, Dahme B, Hasenbring M: The effectiveness of relaxation training in reducing treatment-related symptoms and improving emotional adjustment in acute non-surgical cancer treatment: a meta-analytical review, *Psychol Oncol* 10:490, 2001.

149. Lundgren S, Stenstrom CH: Muscle relaxation training and quality of life in rheumatoid arthritis: a randomized controlled clinical trial, *Scand J Rheumatol* 28:47, 1999.

150. Malone MD, Strube MI, Scogin FR: Meta-analysis of non-medical treatment for chronic pain, *Pain* 34:231, 1988.

151. Man D, Man B, Plosker H: The influence of permanent magnetic field therapy on wound healing in suction lipectomy patients: a double-blind study, *Plast Reconstr Surg* 104:2261, 1999.

152. Management of Cancer Pain Guideline Panel: Management of cancer pain. Clinical practice guideline no 9, AHCPR pub no 94-0592, Agency for Health Care Policy and Research, Public Health Service, Rockville, Md, 1994, US Department of Health and Human Services, 1994.

153. Mannix LK, Chandurkar RS, Rybicki LA, et al: Effect of guided imagery on quality of life for patients with chronic tension-type headache, *Headache* 39:326, 1999.

154. Manyande A, Berg S, Gettins D, et al: Preoperative rehearsal of active coping imagery influences subjective and hormonal responses to abdominal surgery, *Psychosom Med* 57:177, 1995.

155. Marcus DA, Scharff L, Mercer S, et al: Nonpharmacological treatment for migraine: incremental utility of physical therapy with relaxation and thermal biofeedback, *Cephalalgia* 18:266, 1998.

156. Marks RM, Sachar EJ: Undertreatment of medical inpatients with narcotic analgesics, *Ann Intern Med* 78:173, 1973.

157. Matheson JD, Clayton J, Muller MJ: The reduction of itch during burn wound healing, *J Burn Care Rehabil* 22:76, 2001.

158. Mauer MH, Burnett KF, Ouellette EA, et al: Medical hypnosis and orthopedic hand surgery: pain perception, postoperative recovery, and therapeutic comfort, *Int J Clin Exp Hypn* 47:144, 1999.

159. McLintock TT, Aitken H, Downie CF, et al: Postoperative analgesic requirements in patients exposed to positive intraoperative suggestions, *BMJ* 301:788, 1990.

160. Melchart D, Linde K, Fischer P, et al: Acupuncture for idiopathic headache, Cochrane Library 1, 2001.

161. Milne S, Welch V, Brosseau L, et al: Transcutaneous electrical nerve stimulation (TENS) for chronic low back pain, Cochrane Library 1, 2002.

162. Miró J, Raich RM: Effects of a brief and economical intervention in preparing patients for surgery: does coping style matter? *Pain* 83:471, 1999.

163. Mishra KD, Gatchel RJ, Gardea MA: The relative efficacy of three cognitive-behavioral treatment approaches to temporomandibular disorders, *J Behav Med* 23:293, 2000.

164. Montgomery GH, DuHamel KN, Redd WH: A meta-analysis of hypnotically induced analgesia: how effective is hypnosis? *Int J Clin Exp Hypn* 48:138, 2000.

165. Montgomery GH, Weltz CR, Seltz M, et al: Brief presurgery hypnosis reduces distress and pain in excisional breast biopsy patients, *Int J Clin Exp Hypn* 50:17, 2002.

166. Morris KT, Johnson N, Homer L, et al: A comparison of complementary therapy use between breast cancer patients and patients with other primary tumor sites, *Am J Surg* 179:407, 2000.

167. Mueller HH, Donaldson CC, Nelson DV, et al: Treatment of fibromyalgia incorporating EEG-driven stimulation: a clinical outcomes study, *J Clin Psychol* 57:933, 2001.

168. Munshi AK, Hegde AM, Girdhar D: Clinical evaluation of electronic dental anesthesia for various procedures in pediatric dentistry, *J Clin Pediatr Dent* 24:199, 2000.

169. Murphy TP: Medical outcomes studies in peripheral vascular disease, *J Vasc Interv Radiol* 9:879, 1998.

170. Nachemson AL: Newest knowledge of low back pain: a critical look, *Clin Orthop* 279:8, 1992.

171. Nader T, Smith D, Dillbeck M, Schanbacher V et al: A double blind randomized controlled trial of Maharishi Vedic vibration technology in subjects with arthritis, *Front Biosci* 6:H7, 2001.

172. National Cancer Institute Workshop on Cancer Pain, Bethesda, Md, 1990.

173. National Institutes of Health Development Panel on Acupuncture, *JAMA* 280:1518, 1998.

174. National Institutes of Health: Technology assessment statement: Integration of behavioral and relaxation approaches into the treatment of chronic pain and insomnia, Bethesda, Md, 1995.

175. National Institutes of Health: Technology assessment statement: Management of temporomandibular disorders, Bethesda, Md, 1996.

176. Nelson CF, Bronfort G, Evans G, et al: The efficacy of spinal manipulation, amitriptyline and the combination of both therapies for the prophylaxis of migraine headache, *J Manipulative Physiol Ther* 21:511, 1998.

177. Olesen J, Bonica JJ: Headache. In Bonica JJ, editor: *The management of pain,* Malvern, Pa, 1990, Lea & Febiger.

178. Paice JA, Shott S, Oldenburg FP, et al: Efficacy of a vibratory stimulus for the relief of HIV-associated neuropathic pain, *Pain* 84:291, 2000.

179. Palinkas LA, Kabongo ML: The use of complementary and alternative medicine by primary care patients: a SURF*NET study, *J Fam Pract* 49:1121, 2000.

180. Patel M, Gutzwiller F, Paccaud F, et al: A meta-analysis of acupuncture for chronic pain, *Int J Epidemiol* 18:900, 1989

181. Patterson DR, Ptacek JT: Baseline pain as a moderator of hypnotic analgesia for burn injury treatment, *J Counsel Clin Psychol* 65:60, 1997.

182. Pellow JW, Brantingham JW: The efficacy of adjusting the ankle in the treatment of subacute and chronic grade I and grade II ankle inversion sprains, *J Manipulative Physiol Ther* 24:17, 2001.

183. Pfaffenrath V, Wessely P, Meyer C, et al: Magnesium in the prophylaxis of migraine: a double-blind placebo-controlled study, *Cephalalgia* 16:436, 1996.

184. Pittler MH, Ernst E: *Ginkgo biloba* extract for the treatment of intermittent claudication: a meta-analysis of randomized trials, *Am J Med* 108:276, 2000.

185. Pittler MH, Vogler BK, Ernst E: Feverfew for preventing migraine, Cochrane Library 1, 2001.

186. Portenoy RK, Hagen NA: Breakthrough pain: definition, prevalence and characteristics, *Pain* 41:273, 1990.

187. Preyde M: Effectiveness of massage therapy for subacute low-back pain: a randomized controlled trial, *Can Med Assoc J* 162:1815, 2000.

188. Price CIM, Pandyan AD: Electrical stimulation for preventing and treating post-stroke shoulder pain: *Cochrane Stroke Group, Cochrane Database of Systematic Reviews* Issue 3, 2002.

189. Pryse-Phillips WEM, Dodick DW, Edmeads JG, et al: Guidelines for the nonpharmacologic management of migraine in clinical practice, *CMAJ* 159:47, 1998.

190. Rao JK, Mihaliak K, Kroenke K, et al: Use of complementary therapies for arthritis among patients of rheumatologists, *Ann Intern Med* 131:406, 1999.

191. Redd WH, Montgomery GH, DuHamel KN: Behavioral intervention for cancer treatment side effects, *J Natl Cancer Inst* 93:810, 2001.

192. Renzi C, Peticca L, Pescatori M: The use of relaxation techniques in the perioperative management of proctological patients: preliminary results, *Int J Colorectal Dis* 15:313, 2000.

193. Rice BI, Schindler JV: Effect of thermal biofeedback-assisted relaxation training on blood circulation in the lower extremities of a population with diabetes, *Diabetes Care* 15:853, 1992.

194. Richards KC, Gibson R, Overton-McCoy AL: Effects of massage in acute and critical care, *Adv Pract Acute Crit Care* 11:77, 2000.

195. Robinson R, Darlow S, Wright SJ, et al: Is transcutaneous electrical nerve stimulation an effective analgesia during colonoscopy? *Postgrad Med J* 77:445, 2001.

196. Rokicki LA, Holroyd KA, France CR, et al: Change mechanisms associated with combined relaxation/EMG biofeedback training for chronic tension headache, *Appl Psychophys Biofeedback* 22:21, 1997.

197. Rompe JD, Riedel C, Betz U, et al: Chronic lateral epicondylitis of the elbow: a prospective study of low-energy shockwave therapy and low-energy shockwave therapy plus manual therapy, *Arch Phys Med Rehabil* 82:578, 2001.

198. Rosenburg M: *Conceiving the self,* ed 2, Malabar, Fla, 1986, Krieger.

199. Rowlingson JC, Hamill RJ: Concomitant chronic pain syndromes. In Hamill RJ, Rowlingson JC, editors: *Handbook of critical care pain management,* New York, 1992, McGraw-Hill.

200. Rowlingson JC, Kessler RC, Dane JR, et al: Adjunctive therapy for pain. In Hamill RJ, Rowlingson JC, editors: *Handbook of critical care pain management,* New York, 1992, McGraw-Hill.

201. Sarnoch H, Adler F, Scholz OB: Relevance of muscular sensitivity, muscular activity, and cognitive variables for pain reduction associated with EMG biofeedback in fibromyalgia, *Percept Mot Skills* 84:1043, 1997.

202. Sarrell EM, Mandelberg A, Cohen HA: Efficacy of naturopathic extracts in the management of ear pain associated with acute otitis media, *Arch Pediatr Adolesc Med* 155:796, 2001.

203. Sarzi-Puttini P, Comi D, Boccassini L, et al: Diet therapy for rheumatoid arthritis: a controlled double-blind study of two different dietary regimens, *Scand J Rheumatol* 29:302, 2000.

204. Saunders JT, Cox DJ, Teates CD, et al: Thermal biofeedback in the treatment of intermittent claudication in diabetes: a case study, *Biofeedback Self-Regul* 19:337, 1994.

205. Schafer E, Finkensiep H, Kaup M: Effect of transcutaneous electrical nerve stimulation on pain perception threshold of human teeth: a double-blind, placebo-controlled study, *Clin Oral Invest* 4:81, 2000.

206. Schappert SM: National Ambulatory Medical Care Survey: 1992 summary, *Vital Health Stat Adv Data* series 16, 1994.

207. Schiller L: Effectiveness of spinal manipulative therapy in the treatment of mechanical thoracic spine pain: a pilot randomized clinical trial, *J Manipulative Physiol Ther* 24:394, 2001.

208. Schoenberger NE, Shiflett SC, Esty ML, et al: Flexyx neurotherapy system in the treatment of traumatic brain injury: an initial evaluation, *J Head Trauma Rehabil* 16:260, 2001.

209. Schoenen J, Jacquy J, Lenaerts M: Effectiveness of high-dose riboflavin in migraine prophylaxis: a randomized controlled trial, *Neurology* 50:466, 1998.

210. Sharpe L, Sensky T, Timberlake N, et al: A blind, randomized, controlled trial of cognitive-behavioural intervention for patients with recent onset rheumatoid arthritis: preventing psychological and physical morbidity, *Pain* 89:275, 2001.

211. Shekelle PG, Adams AH, Chassin MR, et al: Spinal manipulation for low-back pain, *Ann Intern Med* 117:590, 1992.

212. Shlay JC, Chaloner K, Max MB, et al: Acupuncture and amitriptyline for pain due to HIV-related peripheral neuropathy: a randomized controlled trial, *JAMA* 280:1590, 1998.

213. Gao, S., Zhao, D., Xie, Y: A comparative study on the treatment of migraine headache with combined distant and local acupuncture points versus conventional drug therapy, *Am J Acupunct* 27:27, 1999.

214. Simon EP, Lewis DM: Medical hypnosis for temporomandibular disorders: treatment efficacy and medical utilization outcome, *Oral Surg Oral Med Oral Pathol Oral Radiol Endod* 90:54, 2000.

215. Solomon S, Elkind A, Freitag F, et al: Safety and effectiveness of cranial electrotherapy in the treatment of tension headache, *Headache* 29:445, 1989.

216. Somri M, Vaida SJ, Sabo E, et al: Acupuncture versus ondansetron in the prevention of postoperative vomiting, *Anaesthesia* 56:927, 2001.

217. Spiegel D, Bloom JR: Group therapy and hypnosis reduce metastatic breast carcinoma pain, *Psychosom Med* 45:333, 1983.

218. Stam HJ, McGrath PA, Brooke RI: The effects of a cognitive-behavioral treatment program on temporo-mandibular pain and dysfunction syndrome, *Psychosom Med* 46:534, 1984.

219. Starley IF, Mohmmed P, Schneider G, et al: The treatment of paediatric burns using topical papaya, *Burns* 25:636, 1999.

220. Stener-Victorin E, Waldenstrom U, Nilsson L, et al: A prospective randomized study of electro-acupuncture versus alfentanil as anaesthesia during oocyte aspiration in in-vitro fertilization, *Hum Reprod* 14:2480, 1999.

221. Stephenson NL, Weinrich SP, Tavakoli AS: The effects of foot reflexology on anxiety and pain in patients with breast and lung cancer, *Oncol Nurs For* 27:67, 2000.

222. Stjernberg L, Berglund J: Garlic as an insect repellent, *JAMA* 284:831, 2000.

223. Syrjala KL, Chapko ME: Evidence for a biopsychosocial model of cancer treatment-related pain, *Pain* 61:69, 1995.

224. Syrjala KL, Cummings C, Donaldson GW: Hypnosis or cognitive behavioral training for the reduction of pain and nausea during cancer treatment: a controlled clinical trial, *Pain* 48:137, 1992.

225. Syrjala KL, Donaldson GW, Davis MW, et al: Relaxation and imagery and cognitive-behavioral training reduce pain during cancer treatment: a controlled clinical trial, *Pain* 63:189, 1995.

226. Tanabe P, Thomas R, Paice J, et al: The effect of standard care, ibuprofen, and music on pain relief and patient satisfaction in adults with musculoskeletal trauma, *J Emerg Nurs* 27:124, 2001.

227. Taylor AG, Norris BN, Galper DI, et al: Comparative effects of postoperative massage and vibrational therapy on post-surgical outcomes: a randomized, controlled trial. In *Postoperative massage and vibration*, Charlottesville, 2002, University of Virginia.

228. Taylor H, editor: *The Nuprin pain report*, New York, 1985, Louis Harris & Associates.

229. Ter Riet G, Kleijnen J, Knipschild P: Acupuncture and chronic pain: a criteria-based meta-analysis, *J Clin Epidemiol* 43:1191, 1990.

230. Thompson D, Williams C, Kingsley M, et al: Muscle soreness and damage parameters after prolonged intermittent shuttle-running following acute vitamin C supplementation, *Int J Sports Med* 22:68, 2001.

231. Turk DC, Melzack RD: The measurement of pain and the assessment of people experiencing pain. In Turk DC, Melzack R, editors: *Handbook of pain assessment,* New York, 1992, Guilford Press.

232. Turner JG, Clark AJ, Gauthier DK, et al: The effect of therapeutic touch on pain and anxiety in burn patients, *J Adv Nurs* 28:10, 1998.

233. Tusek DL, Church JM, Strong SA, et al: Guided imagery: a significant advance in the care of patients undergoing elective colorectal surgery, *Dis Colon Rectum* 40:172, 1997.

234. Van Wieringen S, Jansen T, Smits MG, et al: Melatonin for chronic whiplash syndrome with delayed melatonin onset: randomised, placebo-controlled trial, *Clin Drug Invest* 21:813, 2001.

235. Vasudevan SV: Impairment, disability, and functional capacity assessment. In Turk DC, Melzack R, editors: *Handbook of pain assessment,* New York, 1992 Guilford Press.

236. Verhagen AP, de Vet HC, de Bie RA, et al: Balneotherapy for rheumatoid arthritis and osteoarthritis, *Cochrane Musculoskeletal Group, Cochrane Database of Systematic Reviews* Issue 3, 2002.

237. Vickers AJ, Fisher P, Smith C, et al: Homoeopathy for delayed onset muscle soreness: a randomised double blind placebo controlled trial, *Br J Sports Med* 31:304, 1997.

238. Vickers AJ, Fisher P, Smith C, et al: Homoeopathic *Arnica* 30x is ineffective for muscle soreness after long-distance running: a randomised, double-blind, placebo-controlled trial, *Clin J Pain* 14:227, 1998.

239. Vincent CA: A controlled trial of the treatment of migraine acupuncture, *Clin J Pain* 5:305, 1989.

240. Volker D, Fitzgerald P, Major G, et al: Efficacy of fish oil concentrate in the treatment of rheumatoid arthritis, *J Rheumatol* 27:2343, 2000.

241. Walach H, Lowes T, Mussbach D, et al: The long-term effects of homeopathic treatment of chronic headaches: 1 year follow up, *Cephalalgia* 20:835, 2000.

242. Wall PD, Melzack R: *Textbook of pain,* ed 4, New York, 1999, Churchill Livingstone.

243. Wang B, Tang J, White PF, et al: Effect of the intensity of transcutaneous acupoint electrical stimulation on the postoperative analgesic requirement, *Anesth Analg* 85:406, 1997.

244. Wedenberg K, Moen B, Norling A: A prospective randomized study comparing acupuncture with physiotherapy for low-back and pelvic pain in pregnancy, *Acta Obstet Gynecol Scand* 79:331, 2000.

245. Weinstein EJ, Au PK: Use of hypnosis before and during angioplasty, *Am J Clin Hypn* 34:29, 1991.

246. Weitz JI, Byrne J, Clagett P, et al: Diagnosis and treatment of chronic arterial insufficiency of the lower extremities: a critical review, *Circulation* 94:3026, 1996.

247. Welch V, Brosseau L, Shea B, et al: Thermotherapy for treating rheumatoid arthritis, Cochrane database, CD002826, 2001.

248. Werners R, Pynsent PB, Bulstrode CJK: Randomized trial comparing interferential therapy with motorized lumbar traction and massage in the management of low back pain in a primary care setting, *Spine* 24:1579, 1999.

249. White AR, Resch KL, Chan JC, et al: Acupuncture for episodic tension-type headache: a multicenter randomized controlled trial, *Cephalalgia* 20:632, 2000.

250. White PF, Craig WF, Vakharia AS, et al: Percutaneous neuromodulation therapy: does the location of electrical stimulation affect the acute analgesic response? *Anesth Analg* 91:949, 2000.

251. White PF, Li S, Chiu JW: Electroanalgesia: its role in acute and chronic pain management, *Anesth Analg* 92:505, 2001.

252. Wood TG, Colloca CJ, Matthews R: A pilot randomized clinical trial on the relative effect of instrumental (MFMA) versus manual (HVLA) manipulation in the treatment of cervical spine dysfunction, *J Manipulative Physiol Ther* 24:260, 2001.

253. Wright BR, Drummond PD: Rapid induction analgesia for the alleviation of procedural pain during burn care, *Burns* 26:275, 2000.

254. Yi-Kai L, Xueyan A, Fu-Gen W: Silver needle therapy for intractable low-back pain at tender point after removal of nucleus pulposus, *J Manipulative Physiol Ther* 23:320, 2000.

255. Zannetti S, L'Italien GJ, Cambria RP: Functional outcome after surgical treatment for intermittent claudication, *J Vasc Surg* 24:65, 1996.

256. Zurier RB, Rossetti RG, Jacobson EW, et al: Gamma-linolenic acid treatment of rheumatoid arthritis: a randomized, placebo-controlled trial, *Arthritis Rheum* 39:1808, 1996.

SUGGESTED READINGS

Barber J: *Hypnosis and suggestion in the treatment of pain,* New York, 1996, Norton.

Bensky D, Barolet R: *Chinese herbal medicine: formulas and strategies,* Seattle, 1990, Eastland Press.

Blumenthal M, Hall T, Rister R, et al, editors: Therapeutic monographs on medicinal plants for human use. In *The German Commission E monographs,* Austin, Texas, 1996, American Botanical Council.

Boik J: *Cancer and natural medicine: a textbook of basic science and clinical research,* Princeton, Minn, 1995, Oregon Medical Press.

Bonica JJ, editor: *The management of pain,* Malvern, Pa, 1990, Lea & Febiger.

Gatchel RJ, Turk DC, editors: *Psychological approaches to pain management,* New York, 1996, Guilford Press.

Hammill RJ, Rowlingson JC, editors: *Handbook of critical care pain management,* New York, 1994, McGraw-Hill.

Hilgard ER, Hilgard JR. *Hypnosis in the relief of pain,* New York, 1994, Brunner/Mazel.

Huang B, Wang Y: *Thousand formulas and thousand herbs of traditional Chinese medicine,* vol 2, Formulas, Harbin, China, 1993, Heilongjiang Education Press.

Jacobs J: *Encyclopedia of alternative medicine: a complete family guide to complementary therapies,* Boston, 1996, Journey Editions.

McCaffery M, Beebe A: *Pain: clinical manual for nursing practice,* St Louis, 1989, Mosby.

National Institute of Nursing Research: Symptom management: acute pain. In *National Nursing Research Agenda,* vol 6, NIH pub no 94-2421, National Institutes of Health, US Public Health Service, Bethesda, Md, 1994, US Department of Health and Human Services.

Newall CA, Anderson LA, Phillipson JD: *Herbal medicines: a guide for health-care professionals,* London, 1996, Pharmaceutical Press.

Tollison CD, Satterthwaite JR, Tollison JW, editors: *Handbook of pain management,* ed 2, Baltimore, 1994, Lippincott/Williams & Wilkins.

CHAPTER 11

Select Populations: Children

MAY LOO

◥ CAM Therapy Usage in Children

Users of complementary and alternative medicine (CAM) in the general population increased from 34% in 1990 to 42% in 1997.[96] A comprehensive survey in 1994 indicates that the number of children receiving CAM rose rapidly from approximately 2% in 1992 to 11% in 1994.[386] Four recent surveys focused on specific groups rather than the general pediatric population; two surveys revealed a high rate of CAM usage in children with cancer,[123,205] and two others focused on CAM usage in Hispanics, who often combine Western treatment with folk remedies.[312,346] There is growing evidence that the use of CAM has dramatically increased in the pediatric population in the United States, Canada, and western Europe,[25,71,104,130,290] although more recent statistics are not currently available.

Multiple factors influence parents to seek CAM for their children: word-of-mouth recommendations, fear of the side effects of medications, persistence of chronic conditions not well alleviated with conventional treatment, and preference for CAM philosophies and health beliefs.[46,386,425,427] Although most evidence indicates CAM usage in chronic disorders, increasing evidence indicates that CAM therapy also is used as adjunctive treatment for acute pediatric illnesses, from the common cold[312] to hospitalized illnesses,[13] and even for children in the pediatric intensive care unit (PICU).[285] CAM therapy is also given to a wide range of ages, from preterm infants in neonatal intensive care unit (NICU)[154] to adolescents[12,130] and even homeless youths.[40] A review conducted by Tufts University in 2000 indicated that more adolescents are turning to CAM for various conditions, including headaches, asthma, and dietary supplements for athletic events.[130] The autonomy of being able to obtain unregulated products and services is particularly attractive to the teenager.

There is no specific socioeconomic characteristic of CAM therapy patients, who range from affluent, well-educated populations[450] to ethnic, low-income groups.[39,331,445] In a 2001 prospective review of patients seeking consultations from the Center for Holistic Pediatric Education and Research in Boston, children with cancer constitute the majority, usually seeking CAM therapy as an adjunctive management for pain and other discomforts related to the oncologic illness or to medications.[207]

In the general pediatric population, *chiropractic* is the most common form of CAM treatment used by children. Reports indicate that children made up 1% of chiropractic patients in 1977 and 8% in 1985.[303] A survey of the Boston metropolitan area revealed that an estimated 420,000 chiropractic visits were made by children in 1998.[237] Childhood disorders being treated include pain, respiratory and gastrointestinal tract problems, ear infection, enuresis, and hyperactivity.[303] *Homeopathy* was the second most popular form of CAM therapy used by children in Spiegelblatt's 1994 report.[386] In 2001, however, the University of Pittsburgh found that homeopathy was the most common CAM therapy used by children who visited an emergency department (ED).[329] Also, in a 2000 survey of homeopathic practitioners in Massachusetts, children constituted one third of patient visits.[236]

Homeopathic remedies are highly diluted substances that induce self-healing. These remedies are readily available from a variety of sources, including some grocery stores. Although homeopathy may be safe and effective in many childhood conditions, many practitioners believe that homeopathic remedies are best used as adjunctive therapy to conventional medicine in chronic conditions and in acute disorders that respond poorly to conventional therapy.[197,198]

Acupuncture is the third most common therapeutic method used in children[386] but has the largest body of scientific data compared with other CAM therapies.[248] A Harvard survey of 47 patients with a median age of 16 years who received acupuncture treatment, which included needle insertion, moxa/heat, cupping, and magnets, reported that 67% of patients rated the therapy as pleasant and 70% thought treatment helped their symptoms.[209] Electrical stimulation, laser, heat, magnet methods, and acupressure or acumassage[324] are effective alternatives to needles for treating children with needle phobia. Acupuncture and *traditional Chinese medicine* (TCM) have been used in Asia and Europe to treat a wide spectrum of childhood illnesses. Their use in the United States has been recent but is growing rapidly in popularity.

Naturopathy ranks with acupuncture as the third most common complementary therapy used by children,[385] although scientific data are sparse. Currently, evidence-based information is limited about safety and efficacy of herbal remedies, especially in terms of dosage and application in infants and children, who may be more susceptible to some of the adverse effects and toxicities because of differences in physiology and immature metabolic enzyme systems.[293,412]

Other CAM treatments used in children include touch therapy (therapeutic touch), osteopathy, oligotherapy, and hypnosis. Religious practices such as prayer have also become prevalent in the pediatric population.[22] Children have reported the ability to readily feel energy field from touch therapy.[118] The increasing support for *therapeutic touch* (TT)[223,226] has been anecdotal with little scientific data. Approximately 9% of children receiving treatment with CAM therapies seek *osteopaths,*[386] who claim success in treating many common childhood conditions, including colic and otitis.[19] Approximately 4% of pediatric CAM visits are to *oligotherapists,*[386] who administer poorly absorbed trace elements such as copper, manganese, and zinc to improve

TABLE 11–1. **CAM THERAPIES FOR PEDIATRIC CONDITIONS**

Condition	Most Common Therapies	Supportive/Other Data
ADHD	Biofeedback	Improved attention, behavior, and cognition; effects last as long as 10 years[49,246,253,407]
	Acupuncture (laser)	Improved behavior and cognition, but ineffective in severe ADHD (pilot data)[249]
	TCM	Increased urinary neurotransmitter metabolites[464]
	Magnesium supplement	Decreased hyperactivity (200 mg/day)[390]
Allergies	Nutrition	Breast-feeding decreased atopy[451]
	Acupuncture	More effective (greater desensitization) in older teenagers[228]
Asthma	Hypnosis	Asthmatic children were more hypnotizable; reduced physician visits[68,217]
	TCM (oral)	Improved symptoms[170]
	TCM (patch)	Effective in acute atacks; antitussive/antiasthmatic herbal external preventive[400]
Colic	Chiropractic	Controlled colic[215]
	Massage (TT)	Empirically decreased colic[111]
Diarrhea (acute)	Homeopathy	Significant decrease in duration[182]
	Shallow acupuncture	Higher therapeutic effect than drugs[244]
Diarrhea (chronic)	TCM (individualized)	Eliminated symptoms; normalized stools[109]
Enuresis	Hypnotherapy	High success in uncontrolled studies[24,67,74,308-310] Longer dry period than with imipramine[21]
	Acupuncture	Effective alone; more effective with DDAVP[52]
	Chiropractic	Decreased enuretic symptoms[341]
	Oligoantigenic diet	Relapse with reintroduction of foods[281]
Immunization	Homeopathy	Parental preference over vaccination[379]
Otitis media	Homeopathy	Reduced pain; prevented relapses[124]
	Chiropractic	Decreased symptoms (1 chiropractor)[124]
Skin rashes	TCM	Widespread nonexudative eczema[373]
	Acupuncture	Effective for acne[456]
URI	Nutrition	Breast-feeding: less frequent, shorter bouts[251]
	Homeopathy	Ineffective in reducing symptoms[78]
	TCM	Effective in infants[465]

ADHD, Attention deficit–hyperactivity disorder; *TCM*, traditional Chinese medicine, Chinese herbs; *TT*, therapeutic touch; *URI*, upper respiratory tract infection; *DDAVP*, 1-deamino-8-D-arginine vasopressin.

health. *Relaxation training* and *imagery* are forms of hypnosis that have also been effective in children.[309] In fact, children seem to be able to learn relaxation training better and faster than adults.[122] Table 11-1 summarizes the CAM therapies most often used to treat various pediatric conditions. Box 11-1 lists additional and recent surveys and reviews of CAM therapies used to treat pediatric conditions.

◢ Immunizations

Vaccination is an essential component of pediatric well-child care and has both public health and educational ramifications because up-to-date vaccination is required for

---

BOX 11–1. Additional and Recent Surveys, Systematic Reviews, and Cochrane Reviews of CAM and Pediatrics

Fong DP, Fong LK: Usage of complementary medicine among children, *Australian Family Physician* **Apr 31(4):388, 2002.**
Survey data taken from public hospital indicated 33% of parents used CAM for their children. Vitamins were more popular than acupuncture and positive correlations existed between CAM use and inadequate vaccination. No correlation exists with age, complaint, duration of hospital stay, or previous number of admissions.

Glazener CMA, Evans JHC: Simple behavior: physical interventions for nocturnal enuresis in children, Cochrane Library 3, 2002 (Online: Update software).
Reward systems produce fewer wet nights and higher cure rates along with lower relapse rates when compared with controls. Importance of a medication comparison group is noteworthy.

Glazener CMA, Evans JHC: Alarm interventions for nocturnal enuresis in children, Cochrane Library 3, 2002 (Online: Update software).
Most of the studies were poorly done (22 trials selected; $n = 1125$). The groups using the alarm maintained dry condition although tricyclic medication was as effective.

Heuschkel R et al: Complementary medicine use in children and young adults with inflammatory bowel disease, *American Journal of Gastroenterology* **97(2):382, 2002.**
Of children with inflammatory bowel disease, 40% use CAM. Parental use and adverse effects from conventional therapies were best predictors of CAM use.

Moher D et al: Assessing the quality of reports of systematic reviews in pediatric complementary and alternative medicine, *Biomedical Central Pediatrics* **2(1):3, 2002.**
Evaluated quality of reviews ($n = 36$; 17 CAM pediatrics systematic reviews with 19 systematic reviews taken from conventional pediatrics evaluating the same disease.) It was reported that eligibility criteria and evaluation of CAM data were "good," but there was little description of how bias in the selections of major studies was avoided or how "validity" parameters could best be described. Many individual CAM studies failed to randomize subjects, so they were not included in the overall analysis. There seemed to be a disparity between individual CAM trials and their "combined" subsequent integration into any type of review and evaluation. Importantly, the Oxman and Guyatt validated scale was used to evaluate individual aspects of the systematic review, i.e., types of search methods used.[311a]

---

entering school.[50] As with all pharmaceutical products, however, vaccines have risks and can cause rare but serious adverse effects.[99] Controversy is ongoing regarding pediatric immunization schedules[347,375] and effectiveness of multiple-antigen vaccines.[85,105,321] At present, vaccine-preventable disease rates are at their lowest level ever. In 1999 in the United States there were only 86 reported cases of measles, 238 cases of rubella, one case of diphtheria, 33 cases of tetanus, and no wild polio.[103,421]

Vaccine safety is monitored closely. Adverse events are reported to the *Vaccine Adverse Event Reporting System* (VAERS), administered by the Centers for Disease Control and Prevention (CDC) and the U.S. Food and Drug Administration (FDA). Approximately 10,000 adverse cases are reported each year. Data are shared internationally by independent scientific experts on the Joint Committee on Vaccination and Immunization and committees of the Medicines Control Agency. Surveillance results in product withdrawal when there is clear evidence of a safety issue.[300] Currently, several serious pediatric conditions are controversially attributed to vaccination: immune compromise,[377] neurologic sequelae, autism, and Crohn's disease.

The medical community has expressed concern about the effects of vaccination on an immature immune system, especially in neonates.[419] Controversial debates are ongoing regarding the possible connection between vaccination and autoimmune illnesses, such as the association between measles and anti–hepatitis B virus (HBV) vaccines with multiple sclerosis. Tetanus toxoid, influenza vaccines, polio vaccine, and others have been related to autoimmune phenomena ranging from autoantibody production to full-blown illness, such as rheumatoid arthritis and Guillain-Barré syndrome. Recent evidence suggests that autism may be related to the immune system.[273]

The mechanism of autoimmune reactions after immunization has not yet been elucidated. One possibility is molecular similarity between some viral antigen (or other component of the vaccine) and a self-antigen. This similarity may be the trigger to the autoimmune reaction.[16,374]

Before 1991, whole-cell pertussis vaccine was used, composed of a suspension of formalin-inactivated *Bordetella pertussis* B cells. Convulsions occurred in 1 case to 1750 doses administered, and acute encephalopathy occurred rarely, at 10.5 cases per million doses administered. Sudden infant death syndrome (SIDS) and infantile spasms have also been suggested to be associated with diphtheria-pertussis-tetanus (DPT) vaccination.[103] In the 1970s, reports linking pertussis vaccine with infant brain damage attracted media attention,[227] which in turn caused great parental and professional anxiety; the immunization rate fell from 80% to 30%. Between 1976 and 1988, three major pertussis epidemics occurred in the United States, resulting in more than 300,000 hospitalizations and at least 70 deaths.[300] In countries such as Sweden, Japan, United Kingdom, Ireland, Italy, and Australia, antivaccine movements targeted pertussis whole-cell vaccines.[129]

Opponents to the pertussis vaccine have argued that the risks of vaccination outweigh the benefits.[103] The largest study to date conducted by the National Institute of Child Health and Human Development at the National Institutes of Health (NIH) revealed that SIDS was actually less likely to occur in recently vaccinated infants.[165] Another large study showed that the permanent neurologic sequelae due to pertussis vaccine are so rare as to be unquantifiable.[280]

Nevertheless, concerns about brain damage led to the development of *acellular* pertussis vaccine (DTaP) that contains purified, inactivated components of *B. pertussis* cells. This form is associated with a lower frequency of adverse events and is more effective in preventing pertussis disease. DTaP was first licensed for the fourth and fifth doses of the pertussis series in 1991 and for the primary series in 1996. Several studies conducted in Europe and Africa revealed that U.S.-licensed DTaP vaccines have efficacy ranging from 71% to 84%. Currently, only acellular pertussis vaccine is used.[103]

No encephalopathy has been reported. *Hypotonic hyporesponsive episode* (HHE) is the sudden onset of hypotonia, hyporesponsiveness, and pallor or cyanosis that occurs within 48 hours of vaccination, usually after pertussis vaccine administered to children under 2 years of age. HHE occurred in approximately 1 of every 1750 DTa vaccinations. The largest published report of 40,000 cases concluded that although HHE does occur after the administration of DTaP and other non–pertussis-containing vaccines, it is generally benign, self-limited, and nonrecurrent.[92]

The connection of encephalopathy with pertussis vaccine was biologically more plausible than the proposed link between pertussis, measles vaccines, and autism.[300] The incidence of autism has increased from 1 in 10,000 in 1978 to 1 in 300 in 1999 in some U.S. communities. A study of 60 autistic children suggests that autism may be caused by a pertussis toxin found in the DPT vaccine. The toxin separates the G-alpha protein from retinoid receptors, which are critical for vision, sensory perception, language processing, and attention—characteristic problems of autism. Those children most at risk have at least one parent with a preexisting G-alpha protein defect, presenting clinically with night blindness, pseudohypoparathyroidism, or adenoma of the thyroid or pituitary gland. Natural vitamin A may reconnect the retinoid receptors.[273] In recent years, discussion has increasingly centered on the controversy concerning the possible association of the measles-mumps-rubella (MMR) vaccine with autism and Crohn's disease.*

The Chinese were among the first populations to vaccinate, beginning with smallpox vaccine, which was injected intranasally. TCM considers most childhood illnesses to occur at superficial levels, and vaccination actually introduces pathogens, still considered energetically active, into deeper blood levels of the body. In addition, TCM also posits that the body can usually effectively handle only one process at a given time. When two separate processes occur at the same time, the human system could become overwhelmed, especially the tender system of an infant or a young child. Therefore, although multiple vaccines given at the same time are less traumatic for children and save nursing time, they can easily overwhelm an immature immune system and make the child weak and deficient.[352] Although the fear of epidemics motivates the Chinese to vaccinate all their children, TCM practitioners in the West often advise against immunization.[320]

There is discrepancy among the homeopaths regarding recommendation of conventional vaccines. A German questionnaire survey reported that homeopathic physicians generally do not refuse vaccinations but show a preference for the DPT vaccines.[239] A British survey conducted between 1987 and 1993 reported that preference for homeopathic remedies for illnesses and religion were the most common reasons parents refused immunization; 21% believed the risk of diseases to be less than the risk of vaccination and would seek homeopathic treatment if any illness developed in their children, and 17% believed that children "are protected by God and

---

*References 8, 33, 51, 59, 80, 81, 97, 98, 117, 279, 314, 409, 410, 430, 431.

not by vaccines."[379] A U.S. cross-sectional descriptive survey of 42 homeopathic practitioners and 23 naturopathic practitioners in Massachusetts revealed that the majority of the practitioners did not actively recommend immunizations.[236] Many homeopaths recommend homeopathic vaccines, which are not yet supported by scientific data.[399]

A random sample survey by mail of 1% of American chiropractors revealed that one third believe there is no scientific proof that immunization prevents disease, that vaccinations cause more disease than they prevent, and that contracting an infectious disease is safer than immunization.[66] A reported 81% believed that immunization should be voluntary and that spinal adjustment is a viable alternative. A cross-sectional, descriptive survey of 90 chiropractics in the Boston metropolitan area reported that only 30% actively recommended childhood immunization.[237]

The decision of whether or not to immunize a child is difficult for both parents and practitioners. The advantages of vaccination are difficult to refute, but the temporal relationship between immunization and side effects and the controversies surrounding potential risks are disconcerting. Although data are insufficient on CAM approaches to vaccination today, practitioners should be aware of the slow yet steady trend toward alternatives and should properly address parental concerns and questions regarding immunization.[348] Each practitioner needs to inform parents of the most up-to-date pros and cons of vaccination, be as objective as possible, put aside personal belief systems, and be supportive and understanding of whichever decision the parents make. Parents need to become as informed as possible, consider all the pros and cons, weigh the risks and benefits, and realize that ultimately they must live with the outcome of their decision.

▣ Upper Respiratory Tract Infections

The common cold is the most frequent infection in children in the United States and throughout the industrialized world.[394] A preschool-aged child has an average of 4 to 10 colds per year.

The clinical symptoms vary greatly without any correlation with specific viruses.[94,121] The majority of the symptoms are mild, consisting of rhinorrhea, sneezing, nasal congestion and obstruction, postnasal drip, and cough. There may often be additional symptoms of low-grade fever, sore throat, clear eye discharge, digestive discomfort, and general malaise.[180,213,276] Some common viruses that cause upper repiratory tract infections (URIs) include rhinovirus, coronavirus, adenovirus, respiratory syncytial virus (RSV), influenza virus, and parainfluenza virus.[101,121,139] Transmission varies with different viruses. For example, RSV spreads primarily through contact with symptomatic children and contaminated objects, whereas influenza spreads mainly through airborne droplets. The precise route of transmission for rhinovirus remains controversial.[139] The virulence of rhinovirus is maximum in infants before 1 year of age (median age 6.5 months)[327] and in immunocompromised children.[330] Wheezing is associated with RSV in children younger than 2 years of age and with rhinovirus in those over age 2.[338]

Simultaneous infection by more than one virus, such as RSV and adenovirus together, can also occur frequently in the pediatric population. Many children may also have associated bacterial infection, such as *Haemophilus influenzae* conjunctivitis.[327]

The viruses gain entry into host cells through specific viral surface proteins, which cause tissue injury and result in clinical disease.[432] Recent studies suggest that the host's response to the virus, not the virus itself, determines the pathogenesis and severity of the common cold. Proinflammatory mediators, especially the cytokines, appear to be the central component of the response by infected epithelial cells.[158,417] Specific viral diagnosis is not necessary because of the benign, self-limiting nature of the disease[294] and the prevalence of different viruses overlapping from fall to spring, which makes it difficult to determine precisely which virus or viruses are causing the symptoms.[121]

Current medical management of URI remains symptomatic, controversial, and in most cases, ineffective. Fluid, rest, humidifier, and saline nose drops constitute the mainstay of nonpharmacologic treatment. Topical adrenergic agents do not have systemic side effects, but overuse can result in rebound congestion.[84,114] Antihistamine and combinations of antihistamine with decongestants are the ingredients in at least 800 over-the-counter (OTC) cold remedies. The majority of studies have concluded that antihistamines are of marginal or no benefit in treating cold symptoms.[47,110,153,254,383] Dextromethorphan is an antitussive that is abundant in OTC formulations. Although this medication is reportedly safe when taken in the recommended dosages, there have been cases of "recreational" use by teenagers, and deaths by overdose have been reported.[291] Codeine is ineffective in controlling URI cough.[95]

Medications are often overprescribed, leading to higher health care costs[102] and dangerous side effects, such as greater antibiotic resistance.[257] More steroids are prescribed, which leads to a myriad of complications.[274] Although interferon has been shown to produce good protection against infection, the high doses necessary to produce a prophylactic effect are often associated with serious undesirable side effects, including nasal stuffiness, bloody mucus, and mucosal erosions,[213] and the trauma of daily intramuscular injection makes it an unlikely remedy for children.[169]

Research for new medical therapies for the common cold is directed toward increasing resistance to or immunity against the viruses. Histamine antagonists are not indicated in the common cold.[369] Antiinflammatory mediators[417] and specific antiviral agents[361] may be promising. Development of an effective vaccine against the common cold is unlikely because of the large number of viral serotypes.[213] *Rhinovirus*, for example, has at least 100 different immunotypes.[158] Although viral URI is a benign illness of short duration, it can lead to bacterial complications such as otitis media, sinusitis, lower respiratory tract infections, mastoiditis, and even meningitis.[330]

Scientific data on CAM treatment for the common cold are surprisingly sparse. In 1971, Linus Pauling carried out a meta-analysis of four placebo-controlled trials and concluded that vitamin C alleviates cold symptoms, but subsequent reviews indicated that the role of vitamin C in URI is still controversial.[146-148,199]

Although *breast-feeding* has been believed to protect against infection in infants, studies have been inconsistent in demonstrating its efficacy. In a 4-year prospective study that actively tracked breast-feeding and respiratory illnesses in 1202 healthy infants, breast-feeding was found to reduce significantly the duration of respiratory illnesses during the first 6 months of life.[75] A retrospective review from Saudi Arabia of randomly selected charts revealed that a direct correlation exists between duration of breast-feeding and frequency of URI in the first 2 years of life.[1] A hospital-based descriptive recall study from Sri Lanka examined the relationship between breast-feeding and morbidity from respiratory illnesses in infants. Of the 343 infants, 285 were admitted and 58 were controls. An inverse relationship was found between the length of breast-feeding and incidence of respiratory illnesses.[319] A nutritional study of 170 healthy newborns followed for 6 months demonstrated that breast-feeding lowers frequency and duration of acute respiratory tract infection compared with formula feeding.[251] A more recent Japanese study examined the incidence of pathogenic bacteria isolated from the throat of 113 healthy infants fed with different methods.[166] No pathogens were detected in breast-fed and mixed-fed infants, while *H. influenzae* and *Moraxella catarrhalis* were isolated from the oropharynx of formula-fed infants. The investigators suggest that breast milk may inhibit the colonization by respiratory bacterial pathogens of the throat of infants. The mechanism was thought to be enhancement of mucosal immunity against respiratory tract infection.

In addition to the presence of secretory immunoglobulin A (IgA), another mechanism may be the presence of complex carbohydrates in human milk. These glycoconjugates may exert various antipathogenic effects, such as inhibiting the binding of pathogens to the receptors and reducing the production of bacterial toxins.[299] However, a U.S. study that examined nasopharyngeal swabs from 211 infants at 1 month of age and swabs from 173 of these infants at 2 months of age (keeping environmental parameters similar, e.g., number of children in household, number of siblings in day care, proportion with recent URI) revealed that the exclusively breast-fed ($n = 84$) and exclusively formula-fed ($n = 76$) infants did not differ significantly in the number of pathogens.[196] A multicenter randomized trial was conducted in 31 hospitals in the Republic of Belarus.[228] Evaluation within the first year revealed that breast-feeding had no significant reduction in respiratory tract infection compared with the control group. A survey from Singapore of breast-feeding mothers at 6 months postpartum revealed no significant differences in the rates of URI between breast-fed and non–breast-fed infants.[64]

Data are sparse on acupuncture, herbal, and homeopathic remedies for treatment of URI, especially in children. Most data are uncontrolled, clinical reports. Current information on adults supports efficacy of acupuncture for treating the common cold.[172,311,454,462] *Acupuncture* has been shown to increase the velocity of the nasal mucociliary transport in chronic rhinitis patients.[454] One possible use of acupuncture in URI is its potential effect on the immune system.[322] When Chinese herbs were pasted onto acupoints for treating rhinitis and bronchitis in infant, serum immunoglobulin M (IgM), IgG, complement C3, and especially IgA levels increased.[461] Acupuncture has also been shown to increase T lymphocytes.[404] Even massaging local acupoints was effective in relieving symptoms and in enhancing immune functions, with increases in immune indices that persisted for at least 6 months.[466] One report of acu massage of only one point for just 30 seconds resulted in clinical relief from nasal congestion, even though there was no change in nasal airway resistance or airflow.[403] These reports are encouraging for parents because acupressure can be easily learned by nonprofessionals, is well tolerated by children of all ages (including infants), has no side effects, and costs nothing.

A clinical trial administering a nontoxic Chinese herbal mixture to 305 infants demonstrated more than 95.1% effectiveness in treatment of URI.[465] In a single-blind trial using a Chinese herb for acute bronchiolitis with serologic evidence of RSV, 96 hospitalized children were randomized into three treatment groups: herbs, herbs with antibiotics, and antibiotics alone. Herbal treatment was found to decrease symptoms and duration of illness without adverse effects.[218] In a randomized, controlled trial using an herbal mixture, 89 children in the treatment group demonstrated 92% efficacy versus 67% of 61 children in the control group.[255] There was no description in the abstract (original article in Chinese) of what constituted control (e.g., placebo herb, no treatment, conventional drugs) or what constituted efficacy (e.g., improvement in symptoms, duration, of illness). Further rigorous studies are needed to demonstrate safety and efficacy of herbal treatment.

A recent clinical trial that included children over age 12 years and used a fixed-combination homeopathic remedy for a mean 4.1 days of treatment reported that 81.5% reported subjective feelings of being symptom free or significantly improved without complaint of any adverse side effects.[4] A randomized, double-blind, placebo-controlled study from Great Britain of 170 children with a starting median age of 4.2 years in the experimental group and 3.6 years in the placebo group concluded that individually prescribed homeopathic remedies seem to be ineffective in reducing symptoms or decreasing the use of antibiotics in pediatric patients with URI.[78]

⚊ Otitis Media

Otitis media (OM) represents a continuum of conditions that include acute OM, chronic OM with persistent effusion, chronic suppurative OM, recurrent OM, unresponsive OM, and OM with complications.[28]

Acute otitis media (AOM) is most prevalent in young children 8 to 24 months of age. Approximately two thirds of all children will have had at least one episode of AOM before age 3 years, and half of them will have recurrences or chronic serous OM with effusion into early elementary school years.[132] By the time the child reaches adolescence, AOM occurs infrequently.[443] Almost one third of pediatric office visits are for treatment of AOM.[109] The most common etiologic factors are allergic rhinitis[72,336] and ascending bacterial or viral agents from the nasopharynx attributable to eustachian tube dysfunction. The most common viral culprits are RSV,[10] influenza virus,[153] and adenovirus.[108] Two thirds of middle ear infections are caused by bacteria.[109] The predominant organisms are pneumococci, *H. influenzae, M. catarrhalis,*[53,305,358,388] and group B streptococcus.[325] Bacterial pathogens adhere to mucous membranes, and colonization ensues.

The severity of infection or the response to the invading bacteria depends on the health of the child's immune system.[53] The humoral system is especially significant in protecting the middle ear cavity from disease, and the nasopharyngeal lymphoid tissues are the first line of defense against bacterial colonization.[335,359] The sterility of the eustachian tube and tympanic cavity depends on the mucociliary system and on secretion of antimicrobial molecules, such as lysozyme, lactoferrin, and beta-defensins.[313] Evidence indicates that a number of children with recurrent episodes of AOM have minor immunologic defects.[359] *Pneumococcus* is by far the most virulent of AOM bacteria. It causes approximately 6 million cases of OM annually in the United States.[468] Uncontrolled pneumococcal otitis can lead to meningitis.[416] The incidence of AOM is higher in winter and early spring.

Clinically, the child with AOM presents with earache and fever, usually accompanied by upper respiratory symptoms such as rhinorrhea. On otoscopic examination the tympanic membrane varies from hyperemia with preservation of landmarks to a bright-red, tense, bulging, distorted appearance. In advanced stages of suppuration the tympanic membrane ruptures with a gush of purulent or blood-tinged fluid from the ear.[108] Because viral or bacterial OM usually cannot be distinguished by otoscopic examination, AOM is usually treated empirically, using antibiotics such as amoxicillin that have a high concentration in the middle ear fluid.[214,224]

However, the widespread use of antibiotics has resulted in increasing resistance to the more common medications.[53,358] Currently, 10% of children with AOM are recalcitrant to antibiotic therapy.[277] The prevalence of resistant organisms tends to increase in the winter months.[43] Economically, treatment failure due to drug resistance has been responsible for further escalating the billions of dollars spent treating AOM.[287] In addition, antimicrobials suppress normal flora, which is beneficial to the host because the antibiotic can interfere with and therefore prevent pathogenic infections and may enhance recovery from URIs.[43] On the other hand, since the advent of antibiotics, complications such as mastoiditis and intracranial infections have significantly decreased.[297]

The current focus is on prevention of AOM. Breast-feeding confers lifesaving protection against infectious illness, including otitis.[134,156] *Pneumococcal conjugate vaccine* (PCV), approved in 2000 for use in the United States, covers the seven serotypes that account for about 80% of invasive infections in children younger than age 6 years. PCV was demonstrated to have more than 90% efficacy[468] and has resulted in a modest reduction of total episodes of AOM.[317] The goal of PCV is to prevent symptomatic infections in the middle ear and prevent colonization of the pneumococci that can cause subsequent middle ear infections.[41] PCV may eliminate nasopharyngeal carriage of pneumococci.[235] However, because PCV only prevents disease caused by the most common serotypes, there is concern that the nonvaccine serotypes will become more common, especially in children less than 2 years of age.[317]

An effective RSV vaccine for the infant and young child could greatly decrease OM disease.[10] Intranasal spray of attenuated viruses is currently under investigation, in the hope that early antiviral therapy would reduce the risk of OM after URI.[137,153]

Chronic otitis media with effusion (OME) is one of the most common diseases in childhood.[91] OME is associated with infection, eustachian tube obstruction, allergic or immunologic disorders, and enlarged adenoids.[108] The serous fluid still contains bacteria, such as *H. influenzae* and pneumococci.[48] OME has been implicated to be an immune-mediated disease[91] because immune complexes have been demonstrated in the middle ear effusion,[268] and highly organized lymphatic tissue has been found in the middle ear mucosa.[422]

The rationale for treating OME is prevention of recurrence of AOM. Currently, a once-daily antibiotic regimen is the recommended prophylaxis. The benefit is also weighed against the increasing risk of emergence of resistant bacteria.[134] When antibiotics fail to control recurrent OM, a short trial of prednisone may be prescribed. Surgery is recommended when medical treatment fails,[277] especially when the child has hearing loss.[305] Tympanostomy tubes appear to be beneficial in OME but are of less value in chronic suppurative otitis.[134] Increase in hearing loss has been reported with insertion of ventilation tubes.[144] Adenoidectomy is sometimes recommended,[193] especially after tympanostomy tube failure.[134]

Any safe and effective CAM therapy for OM would be an important contribution to the pediatric population. Large-scale, randomized, controlled studies for CAM treatment would need medical collaboration, especially for otoscopic examination and tympanometry.[366] In addition, since AOM has a high rate of spontaneous resolution, any clinical study must also prove that treatment effect is faster than natural improvement.

Although breast-feeding has been found to reduce URI, data concerning its association with frequency or duration of OM have been conflicting. Epidemiologic reports consistently provide evidence of protection of young children from chronic otitis with prolonged breast-feeding.[138] A U.S. study that followed 306 infants at well-baby visits in two suburban pediatric practices reported that the cumulative incidence of first OM episodes increased from 25% to 51% between 6 and 12 months of age in infants exclusively breast-fed versus 54% to 76% in infants formula-fed from birth.[89] There was a two-fold risk of first episodes of AOM or OME in formula-fed babies in the first 6 months. A Danish study that evaluated 500 infants using monthly questionnaires reported no statistical difference in the breast-fed versus formula-fed infants in incidence of OM.[355] An earlier Jewish study comparing 480 infants visiting a pediatric ED with 502 healthy infants found that breast-feeding significantly reduced infectious diseases, including OM in infants under 5 months of age.[76]

A study from Switzerland evaluated 230 children with AOM by administering individualized homeopathic medicine in the pediatric office.[119] If there was insufficient pain reduction after 6 hours, a second (different) homeopathic medicine was given. Antibiotics were given if there was lack of response to the second dose. Pain control was achieved in 39% of the patients after 6 hours, with another 33% after 12 hours. The resolution rate was 2.4 times faster than in placebo controls. No complications were observed in the study group.[119] In a U.S. double-blind, placebo-controlled pilot study, 75 children ages 18 months to 6 years with OME and ear pain and/or fever for more than 36 hours were randomized into individualized homeopathic medicine or placebo group.[181] No statistically significant results were noted. A British nonblinded, randomized pilot study was done with 33 children ages 18 months to 8 years who had OME and hearing loss greater than 20 dB and an abnormal tympanogram.[150] The results revealed that the homeopathy group had more children with a normal tympanogram, fewer referrals to specialists, lower antibiotic consumption, and a higher proportion with a hearing loss less than 20 dB at follow-up. However, the differences were not statistically significant. Further research with larger groups is needed for a definitive trial.

In a prospective, observational study carried out by one homeopath and four conventional ear-nose-throat (ENT) physicians, a single (nonindividualized) homeopathic remedy was compared with nasal drops, antibiotics, and antipyretics.[125] Children between 6 months and 11 years of age were included in the study. Homeopathic treatment was given to 103 children and conventional treatment to 28 children. Homeopathic remedies were found to be significantly more effective in reducing duration of pain and in preventing relapses. Because OM tends to affect predominantly young children, it would be more appropriate for studies to compare results in children of similar age rather than a wide range of ages, from infancy to preadolescence.

A retrospective, nonrandomized study of 46 children under 5 years of age receiving 3 weeks of treatment from a single chiropractor reported a decrease in OM symptoms. The limitations to this study included retrospection and a lack of comparison with the natural course of ear infections.[124]

An Israeli controlled clinical trial examined the efficacy and tolerance of ear drops made with naturopathic extracts in the management of AOM pain.[362] Ranging in age from 6 to 18 years, 103 children were randomized into the treatment group and control group using a conventional anesthetic ear drop. There was statistically significant improvement in both groups, indicating that the naturopathic ear drops were as effective as the anesthetic ear drops. The University of Arizona has initiated a study of the use of *echinacea,* a dietary supplement, in the prevention of recurrent OM.[261] Acupuncture data are lacking on treatment of OM in children.[411] The theoretical potential benefit of acupuncture would appear to be its effect on the immune system, as discussed in the section on URI.

◪ Allergies

Allergic rhinitis affects 5% to 9% of children.[113] *Perennial rhinitis* is related to allergens that children are exposed to continuously, such as animal dander, house dust mites, mold, and feathers. *Seasonal rhinitis* is related to seasonal pollenosis and rarely affects children under age 4 or 5 years.[100] Allergic diseases are major causes of morbidity in children of all ages,[437,447,448] and allergic rhinitis is a significant cause of middle ear effusions.[72,267,336,452] Conventional therapy usually consists of avoidance of allergens, use of air-clearing devices, desensitization shots, and medication with antihistamines and at times steroids, both of which are frequently abused.[179,200] Antihistamines may be beneficial when sneezing and itching are present.[114]

CAM therapy is common among children with allergic diseases in Sweden[155] and is becoming more popular in the United States, although scientific data specifically on children are still lacking. Physicians have become more aware of the importance of nutrition[384,424] and environmental factors in the development of allergic symptomatology in childhood.[289,396,446] A prospective, longitudinal study of healthy infants followed from birth to 6 years of age concluded that recurrent wheezing is less common in nonatopic children who were breast-fed as infants.[450] Hypnosis has been reported anecdotally to be effective in hay fever.[439]

Homeopathic efficacy has received increasing attention in recent years,[342] but data consist of adult studies. An international multicenter study involving 30 investigators in four countries and 500 patients with three diagnoses, including upper and lower respiratory tract allergies, concluded that homeopathy appeared to be at least as effective as conventional medicine.[345] Another multicenter study using a randomized, double-blind, placebo-controlled parallel group design also demonstrated that homeopathic preparations differ from placebo for allergic rhinitis.[408] Homeopathic remedies for allergic children are unsupported by scientific studies at this time.

An adult study using changes in conductance of specific acupuncture points for diagnosis and treatment demonstrated statistically significant changes that correlated with clinical improvement.[195] In a randomized study of 143 patients that included older teenagers, desensitization was compared with specific acupuncture treatment for allergic asthma, allergic rhinitis, or chronic urticaria. The study was ridden with multiple, tedious variables. The conclusion that acupuncture was significantly more effective than desensitization in improving symptoms and in reducing recurrence in all three conditions did not give a breakdown in age groups.[228] In a clinical report of 75 chronic allergic rhinitis cases that included three cases in children 6 to 10 years of age and 17 cases in 11- to 20-year-olds, two different acupuncture treatments were administered according to TCM diagnoses. There was a cumulative 40% cure rate without age differentiation.[454]

◘ Asthma

Asthma is the most common cause of chronic illness in childhood, with approximately 10% of children in the United States carrying the diagnosis.[259,297,442] A significant number of school days are lost because of asthma. A wide variation of incidence is found in different countries, with the highest rates in the United Kingdom, Australia, and New Zealand and the lowest rates in Eastern Europe, China, and India.[296,442] In recent years, prevalence of asthma is increasing worldwide, especially in children under 12 years of age.[17,382]

Although asthma can have onset at any age, 80% to 90% of asthmatic children have their first symptoms before 4 to 5 years of age.[297] Children up to age 4 years have distinct symptoms and require special consideration.[36] They have increased health service utilization, including a higher annual rate of hospitalization,[298] which has almost doubled in the United States from 1980 to 1992 for children 1 to 4 years of age.[17] The same trend is observed by other nations worldwide.[9,18] Among American children ages 5 to 14 years, asthma death rates almost doubled from 1980 to 1995.[17] New Zealand and Canada have observed a similar increase in severity and mortality.[73,387]

Asthma is a diffuse, reversible, obstructive lung disease with three major features: bronchial smooth-muscle spasm, edema and inflammation of the mucous membrane lining the airways, and intraluminal mucus plugs.[442] During the last two decades, chronic airway *inflammation,* rather than smooth muscle contraction alone, has been recognized as playing the key role in the pathogenesis of asthma in adults.[63,131] Although this association is less well established in children, recent guidelines for managing asthma in the pediatric population still have emphasized that treatment be directed toward the inflammatory aspects of the disease.[206,402,440] Chronic inflammation is caused by the local production of inflammatory mediators and an increase in recruitment of inflammatory cells, predominantly eosinophils and mast cells. Studies in young adults suggest that the chronic inflammation may be responsible for long-term pulmonary changes, including bronchial hyperresponsiveness, airway remodeling, and irreversible airflow obstruction. Because of difficulties in conducting studies in infants and young children, pediatric information is incomplete.[230] Limited studies have detected increases in inflammatory cells and thickening of the lung basement membrane in infants and young children and have found that asthmatic children have significantly lower lung function at 6 years of age compared with nonwheezers when both groups of children began with the same baseline at age 6 months. These data support the possible presence of an asthmalike inflammation at a very early age that is associated with nonreversible impairment of lung function.[263]

The excessive inflammatory changes indicate that asthma is caused by a poorly regulated "immunologic runaway response" that, instead of protecting the host, destroys normal structure. Increased concentrations of proinflammatory mediators, such as histamine and leukotrienes, are found in the airways as well as the blood and urine of asthmatic patients[131] during an acute attack and after allergen and exercise challenge.[34] Strong evidence correlates asthma with RSV infection; children who enter day nursery before age 12 months and who are exposed to viruses early in life have built up immunity, with decreased development of allergies.[88] In most children, whose asthma is triggered mainly by respiratory infections at a younger age, asthma symptoms appear to remit by the adolescent years.[263] In older children and teenagers, emotions play a significant role both as the cause of symptoms and as the result of interplay of a chronic illness affecting the child's self-image and family dynamics.[297]

The latest asthma management guidelines classify pediatric asthma into four groups of severity: mild intermittent, mild persistent, moderate persistent, and severe.[206] Mild intermittent asthma can be typified by *exercise-induced asthma,* a common pediatric condition. *Status asthmaticus,* defined as progressive respiratory failure that does not respond to conventional management, is becoming more prevalent in American children.[442]

Conventional treatments for pediatric asthma vary from allergen avoidance to state-of-the-art biochemical therapy. Avoiding allergens has been a successful management of asthma since the sixteenth century. Asthma is a much more complex problem today because of the increasing number of pollutants and chemicals in the environment that are potential allergens for children.[157] Parental education, especially in regard to smoking, can reduce hospital admissions.[449] Because infections that trigger asthma attacks are mostly viral,[31] antibiotics are not routinely indicated.

Medication consists primarily of bronchodilators and inhaled steroids, which are now justified as first-line therapy,[191] both as long-term management[402] and for acute attacks.[231] Because growth suppression due to inhaled corticosteroids has been well documented,[61] it is important to distinguish infants with early-onset asthma from those with transient wheezing.[469]

Recently, the FDA has also approved leukotriene receptor antagonists for use in asthmatic children under 4 years of age.[380] These agents counteract the hyperimmune response, resulting in diminished airway inflammation and decreased eosinophilia in the airway mucosa and peripheral blood.[34]

Parents turn to CAM for their asthmatic children because of drug side effects or fear of taking long-term medication, especially steroids.[11,62] A recent survey from Texas of 48 multicultural parents of children with asthma reported the usage of a variety of CAM therapies, including homeopathy, herbal therapy, vitamins, and massages. Hispanic parents were more likely to use herbal and massage therapies, whereas African-American parents often turned to prayers.[269] The relatively abundant studies on CAM therapy in asthma are on adults and often have flaws in methodology.

Significant improvement[15,308,310] and even complete cure[83] have been demonstrated with hypnosis, although most studies had weak designs. Hypnosis was recommended for children because they were found to be more hypnotizable,[68] but it is unclear whether the efficacy of hypnosis in asthmatic children is a reflection of children's greater suggestibility or a result of a more reversible disease process.[439] In a recent preschool program, 25 children ages 2 to 5 years received treatment with seven hypnotherapy sessions. The number of physician visits was reduced, and parental confidence in self-management skills increased.[217]

TCM has been used to treat asthma for centuries. Asthma epitomizes the Chinese medicine concept of "winter disease, summer cure," which means the best treatment for asthma should be given during the summer, when the child is symptom free. In China, many asthmatic children who were treated with herbal patches applied to acupoints during the summer had minimal or no symptoms during asthmatic seasons.[37,58,320]

Although several recent adult studies used herbs for asthma,[107] only two involved children. A controlled study comparing herbal treatment of 30 children with penicillin and aminophylline treatment of another 30 children revealed no significant difference in the response from the two groups.[242] A multicenter double-blind, placebo-controlled clinical herbal study from Taiwan evaluated 303 asthmatic children using TCM diagnoses.[170] The children were randomized into three different herbal and placebo groups. Although both groups showed improvement, the herbal groups showed greater improvement in symptomatology and in biochemical changes, such as increase in total T cells and decrease in histamine. An animal experiment using a 13-herb concoction revealed 99.1% efficacy in easing bronchial spasm.[170] Another animal study with an herbal preparation demonstrated strong smooth muscle relaxation through inhibition of histamine and acetylcholine.[242]

From the pediatric standpoint, it would be worthwhile to follow the development of external TCM approaches and noninvasive acupuncture. One clinical observation of pasting Chinese herbs to acupuncture points in 72 infants with acute bronchitis showed high cure and improvement rate, especially in infants.[461] Humoral immune substances, especially IgA, were found to be increased after treatment. Another clinical observation reported 78% efficacy in 46 children treated with external application of plasters made of herbal mixtures with antitussive and antiasthmatic properties and 88% efficacy in 17 children treated with antiasthmatic herbal patches. Success was also reported with a different herbal patch for acute attacks. The patches were well received by the children.[401]

Improvement from acupuncture treatment has been reported in asthmatic adults.[392,406,428,463] Despite methodologic weaknesses, it still seems that acupuncture may help asthma, especially drug-induced or allergic asthma.[439] In some European countries, almost a fourth of general practitioners believe in the efficacy of acupuncture in the treatment of asthma.[216] Its role in the United States is still controversial; some physicians accept acupuncture's effectiveness,[426] whereas others criticize data based on poorly conducted studies.[5]

The few current studies and clinical reports on acupuncture treatment of children with asthma are generally favorable.[168,457] A German practitioner reported good results treating asthmatic children using a simple acupuncture regimen in uncontrolled clinical experience.[145] One study demonstrated that although acupuncture did not affect the basal bronchomotor tone, when administered 20 minutes before exercise, acupuncture was shown to be effective in attenuating exercise-induced asthma,[128] which is common in children. One possible mechanism of acupuncture is in reducing the reflex component of bronchoconstriction, but not in influencing direct smooth muscle constriction caused by histamine.[460] For children who are fearful of or who cannot tolerate needles, safe and painless treatments such as cupping and auricular press pellets,[457] laser acupuncture,[288,292] and massage of acupuncture points[168] have also been found to be effective.

The most interesting future role for acupuncture in asthma lies in its potential both in stimulating an immune response and, more importantly, in regulating or modulating a hyperimmune response. At this time, ample biochemical data in the literature support the theory that acupuncture activates both the humoral and the cellular immune systems to protect the host.* Studies have also demonstrated that acupuncture can modulate the synthesis and release of proinflammatory mediators.[192,256,458] Current hypotheses suggest that this is most likely mediated through a common pathway connecting the immune system and the opioids,[30,321,363] which has been well known to be associated with analgesic effects of acupuncture.

Homeopathic remedies have been reported to be remarkably effective in asthma in adults,[120,345,427] and homeopathic doses of allergens have been shown to alleviate allergic symptoms and desensitize patients to allergens.[433] However, there is paucity of scientific data on homeopathy in both children and adults, as well as a lack of consensus among homeopaths as to the appropriate treatment, administration regimen, or

---

*References 86, 192, 306, 349, 360, 363.

potency for asthma.[439] Homeopathic practitioners believe that in chronic conditions such as asthma, homeopathic remedies can stimulate the child's innate healing ability, thereby leading to improvement.[197,198] Two recent large reviews on the role of homeopathy in clinical medicine concluded that, except for the occasionally demonstrated benefit, little scientific evidence exists to support the use of homeopathy in most clinical settings.[159,439] The availability of homeopathic, nutritional, and herbal remedies without a prescription is appealing to the asthmatic adolescent's desire for independence.[12]

In a number of European countries, chiropractic is often used for treatment of asthma.[186] One of the many difficulties in evaluating chiropractic efficacy lies in the varying abilities of the manual therapy practitioners. Natural human differences exist in manual applications and techniques. The practitioners have various training backgrounds, including physiotherapy, respiratory therapy, chiropractic, and osteopathy. A Danish questionnaire survey of 115 families with children up to age 7 years reported that 92% of parents who sought chiropractic help considered the treatment beneficial for their children.[77,423] An Australian survey reported that the most common CAM visits were to chiropractors.[87] A U.S. prospective, observer-blinded, clinical pilot evaluated 36 children from 6 to 17 years of age with mild to moderate persistent asthma for chiropractic treatment in addition to optimal medical management.[42] Children were randomized into treatment and sham spinal manipulative therapy (SMT) for 3 months. The children with combined SMT and medical treatment rated their quality of life substantially higher and their asthma severity substantially lower, and their improvements were maintained at 1-year follow-up. However, there were no significant changes in lung function or hyperresponsiveness. Further research is needed to determine which components of the chiropractic encounter are responsible for the improvements.

A controlled, patient-blinded trial of chiropractic manipulation for 91 children with mild or moderate asthma randomized the children into an active or a simulated chiropractic manipulation for 4 months.[20] Each subject was treated by 1 of 11 participating chiropractors, selected by the family according to location. No significant benefit was observed in the treatment group. A few studies in adults generated statistically insignificant data.[176] One study found subjective but not objective improvements in individuals with asthma who received treatment in a chiropractic clinic.[186] A 2001 systematic review revealed that the majority of the studies on SMT had poor methodology; the two good studies did not demonstrate significant differences between chiropractic SMT and sham maneuver.[167] The reviewers concluded that the evidence is still insufficient at this time to support the use of manual therapies for patients with asthma.

A German pilot study of 15 children ages 5 to 11 years with bronchial asthma combined relaxation using various techniques, including progressive muscle relaxation, autogenic training, fantasy travels, mantras, and periodic music, and demonstrated significant improvement in a number of pulmonary function parameters.[142] However, it is difficult to interpret the results because of the variety of techniques used.[143] A U.S. review of anecdotal reports indicated that massage therapy can improve asthmatic symptoms.[110-112]

◪ Diarrhea

Acute diarrhea is a common occurrence in the pediatric population and a significant cause of pediatric morbidity and mortality in both developed and underdeveloped countries.[79,302,354] Each year an estimated 54,000 to 55,000 U.S. children are hospitalized for diarrhea,[136] and more than 4 million infants and young children worldwide die of acute infectious diarrhea.[354] Infants under 3 months of age have the highest risk for hospitalization and mortality.[304] Children under age 3 years have an average of approximately 2.5 episodes of gastroenteritis per year in the United States.[143,302] Internationally, the average is approximately 3.3 episodes annually.[354] Both diagnosis and treatment continue to be problematic in the pediatric population.[260]

The infectious pathogens that cause acute diarrheal episodes in children include viruses, bacteria, and parasites.[229] Transmission is most likely through the fecal-oral route, from ingesting contaminated food or water,[434] or in infants and toddlers, by mouthing contaminated toys. The nature of food-borne diseases is changing as more mass-produced, minimally processed, and widely distributed foods result in nationwide and international outbreaks of diarrheal disease instead of just a few individuals who shared a meal.[143] A majority of the cases are caused by viral infections. Rotavirus is the most prevalent,[264] and human astrovirus (HAstV) is a significant cause of diarrheal outbreaks.[434] Frequently, children are co-infected by several viruses. Viral diarrhea tends to involve the small bowel, producing large, watery, but relatively infrequent stools.[82] These illnesses usually have short, self-limiting courses,[6] typically lasting 3 to 7 days.[264] However, the diarrheal bouts can be devastating to children with compromised immune systems or structural abnormalities of the gastrointestinal tract.[143]

The most common bacterial agents are enteropathogenic *Escherichia coli*, *Shigella/Salmonella*, and *Campylobacter*.[82,264] These are much more virulent pathogens that usually cause mucocal injury in the small and large intestines, producing frequent, often bloody stools containing leukocytes.[82] *E. coli* has become an important public health problem in recent years, causing more than 20,000 cases of infection and up to 250 deaths per year in the United States.[220,381]

Transmission of infection is most often linked to consumption of contaminated meat, water, unpasteurized milk, leafy lettuce, alfalfa sprouts, and goat's milk,[220,413] and exposure to contaminated water in recreational swimming sites.[413] The most common parasitic infection is *Giardia lamblia,* which often causes secretory diarrhea without blood[264] and frequently leads to chronic diarrhea.[161]

Diagnosis and treatment are still inconsistent. Because most acute diarrheal conditions are self-limited, physicians often do not obtain stool cultures or examination for ova and parasites because the results are not available sometimes for several days. Stool culture can identify different types of bacteria, but detection of specific enteropathogenic strains of *E. coli* requires specific serotyping that is not performed in routine stool cultures.[220] It is expensive, time-consuming, and often not sufficiently specific or sensitive and therefore is not recommended for routine diagnosis.[151]

The primary treatment focus is on correction of *dehydration,*[275] which is the most important cause of morbidity and mortality in acute diarrhea.[243] Oral rehydration treatment (ORT) with solutions containing appropriate concentrations of electrolytes and carbohydrates is recommended by the World Health Organization (WHO) and has significantly reduced mortality.[82,140,367] After rehydration, early refeeding with a lactose-free[82] or normal, age-appropriate diet[229] is important for reducing diarrheal duration, severity, and nutritional impact. Supplementation with specific dietary ingredients that are lost in diarrhea, such as vitamin A, zinc, and folate, is also recommended.[140]

Because most of the acute infectious diarrheal conditions are viral, patients do not require antimicrobial therapy.[326,333] The rotavirus vaccine was put on the market in the United States in October 1998. This vaccine, as the natural infection, decreases the risk of acute rotavirus diarrhea by 50% and the risk of severe diarrhea with dehydration by more than 70%.[367] Improving hygiene such as handwashing is also important, especially in day care.

Breast-feeding is one of the most important preventive measures.[351] Continuation of breast-feeding has been found to control acute diarrheal episodes[140] and lower the frequency and duration of acute diarrhea, especially in infants under 6 months of age.[251] A large-scale randomized trial was conducted in 31 hospitals in the Republic of Belarus. Evaluation within the first year revealed that breast-feeding significantly reduced the risk of gastrointestinal tract infection compared with the control group.[228] However, a survey from Singapore of breast-feeding mothers at 6 months postpartum revealed no significant differences in the rates of diarrheal diseases between breast-fed and non–breast-fed infants.[64]

Treatment with antimicrobial therapy must be instituted carefully and only with specific identification of pathogen and drug sensitivity. With the increasing frequency of antibiotic resistance, common antibiotics may be ineffective in patients with acute diarrhea.[143,351,367] Treatment of salmonellosis with antibiotics can prolong the carrier state and lead to a higher clinical relapse rate.[143] Injudicious antimicrobial therapy may also lead to susceptibility to other infections, enhance colonization of resistant organisms,[29,143] and disrupt the normal intestinal flora, the body's natural defense against infection.[270]

Homeopathy has the most convincing evidence of efficacy in treating diarrhea in children. A randomized, double-blind clinical trial comparing homeopathic medicine with placebo in the treatment of acute childhood diarrhea was conducted in Nicaragua in 1991. Eighty-one children 6 months to 5 years of age were given treatment with individualized homeopathic medicine. Standard ORT was also given. There was a statistically significant decrease in the duration of diarrhea in the treatment group.[182] Although criticisms of the study include homeopathic theory being inconsistent with scientific belief[378] and possible toxicity of the dilute homeopathic remedies,[210] the report was also praised for being an impressive,[54] well-designed[44] study that paves the way for future research into the efficacy of homeopathy and other CAM therapies.[115] Using the predefined measures based on the 1991 study, the same group of researchers more recently carried out a similar study and replicated the same findings of decrease in the duration of diarrhea and number of stools in 126 children in Nepal, ranging in age from 6 months to 5 years.[183]

A few studies have demonstrated effectiveness of *acupuncture* in pediatric diarrhea. The treatment protocols in point selections generally depend on TCM diagnoses, with the majority of points chosen on the two major digestive channels.[109,190,245,398,455] Acupuncture has also been shown to induce favorable anatomic and biochemical changes in improving intestinal peristaltic function and in enhancing both humoral and cellular immunity.[244]

A randomized study comparing *shallow* acupuncture treatment (needles inserted superficially and withdrawn swiftly) with drugs in 761 children ages 1 to 35 months reported significantly higher therapeutic effect in the acupuncture group.[244] The diagnosis and subsequent choice of points were based on TCM principles, not on stool culture results. Unlike the homeopathy study, this investigation grouped together patients with acute and chronic diarrhea. In a clinical trial using one Chinese herbal formula for treatment of acute diarrhea, there was significant reduction of symptoms and duration of diarrhea.[38] A clinical report of 20 years' application of a seven-herb concoction in 419 children demonstrated 96.4% improvement and 90% cure rate.[241] This nonrandomized, nonblinded report used TCM diagnoses that encompassed a variety of diarrheal conditions, including acute, chronic, infectious, and noninfectious diarrhea. The mechanisms were hypothesized as eliminating pathogenicity, improving immunity, accelerating intestinal digestion, and inhibiting intestinal peristalsis. In a clinical report comparing Chinese herbs to Western medicine in 158 children with diarrhea due to rotavirus, the herbs were reported to be superior and had a viral inhibitory rate of 71.43%, but no mention was made of the efficacy of conventional medicine.[435]

Chronic nonspecific diarrhea of childhood differs from acute diarrhea in that it is not associated with significant morbidity. Once potentially serious causes are excluded, appropriate diet can be instituted to minimize complications, and reasonable time is then allowed for spontaneous resolution.[414] In a nonrandomized clinical trial involving 30 children ages 3 months to 8 years with chronic diarrhea of 2 to 4 months' duration that was unresponsive to Western medicine and TCM, individualized acupuncture treatment eliminated symptoms and normalized stools.[109]

◼ Colic

Infantile colic is estimated to affect 20% to 30% of all infants under 4 months of age and remains a medical enigma of nature versus nurture. Colic may represent a heterogeneous expression of developmental variance, unmet biologic needs, psychologic or emotional distress from poor parent-infant interaction, intrinsic temperamental predisposition, colonic hypermotility,[278] or milk allergy.* Although colic is self-limiting by 3 to 4 months of age, treatment is mandated because the psychologic

---

*References 69, 133, 184, 185, 188, 204, 356.

consequences may result in a disturbed mother-infant relationship.[174,355] Evidence suggests that uncontrollable crying is the precipitating factor in many cases of infant abuse.[178,441]

Because the precise etiology is not understood, the therapeutic goal of Western medicine is not aimed at "curing" colic but at containment of the crying.[328] Removing cow's milk protein from the mother's diet, changing formula, and prescribing antispasmodic medications are the mainstays of conventional treatment and may be helpful.[69] Treatment is often directed toward behavioral changes in mothers. Parents may be referred for therapy to learn parenting and coping skills.

CAM treatments yield inconsistent results. Herbs have not yet been proven to be efficacious,[265] although a survey of 51 Hispanic mothers in an urban neighborhood in Texas revealed that herbal teas were commonly used for colic.[346] Evidence is controversial for chiropractic treatment of colic. A multicenter prospective, uncontrolled study of 316 colicky infants involving 73 chiropractors in 50 clinics in the United Kingdom for 3 months demonstrated efficacy with chiropractic SMT in controlling colic, as reported by mothers in 94% of cases.[215] A retrospective questionnaire study in 1985 revealed satisfactory results of chiropractic treatment in 90% of infants.[301] A randomized, blinded, placebo-controlled clinical trial of 100 infants with typical colic reported that chiropractic manipulation was no more effective than placebo.[307] However, a randomized, controlled, 2-week trial comparing SMT with the drug dimethicone demonstrated significantly better results in the chiropractic treatment group.[444]

Craniosacral therapists empirically claim success in treatment of colic.[19] Massage therapists have also found empirically that touch therapy can decrease severity of colic.[111] In a Finnish clinical trial, 58 infants less than 7 weeks of age perceived as colicky by their parents were randomized into an infant massage group ($n = 28$) and a crib vibrator group ($n = 30$).[173] Over 4 weeks there was no difference in the reduction of colicky crying between infants receiving massage and those with a crib vibrator, leading the investigators to conclude that the decrease of crying reflects more the natural course of early infant crying and colic than a specific effect of intervention. Therefore infant massage is not recommended as treatment for colic.

◪ Enuresis

Enuresis is defined as inappropriate or involuntary voiding during the night at an age when urinary control should be achieved.[7] Enuresis is a complex disorder with poorly understood pathogenicity and pathophysiology. It affects children worldwide,[297] with about 5 to 7 million children affected in the United States[281] and as many as 30% of school-age children in Italy.[48]

The condition is classified as *primary nocturnal enuresis* (PNE) when the child has never been dry at night or *secondary nocturnal enuresis* (SNE) when wetting follows a dry period, usually after an identifiable stress.[203,297] By age 8 years, 87% to 90% of children should have nighttime dryness.[65] In 85% of PNE patients, bedwetting is monosymptomatic, with a spontaneous remission rate of 15% per year of age. Both the etiology and the pathophysiology of enuresis are still not well understood.

Multiple factors may interplay: genetic and psychologic predispositions, delayed maturation of the central nervous system, sleep disorders, urinary reservoir abnormalities, detrusor-sphincter incoordination, and urine production disorders.[48]

Although enuresis is benign, treatment is warranted because of adverse personal, family, and psychosocial effects.[281,282] Nocturnal enuresis delays early autonomy and socialization because of a decrease in self-esteem and self-confidence and a fear of detection by peers. The child may be at increased risk for emotional or even physical abuse from family members.[368,438]

The conventional treatment modalities are still controversial. Because the vast majority of PNE cases resolve spontaneously with time, treatment should carry minimal or no risk. The *moisture alarm* is both safe and inexpensive and should be the treatment of choice in most cases[65,286,357] but is often the one least prescribed.[15,258] The medications imipramine and DDAVP were frequently chosen as first-line treatment choices. Adjunctive therapy may include bladder-stretching exercises, which have a success rate of 30%, and behavioral conditioning.[357]

Numerous CAM therapies are available for childhood enuresis; the most common are hypnosis, acupuncture, and biofeedback. Less common CAM therapies are chiropractic and nutrition management.

Hypnotherapy has been recognized by conventional practitioners as a potentially effective therapy.[262,286] Uncontrolled studies have reported high rates of success.[24,67,74,308,310] In one comparative study of imipramine and direct hypnotic suggestion with imagery for functional nocturnal enuresis in 5- to 16-year-old patients, 76% of the imipramine group and 72% of the hypnosis group had positive response.[21] After termination of treatment, the hypnosis group continued practicing self-hypnosis. At 9-month follow-up, 64% of the hypnosis group maintained dryness compared with only 24% of the imipramine group. Hypnosis and self-hypnosis were found to be less effective in younger children (ages 5 to 7 years) compared with imipramine treatment.

Hypnotherapy has the added advantage that nonphysician health care professionals, such as nurse practitioners, can easily learn the technique to help children.[163] A recent review of controlled studies reported promising findings for hypnosis in children with enuresis, but none of the interventions can currently qualify as efficacious. A major limitation is the lack of treatment specification via a manual of its equivalent.[283] The requirement that the child practice the self-hypnosis technique several times a day limits compliance with the program.[286]

Acupuncture has been used as an effective treatment for enuresis since at least the 1950s.[459] Current worldwide literature in general demonstrates its viability as either a primary or an adjunctive therapy for the enuretic child.* A Turkish clinical study on 162 subjects treated with electroacupuncture therapy reported a success rate of 98.2%.[418] Acupuncture has been found to be successful both in decreasing the occurrence of enuresis during treatment and in exerting a long-term effect after treatment.[35,48,370] Parents also report a decrease in sleep arousal threshold.[35] Although the

---

*References 23, 35, 48, 52, 61, 172, 175, 194, 281, 284, 370, 415, 453, 459.

precise mechanism of acupuncture is still unknown, a multidisciplinary approach that included acupuncture demonstrated on electroencephalography (EEG) that treatment normalized activities of the cerebral cortex.[415]

Data from China usually consist of clinical reports of large sample populations. Results in one study of 500 patients treated with acupuncture on only two body points demonstrated cure in 476 patients (98%), improvement in 14, and no response in 10 patients.[459] Number of treatments ranged from one to three in 453 patients and four to six in 23. Another study of 302 enuretic children ages 3 to 15 years (10 over 15 years; oldest 23 years) used TCM diagnosis of organ imbalance and different combinations of acupuncture points, with 10 treatments constituting one course.[453] The results showed that 221 patients were cured, 71 showed marked improvement, and 10 were "effectively" treated. Treatment using scalp acupuncture has also been reported to be successful. In one clinical study, 59 children ages 4 to 17 years were treated for 10 to 15 sessions, and some needed a second course.[61] Cure was obtained in 9 children, marked improvement in 27, improvement in 19, and no response in 4 children.

In all these clinical reports, subjects of a wide range of ages were included in the same study; the discussions were short and generalized, giving very few or no details about the children (e.g., types of enuresis, duration of enuresis, number of wet nights, types of improvement); the methods of treatment were laden with numerous variables (e.g., number of points, treatment courses).

A clinical study from Italy of 20 children with bladder instability due to uninhibited contractions of the detrusor muscle reported that acupuncture treatment was successful in gradual elimination of enuresis in 11 and improvement of symptoms in 7 children. The mechanism was not clarified.[284] A Russian clinical trial of using acupuncture specifically for enuresis due to neurogenic bladder dysfunction demonstrated that acupuncture was beneficial in 17 of 25 children.[194] In a clinical report of 54 enuretic children, short-term success in reducing wet nights was 55% with acupuncture versus 79% with DDAVP, whereas long-term success rates were 40% and 50%, respectively.[48] A Zagreb report of a clinical trial of acupuncture treatment on 37 children with mean age of 8 years who failed psychotherapy demonstrated a statistically significant decrease in enuresis even at 6 months after treatment.[350] A self-controlled regulating device operating on the principles of acupuncture was found to be effective in the treatment of nocturnal enuresis attributable to neurogenic bladder dysfunction.[233] A controlled clinical study of 40 children between 5 and 14 years of age randomly selected into four groups of 10: treatment with DDAVP alone, acupuncture alone, combined DDAVP with acupuncture, and placebo. Efficacy of treatment, expressed as a percentage of dry nights, was high in both DDAVP and acupuncture groups, but the combined-treatment group had the best results.[52]

A Scandinavian clinical trial used traditional Chinese acupuncture for treatment of primary persistent PNE in 50 children ranging in age from 9 to 18 years. The response rate was monitored at 2-week, 4-week, and 3-month intervals.[370] Within 6 months, 43 (86%) of children were completely dry and 2 (10%) were dry on at least 80% of nights, leading the clinicians to conclude that acupuncture is effective, with stable results. Another Scandinavian study investigated the efficacy of electroacupuncture in treating 25 children ranging in age from 7 to 16 years.[35] Twenty treatments were administered over 8 weeks. The number of dry nights consistently increased when the children were reevaluated at 3 weeks, 3 months, and 6 months after treatment. Five children had more than 90% reduction of wet nights at 6 months, and 65% had more dry nights at the 6-month follow-up.

A recent teaching round at the China Academy of Traditional Chinese Medicine in Beijing discussed successful acupuncture treatment of a complicated case of enuresis in a 16-year-old student who had previously failed both Western and Chinese medicines for his physical and emotional sequelae.[171] Using TCM diagnosis of organ imbalances, the treatment combined body acupuncture, scalp acupuncture, and auricular acupressure seed. The patient began improving after three treatments in the first week. He received 3 more weeks of treatment, with no recurrence of enuresis at 6-month follow-up.

Children are often unwilling to undergo needle acupuncture because of fear of pain,[61] prompting researchers to use noninvasive forms of acupuncture. Simple acumassage has been previously reported to be beneficial to the enuretic child.[21] An Austrian prospective, randomized trial evaluated efficacy of laser acupuncture versus desmopressin in 40 children over age 5 years with PNE.[337] At 6-month follow-up, the desmopressin-treated group had 75% success rate with complete resolution of symptoms, an additional 10% had a more than 50% reduction in wet nights, and 20% did not respond. The laser acupuncture group had 65%, 10%, and 15% rates, respectively. The results were not statistically significant. Therefore laser acupuncture should be considered as an alternative, noninvasive, painless, cost-effective, and short-term therapy in children with normal bladder function and high nighttime urine production.

Worldwide reports have demonstrated efficacy in treating enuresis with *biofeedback*,[164,250,318,332] which aims at learning or relearning of influence of involuntary functions.[266] A clinical study from Italy treated 16 boys and 27 girls ages 4 to 14 years with detrusor-sphincter dyssynergy. Biofeedback was successful in all the children, with SNE resolving significantly sooner than PNE and girls responding better than boys. Two-year follow-up still revealed an 87.18% success rate, with 80% at 4 years.[332] In a French study, 120 children with three predominant urinary disorders that included nocturnal enuresis were treated with biofeedback. Detrusor-sphincter discoordination was diagnosed in 33 children. Pelvic floor biofeedback produced excellent results in these children.[323]

Belgian investigators reported a clinical biofeedback study of 24 children with median age of 10.4 years who did not respond to anticholinergics.[164] Seventeen subjects had complete resolution of enuresis, six had a decrease in symptoms, and one child did not respond. At 6-month follow-up, two children in the cured group had recurrence of enuresis. Another study from Belgium also reported success in using biofeedback in 26 children with pseudo-detrusor-sphincter dyssynergy; 17 were completely cured, and 5 improved considerably.[266] A Spanish study used biofeedback to treat unstable detrusor in 65 enuretic children; complete disappearance of symptoms was seen in 70.5%, with improvement in 78.2%.[318]

In a U.S. report of 8 boys and 33 girls ages 5 to 11 years who underwent an average of 6 hours of biofeedback for nocturnal and diurnal enuresis, improvement was noted in 90% of nocturnal enuresis and 89% of diurnal enuresis.[272] Another U.S. clinical study used biofeedback for 21 children with dysfunctional voiding; 17 (81%) had an excellent response, 3 (14%) had a fair response, and 1 (5%) was too inconsistent to rate.[70] The average number of sessions to achieve a consistent urodynamic response was 3.7 (range 2 to 14). Average follow-up was 34 months (range 14 to 51 months). The investigators recommended biofeedback as an effective method that requires only a short period for treating dysfunctional voiding.[70]

All these worldwide studies were clinical reports, not randomized, controlled, blinded studies.

The efficacy of chiropractic manipulation in enuresis has been inconsistent. One clinical report identified an 8-year-old boy with functional enuresis who had successful treatment with manipulation.[37] In an uncontrolled study of 175 children ages 4 to 15 years, with responses monitored by parents, chiropractic manipulation resulted in only 15.5% success.[234] However, a randomized, controlled clinical trial of 57 children demonstrated that 25% of the treatment group had 50% or more reduction in enuretic symptoms, although the pretreatment to posttreatment change in wet night frequency was not statistically significant, and there was no long-term follow-up.[341] A comprehensive review of the literature revealed that SMT was no more effective than the natural regression of enuresis with age.[225]

Food allergy as a cause of enuresis has been in the literature for several decades.[106] A recent study of children with severe migraine or attention deficit disorder (ADD) included 21 children with enuresis. Oligoantigenic diets were successful in curing 12 children and improving enuresis in 4 other children. Relapse of wetting occurred when foods were reintroduced; the substances implicated most often were chocolate, citrus, fruits, and milk from cows.[281] Although no studies are available on naturopathic approaches, which focus on natural remedies (e.g., corn silk and tea, tea and honey), physicians should not dismiss parental opinion that these remedies may be safe and effective.

The future of treatment for enuresis should combine various methods to increase the probability of treatment success and minimize risk to the child.[281]

▧ Skin Rashes

Atopic dermatitis affects almost 10% of all children[56] and 20% of children ages 3 to 11 years.[201,202] It accounts for more than 30% of outpatient pediatric visits.[95] Most children with atopic dermatitis typically come to medical attention with cradle cap and facial and extremity rashes by age 2 to 3 months.[95]

Despite considerable research, the etiology of allergic disease remains poorly understood.[16] Allergic dermatitis can be thought of as an inherited skin "sensitivity" that reacts to various external allergens and changes in psychologic states.[357] Food causes atopic dermatitis in 50% of infants, 20% to 30% of young children, and 10% to 15% of children after puberty.[395] Topical steroids remain the main therapeutic method. Dermatologists tend to prescribe antibiotics and use potent topical steroids,[343] which are more readily absorbed in children and can result in hypothalamic-pituitary-adrenal axis suppression.[179] New immune modulators have shown promise in severe atopic dermatitis.[149,212]

CAM therapies are increasingly used for dermatitis,[127] although most of the information is in clinical reports, and research data are limited. A database review of 272 randomized clinical trials of atopic eczema covering at least 47 different interventions revealed that evidence is still insufficient to make recommendations on maternal allergen avoidance for disease prevention, herbs, dietary restrictions, homeopathy, massage therapy, hypnotherapy, or various topical CAM therapies.[162] A multicenter randomized clinical trial conducted in 31 hospitals in the Republic of Belarus reported that breast-feeding significantly reduced the risk of atopic eczema compared with the control group in the first year of life.[228]

Psoriasis was found to worsen with CAM treatments such as herbs, dietary manipulation, and vitamins.[116] Dietary management with evening primrose oil, rich in gamma-linolenic acid, has been found to be inconsistently effective in small studies. Fish oil supplements (enriched in n-3 polyunsaturated fatty acids) have also been used.[357]

Various herbs offer relief for eczema.[127] A placebo-controlled, double-blind trial used a Chinese herbal prescription specifically formulated for widespread nonexudative atopic eczema. Thirty-seven children were randomly assigned to 8-week active treatment and placebo, with an intervening 4-week "washout" period. The response to active treatment was significantly superior to placebo, without evidence of hematologic, renal, or hepatic toxicity.[373] The same investigators monitored the children over the following 12 months. Eighteen children had at least a 90% reduction in eczema, and five showed lesser degrees of improvement.[374] Two randomized, double-blind placebo-controlled trials from Singapore revealed that a concoction of 10 Chinese herbs was efficacious in the treatment of atopic dermatitis in both children and adults, and that the mechanism may be through the beneficial immunosuppressive effects. Toxicity is a concern, however, because exact dosing of the active derivatives is difficult to achieve.[339]

Acupuncture treatment of acne has been reported to be successful[247] in as many as 91.3% of adolescents given treatment.[456] Other TCM techniques have also been reported to be helpful.[57] A clinical trial treated 20 children with severe, resistant atopic dermatitis with hypnosis.[393] Nineteen showed immediate improvement, 10 maintained improvement in itching, and 9 maintained improvement in sleep disturbance 18 months after treatment.

Homeopathy is frequently used to treat dermatitis. In one homeopathic clinic in Israel, more than 80% of the patients expressed satisfaction with treatment. However, the authors of the survey believed that homeopathic medicine complements conventional medicine and is not an alternative.[316] Chiropractic treatment has also been sought by children for allergic problems.[303]

A small British study tested the hypothesis that massage with essential oils *(aromatherapy)* used as a complementary therapy in conjunction with normal medical treatment would help to alleviate the symptoms of childhood atopic eczema.[9] Eight children were randomized into the treatment group, who were massaged with oil, and the control group, massaged without essential oil. No significant difference was found between the two groups. There was a later deterioration of eczema in the oil massage group, suggesting allergic contact dermatitis provoked by the essential oils themselves.

N Attention Deficit–Hyperactivity Disorder

Attention deficit–hyperactivity disorder (ADHD) is the most common neurodevelopmental disorder of childhood, with a prevalence rate between 2% and 11%,[373] averaging about 5%.[14,371,405] The road constellation of hyperactive, inattentive, and impulsive symptoms combined with the multiple comorbid conditions makes the definition and ADHD controversial and the diagnosis flawed.[405] ADHD is a chronic, heterogeneous condition with academic, social, and emotional ramifications for the school-age child.[371] The disabling symptoms persist into adolescence in approximately 85% of children and into adulthood in approximately 50%.[14,32] There is a developmental pattern in the primary symptoms of the disorder; hyperactivity diminishes while attentional deficits persist or increase with age.[371]

The precise etiology of ADHD is still unknown, and assessment and management remain diverse. Medication continues to be the mainstay of treatment, with methylphenidate (Ritalin) the treatment of choice.[141] The tricyclic antidepressants were added as an alternative medication in the 1970s,[32] with clonidine, buspirone (Buspar), and other antidepressants and neuroleptics added to the list in the 1980s.[55,60] Although it is generally agreed that drugs are beneficial on a short-term basis, there is a paucity of data on the long-term efficacy and safety of medications, especially in children younger than 3 years of age. These drugs have not been shown to produce long-term gains academically or socially.[90]

Besides pharmacotherapy, a multimodal approach using a combination of drugs and other methods, such as *cognitive-behavioral therapy* (CBT), psychotherapy, social skills training, and school interventions, is frequently prescribed for ADHD. CBT represents the most widely used alternative to pharmacotherapy, although previous studies have shown disappointing results.[2,3,45,177] In 1992 the National Institutes of Mental Health (NIMH) began a 14-month, multisite clinical trial, the Multimodal Treatment Study of ADHD (MTA).[160,189] The results indicated that high-quality medication management (with careful titration and follow-up) and a combination of medication and intensive behavioral therapy were substantially superior to behavioral therapy and community medication management. There is slight advantage of combination of medication and behavioral therapy over medication alone. *Psychotherapy* can be an effective adjunct to medication[364,365] but usually requires a long-term commitment to several years of treatment.

Concerns about side effects of medication,[232,391] treatment acceptability,[27,334] and compliance are additional factors that complicate management of the ADHD child. Clearly, there is room to explore safe, acceptable, and relatively easy alternatives. Interest is increasing in more natural, holistic integrative approaches to ADHD.

Studies using CAM therapy for treating ADHD encompass more than the usual research difficulties because of the complexity and heterogeneity of the disorder, as well as subjective evaluation by parents and teachers of a wide range of 18 characteristics that may qualify for several different diagnoses. A majority of the CAM therapies to date continue to have mostly anecdotal and empiric evidence. The few well-designed studies include biofeedback, herbal medicines, dietary modifications or supplements, and acupuncture.[46]

Studies have demonstrated that there is a significant difference in baseline EEG measurements in children with attention deficit disorder (ADD) compared with normal-achieving preadolescent males. These differences occur mainly in the parietal region for on-task conditions[187] and in the cortex and corticothalamic excitatory and inhibitory interactions.[252,255] *Biofeedback* or *neurofeedback* is a technique for modifying neurophysiology for learning.[252] In 1991 a critical review of 36 studies in which biofeedback was used as a treatment for hyperactivity indicated that biofeedback alone had not been effectively evaluated, and methodologic problems limit generalizations that it may be applicable to the entire hyperactive population.[238] A 2001 review continues to indicate that although anecdotal and case reports cite promising evidence, methodologic problems coupled with a paucity of research preclude any definitive conclusions as to the efficacy of enhanced alpha and hemisphere-specific EEG biofeedback training.[340] Some recent studies using more sophisticated technology claim that neurofeedback can improve attention, behavior, and intellectual function in the child with ADD,[49,246,253] with measurable EEG improvement in the frontal/central cortex.[295] Its stabilizing effect has also been found to last as long as 10 years after treatment.[407]

Hypnotherapy and biofeedback do not appear to alter the core symptoms of ADHD but may be helpful in controlling secondary symptoms. These methods allow children to become active agents of their own coping strategies.[26]

DIET THERAPY

A mailed questionnaire survey of 381 children with ADHD with a 76% response rate reported that 69% were using stimulant medication and that 64% of the respondents used or were using a nonprescription therapy. Diet therapies constitute the most common CAM therapy (60%).[397] One review of CAM therapy lends support to individualized dietary management and specific trace element supplementation in some children with ADHD.[26]

Nutritional management of ADD includes elimination diet, megavitamins,[26,372] supplements, and trace element replacement. Simple sugar restriction seems ineffective.[14] The well-known Feingold diet eliminates natural salicylates, food colors, and artificial flavors. Studies have demonstrated mixed results.[211] Megavitamins were demonstrated to be ineffective in the management of ADD in a two-stage study with clinical trial and double-blind crossover. Potential hepatotoxicity is a major concern with use of megavitamins.[152]

In a recent longitudinal, nonrandomized clinical trial, 17 ADHD children were given a glyconutritional product containing saccharides known to be important in healthy functioning and a phytonutritional product containing flash-dried fruits and vegetables.[93] Five children were not receiving methylphenidate (Ritalin), six children were taking prescribed doses of methylphenidate, and the remaining six children had their medications reduced by half after 2 weeks. The glyconutritional supplement was administered for the entire 6 weeks, and the phytonutritional supplement was added after 3 weeks. The teachers and parents rated behavioral items for ADHD, oppositional defiant disorder, and conduct disorder. The conclusion was that the glyconutritional supplement decreased the number and severity of ADHD, associated ODD and CD symptoms, and side effects of medications during the first 2 weeks of the study; there was little further reduction with the addition of the phytonutritional supplement. The three groups did not differ statistically in degree or reduction of symptoms.[93] This 6-week study had too many variables and too few subjects without control for a definitive conclusion, although the concept of simple nutritional supplement is important to explore.

There is increasing interest in abnormality of fatty acid metabolism as the etiology of at least some features of ADHD.[344] These abnormalities can range from genetic abnormalities in the enzymes involved in phospholipid metabolism to symptoms that were reportedly improved after dietary supplementation with long-chain fatty acids.[436] In a randomized, double-blind, placebo-controlled trial of docosahexaenoic acid (DHA) supplementation, 63 children ages 6 to 12 years receiving stimulant medication were randomly assigned to receive DHA supplementation or placebo for 4 months. There was no significant improvement in the treatment group.[429]

Oligotherapy focuses on deficiency of trace elements in children with ADD.[221,389] In a Polish controlled clinical trial, magnesium deficiency was found in blood and in hair of hyperactive children.[390] Fifty 7- to 12-year-old ADD children were given a magnesium supplement of 200 mg/day for 6 months while the control group of 25 children continued on their medical regimen. Increase in magnesium contents in hair correlated with a significant decrease of hyperactivity in the treatment group, whereas hyperactivity actually intensified in the control group. The same investigators also found deficiencies of copper, zinc, calcium, and iron, with magnesium being the most common deficiency, in 116 children with ADHD.[389]

CHINESE HERBAL THERAPY

A thorough literature review of alternative treatments for ADHD identified 24 CAM therapies and reported that Chinese herbal treatment has promising pilot data.[14] A clinical trial using Chinese herbs in the treatment of 66 children with a diagnosis of hyperkinesia based on the American Psychiatric Association's *Diagnostic and Statistical Manual of Mental Disorders,* ed 3 revised (*DSM*-IIIR) criteria demonstrated 84.8% effectiveness in ameliorating hyperactivity and improved attention and school performance.[401] The herbal remedy was prepared according to the TCM diagnosis of common energetic (qi) imbalance found in these children. Clinical observations were substantiated by laboratory findings of significant increase in urinary content of norepinephrine, dopamine, dihydroxyphenylacetic acid, cyclic adenosine monophosphate, and creatinine.[401] In a randomized study, Chinese herbal treatment was found to be comparable to methylphenidate but had fewer side effects.[464] Research is currently being conducted to investigate the efficacy of herbal and homeopathic remedies because current evidence is inconsistent or lacking.[26]

In a prospective, randomized, double-blind pilot study funded by NIH that integrated *DSM*-IV diagnostic criteria, conventional theories of frontal lobe dysfunction, and neurotransmitter abnormalities with traditional Chinese theories of energetic imbalances, laser acupuncture was used in the treatment of ADHD in 7- to 9-year-old children.[249] Preliminary data on the six children in the treatment group showed promise in reducing signs and symptoms of ADHD. Using Conners scale as a weekly follow-up measure, improvement in classroom behavior was reflected by substantial drops in the teachers' scores before and after treatment in five of six children. The parents' scores dropped in three children but did not change in the other three children (Figures 11-1 and 11-2). One child was promoted to the gifted program, and another demonstrated marked improvement in learning disabilities.

HOMEOPATHY AND CHIROPRACTIC

There are no data at this time on homeopathic or chiropractic treatment of ADHD, although many practitioners claim anecdotal success with the use of homeopathic desipramine (Norpramin) and manipulation.

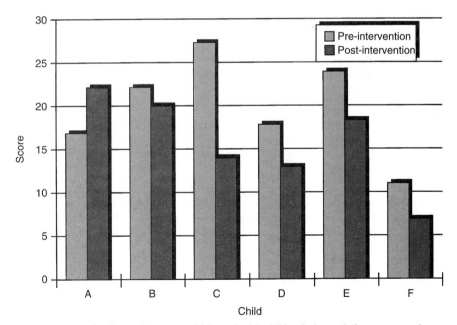

FIGURE 11-1. Teachers' scores (Conners scale) for each of six children before and after treatment of attention deficit–hyperactivity disorder (ADHD) by laser acupuncture.

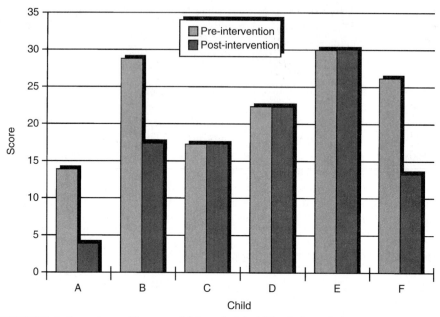

FIGURE 11–2. Parents' scores (Conners scale) for each of six children before and after treatment of ADHD by laser acupuncture.

N Physicians and CAM Therapy in Children

Pediatric use of CAM therapies continues to increase.[385] It is therefore advisable for physicians who treat children to take a thorough history of CAM use, especially in those with chronic disorders, to become knowledgeable about the various alternative therapies that can complement conventional care. This allows practitioners to consider possible adverse effects or interactions of CAM with conventional therapy, to open lines of communication with CAM providers, and even to consider integrating effective CAM therapy into their medical regimen. Although CAM therapy is in general considered safe, there have been a few reports of significant side effects.[219,271] Continuous research is needed to investigate the safety and efficacy of CAM therapies for children; to address explicitly the tremendous heterogeneity between and among the practices, beliefs, and providers of professional and lay services; and to study how CAM may enhance the quality of mainstream health services.[208]

Although children are entitled to new therapies, pediatric research in CAM is further complicated by children's vulnerability to violation of their personal rights and to risk exposure.[420] In children of the same age, varying cognitive capacity can be required for informed consent.[315,353] Differences in physiologic maturation can change the kinetics, end-organ responses, and toxicity of therapy, so data from adult studies cannot be extrapolated for children.[240] Even in conventional medicine, children are often rendered "therapeutic orphans"[376] because of history of abuses in pediatric research, a heightened sensitivity to risks in children—especially since the thalidomide disaster—and a limited market potential.[353] In the United States, 80% of drugs have age limits or contain disclaimers for pediatric use.[135] Therefore protecting children by giving them only scientifically proven therapies is counterbalanced by denying them access to possible safe and effective treatment that may not be proven for many years to come.

A frequently expressed concern is that visits to CAM practitioners may cause delay in diagnosis.[467] A more serious concern is the lack of formal pediatric training in many CAM therapists so that they may fail to recognize potentially serious illnesses, especially in infants.[236] Conventional medicine is endowed with superb technologic support for making physical diagnoses, whereas some CAM practitioners may claim the ability to diagnose a discomfort on an "energetic level" that is not yet defined biomedically. An integration of these disciplines should provide a better understanding of human health and disease. Currently, many medical centers are incorporating courses in CAM. When the gap between conventional medicine and CAM is bridged, delay in diagnosis can be minimized, and the common goal of finding safe and effective treatment for children can be achieved.

REFERENCES

1. Abdulmoneim I, Al-Ghamdi SA: Relationship between breast-feeding duration and acute respiratory infections in infants, *Saudi Med J* 22:347, 2001.
2. Abikoff H: Cognitive training in ADHD children: less to it than meets the eye, *J Learn Disabil* 24:205, 1991.
3. Abikoff H, Gittleman R: Hyperactive children treated with stimulants: is cognitive training a useful adjunct? *Arch Gen Psychiatry* 42:953, 1985.
4. Adler M: Efficacy and safety of a fixed-combination homeopathic therapy for sinusitis, *Adv Ther* 16:103, 1999.
5. Aldrige D, Pietroni PC: Clinical assessment of acupuncture in asthma therapy: discussion paper, *J R Soc Med* 80:222, 1987.
6. American Academy of Pediatrics, Committee on Drugs: Guidelines for the ethical conduct of studies to evaluate drugs in pediatric populations, *Pediatrics* 95:287, 1995.
7. American Academy of Pediatrics, Committee on Children with Disabilities: Counseling families who choose complementary and alternative medicine for their child with chronic illness or disability, *Pediatrics* 107:598, 2001.
8. Amin J, Wong M: Measles-mumps-rubella immunisation, autism, and inflammatory bowel disease: update, *Commun Dis Intell* 23:222, 1999.
9. Anderson C, Lis-Balchin M, Kirk-Smith M: Evaluation of massage with essential oils on childhood atopic eczema, *Phytother Res* 14:452, 2000.
10. Anderson LJ: Respiratory syncytial virus vaccines for otitis media, *Vaccine* 19(suppl 1):59, 2000.
11. Andrews L et al: The use of alternative therapies by children with asthma: a brief report, *J Paediatr Child Health* 34:131, 1998.
12. Angsten JM: Use of complementary and alternative medicine in the treatment of asthma, *Adolesc Med* 11:535, 2000.
13. Armishaw J, Grant CC: Use of complementary treatment by those hospitalised with acute illness, *Arch Dis Child* 81:133, 1999.
14. Arnold LE: Some nontraditional (unconventional and/or innovative) psychosocial treatments for children and adolescents: critique and proposed screening principles, *J Abnorm Child Psychol* 23:125, 1995.

15. Aronoff GM, Aronoff S, Peck LW: Hypnotherapy in the treatment of bronchial asthma, *Ann Allergy* 34:356, 1975.
16. Asher MI et al: International study of asthma and allergies in childhood (ISAAC): rationale and methods, *Eur Resp J* 8:483, 1995.
17. Asthma mortality and hospitalization among children and young adults: United States, 1980–1993, *MMWR* 45:350, 1996.
18. Asthma: United States, 1980–1987, *MMWR* 39:493, 1990.
19. Attlee T: Cranio-sacral therapy and the treatment of common childhood conditions, *Health Visitor* 67:232, 1994.
20. Balon J et al: A comparison of active and simulated chiropractic manipulation as adjunctive treatment for childhood asthma, *N Engl J Med* 339:1013, 1998.
21. Banerjee S, Srivastav A, Palan BM: Hypnosis and self-hypnosis in the management of nocturnal enuresis: a comparative study with imipramine therapy, *Am J Clin Hypn* 36:113, 1993.
22. Barnes LL, Plotnikoff GA, Fox K, Pendleton S: Spirituality, religion, and pediatrics: intersecting worlds of healing, *Pediatrics* 106(4 suppl):899, 2000.
23. Bartocci C, Lucentini M: [Acupuncture and micro-massage in the treatment of idiopathic nocturnal enuresis], *Minerva Med* 72:2237, 1981.
24. Baumann FW, Hinman F: Treatment of incontinent boys with non-obstructive disease, *J Urol* 111:114, 1974.
25. Baumann PH: [Academic medicine and complementary medicine differ from each other in reasoning and evaluation but not in goals], *Schweiz Rundsch Med Praxis* 83:1432, 1994.
26. Baumgaertel A: Alternative and controversial treatments for attention-deficit/hyperactivity disorder, *Pediatr Clin North Am* 46:977, 1999.
27. Bennett DS, Power TJ, Rostain AL, Carr DE: Parent acceptability and feasibility of ADHD interventions: assessment, correlates, and predictive validity, *J Pediatr Psychol* 21:643, 1996.
28. Berman S: Management of acute and chronic otitis media in pediatric practice, *Curr Opin Pediatr* 7:513, 1995.
29. Bernstein DI et al: Evaluation of rhesus rotavirus monovalent and tetravalent reassortant vaccines in U.S. children, *JAMA* 273:1191, 1995.
30. Bianchi M, Jotti E, Sacerdote P, Panerai AE: Traditional acupuncture increases the content of beta-endorphin in immune cells and influences mitogen induced proliferation, *Am J Chin Med* 19:101, 1991.
31. Bibi H et al: [Evaluation of asthmatic children presenting at emergency rooms], *Harefuah* 137:383, 1999.
32. Biederman J et al: A double-blind placebo-controlled study of desipramine in the treatment of ADD. I. Efficacy, *J Am Acad Child Adol Psychiatry* 28:777, 1989.
33. Birmingham K, Cimons M: Reactions to MMR immunization scare, *Nat Med* 4(5 suppl):478, 1998.
34. Bisgaard H: Pathophysiology of the cysteinyl leukotrienes and effects of leukotriene receptor antagonists in asthma, *Allergy* 56:7, 2001.
35. Bjorkstrom G, Hellstrom AL, Andersson S: Electro-acupuncture in the treatment of children with monosymptomatic nocturnal enuresis, *Scand J Urol Nephrol* 34:21, 2000.
36. Blessing-Moore J: Asthma affects all age groups but requires special consideration in the pediatric age group especially in children less than five years of age, *J Asthma* 31:415, 1994.
37. Blomerth PR: Functional nocturnal enuresis, *J Manipulative Phys Ther* 17:335, 1994.
38. Bo MQ, Zhang FR: Xi xie ting in the treatment of infantile diarrhea, *Chung-Kuo Chung Hsi I Chieh Ho Tsa Chih* 13:324, 1993.
39. Boutin PD, Buchwald D, Robinson L, Collier AC: Use of and attitudes about alternative and complementary therapies among outpatients and physicians at a municipal hospital, *J Altern Complement Med* 6:335, 2000.
40. Breuner CC, Barry PJ, Kemper KJ: Alternative medicine use by homeless youth, *Arch Pediatr Adolesc Med* 152:1071, 1998.
41. Briles DE et al: The potential for using protein vaccines to protect against otitis media caused by *Streptococcus pneumoniae*, *Vaccine* 19(suppl 1):87, 2000.

42. Bronfort G, Evans RL, Kubic P, Filkin P: Chronic pediatric asthma and chiropractic spinal manipulation: a prospective clinical series and randomized clinical pilot study, *J Manipulative Phys Ther* 24:369, 2001.

43. Brook I: Microbial factors leading to recurrent upper respiratory tract infections, *Pediatr Infect Dis J* 17(8 suppl):62, 1998.

44. Brown KH: Homeopathy study questions, *Pediatrics* 94:964, 1994 (letter).

45. Brown RT, Wynne ME, Medenis R: Methylphenidate and cognitive therapy: a comparison of treatment approaches with hyperactive boys, *J Abnorm Child Psychol* 13:69, 1985.

46. Brue AW, Oakland TD: Alternative treatments for attention-deficit/hyperactivity disorder: does evidence support their use? *Altern Ther Health Med* 8:68, 2002.

47. Cabenda SI et al: Serous otitis media (SOM): a bacteriological study of the ear canal and the middle ear, *Int J Pediatr Otol* 16:119, 1988.

48. Caione P et al: [Primary enuresis in children: which treatment today?], *Minerva Pediatr* 46:437, 1994.

49. Calhoun G Jr, Fees CK, Bolton JA: Attention-deficit hyperactivity disorder: alternatives for psychotherapy? *Percept Mot Skills* 79:657, 1994.

50. California Department of Health Services, Immunization Branch: New childcare and school entry varicella IZ requirement, January 2001.

51. Calman KC: Measles vaccination as a risk factor for inflammatory bowel disease, *Lancet* 345:1362, 1995.

52. Capozza N et al: [The treatment of nocturnal enuresis: a comparative study between desmopressin and acupuncture used alone or in combination], *Minerva Pediatr* 43:577, 1991.

53. Cappelletty D: Microbiology of bacterial respiratory infections, *Pediatr Infect Dis J* 17(8 suppl):55, 1998.

54. Carlston M: Homeopathic diarrhea trial, *Pediatrics* 1:159, 1995 (letter).

55. Casat CD, Pleasants DZ, Schroeder DH, Parler DW: Bupropion in children with attention deficit disorder, *Psychopharmacol Bull* 25:198, 1989.

56. Charlesworth EN: Practical approaches to the treatment of atopic dermatitis, *Allergy Proc* 15:269, 1994.

57. Chen D, Jiang N, Cong X: Forty-seven cases of acne treated by prick-bloodletting plus cupping, *J Tradit Chin Med* 13:185, 1993.

58. Chen K et al: Two hundred and seventeen cases of winter diseases treated with acupoint stimulation in summer, *J Tradit Chin Med* 20:198, 2000.

59. Chen RT, Destefano F: Vaccine adverse events: causal or coincidental? *Lancet* 351:611, 1998.

60. Chen SW, Vidt DG: Patient acceptance of transdermal clonidine: a retrospective review of 25 patients, *Cleve Clin J Med* 56:21, 1989.

61. Chen Z, Chen L: The treatment of enuresis with scalp acupuncture, *J Tradit Chin Med* 11:29, 1991.

62. Chipps BE, Chipps DR: A review of the role of inhaled corticosteroids in the treatment of acute asthma, *Clin Pediatr (Phila)* 40:185, 2001.

63. Chung KF: Non-invasive biomarkers of asthma, *Pediatr Pulmonol* 18(suppl):41, 1999.

64. Chye JK, Lim CT: Breastfeeding at 6 months and effects on infections, *Singapore Med J* 39:551, 1998.

65. Cochat P, Meunier P, Di Maio M: [Enuresis and benign micturition disorders in childhood. I. Diagnosis and management], *Arch Pediatr* 2:57, 1995.

66. Colley F, Haas M: Attitudes on immunization: a survey of American chiropractors, *J Manipulative Physiol Ther* 17:584, 1994.

67. Collison DR: Hypnotherapy in the management of nocturnal enuresis, *Med J* 1:52, 1970.

68. Collison DR: Which asthmatic patients should be treated by hypnotherapy? *Med J Aust* 1:776, 1975.

69. Colon AR, DiPalma JS: Colic: removal of cow's milk protein from the diet eliminates colic in 30% of infants, *Am Fam Physician* 40:122, 1989.

70. Combs AJ, Glassberg AD, Gerdes D, Horowitz M: Biofeedback therapy for children with dysfunctional voiding, *Urology* 52:312, 1998.

71. Cooper RA, Stoflet SJ: Trends in the education and practice of alternative medicine clinicians, *Health Affairs* 15:226, 1996.

72. Corey JP, Adham RE, Abbass AH, Seligman I: The role of IgE-mediated hypersensitivity in otitis media with effusion, *Am J Otolaryngol* 15:138, 1994.

73. Crane J et al: Prescribed fenoterol and death from asthma in New Zealand, 1981–83: case control study, *Lancet* 1:917, 1989.

74. Crasilneck HB, Hall JA: *Clinical hypnosis: principles and applications,* New York, 1996, Grune & Stratton, p 245.

75. Cushing AH et al: Breastfeeding reduces risk of respiratory illness in infants, *Am J Epidemiol* 147:863, 1998.

76. Dagan R, Pridan H: Relationship of breast feeding versus bottle feeding with emergency room visits and hospitalization for infectious diseases, *Eur J Pediatr* 139:192, 1982.

77. Danish Public Health Insurance statistics on chiropractic treatment. In *Sygesikringens Forhandlingsudvalg,* Copenhagen, 1980, Amstraadsforeningen.

78. De Lange de Klerk ES et al: Effect of homoeopathic medicines on daily burden of symptoms in children with recurrent upper respiratory tract infections, *BMJ* 309:1329, 1994.

79. DeSousa JS: [Acute infectious diarrhea in children], *Acta Med Port* 9:347, 1996.

80. DeStefano F, Chen RT: Autism and measles, mumps, and rubella vaccine: no epidemiological evidence for a causal association, *J Pediatr* 136:125, 2000.

81. DeStefano F, Chen RT: Negative association between MMR and autism, *Lancet* 353:1987, 1999.

82. DeWitt TG: Acute diarrhea in children, *Pediatr Rev* 11:6, 1989.

83. Diamond HH: Hypnosis in children: complete cure of forty cases of asthma, *Am J Hypn* 1:124, 1959.

84. Diamond L et al: A dose-response study of the efficacy and safety of ipratropium bromide nasal spray in the treatment of the common cold, *J Allergy Clin Immunol* 95:1139, 1995.

85. Dionne M et al: [Lack of conviction about vaccination in certain Quebec vaccinators], *Can J Public Health* 92:100, 2001.

86. Dong L et al: [Effect of HE-NE laser acupuncture on the spleen in rats], *Zhen Ci Yan Jiu* 21:64, 1996.

87. Donnelly WJ, Spykerboer JE, Thong YH: Are patients who use alternative medicine dissatisfied with orthodox medicine? *Med J Aust* 142:439, 1985.

88. Dubus JC, Bosdure E, Mates M, Mely L: [Virus and respiratory allergy in children], *Allergy Immunol (Paris)* 33:78, 2001.

89. Duffy LC et al: Exclusive breastfeeding protects against bacterial colonization and day care exposure to otitis media, *Pediatrics* 100:E7, 1997.

90. Dulcan MK: Using psychostimulants to treat behavioral disorders of children and adolescents, *J Child Adolesc Psychopharmacol* 1:7, 1990.

91. Dunne AA, Werner JA: [Status of the controversial discussion of the pathogenesis and treatment of chronic otitis media with effusion in childhood], *Laryngorhinootologie* 80:1, 2001.

92. DuVernoy TS, Braun NM: Hypotonic-hyporesponsive episodes reported to the Vaccine Adverse Event Reporting System (VAERS), 1996-1998, *Pediatrics* 106:E52, 2000.

93. Dykman KD, Dykman RA: Effect of nutritional supplements on attentional-deficit hyperactivity disorder, *Integr Physiol Behav Sci* 33:49, 1998.

94. Eccles R: Codeine, cough and upper respiratory infection, *Pulm Pharmacol* 9:293, 1996.

95. Eichinwald H, editor: *Pediatric therapy,* St Louis, 1993, Mosby.

96. Eisenberg DM et al: Trends in alternative medicine use in the United States, 1990-1997, *JAMA* 280(18):1569, 1998.

97. Ekbom A, Daszak P, Kraaz W, Wakefield AJ: Crohn's disease after in-utero measles virus exposure, *Lancet* 348:515, 1996.

98. Ekbom A, Wakefield AJ, Zack M, Adami HO: Perinatal measles infection and subsequent Crohn's disease, *Lancet* 344:508, 1994.

99. Ellenberg SS, Chen RT: The complicated task of monitoring vaccine safety, *Public Health Rep* 112:10, 1997.

100. Elliot FE, Ugazio AG: Allergies. In Eichinwald H, editor: *Pediatric therapy,* St Louis, 1993, Mosby.

101. El-Sahly HM, Atmar RL, Glezen WP, Greenberg SB: Spectrum of clinical illness in hospitalized patients with "common cold" virus infections, *Clin Infect Dis* 31:96, 2000.

102. English JA, Bauman KA: Evidence-based management of upper respiratory infection in a family practice teaching clinic, *Fam Med* 29:38, 1997.

103. *Epidemiology and prevention of vaccine-preventable diseases (The pink book),* ed 6, Waldorf, Md, 2001, Public Health Foundation.

104. Ernst E: Prevalence of complementary/alternative medicine for children: a systematic review, *Eur J Pediatr* 158:7, 1999.
105. Eskola J: Epidemiological views into possible components of pediatric combined vaccines in 2015, *Biologicals* 22:323, 1994.
106. Esperanca M, Gerrard JW: Nocturnal enuresis: comparison of the effect of imipramine and dietary restriction on bladder capacity, *Can Med Assoc J* 101:721, 1969.
107. Fedoseev GB et al: The correction of biological defects in bronchial asthma patients by the methods of Chinese medicine, *Terapevticheskii Arkhiv* 68:52, 1996.
108. Feigin R, Cherry JD: *Textbook of pediatric infectious diseases,* ed 3, Philadelphia, 1992, Saunders.
109. Feng WL: Acupuncture treatment for 30 cases of infantile chronic diarrhea, *J Tradit Chin Med* 9:106, 1989.
110. Field T: Massage therapy, *Med Clin North Am* 86:163, 2002.
111. Field T: Massage therapy for infants and children, *J Dev Behav Pediatr* 16:105, 1995.
112. Field TM: Massage therapy effects, *Am Psychol* 53:1270, 1998.
113. Fireman P: Diagnosis of allergic disorder, *Pediatr Rev* 16:178, 1995.
114. Fireman P: Pathophysiology and pharmacotherapy of common upper respiratory diseases, *Pharmacotherapy* 13:101S, 1993.
115. Fisher P et al: Homeopathic treatment of childhood diarrhea, *Pediatrics* 97:776, 1996 (letter).
116. Fleischer AB Jr et al: Alternative therapies commonly used within a population of patients with psoriasis, *Cutis* 58:216, 1996.
117. Fombonne E: Are measles infections or measles immunizations linked to autism? *J Autism Dev Disord* 29:349, 1999.
118. France NE: The child's perception of the human energy field using therapeutic touch, *J Holist Nurs* 11:319, 1993.
119. Frei H, Thurneysen A: Homeopathy in acute otitis media in children: treatment effect or spontaneous resolution? *Br Homeopath J* 90:180, 2001.
120. Frenkel M, Hermoni D: Effects of homeopathic intervention on medication consumption in atopic and allergic disorders, *Altern Ther Health Med* 8:76, 2002.
121. Freymuth F et al: [Epidemiology of respiratory virus infections], *Allergy Immunol (Paris)* 33:66, 2001.
122. Friebel V: Relaxation training for children—a review of the literature (German), *Praxis Kinderpsychol Kinderpsychiatrie* 43:16, 1994.
123. Friedman T et al: Use of alternative therapies for children with cancer, *Pediatrics* 100:E1, 1997
124. Friese KH, Kruse S, Moeller H: Acute otitis media in children, comparison between conventional and homeopathic therapy, *HNO (German)* 44:462, 1996.
125. Friese KH, Kruse S, Ludtke R, Moeller H: The homoeopathic treatment of otitis media in children: comparisons with conventional therapy, *Int J Clin Pharmacol Ther* 35:296, 1997.
126. Froehle RM: Ear infection: a retrospective study examining improvement from chiropractic care and analyzing for influencing factors, *J Manipulative Physiol Ther* 19:169, 1996.
127. Frost J: Complementary treatments for eczema in children, *Prof Nurse* 9:330, 1994.
128. Fung KP, Chow OK, So SY: Attenuation of exercise-induced asthma by acupuncture, *Lancet* 2:1419, 1986.
129. Gangarosa EJ et al: Impact of anti-vaccine movements on pertussis control: the untold story, *Lancet* 351:356, 1998.
130. Gardiner P, Wornham W: Recent review of complementary and alternative medicine used by adolescents, *Curr Opin Pediatr* 12:298, 2000.
131. Gaston B: Managing asthmatic airway inflammation: what is the role of expired nitric oxide measurement? *Curr Probl Pediatr* 28:245, 1998.
132. *Gellis & Kagan's current pediatric therapy,* vol 14, Philadelphia, 1993, Saunders.
133. Gerrard JW: Allergies in breastfed babies to foods ingested by the mother, *Clin Rev Allergy* 2:143, 1984.
134. Giebink GS: Otitis media prevention: non-vaccine prophylaxis, *Vaccine* 19(suppl 1):129, 2000.
135. Gilman J, Gal P: Pharmacokinetic and pharmacodynamic data collection in children and neonates, *Clin Pharmacokinet* 23:1, 1992.
136. Glass RC et al: The epidemiology of rotavirus diarrhea in the United States: surveillance and estimates of disease burden, *J Infect Dis* 174(suppl 1):5, 1996.

137. Glezen WP: Prevention of acute otitis media by prophylaxis and treatment of influenza virus infections, *Vaccine* 19(suppl 1):56, 2000.

138. Golding J, Emmett PM, Rogers IS: Does breast feeding protect against non-gastric infections? *Early Hum Dev* 49(suppl):105, 1997.

139. Goldmann DA: Transmission of viral respiratory infections in the home, *Pediatr Infect Dis J* 19(10 suppl):97, 2000.

140. Gracey M: Nutritional effects and management of diarrhoea in infancy, *Acta Pediatr Suppl* 88:110, 1999.

141. Greenhill LL: Pharmacologic treatment of attention deficit hyperactivity disorder: pediatric psychopharmacology, *Psychiatr Clin North Am* 15:1, 1992.

142. Groller B: [Effectiveness of combined relaxation exercises for children with bronchial asthma], *Kinderarztl Prax* 60:12, 1992.

143. Guerrant RL et al: Practice guidelines for the management of infectious diarrhea: Infectious Diseases Society of America, *Clin Infect Dis* 32:331, 2001.

144. Gundersen T et al: Ventilating tubes in the middle ear: long-term observations, *Arch Otolaryngol* 110:783, 1984.

145. Haidvogl M: [Alternative treatment possibilities of atopic diseases], *Padiatr Padol* 25:389, 1990.

146. Hamila H: Vitamin C and common cold incidence: a review of studies with subjects under heavy physical stress, *Int J Sports Med* 17:379, 1996.

147. Hamila H: Vitamin C intake and susceptibility to the common cold, *Br J Nutr* 77:59, 1997.

148. Hamila H: Vitamin C supplementation and common cold symptoms: problems with inaccurate reviews, *Nutrition* 12:804, 1996.

149. Hanifin JM et al: Recombinant interferon gamma therapy for atopic dermatitis, *J Am Acad Dermatol* 28:189, 1993.

150. Harrison H, Fixsen A, Vickers A: A randomized comparison of homoeopathic and standard care for the treatment of glue ear in children, *Complement Ther Med* 7:132, 1999.

151. Hart CA, Batt RM, Saunders JR: Diarrhoea caused by *Escherichia coli*, *Ann Trop Pediatr* 13:121, 1993.

152. Haslam RA, Dalby JT, Rademaker AW: Megavitamin therapy and attention deficit disorders, *Pediatrics* 74:103, 1984.

153. Hayden FG: Influenza virus and rhinovirus-related otitis media: potential for antiviral intervention, *Vaccine* 19(suppl 1):66, 2000.

154. Hayes JA, Cox CL: The integration of complementary therapies in North and South Thames Regional Health Authorities' critical care units, *Complement Ther Nurs Midwifery* 5:103,1999.

155. Hedros CA: [Alternative therapy is common among children with allergic diseases], *Lakartidningen* 85:3580, 1988.

156. Heinig MJ: Host defense benefits of breastfeeding for the infant: effect of breastfeeding duration and exclusivity, *Pediatr Clin North Am* 48:105, 2001.

157. Helfaer MA, Nichols DG, Rogers MC: Lower airway disease: bronchiolitis and asthma. In Rogers MC, Nichols DG, editors: *Textbook of pediatric intensive care*, ed 3, Baltimore, 1996, Williams & Wilkins, p 127.

158. Hendley JO: Clinical virology of rhinoviruses, *Adv Virus Res* 54:453, 1999.

159. Hill C, Doyon F: Review of randomised trials in homeopathy, *Rev Epidemiol Sante Publ* 38:138, 1990.

160. Hinshaw SP et al: Comprehensive assessment of childhood attention-deficit hyperactivity disorder in the context of a multisite, multimodal clinical trial, *J Atten Deficit* 1:217, 1997.

161. Hjelt K, Paerregaard A, Krasilnikoff PA: [Giardiasis in children with chronic diarrhea: incidence, growth, clinical symptoms and changes in the small intestine], *Ugeskr Laeger* 155:4083, 1993.

162. Hoare C, Li Wan Po A, Williams H: Systematic review of treatments for atopic eczema, *Health Technol Assess* 4:1, 2000.

163. Hobbie C: Relaxation techniques for children and young people, *J Pediatr Health Care* 3:83, 1989.

164. Hoekx L, Wyndaele JJ, Vermandel A: The role of bladder biofeedback in the treatment of children with refractory nocturnal enuresis associated with idiopathic detrusor instability and small bladder capacity, *J Urol* 160:858, 1998.

165. Hoffman HJ et al: Diphtheria-tetanus-pertussis immunization and sudden infant death: results of the National Institutes of Child Health and Human Development Cooperative Epidemiological study of sudden infant death syndrome risk factors *Pediatrics* 79(4):598, 1987.

166. Hokama T, Yara A, Hirayama K, Takamine F: Isolation of respiratory bacterial pathogens from the throats of healthy infants fed by different methods, *J Trop Pediatr* 45:173, 1999.

167. Hondras MA, Linde K, Jones AP: Manual therapy for asthma, *Cochrane Database Syst Rev* 1, CD001002, 2001.

168. Hossri CM: The treatment of asthma in children through acupuncture massage, *J Am Soc Psychosom Dent Med* 23:3, 1976.

169. Houglum JE: Interferon: mechanisms of action and clinical value, *Clin Pharmacol* 2:20, 1983.

170. Hsieh KH: Evaluation of efficacy of traditional Chinese medicines in the treatment of childhood bronchial asthma: clinical trial, immunological tests and animal study. Taiwan Asthma Study Group, *Pediatr Allergy Immunol* 7:130, 1996.

171. Hu J: Acupuncture treatment of enuresis, *J Tradit Chin Med* 20:158, 2000.

172. Hu J: Acupuncture treatment of common cold, *J Tradit Chin Med* 20:227, 2000.

173. Huhtala V, Lehtonen L, Heinonen R, Korvenranta H: Infant massage compared with crib vibrator in the treatment of colicky infants, *Pediatrics* 105:E84, 2000.

174. Hunziker UA, Barr RG: Increased carrying reduces infant crying: a randomized controlled trial, *Pediatrics* 77:641, 1986.

175. Huo JS: Treatment of 11 cases of chronic enuresis by acupuncture and massage, *J Tradit Chin Med* 8:195, 1988.

176. Hviid C: A comparison of the effect of chiropractic treatment on respiratory function in patients with respiratory distress symptoms and patients without, *Bull Eur Chiro Union* 26:17, 1978.

177. Ialongo NS et al: The effects of a multimodal intervention with attention deficit hyperactivity disorder children: a 9-month follow-up, *J Am Acad Child Adolesc Psychiatry* 32:182, 1993.

178. Illingworth RS: Infantile colic revisited, *Arch Dis Child* 60:981, 1985.

179. Imam AP, Halpern GM: Uses, adverse effects of abuse of corticosteroids. Part II, *Allergol Immunopathol* 23:2, 1995.

180. Isaacson G: Sinusitis in childhood, *Pediatr Clin North Am* 436:1297, 1996.

181. Jacobs J, Springer DA, Crothers D: Homeopathic treatment of acute otitis media in children: a preliminary randomized placebo-controlled trial, *Pediatr Infect Dis J* 20:177, 2001.

182. Jacobs J et al: Treatment of acute childhood diarrhea with homeopathic medicine: a randomized clinical trial in Nicaragua, *Pediatrics* 93:719, 1994.

183. Jacobs J et al: Homeopathic treatment of acute childhood diarrhea: results from a clinical trial in Nepal, *J Altern Complement Med* 6:131, 2000.

184. Jakobsson I, Lindberg T: Cow's milk as a cause of infantile colic in breast-fed infants, *Lancet* 2:437, 1978.

185. Jakobsson I, Lindberg T: Cow's milk proteins cause infantile colic in breast-fed infants: a double-blind crossover study, *Pediatrics* 71:268, 1983.

186. Jamison JR et al: Asthma in chiropractic clinic: a pilot study, *J Aust Chiro Assoc* 16:137, 1986.

187. Janzen T et al: Differences in baseline EEG measures for ADD and normally achieving preadolescent males, *Biofeedback Self Regul* 20:65, 1995.

188. Jenkins GH: Milk-drinking mothers with colicky babies, *Lancet* 2:261, 1981.

189. Jensen PS et al: Findings from the NIMH Multimodal Treatment Study of ADHD (MTA): implications and applications for primary care providers, *J Dev Behav Pediatr* 22:60, 2001.

190. Jiang R: Analgesic effect of acupuncture on acute intestinal colic in 190 cases, *J Tradit Chin Med* 10:20, 1990.

191. Johnston SL: The role of viral and atypical bacterial pathogens in asthma pathogenesis, *Pediatr Pulmonol Suppl* 18:141, 1999.

192. Joos S et al: Immunomodulatory effects of acupuncture in the treatment of allergic asthma: a randomized controlled study, *J Altern Complement Med* 6:519, 2000.

193. Jund R, Grevers G: [Rhinitis, sore throat and otalgia: benign common cold or dangerous infection?] *MMW Fortschr Med* 142:32, 2000.

194. Kachan AT, Trubin MI, Skoromets AA, Shmushkevich AI: [Acupuncture reflexotherapy of neurogenic bladder dysfunction in children with enuresis], *Zh Nevropatol Psikhiatr Korsakova* 93:40, 1993.
195. Kail K: Clinical outcomes of a diagnostic and treatment protocol in allergy/sensitivity patients, *Altern Med Rev* 6:188, 2001.
196. Kaleida PH, Nativio DG, Chao HP, Cowden SN: Prevalence of bacterial respiratory pathogens in the nasopharynx in breast-fed versus formula-fed infants, *J Clin Microbiol* 31:2674, 1993.
197. Kaplan B: Homeopathy: in pregnancy and for the under-fives, *Prof Care Mother Child* 4:185, 1994.
198. Kaplan B: Homeopathy: everyday uses for all the family, *Prof Care Mother Child* 4:212, 1994.
199. Kasa RM: Vitamin C: from scurvy to the common cold, *Am J Med Technol* 49:23, 1983.
200. Katcher ML: Cold, cough, and allergy medications: uses and abuses, *Pediatr Rev* 17:12, 1996.
201. Kay AB: Alternative allergy and the General Medical Council, *BMJ* 306(6870):122, 1993.
202. Kay J, Gawkrodger DJ, Mortimer MJ, Jaron AG: The prevalence of childhood atopic eczema in a general population, *J Am Acad Dermatol* 30:35, 1994.
203. Keatin JC Jr: Functional nocturnal enuresis, *J Manipulative Physiol Ther* 18:44, 1995 (letter).
204. Keefe MR, Kotzer AM, Froese-Fretz A, Curtin M: A longitudinal comparison of irritable and nonirritable infants, *Nurs Res* 45:4, 1996.
205. Kelly KM et al: Use of unconventional therapies by children with cancer at an urban medical center, *J Pediatr Hematol Oncol* 22:412, 2000.
206. Kemp JP: Role of leukotriene receptor antagonists in pediatric asthma, *Pediatr Pulmonol* 30:177, 2000.
207. Kemper KJ, Wornham WL: Consultations for holistic pediatric services for inpatients and outpatient oncology patients at a children's hospital, *Arch Pediatr Adolesc Med* 155:449, 2001.
208. Kemper KJ, Cassileth B, Ferris T: Holistic pediatrics: a research agenda, *Pediatrics* 103:902, 1999.
209. Kemper KJ et al: On pins and needles? Pediatric pain patients' experience with acupuncture, *Pediatrics* 105:941, 2000.
210. Kerr HD: Homeopathy study questions, *Pediatrics* 94:964, 1994 (letter).
211. Kien CL: Current controversies in nutrition, *Curr Probl Pediatr* 22:351, 1990.
212. Kimata H: High dose gamma-globulin treatment for atopic dermatitis, *Arch Dis Child* 70:335, 1994.
213. Kirkpatrick GL: The common cold: Primary Care, *Clin Off Prac* 23(4):657, 1996.
214. Klimek JJ et al: Comparison of concentrations of amoxicillin and ampicillin in serum and middle ear fluid of children with chronic otitis media, *J Infect Dis* 135:999, 1977.
215. Klougart N, Nilsson N, Jacobsen J: Infantile colic treated by chiropractors: a prospective study of 316 cases, *J Manipulative Physiol Ther* 12:281, 1989.
216. Knipschild P: Systematic reviews: some examples, *BMJ* 309:719, 1994.
217. Kohen DP, Wynne E: Applying hypnosis in a preschool family asthma education program: uses of storytelling, imagery, and relaxation, *Am J Clin Hypn* 39:169, 1997.
218. Kong XT et al: Treatment of acute bronchiolitis with Chinese herbs, *Arch Dis Child* 68:468, 1993.
219. Korkmaz A, Sahiner U, Yurdakok M: Chemical burn caused by topical vinegar application in a newborn infant, *Pediatr Dermatol* 17:34, 2000.
220. Koutkia P, Mylonakis E, Flanigan T: Enterohemorrhagic *Escherichia coli* O157:H7—an emerging pathogen, *Am Fam Physician* 56:853, 1997.
221. Koziclec T, Starobrat-Hermelin B, Kotkoiak L: [Deficiency of certain trace elements in children with hyperactivity], *Psychiatria Polska* 28:345, 1994.
222. Kramer MS et al: Promotion of Breastfeeding Intervention Trial (PROBIT): a randomized trial in the Republic of Belarus, *JAMA* 285:413, 2001.
223. Kramer NA: Comparison of therapeutic touch and casual touch in stress reduction of hospitalized children, *Pediatr Nurs* 16:483, 1990.
224. Krause PJ et al: Penetration of amoxicillin, cefaclor, erythromycin-sulfisoxazole, and trimethoprim-sulfamethoxazole into the middle ear fluid of patients with chronic serous otitis media, *J Infect Dis* 145:815, 1982.
225. Kreitz BG, Aker PD: Nocturnal enuresis: treatment implications for the chiropractor, *J Manipulative Physiol Ther* 17:465, 1994.
226. Krieger D: *Therapeutic touch: how to use your hands to help or heal*, Englewood Cliffs, NJ, 1979, Prentice-Hall.

227. Kulenkampff M, Schwartzman JS, Wilson J: Neurological complications of pertussis inoculation, *Arch Dis Child* 49:46, 1974.
228. Lai X: Observation on the curative effect of acupuncture on type I allergic diseases, *J Tradit Chin Med* 13:243, 1993.
229. Laney DW Jr, Cohen MB: Approach to the pediatric patient with diarrhea, *Gastroenterol Clin North Am* 22:499, 1993.
230. Larsen GL: Differences between adult and childhood asthma, *Dis Mon* 47:34, 2001.
231. Laurie S, Khan D: Inhaled corticosteroids as first-line therapy for asthma: why they work—and what the guidelines and evidence suggest, *Postgrad Med* 109:44, 2001.
232. Lawrence JD, Lawrence DB, Carson BS: Optimizing ADHD therapy with sustained release methylphenidate, *Am Fam Physician* 55:1705, 1997.
233. Lebedev VA: [The treatment of neurogenic bladder dysfunction with enuresis in children using the SKENAR apparatus (self-controlled energy-neuroadaptive regulator), Voprosy Kurortologii], *Fizioterap Lechebn Fizichesk Kultur* 4:25, 1995.
234. Leboeuf C et al: Chiropractic care of children with nocturnal enuresis: a prospective outcome study, *J Manipulative Physiol Ther* 14:110, 1991.
235. Ledwith M: Pneumococcal conjugate vaccine, *Curr Opin Pediatr* 13:70, 2001.
236. Lee AC, Kemper KJ: Homeopathy and naturopathy: practice characteristics and pediatric care, *Arch Pediatr Adolesc Med* 154:75, 2000.
237. Lee AC, Li DH, Kemper KJ: Chiropractic care for children, *Arch Pediatr Adolesc Med* 154:401, 2000.
238. Lee SW: Biofeedback as a treatment for childhood hyperactivity: a critical review of the literature, *Psychol Rep* 68:163, 1991.
239. Lehrke P, Nuebling M, Hofmann F, Stoessel U: Attitudes of homoeopathic physicians towards vaccination, *Vaccine* 19:4859, 2001.
240. Levine R: *Ethics and regulation of clinical research*, ed 2, New Haven, Conn, 1986, Yale University Press.
241. Li YL: [Clinical and experimental study on the treatment of children diarrhea by granule of children-diarrhea fast-stopping], *Zhongguo Zhong Xi Yi Jie He Za Zhi* 11:79, 1991.
242. Li YQ, Yuan W, Zhang SL. [Clinical and experimental study of xiao er ke cuan ling oral liquid in the treatment of infantile bronchopneumonia], *Zhongguo Zhong Xi Yi Jie He Za Zhi* 12:719, 1992.
243. Liebelt EL: Clinical and laboratory evaluation and management of children with vomiting, diarrhea, and dehydration, *Curr Opin Pediatr* 10:461, 1998.
244. Lin Y et al: Clinical and experimental studies on shallow needling technique for treating childhood diarrhea, *J Tradit Chin Med* 13:107, 1993.
245. Lin YC: Observation of the therapeutic effects of acupuncture treatment in 170 cases of infantile diarrhea, *J Tradit Chin Med* 7:203, 1987.
246. Linden M, Habib T, Radojevic V: A controlled study of the effects of EEG biofeedback on cognition and behavior of children with attention deficit disorder and learning disabilities, *Biofeedback Self Regul* 21:35, 1996.
247. Liu J: Treatment of adolescent acne with acupuncture, *J Tradit Chin Med* 13:187, 1993.
248. Loo M: *Pediatric acupuncture*, London, 2002, Churchill Livingstone.
249. Loo M, Naeser MA, Hinshaw S, Bay RB: Laser acupuncture treatment for ADHD. NIH Grant 1 RO3 MH56009-01. Presented at 1998 Annual American Academy of Medical Acupuncture (AAMA) Symposium, San Diego (recipient of Medical Acupuncture Research Foundation [MARF] First Place Research Award).
250. Lopez A. [Unstable detrusor: usefulness of biofeedback], *Acta Urol Esp* 20:640, 1996.
251. Lopez-Alarcon M, Villalpando S, Fajardo A: Breast-feeding lowers the frequency and duration of acute respiratory infection and diarrhea in infants under six months of age, *J Nutr* 127:436, 1997.
252. Lubar JF: Neocortical dynamics: implications for understanding the role of neurofeedback and related techniques for the enhancement of attention, *Appl Psychophysiol Biofeedback* (2):111, 1997.
253. Lubar JF, Swartwood MO, Swartwood JN, O'Donnell PH: Evaluation of the effectiveness of EEG neurofeedback training for ADHD in a clinical setting as measured by changes in TOVA scores, behavioral ratings, and WISC-R performance, *Biofeedback Self Regul* 20:83, 1995.

254. Luks D, Anderson MR: Antihistamines and the common cold: a review and critique of the literature, *J Gen Intern Med* 11:240, 1996.
255. Luo H: [Treatment of upper respiratory infection with mixture 716 compound], *Zhongguo Zhong Xi Yi Jie He Za Zhi* 13:730, 1993.
256. Ma Z, Wang Y, Fan Q. [The influence of acupuncture on interleukin 2–interferon: natural killer cell regulatory network of kidney-deficiency mice], *Zhen Ci Yan Jiu* 17:139, 1992.
257. Mainous AG III, Hueston WJ, Clark JR: Antibiotics and upper respiratory infection: do some folks think there is a cure for the common cold? *J Fam Pract* 42:357, 1996.
258. Maizels M, Gandhi K, Keating B, Rosenbaum D: Diagnosis and treatment for children who cannot control urination, *Curr Probl Pediatr* 23:402, 1993.
259. Mannino DM et al: Surveillance for asthma: United States, 1960–1995, *MMWR* 47:1, 1998.
260. Marbet UA: [Diagnosis and therapy of diarrhea], *Schweiz Med Wochenschr* 124:439, 1994.
261. Mark JD, Grant KL, Barton LL: The use of dietary supplements in pediatrics: a study of echinacea, *Clin Pediatr (Phila)* 40:265, 2001.
262. Martens M: [Enuresis as an individual symptom and systemic manifestation: considerations on using hypnotherapy in family dynamic interventions], *Prax Kinderpsychol Kinderpsychiatr* 43:54, 1994.
263. Martinez FD: Links between pediatric and adult asthma, *J Allergy Clin Immunol* 107(5 suppl):449, 2001.
264. Mason JD: The evaluation of acute abdominal pain in children: gastrointestinal emergencies. Part I, *Emerg Med Clin North Am* 14:629, 1996.
265. Matheson I: [Infantile colic: what will help?], *Tidsskr Nor Laegeforen* 115:2386, 1995.
266. Mattelaer P et al: Biofeedback in the treatment of voiding disorders in childhood, *Acta Urol Belg* 63:5, 1995.
267. Mattucci KF, Greenfield BJ: Middle ear effusion–allergy relationships, *Ear Nose Throat J* 74:752, 1995.
268. Maxim PE et al: Chronic serous otitis media: an immune complex disease, *Trans Am Acad Ophthalmol Otolaryngol* 84:234, 1977.
269. Mazur LJ, De Ybarrondo L, Miller J, Colasurdo G: Use of alternative and complementary therapies for pediatric asthma, *Tex Med* 97:64, 2001.
270. McFarland LV: Microecologic approaches for traveler's diarrhea, antibiotic-associated diarrhea, and acute pediatric diarrhea, *Curr Gastroenterol Rep* 1:301, 1999.
271. McGuire JK, Kulkarni MS, Baden HP: Fatal hypermagnesemia in a child treated with megavitamin/megamineral therapy, *Pediatrics* 105:E18, 2000.
272. McKenna PH, Herndon CD, Connery S, Ferrer FA: Pelvic floor muscle retraining for pediatric voiding dysfunction using interactive computer games, *J Urol* 162:1056, 1999.
273. Megson MN: Is autism a G-alpha protein defect reversible with natural vitamin A? *Med Hypotheses* 54:979, 2000.
274. Meltzer EO et al: A pharmacologic continuum in the treatment of rhinorrhea: the clinician as economist, *J Allergy Clin Immunol* 95:1147, 1995.
275. Meyers A: Modern management of acute diarrhea and dehydration in children, *Am Fam Physician* 51:1103, 1995.
276. Middleton DB: An approach to pediatric upper respiratory infections, *Am Fam Physician* 44 (5 suppl):33, 1991.
277. Middleton DB: Pharyngitis, *Prim Care* 23:719, 1996.
278. Miller AR, Barr RG: Infantile colic: is it a gut issue? *Pediatr Clin North Am* 38:1407, 1991.
279. Miller D, Wadsworth J, Diamond J, Ross E: Measles vaccination and neurological events, *Lancet* 349:730, 1997.
280. Miller D et al: Pertussis immunization and serious acute neurological illness in children, *BMJ* 307:1171, 1993.
281. Miller K: Concomitant nonpharmacologic therapy in the treatment of primary nocturnal enuresis, *Clin Pediatr (Phila)* Special:32, 1993.
282. Miller WD: Treatment of visceral disorders by manipulative therapy. In Goldstein M, editor: *The research status of spinal manipulative therapy,* NINCDS monograph, Bethesda, Md, 1975, US Department of Health, Education, and Welfare, p 295.

283. Milling LS, Costantino CA: Clinical hypnosis with children: first steps toward empirical support, *Int J Clin Exp Hypn* 48:113, 2000.

284. Minni B et al: [Bladder instability and enuresis treated by acupuncture and electro-therapeutics: early urodynamic observations], *Acupunct Electrother Res* 15:19, 1990.

285. Moenkhoff M, Baenziger O, Fischer J, Fanconi S: Parental attitude towards alternative medicine in the paediatric intensive care unit, *Eur J Pediatr* 158:12, 1999.

286. Moffatt ME: Nocturnal enuresis: a review of the efficacy of treatments and practical advice for clinicians, *J Dev Behav Pediatr* 18:49, 1997.

287. Mogyoros M: Challenges of managed care organizations in treating respiratory tract infections in an age of antibiotic resistance, *Am J Managed Care* 7(6 suppl):163, 2001.

288. Morton AR, Fazio SM, Miller D: Efficacy of laser-acupuncture in the prevention of exercise-induced asthma, *Ann Allergy* 70:295, 1993.

289. Mudd KE: Indoor environmental allergy: a guide to environmental controls, *Pediatr Nurs* 21:534, 1995 (review).

290. Murray RH, Rubel AJ: Physicians and healers—unwitting partners in health care, *N Engl J Med* 326:61, 1992.

291. Murray S, Brewerton T: Abuse of over-the-counter dextromethorphan by teenagers, *South Med J* 86:1151, 1993.

292. Naeser MA, Wei XB: *Laser acupuncture: an introductory textbook,* Boston, 1994, Boston Chinese Medicine.

293. Nagel GA: [Naturopathy as metaphor], *Schweiz Rund Med Praxis* 82:735, 1993.

294. Nahmias A, Yolken R, Keyserling H: Rapid diagnosis of viral infections: a new challenge for the pediatrician, *Adv Pediatr* 32:507, 1985.

295. Nash JK: Treatment of attention deficit hyperactivity disorder with neurotherapy, *Clin Electroencephalogr* 31:30, 2000.

296. National Center for Health Statistics: Asthma: United States, 1980–1987, *MMWR* 39:493, 1990.

297. Nelson WE et al, editors: *Nelson's textbook of pediatrics,* ed 15, Philadelphia, 1996, Saunders.

298. Neville RG, McCowan C, Hoskins G, Thomas G: Cross-sectional observations on the natural history of asthma, *Br J Gen Pract* 51:361, 2001.

299. Newburg DS: Human milk glycoconjugates that inhibit pathogens, *Curr Med Chem* 6:117, 1999.

300. Nicoll A, Elliman D, Ross E: MMR vaccination and autism 1998: deja vu—pertussis and brain damage 1974? *BMJ* 316:715, 1998.

301. Nilsson N: Infantile colic and chiropractic, *Eur J Chiro* 33:264, 1985.

302. Northrup RS, Flanigan TP: Gastroenteritis, *Pediatr Rev* 15:461, 1994.

303. Nyiendo J, Olsen E: Visi characteristics of 217 children attending a chiropractic college teaching clinic, *J Manipulative Physiol Ther* 2:78, 1988.

304. Oguz F et al: The impact of systematic use of oral rehydration therapy on outcome in acute diarrheal disease in children, *Pediatr Emerg Care* 10:326, 1994.

305. Oh HM: Upper respiratory tract infections: otitis media, sinusitis and pharyngitis, *Singapore Med J* 36:428, 1995.

306. Okumura M et al: Effects of acupuncture on peripheral T lymphocyte subpopulation and amounts of cerebral catecholamines in mice, *Acupunct Electrother Res* 24:127, 1999.

307. Olafsdottir E, Forshei S, Fluge G, Markestad T: Randomised controlled trial of infantile colic treated with chiropractic spinal manipulation, *Arch Dis Child* 84:138, 2001.

308. Olness K: The use of self-hypnosis in the treatment of childhood nocturnal enuresis: a report on forty patients, *Clin Pediatr* 14:273, 1975.

309. Olness KN: Hypnotherapy in children: new approach to solving common pediatric problems, *Postgrad Med* 79:95, 1986.

310. Olness K, Kohen DP: *Hypnosis and hypnotherapy with children,* ed 3, New York, 1996, Guilford Press.

311. Oskolkova MK et al: [Acupuncture and electropuncture in the overall therapy of diseases in children], *Pediatriia* 3:53, 1980.

311a. Oxman AD, Guyatt GH: Validation of an index of the quality of review articles, *J Clin Epidemiol* 44:1271, 1991.

312. Pachter LM et al: Home-based therapies for the common cold among European American and ethnic minority families: the interface between alternative/complementary and folk medicine, *Arch Pediatr Adolesc Med* 152:1083, 1998.

313. Park K, Lim DJ: Development of secretory elements in murine tubotympanum: lysozyme and lactoferrin immunohistochemistry, *Ann Otol Rhinol Laryngol* 102:385, 1993.

314. Passwell JH: MMR vaccination, Crohn's disease, and autism: a real or imagined "stomachache/headache?" *Isr Med Assoc J* 1:176, 1999.

315. Paul M: Informed consent in medical research: children from the age of 5 should be presumed competent, *BMJ* 314:1480, 1997 (letter).

316. Peer O, Bar Dayan Y, Shoenfeld Y: Satisfaction among patients of a homeopathic clinic, *Harefuah* 130:86, 1996.

317. Pelton SI: Acute otitis media in the era of effective pneumococcal conjugate vaccine: will new pathogens emerge? *Vaccine* 19(suppl 1):96, 2000.

318. Pena-Outeirino JM et al: [Unstable detrusor: usefulness of biofeedback], *Acta Urol Esp* 20:640, 1996.

319. Perera BJ, Ganesan S, Jayarasa J, Ranaweera S: The impact of breastfeeding practices on respiratory and diarrhoeal disease in infancy: a study from Sri Lanka, *J Trop Pediatr* 45:115, 1999.

320. Personal observation: TCM Pediatric Ward, Xinhua Hospital, Shanghai, 1999.

321. Petry LJ: Immunization controversies, *J Fam Pract* 36:141, 1993 (editorial).

322. Petti F et al: Effects of acupuncture on immune response related to opioid-like peptides, *J Tradit Chin Med* 18:55, 1998.

323. Pfister C et al: The usefulness of a minimal urodynamic evaluation and pelvic floor biofeedback in children with chronic voiding dysfunction, *BJU Int* 84:1054, 1999.

324. Phillips K, Gill L: Acupressure: a point of pressure, *Nurs Times* 89:44, 1993.

325. Pichichero ME: Group A beta-hemolytic streptococcal infections, *Pediatr Rev* 19:291, 1998.

326. Pickering LK: Therapy for acute infectious diarrhea in children, *J Pediatr* 118:118, 1991.

327. Pierres-Surer N et al: [Rhinovirus infections in hospitalized children: a 3-year study], *Arch Pediatr* 5:9, 1998.

328. Pinyerd BJ: Strategies for consoling the infant with colic: fact or fiction? *J Pediatr Nurs* 7:403, 1992.

329. Pitetti R et al: Complementary and alternative medicine use in children, *Pediatr Emerg Care* 17:165, 2001.

330. Pitkaranta A, Hayden FG: Rhinoviruses: important respiratory pathogens, *Ann Med* 30:529, 1998.

331. Planta M, Gundersen B, Petitt JC: Prevalence of the use of herbal products in a low-income population, *Fam Med* 32:252, 2000.

332. Porena M, Costantini E, Rociola W, Mearini E: Biofeedback successfully cures detrusor-sphincter dyssynergia in pediatric patients, *Paediatr Nurs* 12:14, 2000.

333. Powell DW, Szauter KE: Nonantibiotic therapy and pharmacotherapy of acute infectious diarrhea, *Gastroenterol Clin North Am* 22:683, 1993.

334. Power TJ, Hess LE, Bennett DS: The acceptability of interventions for attention-deficit hyperactivity disorder among elementary and middle school teachers, *J Dev Behav Pediatr* 16:238, 1995.

335. Prellner K et al: Complement and C1q binding substances in otitis media, *Ann Otol Rhinol Laryngol Suppl* 89:129, 1980.

336. Pulec JL: Allergy: a commonly neglected etiology of serous otitis media, *Ear Nose Throat J* 74:739, 1995 (editorial).

337. Radmayr C, Schlager A, Studen M, Bartsch G: Prospective randomized trial using laser acupuncture versus desmopressin in the treatment of nocturnal enuresis, *Eur Urol* 40:201, 2001.

338. Rakes GP et al: Rhinovirus and respiratory syncytial virus in wheezing children requiring emergency care: IgE and eosinophil analyses, *Am J Respir Crit Care Med* 159:785, 1999.

339. Ramgolam V et al: Traditional Chinese medicines as immunosuppressive agents, *Ann Acad Med Singapore* 29:11, 2000.

340. Ramirez PM, Desantis D, Opler LA: EEG biofeedback treatment of ADD: a viable alternative to traditional medical intervention? *Ann NY Acad Sci* 931:342, 2001.

341. Reed WR, Beavers S, Reddy SK, Kern G: Chiropractic management of primary nocturnal enuresis, *J Manipulative Physiol Ther* 17:596, 1994.

342. Reilly DT, Taylor MA, McSharry C, Atchison T: Is homeopathy a placebo response? Controlled trial of homeopathic potency, with pollen in hayfever as model, *Lancet* 2(8512):881, 1986.

343. Resnick SD, Hornung R, Konrad TR: A comparison of dermatologists' and generalists' management of childhood atopic dermatitis, *Arch Dermatol* 132:1047, 1996.

344. Richardson AJ, Puri BK: The potential role of fatty acids in attention-deficit/hyperactivity disorder, *Prostagland Leukot Essent Fatty Acids* 63:79, 2000.

345. Riley D et al: Homeopathy and conventional medicine: an outcomes study comparing effectiveness in a primary care setting, *J Altern Complement Med* 7:149, 2001.

346. Risser AL, Mazur LJ: Use of folk remedies in a Hispanic population, *Arch Pediatr Adolesc Med* 149:978, 1995.

347. Robbins AS: Controversies in measles immunization recommendations, *West J Med* 158:36, 1993.

348. Roden J: Childhood immunization, homeopathy and community nurses, *Contemp Nurs* 3:34, 1994.

349. Rogers PA, Schoen AM, Limehouse J: Acupuncture for immune-mediated disorders: literature review and clinical applications, *Probl Vet Med* 4:162, 1992.

350. Roje-Starcevic M: The treatment of nocturnal enuresis by acupuncture, *Neurologija* 39:179, 1990.

351. Roncoroni AJ Jr, de Cortigianni MR, Garcia Damiano MC: [Cost and effectiveness of fecal culture in the etiologic diagnosis of acute diarrhea], *Bol Oficina Sanit Panam* 107:381, 1989.

352. Rosenberg Z: Lectures and personal communications: Immunizations, Pacific College of Oriental Medicine, San Diego, 1999.

353. Rowell M, Zlotkin S: The ethical boundaries of drug research in pediatrics, *Pediatr Clin North Am* 44:27, 1997.

354. Roy CC, Silverman A, Alagille D: *Pediatric clinical gastroenterology,* ed 4, St Louis, 1995, Mosby.

355. Rubin DH et al: Relationship between infant feeding and infectious illness: a prospective study of infants during the first year of life, *Pediatrics* 85:464, 1990.

356. Rubin SP, Pendergast M: Infantile colic: incidence and treatment in a Norfolk community, *Child Care Health Dev* 10:219, 1984.

357. Rudolph AM: *Rudolph's pediatrics,* ed 20, Stamford, 1996, Appleton & Lange.

358. Ruoff G: Upper respiratory tract infections in family practice, *Pediatr Infect Dis J* 17(8 suppl):73, 1998.

359. Rynnel-Dagoo B, Agren K: The nasopharynx and the middle ear: inflammatory reactions in middle ear disease, *Vaccine* 19(suppl 1):26, 2000.

360. Sakic B, Kojic L, Jankovic BD, Skokljev A: Electro-acupuncture modifies humoral immune response in the rat, *Acupunct Electrother Res* 14:115, 1989.

361. Saroea HG: Common colds: causes, potential cures, and treatment, *Can Fam Physician* 39:2215, 1993.

362. Sarrell EM, Mandelberg A, Cohen HA: Efficacy of naturopathic extracts in the management of ear pain associated with acute otitis media, *Arch Pediatr Adolesc Med* 155:796, 2001.

363. Sato T et al: Acupuncture stimulation enhances splenic natural killer cell cytotoxicity in rats, *Jpn J Physiol* 46:131, 1996.

364. Satterfield JH, Cantwell DP, Satterfield BT: Multimodality treatment: a two year evaluation of 61 hyperactive boys, *Arch Gen Psychiatry* 36:965, 1980.

365. Satterfield JH et al: Three year multimodality treatment study of 100 hyperactive boys, *J Pediatr* 98:650, 1981.

366. Sawyer CE et al: A feasibility study of chiropractic spinal manipulation versus sham spinal manipulation for chronic otitis media with effusion in children, *J Manipulative Physiol Ther* 22:292, 1999.

367. Schmitz J: [Anti-rotavirus vaccinations], *Arch Pediatr* 6:979, 1999.

368. Schulman SL, Colish Y, von Zuben FC, Kodman-Jones C: Effectiveness of treatments for nocturnal enuresis in a heterogeneous population, *Clin Pediatr (Phila)* 39:359, 2000.

369. Seidenberg J: [Antihistamines in pediatrics], *Monatsschr Kinderheilkd* 137:54, 1989.

370. Serel TA et al: Acupuncture therapy in the management of persistent primary nocturnal enuresis: preliminary results, *Scand J Urol Nephrol* 35:40, 2001.

371. Shaywitz B, Fletcher JM, Shaywitz SE: Attention deficit hyperactivity disorder, *Adv Pediatr* 44:331, 1997.

372. Shaywitz B, Siegel NJ, Pearson HA: Megavitamins for minimal brain dysfunction: a potentially dangerous therapy, *JAMA* 238:1749, 1977.

373. Sheehan MP, Atherton DJ: A controlled trial of traditional Chinese medicinal plants in widespread non-exudative atopic eczema, *Br J Dermatol* 126:179, 1992.

374. Sheehan MP, Atherton DJ: One-year follow up of children treated with Chinese medicinal herbs for atopic eczema, *Br J Dermatol* 130:488, 1994.

375. Shields JH: Childhood immunizations: controversy and change, *Pa Nurse* 48:6, 1993.

376. Shirkey H: Therapeutic orphans, *J Pediatr* 72:119, 1968.

377. Shoenfeld Y, Aron-Maor A: Vaccination and autoimmunity—"vaccinosis": a dangerous liaison? *J Autoimmun* 14:1, 2000.

378. Shoultz DA: Homeopathic diarrhea trial, *Pediatrics* 95:160, 1995 (letter).

379. Simpson N, Lenton S, Randall R: Parental refusal to have children immunized: extent and reasons, *BMJ* 310:227 (erratum, 777), 1995.

380. Skoner DP: Management and treatment of pediatric asthma: update, *Allergy Asthma Proc* 22:71, 2001.

381. Slutsker L et al: *Escherichia coli* 0157:H7 diarrhea in the United States: clinical and epidemiologic features, *Ann Intern Med* 126:505, 1997.

382. Sly RM: Changing prevalence of allergic rhinitis and asthma, *Ann Allergy Asthma Immunol* 82:233, 1999.

383. Smith MB, Feldman W: Over-the-counter cold medications: a critical review of clinical trials between 1950 and 1991, *JAMA* 269:2258, 1993.

384. Solomon WR: Prevention of allergic disorders, *Pediatr Rev* 15:301, 1994.

385. Spiegelblatt LS: Alternative medicine: should it be used by children? *Curr Probl Pediatr* 25:180, 1995.

386. Spiegelblatt LS: The use of alternative medicine by children, *Pediatrics* 94:811, 1994.

387. Spitzer WO et al: The use of β-agonists and the risk of death and near death from asthma, *N Engl J Med* 326:501, 1992.

388. St Geme JW III: The pathogenesis of nontypable *Haemophilus influenzae* otitis media, *Vaccine* 19(suppl 1):41, 2000.

389. Starobrat-Hermelin B: [The effect of deficiency of selected bioelements on hyperactivity in children with certain specified mental disorders], *Ann Acad Med Stetin* 44:297, 1998.

390. Starobrat-Hermelin B, Kozielec T: [The effects of magnesium physiological supplementation on hyperactivity in children with attention deficit hyperactivity disorder (ADHD): positive response to magnesium oral loading test], *Magnes Res* 10:149, 1997.

391. Stein MA et al: Methylphenidate dosing: twice daily versus three times daily, *Pediatrics* 98:748, 1996.

392. Sternfield M, Fink A, Bentwich Z, Eliraz A: The role of acupuncture in asthma: changes in airway dynamics and LTC4-induced LAI, *Am J Clin Med* 17:129, 1989.

393. Stewart AC, Thomas SE: Hypnotherapy as a treatment for atopic dermatitis in adults and children, *Br J Dermatol* 132:778, 1995.

394. Stickler GB, Smith TF, Broughton DD: The common cold, *Eur J Pediatr* 144:4, 1985.

395. Stogman W, Kurz H: [Atopic dermatitis and food allergy in infancy and children], *Wiener Medizinische Wochenschrift* 146:411, 1996.

396. Strachan DP, Anderson HR, Johnston ID: Breastfeeding as prophylaxis against atopic disease, *Lancet* 346:1714, 1995 (letter).

397. Stubberfield T, Parry T: Utilization of alternative therapies in attention-deficit hyperactivity disorder, *J Paediatr Child Health* 35:450, 1999.

398. Su Z: Acupuncture treatment of infantile diarrhea: a report of 1050 cases, *J Tradit Chin Med* 12:120, 1992.

399. Sulfaro F, Fasher B, Burgess MA: Homoeopathic vaccination: what does it mean? Immunisation Interest Group, Royal Alexandra Hospital for Children, *Med J Aust* 161:305, 1994.

400. Sun Y: External approach to the treatment of pediatric asthma, *J Tradit Chin Med* 15:290, 1995.

401. Sun Y et al: Clinical observation and treatment of hyperkinesia in children by traditional Chinese medicine, *J Tradit Chin Med* 14:105, 1994.

402. Szefler SJ, Nelson HS: Alternative agents for anti-inflammatory treatment of asthma, *J Allergy Clin Immunol* 102:23, 1998.

403. Takeuchi H, Jawad MS, Eccles R: The effects of nasal massage of the "yingxiang" acupuncture point on nasal airway resistance and sensation of nasal airflow in patients with nasal congestion associated with acute upper respiratory tract infection, *Am J Rhinol* 13:77, 1999.

404. Tan D: Treatment of fever due to exopathic wind-cold by rapid acupuncture, *J Tradit Chin Med* 12:267, 1992.
405. Tan G, Schneider SC: Attention deficit hyperactivity disorder: pharmacotherapy and beyond, *Postgrad Med* 101:201, 1997.
406. Tandon MK, Soh PF, Wood AT: Acupuncture for bronchial asthma? A double-blind crossover study, *Med J Aust* 154:9, 1991.
407. Tansey MA: Ten-year stability of EEG biofeedback results for a hyperactive boy who failed fourth grade perceptually impaired class, *Biofeedback Self Regul* 18:33, 1993.
408. Taylor MA et al: Randomised trial of homoeopathy versus placebo in perennial allergic rhinitis with overview of four trial series, *BMJ* 321:471, 2000.
409. Tettenborn MA: Autism, inflammatory bowel disease, and MMR vaccine, *Lancet* 351:1357, 1998.
410. Thompson NP, Montgomery SM, Pounder RE, Wakefield AJ: Is measles vaccination a risk factor for inflammatory bowel disease? *Lancet* 345:1071, 1995.
411. Tian ZM: Acupuncture treatment for aerotitis media, *J Tradit Chin Med* 5:259, 1985.
412. Tomassoni AJ, Simone K: Herbal medicines for children: an illusion of safety? *Curr Opin Pediatr* 13:162, 2001.
413. Trachtman H, Christen E: Pathogenesis, treatment, and therapeutic trials in hemolytic uremic syndrome, *Curr Opin Pediatr* 11:162, 1999.
414. Treem WR: Chronic non-specific diarrhea of childhood, *Clin Pediatr* 31:413, 1992.
415. Tret'iakova EE, Komissarov VI: [Characteristics of the electric activity of the projection areas of the large hemispheres in children with enuresis], *Zh Nevropatol Psikhiatr Korsakova* 90:41, 1990.
416. Tuomanen EI: Pathogenesis of pneumococcal inflammation: otitis media. *Vaccine* 19(suppl 1):38, 2000.
417. Turner RB: Epidemiology, pathogenesis, and treatment of the common cold, *Ann Allergy Asthma Immunol* 78:531, 1997.
418. Tuzuner F, Kecik Y, Ozdemir S, Canakci N: Electro-acupuncture in the treatment of enuresis nocturna, *Acupunct Electrother Res* 14:211, 1989 (abstract).
419. Ugazio AG, Plebani A: Vaccinations in childhood: when and why, *Rec Prog Med* 84:864, 1993.
420. United Nations General Assembly: 1960 Declaration of the Rights of the Child, New York, 1959, United Nations.
421. US Department of Health and Human Services, Centers for Disease Control and Prevention: Vaccine information statement: Varicella, February 2001.
422. Van der Baan S et al: Serous otitis media and immunological reactions in the middle ear mucosa, *Acta Otolaryngol* 106:428, 1988.
423. Vange B: [Contact between preschool children with chronic diseases and the authorized health services and forms of alternative therapy], *Ugeskr Laeger* 151:1815, 1989.
424. Vidailhet M: Towards preventive dietetics in children, *Revue du Praticien* 43:171, 1993.
425. Vincent C, Furnham A: Why do patients turn to complementary medicine? An empirical study, *Br J Clin Psychol* 35:37, 1996.
426. Vincent CA, Richardson PH: Acupuncture for some common disorders: a review of evaluative research, *J R Coll Gen Pract* 37:77, 1987.
427. Vincenzo F: A clinical case: asthma and *Staphysagria* and homeo-mesotherapy, *Homeopath Int* 1(2):13, 1987.
428. Virsik K, Kritufek D, Bangha O, Urban S: The effect of acupuncture on bronchial asthma, *Prog Respir Res* 14:271, 1980.
429. Voigt RG et al: A randomized, double-blind, placebo-controlled trial of docosahexaenoic acid supplementation in children with attention-deficit/hyperactivity disorder, *J Pediatr* 139:189, 2001.
430. Wakefield AJ: National Vaccine Information Centre: First international public conference on vaccination, Alexandria, Va, 1997.
431. Wakefield AJ et al: Ileal-lymphoid-nodular hyperplasia, non-specific colitis and pervasive developmental disorder in children, *Lancet* 351:637, 1998.
432. Walker TA, Khurana S, Tilden SJ: Viral respiratory infections, *Pediatr Clin North Am* 41:1365, 1994.
433. Wallace KR: The homeopathic treatment of asthma and allergies, *Br Homeopath J* 75:218, 1986.

434. Walter JE, Mitchell DK: Role of astroviruses in childhood diarrhea, *Curr Opin Pediatr* 12:275, 2000.

435. Wang Y: [Clinical therapy and etiology of viral diarrhea in children], *Zhongguo Zhong Xi Yi Jie He Za Zhi* 10:25, 1990.

436. Ward PE: Potential diagnostic aids for abnormal fatty acid metabolism in a range of neurodevelopmental disorders, *Prostagland Leukot Essent Fatty Acids* 63:65, 2000.

437. Warner JO: Worldwide variations in the prevalence of atopic symptoms: what does it all mean? *Thorax* 54:S46, 1999.

438. Warzak WJ: Psychosocial implications of nocturnal enuresis, *Clin Pediatr (Phila)* Special:38, 1993.

439. Watkins AD: The role of alternative therapies in the treatment of allergic diseases, *Clin Exper Allergy* 24:813, 1994.

440. Weisberg SC: Pharmacotherapy of asthma in children, with special reference to leukotriene receptor antagonists, *Pediatr Pulmonol* 29:46, 2000.

441. Weissbluth M, Christoffel KK, Davis AT: Treatment of infantile colic with diclyclomine hydrochloride, *J Pediatr* 104:951, 1984.

442. Werner HA: Status asthmaticus in children : a review, *Chest* 119:1913, 2001.

443. White CB, Foshee WS: Upper respiratory tract infections in adolescents, *Adolesc Med* 11:225, 2000.

444. Wiberg JM, Nordsteen J, Nilsson N: The short-term effect of spinal manipulation in the treatment of infantile colic: a randomized controlled clinical trial with a blinded observer, *J Manipulative Physiol Ther* 22:517, 1999.

445. Wolsko P et al: Alternative/complementary medicine: wider usage than generally appreciated, *J Altern Complement Med* 6:321, 2000.

446. Wood RA: Environmental control in the prevention and treatment of pediatric allergic diseases, *Curr Opin Pediatr* 5:692, 1993.

447. Wood RA: Prospects for the prevention of allergy in children, *Curr Opin Pediatr* 8:601, 1996.

448. Wood RA, Doran TF: Atopic disease, rhinitis and conjunctivitis, and upper respiratory infections, *Curr Opin Pediatr* 7:615, 1995.

449. Woodcock A, Custovic A: Allergen avoidance: does it work? *Br Med Bull* 56:1071, 2000.

450. Wooten JC, Sparber A: Surveys of complementary and alternative medicine. I. General trends and demographic groups, *J Altern Complement Med* 2:195, 2001.

451. Wright AL, Holberg CJ, Taussig LM, Martinez FD: Relationship of infant feeding to recurrent wheezing at age 6 years, *Arch Pediatr Adolesc Med* 149:758, 1995.

452. Wright DN, Huang SW: Current treatment of allergic rhinitis and sinusitis, *J Fla Med Assoc* 83:389, 1996.

453. Xu B: 302 cases of enuresis treated with acupuncture, *J Tradit Chin Med* 11:121, 1991.

454. Xu J: [Influence of acupuncture on human nasal mucociliary transport], *Zhonghua Er Bi Yan Hou Ke Za Zhi* 24:90, 1989.

455. Xu JH, Lin LH, Zhang PY: [Treatment of infantile diarrhea with anisodamine by the injection method of Zu San Li acupuncture points], *Zhonghua Hu Li Za Zhi* 31:345, 1996.

456. Xu Y: Treatment of acne with ear acupuncture—a clinical observation of 80 cases, *J Tradit Chin Med* 9:238, 1989.

457. Yan S: 14 cases of child bronchial asthma treated by auricular plaster and meridian instrument, *J Tradit Chin Med* 8:202, 1998.

458. Yan WX, Wang JH, Chang QQ: [Effect of *leu*-enkephalin in striatum on modulating cellular immune during electropuncture], *Sheng Li Xue Bao* 43:451, 1991.

459. Yang CP: Acupuncture of guanyuan (Ren 4) and Baihui (Du 20) in the treatment of 500 cases of enuresis, *J Tradit Chin Med* 8:197, 1988.

460. Yu DY, Lee SP: Effect of acupuncture on bronchial asthma, *Clin Sci Mol Med* 51:503, 1976.

461. Yu P, Hao X, Zhao R, Qin M: [Pasting acupoints with Chinese herbs applying in infant acute bronchitis and effect on humoral immune substances], *Zhen Ci Yan Jiu* 17:110, 1992.

462. Yu S, Cao J, Yu Z: Acupuncture treatment of chronic rhinitis in 75 cases, *J Tradit Chin Med* 13:103, 1993.

463. Zang J: Immediate antiasthmatic effect of acupuncture in 192 cases of bronchial asthma, *J Tradit Chin Med* 10:89, 1990.

464. Zhang H, Huang J: [Preliminary study of traditional Chinese medicine treatment of minimal brain dysfunction: analysis of 100 cases], *Chung Hsi I Chieh Ho Tsa Chih* 10:278, 1990.

465. Zhang XP: [Clinical and experimental study on yifei jianshen mixture in preventing and treating infantile repetitive respiratory infection], *Chung-kuo Chung Hsi Chieh Ho Tsa Chih* 13:23, 1993.

466. Zhu S et al: Clinical investigation on massage for prevention and treatment of recurrent respiratory tract infection in children, *J Tradit Chin Med* 18:285, 1998.

467. Zimmer G, Miltner E, Mattern R: [Life threatening complications in alternative medicine—problems in patient education], *Versicherungsmedizin* 46:171, 1994.

468. Zimmerman RK: Pneumococcal conjugate vaccine for young children, *Am Fam Physician* 63:1991, 2001.

469. Zorc JJ, Pawlowski NA: Prevention of asthma morbidity: recent advances, *Curr Opin Pediatr* 12:438, 2000.

CHAPTER 12

Select Populations: Women

FREDI KRONENBERG, PATRICIA AIKINS MURPHY,
and CHRISTINE WADE

$\mathbf{W}$omen's health is studied by a broad spectrum of medical and social science disciplines, but as a discrete topic it is difficult to define. A reductive view limits the discussion of women's health to reproductive function, whereas a broader perspective encompasses not only disease states but also normal life events. Women's health is affected by major causes of mortality, morbidity, and disability (e.g., cardiovascular disease, cancer), but women also seek health care in connection with menstruation, pregnancy, childbirth, menopause, and aging.

Medical treatment of women has been characterized by both overintervention and neglect, and research on many topics in women's health is often sparse. In an effort to correct this situation, the National Institutes of Health (NIH) established an Office of Research on Women's Health (ORWH) in 1990 to ensure that appropriate research is conducted to fill gaps in knowledge. Resources are now being brought to bear to implement a research agenda in women's health to better understand and promote health, prevent illness, and effectively treat disease.

◼ CAM Usage by Women

Women are the primary users of complementary and alternative medicine (CAM), as they are of conventional medicine.[11,42] As caregivers for their families and often their communities, for centuries women have used "folk medicine" and "home remedies" now being called CAM. These remedies are currently the subject of biomedical research to determine what works, for whom, under what conditions, and at what dose. Although women constitute 52% of the U.S. population, they make 57% of visits to physicians, are prescribed 60% of all prescription medication, and undergo 59% of hospital procedures.[33,34,121] The two leading surgeries in the United States are exclusive to women: cesarean section (birth) and hysterectomy.[102] Women make 75% of health care decisions and spend two of every three health care dollars.[33,34]

Women use conventional medicine services more often than men and also use CAM more extensively.[11,42] The follow-up to a 1993 U.S. national survey found that gender predicted CAM use (women 48.9%; men 37.8%).[42] In the first national survey of CAM use exclusively among U.S. women, 53% of women reported using at least one CAM modality for a women's health condition in the past year.[80] A number of previous studies supported these results. Research in Germany found that more women than men (44% vs. 32%) were given CAM, and more women than men preferred CAM to mainstream medicine (62% vs. 52%).[62] A study of Chinese medicine practitioners in New York City found more women than men among non-Asian patients (59% vs. 41%).[60] Women are also greater users of homeopathic remedies (66%).[13]

Why do women choose CAM? Despite the achievements of contemporary conventional medicine, the answers are numerous and vary with the study.[41] Reasons include a preference for more "natural" treatment, belief in unconventional medicine, concern about the side effects of conventional treatments, and dissatisfaction with or lack of confidence in conventional medicine.[89] Studies of people who choose alternatives suggest that most are not poorly educated or gullible. Indeed, they have been shown to be relatively well educated and middle class.[30,43] McGregor and Peay[89] demonstrated that CAM patients have a substantially lower level of confidence in the efficacy of conventional medicine; however, they clearly were not dissatisfied with their medical practitioners. People who choose alternatives speak of conventional medicine's limitations and "narrow-mindedness," as well as their desire for control over their health and health care. Although this is certainly changing, patients still most often use CAM without informing their conventional medical physicians.[43]

In addition to these general reasons, women may turn to CAM when faced with problems for which Western biomedicine offers treatments that may produce undesirable and sometimes unacceptable effects. For example, pregnant women may want to avoid drugs that could interfere with fetal development. During menopause, although hormone therapy typically provides effective relief of symptoms such as hot flashes, it may be contraindicated for some individuals, and others may desire a more natural approach.

Women also seek alternative approaches in an effort to avoid surgery. Hysterectomy is the most common non–pregnancy-related surgical procedure for U.S. women; one third of all women will have had a hysterectomy by 65 years of age.[129] Uterine fibroids are the primary indication in almost two thirds of black women and in one third of white women who have hysterectomies. In light of the cost and risk associated with surgery, evaluation of the effectiveness of CAM in reducing the need for surgery is an important issue in women's health.

A survey of three ethnic groups of women in New York City found that 58% used CAM and about 40% have visited at least one CAM practitioner.[48] In addition to seeking the care of CAM practitioners, many women self-medicate in search of suitable remedies. They do so with insufficient information on safety and efficacy to guide them. Not only does this waste time and money, but some types of experimentation may put certain women at risk. For example, herbs are often considered "natural" and assumed to be nontoxic, but they have numerous physiologically active components, some of which may be contraindicated for individuals with particular medical conditions. Remedies taken by pregnant women may have unknown consequences for fetal growth and development.

It is often argued that CAM remedies are natural and therefore safe. Some CAM methods have been used in traditional cultures for centuries without apparent ill effects. Historical use does not necessarily mean safety, however, and these arguments do not eliminate the need for a research agenda on CAM and women's health that includes well-designed studies on safety and efficacy.

Ideally, clinical decisions should be based on systematic and scientific observations drawn from well-designed research studies.[47] In both conventional medicine and CAM, evidence about the risks, benefits, and efficacy of various treatment choices is lacking in many areas.[96] CAM treatments for women's health problems are particularly in need of research.

N CAM Methods for Women's Health

Most CAM methods find application across the range of women's health concerns, and women are using many of them. However, certain CAM modalities are particularly promising with respect to women's health. The following brief overview of CAM methods covers important indications and applications but is by no means complete.

Medical systems from other countries, so-called ethnomedicines or traditional medicines, are particularly promising for treatment of women's gynecologic conditions. Some of these systems, such as Ayurveda, traditional Chinese medicine (TCM), and Tibetan medicine, have complex theoretic structures and empiric, literature-based traditions and have been practiced as medical systems for thousands of years. They have classic gynecologic texts, materia medica with specific herbs for gynecologic conditions, and modern practitioners who claim success in treating women's reproductive and gynecologic problems. Other traditions are primarily oral and are passed along through apprenticeship.

These systems use different diagnostic techniques than Western medicine. For example, TCM uses pulse and tongue diagnosis with other observations to identify patterns in the individual that indicate imbalances. Herbal formulas, acupuncture, and other techniques are used to restore balance. Treatment of *preconditions* to disease, as evident in pattern diagnosis, is an important aspect of these systems. For example, careful attention is paid within these medical systems to length, regularity, flow, blood qualities, and other aspects of the menstrual cycle to prevent development of chronic disease. This type of diagnosis is not typical in Western gynecologic practice. Research is needed on its relevance to women's health outcomes.

Folk herbalism has a long history of use for women's health conditions. There are many ethnic expressions of the tradition of folk herbalism, including practices from countries worldwide. The tradition of female folk herbalists is sometimes known as the "wise woman" tradition and has within its practice remedies for women's health conditions that are promising for research. Herbalism, especially as practiced by midwives, is undergoing a revival in the United States. Almost daily, the popular press and other media are deluging women with articles and other reports on herbal medicine.

A profusion of new products confront and confuse the consumer. For women to make better-informed choices, it is incumbent on researchers to study the safety and efficacy of these therapies, dosing schemes, and subpopulations for whom a therapy may be more or less effective.

Mind-body therapies include a vast array of disciplines ranging from biofeedback and hypnosis to guided imagery. Many women use mind-body therapies primarily as complements to biomedicine and to prevent disease. These therapies are also being explored as treatments for conditions such as hot flashes, immune dysfunction, chronic pain, diabetes, infertility, and complications of pregnancy. These methods usually have minimal side effects, and research has demonstrated the efficacy of these methods for many conditions not specific to women's health.

It is now recognized that nutrition plays a role in maintaining health and possibly in the treatment of disease. Although specific details continue to be researched, several dietary topics are emerging as important to women's health. *Dietary estrogens* are plant-based sources of estrogenic substances found in many foods and herbs. The mechanism of these *phytoestrogens* and their potential role in women's hormone-dependent diseases, such as uterine fibroids and breast cancer, are areas of current interest and increased research. Phytoestrogens are found in fruits, vegetables, and legumes such as soy (see later discussions of menopause and breast cancer).

CAM and Women's Health Conditions

This section is a summary of CAM research published in the Western scientific literature in three areas of women's health: menopausal hot flashes, nausea and vomiting in pregnancy, and breast cancer. Two of these conditions are self-limiting and, although not life threatening, are common and can cause women appreciable distress. At times, for some women, nausea and vomiting during pregnancy and menopausal hot flashes can be functionally incapacitating. Breast cancer is a serious illness with considerable associated mortality and morbidity. The research literature in these three areas is of varying quantity and quality. For many women's health problems, such as fibroids and endometriosis, our searches of the English-language literature have yielded results too meager to summarize.

MENOPAUSAL HOT FLASHES

Women in the perimenopausal and postmenopausal years may have a number of problems that either occur for a limited time before resolving or may increase in magnitude over years after menopause. Other problems continue for years at levels ranging from barely perceptible to annoying to intolerable. Women have increasingly been seeking modes of therapy other than the standard hormone therapy for several complaints associated with the menopausal period, including hot flashes, sleep problems, vaginal dryness, joint pain, weight gain, mood swings, and fatigue.

Hot flashes are the primary complaint for which women seek treatment. Hormone therapy (estrogen with or without progesterone) is extremely efficacious in the treatment of hot flashes. It significantly ameliorates and often eliminates hot flashes for a large percentage of women. Some women need or desire other options, however, because they have medical conditions or risk factors for which estrogen is contraindicated, have some adverse reaction to hormone therapy, or choose not to take hormones.

Women have been exploring a number of nonpharmacologic approaches to hot flashes on their own. These therapies include vitamins (in particular vitamin E), behavioral therapies (e.g., yoga, relaxation, biofeedback), lifestyle changes (e.g., exercise, alcohol use, dietary changes), herbal remedies (e.g., black cohosh, ginseng, dong quai), traditional systems of medicine (e.g., TCM, Ayurveda, Tibetan), homeopathy, and acupuncture. The efficacy of these approaches has not been demonstrated, but because of the popularity of CAM since 1994, investigators are now developing studies of CAM therapies for menopausal problems, particularly hot flashes.

Medicinal Herbs

Women of many cultures have used herbs to reduce the discomfort of hot flashes. This usage includes a history of herbal therapy in Western countries. For most herbal remedies, few clinical studies are available for treatment recommendations. We do know that many herbs contain substances that have potent physiologic effects.

Native American women have traditionally used black cohosh *(Cimicifuga racemosa)* to treat gynecologic and other conditions.[49] Black cohosh has been used in German medicine for about 50 years and is approved by the German Commission E (comparable to the U.S. Food and Drug Administration [FDA]) for use in premenstrual discomfort, dysmenorrhea, and menopausal symptoms. It is increasing in popularity in the United States. Most clinical studies of black cohosh have been conducted in Germany using the product Remifemin. Of five randomized controlled trials, one was placebo controlled,[72] one used both a treatment and a placebo control,[117] and two were treatment controlled.[84,125] Most controlled trials have shown a benefit for black cohosh, with few reported side effects. Neither the identity of active compound(s) nor the mechanism of action of black cohosh is known. Although formononetin, an estrogenic isoflavone, was reported to have been isolated from black cohosh extract,[73] a recent systematic study of black cohosh samples found no formononetin.[76] Further work is needed to understand the biologic activity of black cohosh.

Safety is a concern with black cohosh, particularly with long-term use and for women with breast cancer who cannot take estrogen. In vitro and in vivo studies are inconsistent and insufficient, although a body of data is developing. Initial small studies found that black cohosh binds to estrogen receptors, and researchers have postulated that the herb has estrogenic effects.[37,73] Recently published works showed no activity of black cohosh in several estrogen receptor binding assays and other in vitro assays assessing estrogenic activity.[87,99]

Investigators are now developing studies of CAM therapies for menopausal problems, particularly hot flashes. A review of clinical studies of herbal and phytoestrogenic therapies for menopausal symptoms yielded 29 randomized, controlled trials. The scientific data are still thin for most herbal remedies, with black cohosh holding the most promise at this time. The data on soy and soy isoflavones appear to be only modest for the treatment of hot flashes.[78a] The important studies are summarized in the following paragraphs.

Dong quai *(Angelica sinensis)* is a Chinese herb used by menopausal women, some of whom report that it helps relieve hot flashes.[79] In the first randomized, placebo-controlled clinical trial of *dong quai* for the treatment of menopausal symptoms (in 71 postmenopausal women), investigators found no statistically significant difference in the number of hot flashes, vaginal maturation index, or Kupperman index (a combined index of 11 menopausal complaints).[63] The authors concluded that dong quai, when used alone, is not helpful in relieving menopausal symptoms. Dong quai is typically used as one of several components of traditional Chinese herbal formulas as a tonic for women; it is not used alone in TCM and would not be prescribed for all women with menopausal symptoms. Dong quai is sold as a single herbal remedy in U.S. health food stores; women buy it for the treatment of menopausal problems, and some find it helpful. Additional studies are needed to clarify the role of dong quai, either singly or in herbal mixtures, for treatment of menopausal complaints.

Ginseng *(Panax ginseng)* has estrogenic actions that have been demonstrated in humans.[65,104] *Ginseng* is reported by women to be effective in relieving menopausal symptoms. In a recent placebo-controlled trial ginseng (Ginsana G115) provided some symptomatic relief, particularly for depressed mood, and improved self-reported general health and well-being. It was less satisfactory for relief of hot flashes.[86,126] Ginseng has been used for centuries in Asia as a tonic.

Dietary Phytoestrogens

Although particular foods (e.g., coffee, spicy foods) are reported by some women to trigger individual hot flashes, long-term consumption or emphasis on certain foods in the diet may influence hormone levels and thereby affect whether hot flashes occur at all. Many food plants contain physiologically active estrogenic substances (phytoestrogens). The major classes of phytoestrogens are isoflavones, lignans, coumestans, and resorcylic acid lactones; these are *phenolic* rather than steroidal compounds. *Isoflavones* are found in legumes such as soy, clover, and alfalfa. *Lignans* are found in whole grains, seeds, fruits, vegetables (especially flaxseed/linseed), rye, millet, and legumes.[6]

Grains and soybeans are the most common foods with estrogenic activity, but other plants that contain phytoestrogens include chick peas, pinto beans, french beans, pomegranates, lima beans, and clover.[103] Plant lignans found in the grains and seeds are broken down by bacteria in the gut to enterolactone and enterodiol (also called mammalian lignans). Bacteria also remove a glycoside from isoflavone precursors to create the active mammalian isoflavones genistein, daidzein, and equol. Many whole grains, including wheat, oats, corn, and rye, contain a fungus *(Fusarium)* that produces estrogenic substances called zearalenol and zearalenone,[103] which are much stronger phytoestrogens than those produced by the plants themselves, although still weaker than endogenous estrogens.

It is now well established that ingestion of plants containing phytoestrogens can cause reproductive disorders in mammals.[110,111] A diet with substantial intake of these foods can produce estrogen-like effects in women as well. For example, ingestion of estrogenic food plants (e.g., linseed, clover sprouts) by postmenopausal women produced changes in vaginal maturation values in an Australian study.[128] A U.S. study of a dietary soy intervention in postmenopausal women found a slight but not statistically significant estrogenic effect on vaginal epithelium.[16] It is not surprising that results differ among these studies, since the food plants involved contain different classes of estrogenic compounds (e.g., lignans in grasses, oilseeds and isoflavones in soy) with differing degrees of estrogenicity.

Some phytoestrogens are weakly estrogenic, but they are often found in very high levels in the body. In a study comparing American and Finnish women consuming three diets (omnivorous, lactovegetarian, macrobiotic), excretion of the most abundant phytoestrogen was found to be highest in the macrobiotic group and lowest in the omnivorous group.[4] Postmenopausal women in Japan eating a traditional low-fat diet were found to have 100 to 1000 times higher levels of several urinary phytoestrogens than levels of the endogenous estrogens in the urine of American or Finnish women eating an omnivorous diet.[7] The Asian diets are associated with a high intake of soy products. The high levels of dietary phytoestrogens may offer an explanation for the low level of hot flashes reported by many Japanese women.

In a study designed to examine the effect of soy on hot flashes more directly, Murkies et al.[93] compared the effect of soy flour with wheat flour supplementation in a randomized, double-blind trial. Hot flashes decreased significantly in the soy group by week 6 and in both groups by week 12. There was no change in vaginal maturation index in either group. Excretion of urinary daidzein, an estrogenic isoflavone in soy, had increased significantly at 12 weeks in the soy group, and there was no significant increase in excretion of urinary phytoestrogens in the wheat group. Interpretation of these results is not clear. Wheat flour also contains phytoestrogens, but with less estrogenic potency than soy phytoestrogens. Milling supposedly removes most of the phytoestrogens from wheat (thus the choice for placebo).

Nine clinical trials are now examining soy supplementation for hot flashes.[93] Two of the seven studies that lasted longer than 6 weeks showed statistically significant improvement in hot flashes at the end of the study. Products tested varied across the studies. The overall conclusion one can draw at this date is that soy seems to have only modest effects on hot flashes, and most benefits disappeared after 6 weeks. Additional studies of menopausal symptoms would be valuable to determine whether whole foods, soy protein, and isolated isoflavones have different degrees of efficacy. Although soy has been consumed as a food for centuries and is presumed safe, the same cannot be presumed for isolated isoflavones, increasingly being offered over the counter at often high, untested doses.

Clearly, diet plays a role in modulating endocrine actions in the body. As data accumulate to provide evidence that the phytoestrogen content of some foods may affect physiologic function, diet may be found to influence an individual's hot flash pattern and even whether a woman has hot flashes at all. The extent of diet's role and whether biologic (genetic) differences exist among populations and result in observed differences in hot flash prevalence remain to be determined.

Vitamin E

There are anecdotal reports of vitamin E's effectiveness for treating hot flashes, but few objective data. A few clinical trials were conducted in the 1940s and 1950s, and some found vitamin E to be of value in treating hot flashes. Considering that most drug studies of hot flash therapies have a placebo effect, however, the studies usually were not double blind, placebo controlled, or of adequate duration. In Blatt's much- cited 1953 study,[24] a double-blind design (no crossover) was used to compare the effect of vitamin E, estrogen, and a placebo on a combined group of 11 symptoms (not on hot flashes specifically). Vitamin E was no more effective than placebo in treating this symptom complex. This study is cited as demonstrating lack of effectiveness of vitamin E for treating hot flashes, a conclusion not justified from these data.

A more recent, randomized, placebo-controlled study of breast cancer patients with hot flashes tested vitamin E (400 IU twice daily) for 4 weeks, an insufficient length of time for a study of therapeutic efficacy for hot flashes. The result of one hot flash less per day for those on vitamin E, while statistically significant, was not of clinical importance.[18]

Acupuncture

Wyon et al.[130] administered 8 weeks of acupuncture (one or two times per week for 30 minutes) to 24 naturally menopausal women with hot flashes. The authors compared two forms of acupuncture and found that both significantly reduced the daily number of hot flashes. They also found a decrease in urinary calcitonin gene-related peptide (a potent endothelium-dependent vasodilator of systemic blood vessels). Although there is controversy in the acupuncture field about the appropriateness of the controls used, this study is an important first step in the scientific examination of acupuncture for the treatment of menopausal symptoms.

Behavioral Therapies

Behavioral methods for moderating hot flashes have received limited study. Freedman and Woodward[52] compared paced respiration with muscle relaxation and alpha electroencephalogam (EEG) biofeedback and found that paced respiration training reduced the frequency of hot flashes by about 40% compared with women who received progressive muscle relaxation training or controls (11 women in each group). Freedman et al.[53] obtained similar results in a more recent study with a larger subject population ($n = 24$). Elucidation of the relaxation response for 7 weeks in a randomized, controlled study resulted in significant reductions in hot flash intensity but not in hot flash frequency.[70] The results from these studies suggest the need for additional research in behavioral therapy.

Exercise

Several groups have presented preliminary data suggesting that exercise moderates at least the severity, if not the frequency, of hot flashes. Because exercise has demonstrated effects on sex steroids, it might influence hot flashes as well. In a study of the relationship between menopausal symptoms and aerobic fitness in healthy volunteers, Wilbur et al.[127] found that of their 375 subjects (mean age 47 years), 27% reported through a symptom checklist that they were having hot flashes or night sweats. Joint pains and backaches were the most frequently reported symptom. A bicycle ergometric test of aerobic fitness indicated that 54% of the sample had above-average or average, 27% had average, and 19% had low fitness levels. Hot flashes and night sweats were highest in perimenopausal women. Aerobic fitness was negatively related to hot flashes (although the finding was not statistically significant). Hammar et al.[59] reported that women who belonged to a gymnastic club had fewer hot flashes than women who did not belong, but whose physical activity was not reported.

Although these data are weak and no study has demonstrated that physical activity is a substitute for hormone therapy in relieving hot flashes, exercise may help ameliorate hot flashes.

NAUSEA AND VOMITING IN PREGNANCY

Nausea and vomiting are among the most common complaints during early pregnancy. The symptoms affect more than 50% of women in Western societies. For most women the condition is self-limiting, with symptoms most common and troublesome in early pregnancy and resolving by the beginning of the second trimester. In some women, severe symptoms may lead to dehydration, weight loss, and acidosis, requiring hospitalization for fluid replacement. Whether or not the condition becomes this severe, nausea and vomiting can cause considerable distress and temporary disability. Almost half of employed women believe their work efficiency is reduced by this problem, and as many as 25% require time off from work.[122]

Pharmacologic treatments exist for nausea and vomiting during pregnancy, but concerns about the potential teratogenic effects of medication taken during the critical embryogenic stage limit their use. Most available drugs are listed as FDA category C, which means either that adverse effects have been noted in animal studies and no human studies are available or that there are no human or animal studies. Other recommendations include dietary advice (e.g., avoidance of fatty or spicy foods) and lifestyle change (e.g., avoiding cooking), but few women report complete relief with these recommendations.[97] Consequently, many pregnant women turn to CAM therapies to treat nausea and vomiting.

A review of both pregnancy self-help books and lay CAM publications indicates that women use a host of alternatives, including vitamins, herbal products, homeopathic agents, acupressure, and acupuncture. Western scientific evidence is sparse about the efficacy of these remedies. This review summarizes the available clinical research.[94]

Acupressure, Acupuncture, and Related Methods

Acupressure (use of the fingers or other devices, rather than needles, to stimulate specific points) is the best-studied CAM measure for the treatment of nausea and vomiting of pregnancy. The specific intervention involves stimulation of or pressure on an acupuncture point known as *pericardium 6* (P6), or the *Nei Guan point*, which is on the volar surface of the forearm, two to three finger breadths above the wrist. P6 has been shown in other studies of postoperative emesis, chemotherapy-associated emesis, and motion sickness to be important in the relief of nausea and vomiting.[123] In many studies a commercially available wristband designed to prevent motion sickness has been used. These devices (Sea Bands), when properly placed, are designed to apply pressure over the Nei Guan point.

Seven clinical trials of acupressure for treating nausea and vomiting of early pregnancy have compared women using acupressure over the Nei Guan point with a variety of groups (Table 12-1). In five of the seven trials, significant reductions in nausea and vomiting were noted in the women using acupressure. However, it may not be possible to perform a true double-blind, placebo-controlled trial (the gold standard of clinical research) because of the nature of the intervention. The potential exists for a strong "placebo effect" in such studies, given the subjective nature of grading the presence and severity of outcome variables such as nausea and vomiting. Some studies used no alternate intervention, which raises a concern that any benefit attributable to acupressure could have been the result of the placebo effect. In other studies, acupressure was applied to a sham or *dummy* point (one other than the point thought to be important). The correct point, however, can be identified easily in any number of self-help books, so there remains a concern about a placebo effect. In addition, in two studies the group receiving acupressure was further along in pregnancy than the control subjects; because the condition in question resolves spontaneously as pregnancy advances, the observed benefits could have been caused by the normal evolution of pregnancy. In two other studies there was a significant loss (30% to 50%) of study subjects, which also compromises findings. The largest clinical trial, which compared acupressure to sham acupressure and to no intervention, found no beneficial effects. Thus the literature is equivocal.

One study evaluated a related method, *sensory afferent stimulation,* which delivers a continuous electric current to the volar surface of the wrist.[45] The exact location of the stimulation was not described but was verified in another report to have been the P6 point.[123] Such electrical stimulation has been characterized as a form of "electroacupuncture." Those using the device reported significantly more improvement in symptoms of nausea and vomiting than those wearing the placebo unit. However, a subject probably could determine which was the active unit, because it produced a tingling sensation in the wrist or hand; thus benefits could have been caused by a placebo-type effect. Other observational studies have been made but do not meet criteria for randomized, controlled clinical trials.

The clinical trial research on the use of acupressure or related methods has not produced consistent or methodologically sound findings. However, these studies clearly show that acupressure of the Nei Guan point benefits many women. In studies that did not provide an intervention to the control group or arm of the trial, positive findings might result only from the placebo effect. However, there may be value in mobilizing such a mind-body interaction if the intervention is simple and inexpensive, if it results in reduction of symptoms, and if it is not associated with any risk.

Acupuncture (use of needles rather than pressure to stimulate points) has not been studied in controlled trials as extensively as acupressure. Two Chinese case series described such treatment for nausea and vomiting in early pregnancy,[131,132] but there

TABLE 12–1. **RANDOMIZED CLINICAL TRIALS OF ACUPRESSURE FOR NAUSEA AND VOMITING IN PREGNANCY**

Study/No.	Intervention/Duration	Results
Dundee et al.[38] (1988); 350	Manual acupressure over pericardium 6 (P6) or dummy point vs. control (no intervention); 4 days*	"Severe" or "troublesome" morning sickness in 24% using P6, 37% using dummy, 56% of control (p <.005)
Hyde[68] (1989); 16	Acupressure wristbands vs. no intervention; 5 days, followed by crossover to other group for 5 days	Relief of morning sickness in 75% using wristbands (p <.025) Reduction in anxiety, depression, and behavioral dysfunction, as measured by standard psychometric tools (p <.05)
De Aloysio, Penacchioni[36] (1992); 60	Unilateral (right or left wrist) or bilateral acupressure wristbands* vs. placebo bands (no pressure exerted on P6); 3 days in crossover design	Reduction or elimination of symptoms in 65%-69% using acupressure vs. 29%-31% using placebo (p <.05)
Bayreuther et al.[20] (1994); 16	Acupressure wristbands* vs. placebo bands applied over dummy point; 7 days, followed by crossover to alternate intervention for 7 days	Nausea score (visual analog scale) lower in acupressure group vs. placebo group (p = .019) No effect on vomiting
Belloumini et al.[22] (1994); 60	Manual acupressure on P6 vs. pressure on dummy point; 3 days	Nausea significantly decreased in treatment group (p = .0021) No difference in severity or frequency of vomiting
O'Brien et al.[98] (1996); 161	Acupressure wristbands* vs. bands over dummy point vs. control with no intervention; 7 days	No difference across groups in nausea or vomiting
Evans et al.[45] (1993); 23	Continuous electrical current stimulation at P6 vs. no stimulation; 48 hours, followed by crossover to alternate intervention	Improvement in symptoms of nausea and vomiting in 87% of experimental group vs. 43% of control group (p <.05)

Modified from American College of Obstetricians and Gynecologists: *Obstet Gynecol* 91:151, 1998.
*Sea Bands, Sea Band International, Greensboro, NC.

were no control groups or discussion of outcome measurements. A Swedish trial randomized 40 women admitted to the hospital for severe vomiting *(hyperemesis gravidarum).*[29] In this randomized, single-blind, crossover trial, "deep" acupuncture was given by specially trained midwives at the P6 point and compared to "shallow" (placebo) acupuncture at a different point. Subjects received treatment for 2 days, and after a washout period of 2 days, they were crossed over to the other treatment. Treatments were three times a day for 30 minutes each. Routine medical care for hyperemesis was given concurrently. Thirty-three women completed the trial; both nausea and vomiting were reduced in the "deep" acupuncture group.

A 2001 study compared traditional acupuncture to a control intervention that involved tapping a blunt stick over a bony prominence near the acupuncture point.[77] The subject/observer-masked trial evaluated 55 women between 6 and 10 weeks' gestation; women with symptoms severe enough to require hospitalization were excluded. Women received three or four treatments over 3 weeks. Although there were profound reductions in nausea scores in both groups, no differences were found between groups. A traditional Chinese medical diagnosis was done, and subjects received treatment at the points suggested by this diagnosis. Thus treatment was not identical for all subjects, but it was appropriate for the TCM diagnosis. The protocol did not allow for variations in treatment after the initial visit in subjects who failed to respond; the authors suggested this might have rendered the active treatment less than ideal.[77] Finally, the sham procedure may not have been completely without effect because evidence suggests that "sham" treatment can produce improvement in symptoms.

Another trial randomized 593 women to four groups: traditional acupuncture, based on a traditional Chinese medicine diagnosis; P6 acupuncture, with treatment only at the Nei Guan point (as used in the acupressure studies); sham acupuncture, with treatment at points near but not on four specific acupoints; and no treatment (control).[114] Subjects in the control group received advice on diet, lifestyle, and the use of vitamin B_6, as well as weekly telephone calls to assess their well-being. In the 4-week trial, women in the two acupuncture groups and the sham acupuncture group were treated twice during the first week, then weekly. Data were available for 90% of subjects after the first week and for 75% by the end of the trial.

The traditional acupuncture group had less nausea throughout the trial, with less nausea in the P6 acupuncture group from the second week and in the sham acupuncture group from the third week.[114] Less dry retching was reported in the traditional acupuncture group from the second week and in the P6 and sham acupuncture groups from the third week. All comparisons were with the no-acupuncture group, and all reductions in symptoms were statistically significant. There were no differences in vomiting among groups at any time during the trial, although the frequency of treatments in this trial may not have been optimized for treatment of vomiting. Women's health status was also measured using the MOS 36 Short Form Health Survey, a standardized outcome measure that evaluates physical, emotional, and social functioning; bodily pain; mental health; and general health perceptions.

Results suggested an improvement in women's health status over the course of the study, with most improvement in the traditional acupuncture group.[114] The authors of this study did not specify whether treatment in the traditional acupuncture group was allowed to vary depending on the subject's response. They suggested that a difference in data collection tools may explain the difference in findings.

In summary, despite differences in study design, patient populations, treatment, and outcome measures, evidence suggests that both traditional (based on TCM diagnosis) and P6 acupuncture may be of benefit for nausea and vomiting of pregnancy. Optimal frequency of treatments, as related to outcome, needs to be better characterized in further research. Because this is not a self-administered intervention, as is manual acupressure, the actual benefits of such treatment in the population of pregnant women will also depend on the availability of practitioners and the overall costs of treatment (practitioner fees, time, and travel).

The issue of fetal risk has not been addressed in studies. No theoretic risk of teratogenesis seems to exist from acupressure, acupuncture, or related methods. However, certain acupoints are contraindicated in pregnancy because of their potential to produce uterine contractions; these are not near the Nei Guan point.

Ginger

Ginger root is a remedy used in many traditional cultures as a treatment for nausea. It is frequently mentioned in self-help books as a treatment for nausea and vomiting of pregnancy. Ginger's efficacy is thought to result from its aromatic, carminative, and absorbent properties. Studies of its use with other types of nausea and vomiting (e.g., motion sickness) confirm its potential as a treatment.[44]

Two trials have examined the efficacy of ginger in pregnancy.[51,124] In the first trial, women who had been admitted to the hospital for treatment of hyperemesis gravidarum were randomly assigned to treatment with either 250 mg of ginger in a capsule four times a day or a placebo. Significant improvement was associated with ginger, with a reduction in the degree of nausea and the number of vomiting attacks.[51] The second trial, a double-blind, controlled study, evaluated a larger group of women with less severe symptoms than the hospitalized women in the first study. Seventy women were randomized to receive either oral ginger (1 g/day in divided doses) or an identical placebo for 4 days. Significant decreases in both nausea scores and vomiting episodes were associated with the use of ginger.[124]

A caution was raised by one scientist, who suggested that because ginger is a thromboxane synthetase inhibitor, it could theoretically affect sex steroid differentiation of the fetal brain.[14] In both trials a cumulative total of 59 subjects received ginger, and no adverse effects on pregnancy outcome were detected.[51,124] Although some problems may be too subtle to detect in such a small sample, the amount of ginger used in these trials was very small and well within the range of common dietary sources of ginger.

In addition, some herbalists describe ginger as a traditional "menstruation promoter"; whether this means it has potential as an abortifacient is unclear. TCM advises caution in the use of dried ginger in pregnancy. However, Bergner[23] pointed out that typical doses in TCM are larger, perhaps 3 g a day or more. The dose used in the study was 1 g, roughly equivalent to an 8-ounce glass of ginger ale or 4 cups of ginger tea.

There has been little research assessment of ginger as a remedy widely used traditionally and across cultures. Based on work in other areas and the one trial reported here, it is likely that ginger will be of benefit to some women. Concerns have been raised about its teratogenic potential, but directed investigation of this hypothesis has not been performed. Prudence might indicate avoiding intake of ginger in excess of 1 g daily.

Vitamin B$_6$

Vitamin B$_6$ *(pyridoxine)* was included in the original formulation of the drug Bendectin (Merrell Dow Pharmaceuticals, Cincinnati), which was the only drug approved by the FDA for treatment of nausea and vomiting in pregnancy. Bendectin, consisting of 10 mg doxylamine and 10 mg pyridoxine, was withdrawn from the market by its manufacturer after several lawsuits alleging birth defects related to its use. Further epidemiologic study has failed to corroborate allegations of teratogenesis from the use of this drug combination.[12,100]

Some clinicians questioned whether the benefit seen from Bendectin may have resulted from its vitamin content, and two studies have addressed the efficacy of pyridoxine treatment of nausea and vomiting in early pregnancy. Sahakian et al.[107] compared vitamin B_6 to a placebo; women received 25 mg of pyridoxine every 8 hours for 3 days. Although symptoms differed little in patients with mild to moderate nausea, significant improvement was seen in women with severe nausea, with a significant overall reduction in vomiting episodes. In another study, women took either 30 mg of pyridoxine daily or a placebo in a randomized, double-blind trial.[124a] There was a significant decrease in nausea, as well as a nonsignificant trend toward reduction in episodes of vomiting, associated with vitamin use. Of interest is a study that was unable to demonstrate a relationship between serum vitamin B_6 levels and the prevalence or degree of morning sickness.[111] This finding suggests that if pyridoxine supplementation is efficacious, the mechanism may not be related to levels of pyridoxine in the blood but to some other factor.

Vitamin B_6 is also a common, available, and inexpensive remedy. It apparently benefits some women in doses of 30 to 75 mg/day, which is higher than the recommended daily allowance (RDA) of 2.2 mg/day.[95] Little evidence supports a teratogenic effect from this supplement in doses up to 40 mg/day. However, issues of appropriate dosage in pregnancy should be addressed because pyridoxine has been shown to cause neurologic problems in nonpregnant adults when taken in excessive doses.[32,106,109]

Hypnosis, Hypnotherapy, and Behavior Modification

Some authors characterize nausea and vomiting of pregnancy as a psychologic or behavioral disorder, for which hypnosis is one treatment technique. Several published reports have addressed the treatment of nausea and vomiting in early pregnancy using hypnotherapy or behavior modification.[54,61,88,113,119] Most are case series dealing with severely ill women (many were hospitalized). Symptoms improved after hypnotherapy, but it is difficult to separate the effects of treatment from longitudinal improvement as pregnancy advances. Thus the benefits of this intervention are unclear.

Overall Considerations

There is a dearth of research literature to support or refute the efficacy of a number of common remedies for the common problem of nausea and vomiting during pregnancy. The best-studied remedy seems to be acupressure over the Nei Guan point. A systematic review of this literature (excluding studies of poor methodologic quality and those with data that could not be combined) found the effects of acupressure to be comparable to those of antiemetic medications but cautioned that the evidence is equivocal.[74] Herbal remedies are often advised for nausea and vomiting in pregnancy, and the more common preparations are readily available over the counter in health food stores and many pharmacies. Many have pharmacologic effects in the body, and some remedies are contraindicated in pregnancy. Of the many suggestions encountered in various lay publications, only ginger has been studied, and only in one trial.

Women seeking alternative, nonpharmacologic therapies for nausea and vomiting of early pregnancy may be advised to try acupressure over the Nei Guan point.

This can be achieved through the use of commercial wristbands or by applying manual pressure to the appropriate spot on the volar surface of the wrist. Ginger may be recommended as well, in prudent doses. Vitamin B$_6$ may also be efficacious in doses that do not exceed 75 mg a day. Apart from these few studies, however, little evidence exists to support or refute the benefits or risks of other remedies. Given the prevalence of the problem of nausea and vomiting for pregnant women and the potential for adverse effects from the use of teratogenic or abortifacient remedies, more research in this field is needed.

BREAST CANCER

The most common cancers affecting women in the United States are breast cancer, colorectal cancer, cancers of the reproductive organs, and lung cancer. Breast cancer accounts for more than 30% of newly diagnosed cancer in women and almost 20% of cancer deaths.[8] It is the leading cause of cancer death in women ages 40 to 55 years. Recently, breast cancer incidence has leveled off at a rate of about 110 new cases per 100,000 women per year.[9] Currently identified risk factors account for only a minority of cases and are generally not modifiable through preventive behavior.[75] Secondary prevention strategies through screening are the current means for improving survival. Breast cancer is a major health issue for women not only because it is the most common of women's cancers, but also because of its impact on survival, lifestyle, self-image, and quality of life.[66] Research on both prevention and improving survival is a priority of the current health agenda in the United States.

Dietary Estrogens: Estrogens and Antiestrogens for Hormone-dependent Cancer

Exposure to estrogens, whether environmental or endogenous, may increase risk for breast cancer, other hormone-dependent cancers, and other hormone-dependent conditions in women, such as uterine fibroids. Eating soybeans and other plants containing estrogenic substances may lower the risk of developing breast and other cancers.[57] Asians who follow traditional diets have lower breast cancer rates than those who adopt a Western diet.[2] Asians eat much less fat and protein, more fiber, and more carbohydrates and consume high amounts (10 to 30 g) of soy products compared with the American diet.[64] Adlercreutz et al.[5] reported that the mean consumption of soy products in the traditional Japanese diet of men was 39.2 g daily. The increasing popularity of soy and other phytoestrogenic foods in the American diet, especially in certain subgroups such as vegetarians, may soon reach (or may have reached for some women) biologically active levels. The intake of soy products by Americans has increased approximately 40% between 1980 and 1990.[90]

At present, women in Western countries are exposed to higher levels of estrogen over their lifetimes than their ancestors. Part of the reason is that they produce more estrogen over their lifetimes; they weigh more (fat increases estrogen levels through peripheral aromatization), begin to menstruate at a younger age, bear fewer children, breast-feed for shorter periods (if at all), and lead relatively sedentary lives. They also eat many animal products; high-fat diets also appear to increase estrogen levels. This higher lifetime exposure to endogenous estrogens has been postulated to be one reason for high breast cancer incidence in Western countries.[101]

It is hypothesized that ingestion of plant estrogens may reduce risk because plant estrogens tend to be weak estrogens, the strongest being only 1/200th as strong as human estrogens.[103] These weak estrogens may perform some of the same beneficial functions as endogenous estrogens and may turn down endogenous estrogen production through a negative feedback effect on the production of hypothalamic and pituitary hormones. Thus women who eat plant estrogens every day may have a constantly lower rate of estrogen production, which may lower their risk of breast cancer. An epidemiologic study of Chinese women in Singapore found that women who ate a diet high in soy had a lower rate of premenopausal (but not postmenopausal) breast cancer.[83] Dietary intake of red meat increased risk, and polyunsaturated fatty acids, beta-carotenes, and soy protein reduced risk.

The best-studied phytoestrogen is *genistein,* which decreases tyrosine kinase (involved in cell cycle regulation and control of mitogenesis) and inhibits angiogenesis.[78] One study found that baby rats exposed to a carcinogen had a 40% lower cancer rate if they also received genistein.[81] Genistein may be an active ingredient, but whole soybeans work as well; a previous study showed that rats fed soybean chips had lower rates of mammary tumors.[17]

Several studies have explored possible associations between aspects of the traditional Asian diet and low risk for hormone-based cancers and other hormone-dependent conditions in women.[6,7] In addition to lower fat content, higher fiber-to-protein ratios are also characteristic of traditional Asian diets when compared with typical diets in the West.

Thus dietary factors may influence hormone levels in women and may play a role in the etiology of hormone-dependent disease. Western diets elevate sex hormones and decrease sex hormone binding globulin (SHBG) concentration, thus increasing the availability of the endogenous steroids to peripheral tissues.[6] Increased fat intake decreases fecal excretion of endogenous estrogen, which may contribute to elevated serum levels and increase availability of endogenous estrogen at peripheral sites.[7] Increased fiber intake increases fecal excretion of endogenous estrogen, thus lowering serum levels.[3] High-fiber diets are associated with increased urinary lignans and isoflavones.[5]

ADVERSE EFFECTS. Phytoestrogens, including those contained in soy, have been associated with infertility in animals. In Australia in the 1940s, infertility that decimated the sheep industry was subsequently linked to clover forage containing phytoestrogens.[110] Captive cheetahs were found to be infertile after being fed a soy-based diet.[112] Whether phytoestrogens could cause infertility, precocious puberty in children, or cancer is an obvious question. To date, the data and observations do not provide an affirmative answer. In Asia, people of all ages consume considerable quantities of soy-based foods. Asians have lower rates of breast and prostate cancers, as well as later onset of puberty and no more infertility than Westerners. Additional research is needed to confirm the long-term safety of dietary phytoestrogens.

Despite these safety issues, studies on the role of phytoestrogens in the prevention and treatment of hormone-dependent cancers have a clear place in a research agenda on CAM and women's health.

Overview of CAM Therapies and Outcomes

A search of the Western scientific literature since 1970 found more than 100 studies that examined CAM methods and breast cancer.[71] Sixty-eight of these were studies of treatments in women; the rest were in animals or in vitro. The biomedical literature since 1980 describes mostly favorable results in the in vitro and animal studies of a variety of agents, but it is important to remind patients that these may not result in safe and effective treatments in humans.[71] These laboratory studies are not described in this chapter. Many studies in human subjects were case reports or case series and also are not described. Of the 68 studies in humans, only 15 controlled clinical trials randomly assigned patients to treatment groups.

The outcomes described in this literature include effects on relief of general symptoms, postmastectomy symptoms, side effects of chemotherapy and radiation, immune function, and survival. The treatments tested include herbs, nutrition, chemical treatments, acupuncture, mind-body techniques, manual therapies, and psychosocial interventions. By no means do the methods studied represent the range of CAM used by breast cancer patients. Breast cancer patients use many CAM treatments even though no studies have been done in breast cancer populations.

Diet Therapy

There is much speculation on the role of diet in prevention and treatment of cancer. Only one published study has examined the effect of a dietary program for breast cancer patients. In a study of 795 patients, those enrolled in the Bristol Cancer Help Center diet and counseling program had poorer survival than the control patients, who received only conventional treatment.[15] Differences between the Bristol patients and control subjects at baseline may account for this finding, which remains controversial. A review of 73 studies of dietary fat intake concluded that linoleic acid and its metabolic derivative arachidonic acid enhance metastasis in breast cancer.[105] This finding may have implications for both primary prevention and prevention of disease recurrence.

Another study assessed diet before cancer diagnosis as a predictor of survival in breast cancer patients and found that beta-carotene and fruit were associated with enhanced survival.[69] Among 100 patients given treatment with ascorbic acid, mean survival time was 300 days longer than among untreated controls.[27] A review of eight studies of ascorbic acid found no clear benefits, although an earlier review of 71 studies suggested substantial benefits.[19,28]

Psychosocial and Mind-Body Therapies

Two retrospective cohort studies found that patients in a breast cancer support group did not survive longer than control subjects.[56,92] A 10-year follow-up of a randomized, controlled trial, however, found that self-hypnosis and support group meetings significantly increased the mean survival time by 18 months.[116]

Relaxation techniques, cognitive therapy, biofeedback, music therapy, breathing exercises, hypnosis, and support groups and their effect on pain control, mood control, reduced anxiety, and adaptation have been examined in studies of varied designs.* A randomized clinical trial of biofeedback and cognitive therapy in 12 patients found that cognitive therapy decreased urinary cortisol levels, a biomarker for stress response.[34] Two studies of mind-body interventions reported reduction of cancer-related pain in the treatment groups.[10,115] A nonrandomized, crossover study found that relaxation, guided imagery, and biofeedback improved various measures of immune function (natural killer cell activity, mixed lymphocyte responsiveness, number of peripheral blood lymphocytes) in 13 patients.[58] These investigations indicate that these types of methods may be very important for the cancer patient, although the results of these studies are not comparable by method or end points, and no one study is particularly compelling.

Acupuncture

Acupuncture provides some relief from symptoms associated with conventional cancer treatment, in particular, nausea and vomiting associated with chemotherapy.[123] Acupuncture to relieve chemotherapy-induced nausea and vomiting has seldom been studied among breast cancer patients. One nonrandomized, controlled, crossover study found that 63% of patients receiving electroacupuncture treatment had reduced vomiting within 8 hours of treatment.[38] Almost half the subjects in the study were breast cancer patients. A preacupuncture and postacupuncture treatment study found that symptoms were reduced in 52% of breast cancer patients and that 47% had reduced pain.[50] There is considerable literature on the use of acupuncture to control chronic pain, including meta-analyses.[118] Research is needed to determine how well acupuncture can reduce symptoms in breast cancer patients.

In a nonrandomized, controlled study of immune function in 49 patients, 10 of whom had breast cancer, microwave acupuncture raised white blood cell counts slightly.[31]

Herbal Therapy

A number of herbal agents used for cancer treatment side effects appear promising enough to warrant further research, although they are not necessarily ready for formal clinical trials.[71]

Mistletoe *(Viscum album),* also called Iscador, has been found to stimulate immune function. A 1973 review of 11 studies found *mistletoe* promising for decreasing tumor size and extending survival.[46] A more recent review of three studies found no evidence of mistletoe's effect on immune function.[55] The relationship between immune function and cancer survival in humans is complex. A well-controlled observational study of survival among patients who use mistletoe might begin to address this question.

---

*References 21, 25, 35, 39, 82, 91, 108.

A randomized, controlled trial found that lymphocyte transformation was enhanced in patients who received a Chinese herb formula containing gymnostemma, pentphyllum, makino, and radix atragali seu heysari in addition to conventional treatment.[67] However, the number of patients was small, tumor types varied, and conventional treatments were not described. Another Chinese herbal formula, identified as Yi Qi Sheng Xue, was also found to improve white blood cell counts in the morning in a randomized, controlled trial that studied time of day of administration.[85] Again, chemotherapy regimens were not reported.

Whether there are botanic medicine treatments that enhance immune function after chemotherapy is worthy of further study. The effects of these agents on compliance with treatment schedules, other side effects and symptoms of treatment, disease recurrence, and survival are important research questions. In the study of the immune system, variables important to breast cancer patients will have to be identified as outcome measures in studies of botanicals in order to develop the science in this area.

SUMMARY

The research to date on CAM and breast cancer, menopausal hot flashes, and nausea and vomiting of pregnancy does not provide sufficient information about safety and efficacy to make clear clinical recommendations to patients. Although cancer survival has improved, cancer patients are increasingly turning to unconventional therapies in addition to conventional treatment or after exhausting conventional treatment.[1,26] Where conventional intervention is limited, as for nausea and vomiting during pregnancy, pregnant women are seeking alternatives that provide relief and are safe for developing fetuses.

Where women are dissatisfied with standard treatment or fear ways in which it may put them at risk, as in hormone replacement therapies for menopausal symptoms or hysterectomy for uterine fibroids, they will continue to seek and use CAM. Patients are reading about CAM therapies in the popular press, hearing about them from friends and relatives, learning about them at workshops on women's health, and choosing products at the health food store or even at the local drug store. Many patients are interested in dietary modification, nutritional supplementation, and mind-body approaches such as yoga, meditation, guided imagery, and support groups. Others are using herbs that may be unfamiliar to their physician, agents such as shark cartilage and antineoplastons, and detoxification techniques such as fasts or enemas.

Women are also seeking help from many types of CAM practitioners. They pursue treatment from practitioners of herbal medicine such as TCM, from Ayurveda doctors, and from Western herbalists, as well as homeopaths and naturopaths. Patients also turn to chiropractors, massage therapists, and other manual therapists.

Because so little scientific information exists on the safety and efficacy of these approaches, advising patients who seek or use CAM presents a professional challenge to conventional medicine providers. A step-by-step approach for proactively discussing the use of these therapies can be employed.[40] Such a strategy involves listening to patients as well as advising them, and this type of consultation requires time. The responsibility to do so is the same as discussing other issues essential to medical care, such as alcohol or drug use or a patient's preference for resuscitation. As treatment options broaden, partnership between care providers and patients in making treatment decisions is crucial for optimal health care.

REFERENCES

1. Abu-Realh MH et al: The use of complementary therapies by cancer patients, *Nurs Connect* 9:3, 1996 (review, 30 references).
2. Adlercreutz H, Honjo H, Higashi A: Urinary excretion of lignans and isoflavonoid phytoestrogens in Japanese men and women consuming a traditional Japanese diet, *Am J Clin Nutr* 54:1093, 1991.
3. Adlercreutz H et al: Excretion of the lignans enterolactone and enterodiol and of equol in omnivorous and vegetarian postmenopausal women and in women with breast cancer, *Lancet* 2:1295, 1982.
4. Adlercreutz H et al: Urinary estrogen profile determination in young Finnish vegetarian and omnivorous women, *J Steroid Biochem* 24:289, 1986.
5. Adlercreutz H et al: Effect of dietary components, including lignans and phytoestrogens, on enterohepatic circulation and liver metabolism of estrogens and on sex hormone binding globulin (SHBG), *J Steroid Biochem* 27:1135, 1987.
6. Adlercreutz H et al: Dietary phytoestrogens and cancer: in vitro and in vivo studies, *J Steroid Biochem Mol Biol* 41:331, 1992.
7. Adlercreutz H et al: Dietary phytoestrogens and the menopause in Japan, *Lancet* 339:1233, 1992.
8. American Cancer Society: *Cancer facts and figures,* Atlanta, 1994, The Society.
9. American Cancer Society: *Cancer facts and figures,* Atlanta, 1997, The Society (website).
10. Arathuzik D: Effects of cognitive-behavioral strategies on pain in cancer patients, *Cancer Nurs* 17:207, 1994.
11. Astin JA: Why patients use alternative medicine: results of a national study. *JAMA* 279:1548, 1998.
12. Atanackovic G, Navioz Y, Moretti ME, Koren G: The safety of higher than standard dose of doxylamine-pyridoxine (Diclectin) for nausea and vomiting of pregnancy, *J Clin Pharm* 41:842, 2001.
13. Avina RL, Schneiderman LJ: Why patients choose homeopathy, *West J Med* 128:366, 1978.
14. Backon J: Ginger in preventing nausea and vomiting of pregnancy; a caveat due to its thromboxane synthetase activity and effect on testosterone binding, *Eur J Obstet Gynecol Reprod Biol* 42:163, 1991.
15. Bagenal FS et al: Survival of patients with breast cancer attending Bristol Cancer Help Centre, *Lancet* 336:606, 1990.
16. Baird D et al: Dietary intervention study to assess estrogenicity of dietary soy among postmenopausal women, *J Clin Endocrinol Metab* 80:1685, 1995.
17. Barnes S et al: Soybeans inhibit mammary tumors in models of breast cancer, *Prog Clin Biol Res* 347:239, 1990.
18. Barton DL et al: Prospective evaluation of vitamin E for hot flashes in breast cancer survivors, *J Clin Oncol* 16:495, 1998.
19. Basu TK: The significance of ascorbic acid, thiamin and retinol in cancer, *Int J Vitam Nutr Res Suppl* 24:105, 1983.
20. Bayreuther J, Lewith GT, Pickering R: A double-blind cross-over study to evaluate the effectiveness of acupressure at pericardium 6 (P6) in the treatment of early morning sickness (EMS), *Complement Ther Med* 2:70, 1994.
21. Beck SL: The therapeutic use of music for cancer-related pain, *Oncol Nurs Forum* 18:1327, 1991.
22. Belluomini J et al: Acupressure for nausea and vomiting of pregnancy: a randomized, blinded study, *Obstet Gynecol* 84:245, 1994.
23. Bergner P: Is ginger safe in pregnancy? *Med Herb* 3:3, 1991.
24. Blatt MHG, Wiesbader H, Kupperman HS: Vitamin E and climacteric syndrome, *Arch Intern Med* 91:792, 1953.
25. Bridge LR et al: Relaxation and imagery in the treatment of breast cancer, *Br Med J* 297:1169, 1988.
26. Brigden ML: Unproven (questionable) cancer therapies, *West J Med* 163:463, 1995.

27. Cameron E, Pauling L: Supplemental ascorbate in the supportive treatment of cancer: reevaluation of the prolongation of survival times in terminal human cancer, *Proc Natl Acad Sci USA* 75:4538, 1978.
28. Cameron E, Pauling L, Leibovitz B: Ascorbic acid and cancer: a review, *Cancer Res* 39:663, 1979.
29. Carlsson CPO et al: Manual acupuncture reduces hyperemesis gravidarum: a placebo-controlled, randomized, single-blind, crossover study, *J Pain Symptom Manage* 20:273, 2000.
30. Cassileth BR et al: Contemporary unorthodox treatments in cancer medicine, *Ann Int Med* 101:105, 1984.
31. Chengjiang H et al: Effects of microwave acupuncture on the immunological function of cancer patients, *J Tradit Chin Med* 7:9, 1987.
32. Cohen M, Bendich A: Safety of pyridoxine: a review of human and animal studies, *Toxicol Lett* 34:129, 1986.
33. Commonwealth Fund: *Selected facts on U.S. women's health,* New York, 1997, The Fund.
34. Commonwealth Fund with Falik M, Collins K, editors: *Women's health: Commonwealth Fund survey,* Baltimore, 1996, Johns Hopkins University Press.
35. Davis H IV: Effects of biofeedback and cognitive therapy on stress in patients with breast cancer, *Psychol Rep* 59:967, 1986.
36. De Aloysio D, Penacchioni P: Morning sickness control in early pregnancy by Nei Guan point acupressure, *Obstet Gynecol* 80:852, 1992.
37. Duker EM et al: Effects of extracts from *Cimicifuga racemosa* on gonadotropin release in menopausal women and ovariectomized rats, *Planta Med* 57:420, 1991.
38. Dundee JW, Sourial FB, Bell PF: P6 acupressure reduces morning sickness: acupuncture prophylaxis of cancer chemotherapy-induced sickness, *J R Soc Med* 81:456, 1988.
39. Edgar L, Rosberger Z, Nowlis D: Coping with cancer during the first year after diagnosis: assessment and intervention, *Cancer* 69:817, 1992.
40. Eisenberg DM: Advising patients who seek alternative medical therapies, *Ann Int Med* 127:61, 1997.
41. Eisenberg DM et al: Unconventional medicine in the United States: prevalence, costs, and patterns of use, *N Engl J Med* 328:246, 1993.
42. Eisenberg DM et al: Trends in alternative medicine use in the United States, 1990–1997: results of a follow-up national survey, *JAMA* 280:1569, 1998.
43. Elder NC, Gillcrist A, Minz R: Use of alternative health care by family practice patients, *Arch Fam Med* 6:181, 1997.
44. Ernst E, Pittler MH: Efficacy of ginger for nausea and vomiting: a systematic review of randomized clinical trials, *Br J Anaesth* 84:367, 2000.
45. Evans AT et al: Suppression of pregnancy-induced nausea and vomiting with sensory afferent stimulation, *J Reprod Med* 38:603, 1993.
46. Evans MR, Preece AW: *Viscum album*: a possible treatment for cancer? *Bristol Med Chir J* 88:17, 1973.
47. Evidence-Based Work Group: Evidence-based medicine: a new approach to teaching the practice of medicine, *JAMA* 268:2420, 1997.
48. Factor-Litvak P et al: Complementary and alternative medicine use for women's health conditions: a pilot survey, 1997 (unpublished work).
49. Felter H, Lloyd J: *King's American dispensatory,* 1898, Sandy, Ore, 1992, Eclectic Medical Publishing.
50. Filshie J, Redman D: Acupuncture and malignant pain problems, *Eur J Surg Oncol* 11:389, 1985.
51. Fischer-Rasmussen W et al: Ginger treatment of hyperemesis gravidarum, *Eur J Obstet Gynecol Reprod Biol* 38:19, 1991.
52. Freedman RR, Woodward S: Behavioral treatment of menopausal hot flushes: evaluation by ambulatory monitoring, *Am J Obstet Gynecol* 167:436, 1992.
53. Freedman RR et al: Biochemical and thermoregulatory effects of behavioral treatment for menopausal hot flashes, *Menopause* 2:211, 1995.
54. Fuchs K et al: Treatment of hyperemesis gravidarum by hypnosis, *Int J Clin Exp Hypn* 28:313, 1980.
55. Gabius HJ et al: From ill-defined extracts to the immunomodulatory lectin: will there be a reason for oncological application of mistletoe? *Planta Med* 60:2, 1994.

56. Gellert GA, Maxwell RM, Siegel BS: Survival of breast cancer patients receiving adjunctive psychosocial support therapy: a 10-year follow-up study, *J Clin Oncol* 11:66, 1993.

57. Goodman MT et al: Association of soy and fiber consumption with the risk of endometrial cancer, *Am J Epidemiol* 146:294, 1997.

58. Gruber BL et al: Immunological responses of breast cancer patients to behavioral interventions, *Biofeedback Self Regul* 18:1, 1993.

59. Hammar M, Berg G, Lindgren R: Does physical exercise influence the frequency of postmenopausal hot flushes? *Acta Obstet Gynecol Scand* 69:409, 1990.

60. Hare ML: The emergence of an urban U.S. Chinese medicine, *Med Anthropol Q* 7:30, 1993.

61. Henker FO III: Psychotherapy as adjunct in treatment of vomiting during pregnancy, *South Med J* 69:1585, 1976.

62. Himmel W, Schulte M, Kochen MM: Complementary medicine: are patients' expectations being met by their general practitioners? *Br J Gen Pract* 43:232, 1993.

63. Hirata J et al: Does Dong Quai have estrogenic effects in postmenopausal women? A double-blind, placebo-controlled trial, *Menopause* 4:4, 1997.

64. Holt S: *Soya for health: the definitive medical guide,* New York, 1996, Liebert.

65. Hopkins MP, Androff L, Benninghoff AS: Ginseng face cream and unexplained vaginal bleeding, *Am J Obstet Gynecol* 159:1121, 1988.

66. Horton J, editor: *The women's health data book: a profile of women's health in the United States,* New York, 1992, Elsevier Science.

67. Hou J et al: Effects of gynostemma pentaphyllum makino on the immunological function of cancer patients, *J Tradit Chin Med* 11:47, 1991.

68. Hyde E: Acupressure therapy for morning sickness: a controlled clinical trial, *J Nurse Midwife* 34:171, 1989.

69. Ingram D: Diet and subsequent survival in women with breast cancer, *Br J Cancer* 69:592, 1994.

70. Irvin JH et al: The effects of relaxation response training on menopausal symptoms, *J Psychosom Obstet Gynaecol* 17:202, 1996.

71. Jacobson J, Workman S, Kronenberg F: Complementary and alternative therapies for breast cancer: a review of the biomedical literature, 1997 (unpublished work).

72. Jacobson JS et al: Randomized trial of black cohosh for the treatment of hot flashes among women with a history of breast cancer, *J Clin Oncol* 19:2739, 2001.

73. Jarry H, Harnischfeger G: Untersuchungen zur endokrinen wirksamkeit von inhaltsstoffen aus *Cimicifuga racemosa, Planta Med* 46, 1985.

74. Jewell D et al: Pregnancy and childbirth module, *Cochrane Database Syst Rev* 1, Oxford, 1997 (CD-ROM).

75. Kelsey J, Bernstein L: Epidemiology and prevention of breast cancer, *Annu Rev Public Health* 17:47, 1996.

76. Kennelly EJ et al: Analysis of thirteen populations of black cohosh for formononetin, *Phytomedicine,* 9:461, 2002.

77. Knight B et al: Effect of acupuncture on nausea of pregnancy: a randomized, controlled trial, *Obstet Gynecol* 97:184, 2001.

78. Knight D, Eden J: Phytoestrogens: a short review, *Maturitas* 22:167, 1995.

78a. Kronenberg F, Fugh-Berman A: Complementary and alternative medicine (CAM) for menopausal symptoms: a review of randomized controlled trials, *Ann Int Med* 137 (10): 805, 2002.

79. Kronenberg F, O'Leary Cobb J, McMahon D: Alternative medicine for menopausal problems: results of a survey, *Menopause* 1:171, 1994.

80. Kronenberg F et al: Complementary and alternative medicine use among American women in four race/ethnic groups, International Scientific Conference on Complementary, Alternative, and Integrative Medicine Research, Boston, 2002 (abstract to be published).

81. Lamartiniere C: Genistein programs against mammary cancer. Presented at Dietary Phyto-estrogens: Cancer Cause or Prevention? (conference), Herndon, Va, 1994, National Cancer Institute.

82. Larsson G, Starrin B: Relaxation training as an integral part of caring activities for cancer patients: effects on well-being, *Scand J Caring Sci* 6:179, 1992.

83. Lee H et al: Dietary effects on breast-cancer risk in Singapore, *Lancet* 337:1197, 1991.

84. Lehmann-Willenbrock E, Riedel HH: Clinical and endocrinological examinations concerning therapy of climacteric symptoms following hysterectomy with remaining ovaries, *Zent Bl Gynakol* 110:611, 1988.

85. Li Y, Yu G: A comparative clinical study on prevention and treatment with selected chronomedication of leukopenia induced by chemotherapy, *J Tradit Chin Med* 13:257, 1993.

86. Lindgrin R et al: Effects of gingseng on quality of life in postmenopausal women, *Menopause* 4:4, 1997.

87. Liu J et al: Evaluation of estrogenic activity of plant extracts for the potential treatment of menopausal symptoms, *J Agric Food Chem* 49:2472, 2001.

88. Long MAD, Simone SS, Tucher JJ: Outpatient treatment of hyperemesis gravidarum with stimulus control and imagery procedures, *J Behav Ther Exp Psychiatry* 17:105, 1986.

89. McGregor KJ, Peay ER: The choice of alternative therapy for health care: testing some propositions, *Soc Sci Med* 43:1317, 1996.

90. Messina M, Barnes S: The role of soy products in reducing risk of cancer, *J Natl Cancer Inst* 83:541, 1991.

91. Mock V et al: A nursing rehabilitation program for women with breast cancer receiving adjuvant chemotherapy, *Oncol Nurs Forum* 21:899, 1994.

92. Morgenstern H et al: The impact of a psychosocial support program on survival with breast cancer: the importance of selection bias in program evaluation, *J Chron Dis* 37:273, 1984.

93. Murkies AL et al: Dietary flour supplementation decreases post-menopausal hot flushes: effect of soy and wheat, *Maturitas* 21:189, 1995.

94. Murphy PA: Alternative therapies for nausea and vomiting of pregnancy, *Obstet Gynecol* 91:149, 1997.

95. National Research Council: *Recommended daily allowances*, ed 10, Washington, DC, 1989, National Academy Press.

96. Naylor CD: Grey zones of clinical practice: some limits to evidence-based medicine, *Lancet* 345:840, 1995.

97. O'Brien B, Naber S: Nausea and vomiting during pregnancy: effects on the quality of women's lives, *Birth* 19:138, 1992.

98. O'Brien B, Relyea MJ, Taerum T: Efficacy of P6 acupressure in the treatment of nausea and vomiting during pregnancy, *Am J Obstet Gynecol* 174:708, 1996.

99. Oketch-Rabah HA, Mehemi I, Tsai MS et al: Black cohosh *(Cimicifuga racemosa)* does not contain estrogenic activity, 2002 (in press).

100. Ornstein M, Einarson A, Koren G: Bendectin/Diclectin for morning sickness: a Canadian follow-up of an American tragedy, *Reprod Toxicol* 9:1, 1995.

101. Pike M, Spicer D: The chemoprevention of breast cancer by reducing sex steroid exposure: perspectives from epidemiology, *J Cell Biochem* 17G(suppl):26, 1993.

102. Pinn V: *Unnecessary hysterectomies: the second most common major surgery in the United States*, Washington, DC, 1993, US Committee on Labor and Human Resources, Subcommittee on Aging.

103. Price KR, Fenwick GR: Naturally occurring oestrogens in foods: a review, *Food Addit Contam* 2:73, 1985.

104. Punnonen R, Lukola A: Oestrogen-like effect of ginseng, *Br Med J* 281:1110, 1980.

105. Rose DP, Hatala MA: Dietary fatty acids and breast cancer invasion and metastasis, *Nutr Cancer* 21:103, 1994.

106. Rudman D, Williams PJ: Megadose vitamins: use and misuse, *N Engl J Med* 309:488, 1983.

107. Sahakian V et al: Vitamin B_6 is effective therapy for nausea and vomiting of pregnancy: a randomized, double-blind placebo-controlled study, *Obstet Gynecol* 78:33, 1991.

108. Samarel N, Fawcett J, Tulman L: The effects of coaching in breast cancer support groups: a pilot study, *Oncol Nurs Forum* 20:795, 1993.

109. Schaumburg H et al: Sensory neuropathy from pyridoxine abuse: a new megavitamin syndrome, *N Engl J Med* 309:445, 1983.

110. Schinckel P: Infertility in ewes grazing subterranean clover pastures: observations on breeding behavior following transfer to "sound" country, *Aust Vet J* 24:289, 1948.

111. Schuster K et al: Morning sickness and vitamin B_6 status of pregnant women, *Hum Nutr Clin Nutr* 39:75, 1985.

112. Setchell K et al: Dietary estrogens: a probable cause of infertility and liver disease in captive cheetahs, *Gastroenterology* 93:225, 1987.

113. Smith BJ: Management of the patient with hyperemesis gravidarum in family therapy with hypnotherapy as an adjunct, *J N Y State Nurses Assoc* 13:17, 1982.

114. Smith C, Crowther C, Beilby J: Acupuncture to treat nausea and vomiting in early pregnancy: a randomized controlled trial, *Birth* 29:1, 2002.

115. Spiegel D, Bloom JR: Group therapy and hypnosis reduce metastatic breast carcinoma pain, *Psychosom Med* 45:333, 1983.

116. Spiegel D, Bloom JR: Effect of psychosocial treatment on survival of patients with metastatic breast cancer, *Lancet* 2(8668): 888, 1989.

117. Stoll W: [Phytopharmacon influences atrophic vaginal epithelium: double-blind study—*Cimicifuga* vs. estrogenic substances], *Therapeutikon* 1:23, 1987.

118. Ter Riet G, Kleijnen J, Knipschild P: Acupuncture and chronic pain: a criteria-based meta-analysis, *J Clin Epidemiol* 43:1191, 1990.

119. Torem MS: Hypnotherapeutic techniques in the treatment of hyperemesis gravidarum, *Am J Clin Hypn* 37:1, 1994.

120. Updates: Report on '84 drug sales, *FDA Consumer* 20:2, 1986.

121. US Department of Health and Human Services: *Racial and ethnic disparities in health: response to the President's Initiative on Race,* Washington, DC, 1988, US Government Printing Office.

122. Vellacott ID, Cooke EJ, James CE: Nausea and vomiting in early pregnancy, *Int J Gyneacol Obstet* 27:27, 1988.

123. Vickers AJ: Can acupuncture have specific effects on health? A systematic review of acupuncture antiemesis trials, *J R Soc Med* 89:303, 1996.

124. Vutyavanich T, Kraisarin T, Ruangsri R: Ginger for nausea and vomiting in pregnancy: randomized, double-masked, placebo-controlled trial, *Obstet Gynecol* 97:577, 2001.

124a. Vutyavanich T, Wongtra-ngan S, Ruangsri R: Pyridoxine for nausea and vomiting of pregnancy: a randomized, double-blind, placebo-controlled trial, *Am J Obstet Gynecol* 173:881, 1995.

125. Warnecke G: Beeinflussung klimakterischer beschwerden durch ein phytotherapeutikum: erfolgreiche therapie mit cimicifuga-monoextrakt, *Medwelt* 36:871, 1985.

126. Wiklund IK, Mattsson LA, Lindgren R, Limoni C: Effects of a standardized ginseng extract on quality of life and physiological parameters in symptomatic postmenopausal women: a double-blind, placebo-controlled trial, *Int J Clin Pharmacol Res* 19:89, 1999.

127. Wilbur J et al: The relationship among menopausal status, menopausal symptoms, and physical activity in midlife women, *Fam Community Health* 13:67, 1990.

128. Wilcox G et al: Oestrogenic effects of plant foods in postmenopausal women, *BMJ* 301:905, 1990.

129. Wilcox LS, Koonin LM, Pokras R, et al: Hysterectomy in the United States, *Obstet Gynecol* 83:549, 1994.

130. Wyon Y et al: Effects of acupuncture on climacteric vasomotor symptoms, quality of life, and urinary excretion of neuropeptides among postmenopausal women, *Menopause* 2:3, 1995.

131. Zhao CX: Acupuncture treatment of morning sickness, *J Tradit Chin Med* 8:228, 1988.

132. Zhao RJ: 39 cases of morning sickness treated with acupuncture, *J Tradit Chin Med* 7:25, 1987.

SUGGESTED READING

Tiran D, Mack S: *Complementary therapies for pregnancy and childbirth,* London, 1995, Balliere Tindall.

ACKNOWLEDGMENT

Partial support was received from National Institutes of Health, National Center for Complementary and Alternative Medicine grant P50-AT00090.

CHAPTER 13

Select Populations: Elderly Patients

FREDERIC M. LUSKIN, ELLEN M. DINUCCI,
KATHRYN A. NEWELL, and WILLIAM L. HASKELL

Although elderly persons may not use complementary and alternative medicine (CAM) as frequently as the rest of the population, CAM usage by the elderly is significant. CAM therapy for elderly persons has not been extensively reviewed in published surveys, and therefore all the data are recent. A national study found that 30% of Americans over age 65 used some form of CAM at least once in the previous year.[41] In contrast, 46% of people under age 65 used CAM therapies. Chiropractic and herbal medicines were the therapies most often used. Astin et al.[9] found similar numbers in a survey of Medicare recipients in California. Another survey found that 58% of the elderly cohort used CAM.[25] Usage was strongly correlated with female gender, higher level of education, and prevalence of arthritis. Interestingly, in both national telephone surveys conducted by Eisenberg et al.,[33,34] arthritis was a common reason for people to turn to CAM methods.

In this chapter we evaluate the use of CAM approaches to the treatment of Alzheimer's disease and osteoarthritis. We have chosen these two chronic conditions because they are responsible for disability in a great number people age 65 and over, and because current medical management is often inadequate. There is neither a cure nor a clearly proven treatment for either condition. Therefore these conditions can lead to costly medical care that is often palliative at best, and each deserves a careful exploration of the efficacy of alternative treatment methods.

◣ Alzheimer's Disease

Alzheimer's disease (AD) is a degenerative disorder that alters memory, cognition, and behavior. About 10% of Americans ages 65 and older have AD, and up to 50% of those 85 and older have some form of the disease.[4] In 1995, approximately 4 million

Americans had AD, a prevalence expected to triple by the year 2050. Current U.S. costs for the care of AD patients are calculated at $90 to $100 billion annually.[86]

AD is the most common form of *dementia,* which is a cluster of symptoms that create an escalating inability to use intellectual capabilities to carry out regular daily activities. There is no cure for AD, and the causes are still unknown.

DIAGNOSIS

The only definitive method for diagnosing AD is through patient autopsy. During autopsy, brain tissue is examined for the presence of neurofibrillary tangles and neuritic plaques. Diagnosis is difficult because such plaques and tangles also exist, in smaller amounts, in normal elderly persons. In patients with Alzheimer's brain tissue, plaque may be composed of unusual formations or may contain an overabundance of proteins, such as microtubule-associated protein (MAP), tau protein, and amyloid protein. In addition to brain tissue abnormalities, lower quantities of neurotransmitters, such as serotonin, acetylcholine, norepinephrine, somatostatin, and corticotropin-releasing factor, are often found. Finally, in some AD patients, larger-than-normal quantities of aluminum have been discovered in the brain. It has not been proven, however, that prolonged exposure to aluminum is the cause of AD.[79]

According to the *Diagnostic and Statistical Manual of Mental Disorders* (fourth edition, *DSM*-IV) of the American Psychiatric Association,[31] the criteria for determining the presence of AD include the following:

- Cognitive impairment, as evidenced by inadequate memory
- One or more of these conditions: aphasia, apraxia, agnosia, and inability to plan and organize life
- Inability to function in social or occupational settings
- Slow onset and steady decrease in cognitive abilities
- No diagnosis of other diseases, such as Parkinson's brain tumor, nutritional deficiencies, hypothyroidism, and substance abuse

Normally there are three stages in the progression of AD. As with most diseases that occur in stages, progress from one stage to another is not inevitable and is often uneven. The *first stage* includes such symptoms as recent memory impairment impacting work-related duties, confusion about directions to frequently traveled locations, and changes in behavior and mood. During the *second stage,* AD patients may experience auditory or visual hallucinations, difficulty in reading and writing, and behaviors that require that they be constantly monitored. In the *third stage,* patients may become mute, may lose control of their excretory processes, and may have limited capability in caring for their own well-being.[53]

A person's genes have been linked to the development of AD. People whose parents have AD are at higher risk for developing the disease. Apolipoprotein E (apo E) gene on chromosome 19 has been associated with a risk for developing AD.[8] However, even if a person has one or more family members who have the disease, this does not necessarily mean that person will develop AD. In addition to genetic predisposition, other risk factors include aging, past serious head trauma that produced an unconscious state,[14] Down syndrome, and little or no formal education.

In a study using Catholic nuns as subjects, the importance of prevention and lifestyle factors on the manifestation of AD is suggested.[104] Some nuns who exhibited the tangles and plaques associated with AD on autopsy never developed the disease while alive. The critical finding was that nuns who had had a stroke were more likely to show AD symptoms. Corollary evidence also links atherosclerosis with the development of AD.[7]

Interestingly, the rate of AD tends to be higher in those who are less educated, suggesting that cognitive abilities developed earlier in life may protect older individuals from the ravages of the disease. In the study with Catholic nuns, researchers examined their early adult diaries. Nuns who used less complex sentences and less descriptive prose showed a decline in cognitive abilities and a concomitant tendency to develop AD later in life.

CONVENTIONAL MEDICAL MANAGEMENT

Although there is no cure for AD, conventional treatments alleviate some memory difficulties as well as other symptoms in patients with mild to moderate forms of the disease. The four drugs approved by the U.S. Food and Drug Administration (FDA) specifically for AD carry significant risk for side effects.[5–7a]

Other conventional treatments include hormone replacement therapy (HRT) in women and the use of antiinflammatory drugs such as ibuprofen. The research on HRT has shown some positive results in limiting dementia, but the number of randomized, controlled trials (RCTs) is insufficient, and none has established the relative risk of dementia.[73] To treat behavioral disturbance and psychotic symptoms, neuroleptic drugs are typically used.[30] However, a 2-year prospective, longitudinal study reported that use of neuroleptic substances may accelerate cognitive deterioration in those with dementia.[82]

Nonpharmacologic treatment of AD patients includes behavioral therapies, physical and mental stimulation, reality orientation therapy, memory training programs, psychotherapy, and physical stimulation through physical exercise, occupational therapy, and positive interactions therapy.[18]

CAM THERAPIES WITH SCIENTIFIC EFFICACY

A survey of CAM therapy usage for AD questioned 101 primary caregivers of AD patients and those who attended support groups and found that 55% administered at least one alternative therapy to enhance memory of the patient and that 20% tried three or more treatments, including vitamins (84%), health foods (27%), herbal medicines (11%), "smart pills" (9%), and home remedies (7%).[26]

This section reviews the CAM therapies that have the best research to substantiate their continued use. For AD the three with the greatest scientific efficacy are *Ginkgo biloba*, vitamin E, and music therapy. At present, all three treatments appear useful for different aspects of the disease, and each has minimal side effects compared with conventional drug treatments.

Ginkgo biloba

Ginkgo biloba extract is a prevalent, legal, over-the-counter (OTC) medicine in Europe. In 1994 the German government approved *G. biloba* for use with dementia patients. In the United States, however, the extract has not yet been approved by the FDA, although it can be bought in the United States as an OTC medication at health food and grocery stores. *G. biloba* extract (GBE) is derived from the leaves of the ginkgo, a fruit-bearing tree that is indigenous to eastern China.

Research suggests that GBE is effective in enhancing the cognitive abilities of AD patients. With one significant exception, evidence suggests that GBE is useful for patients with mild to moderate AD. GBE (EGb 761) was tested in a randomized, placebo-controlled study on 40 patients with AD of medium severity.[58] Attention, memory, psychopathology, functional performance, and psychomotor ability improved in the treatment group after 1 month. No adverse reactions to the extract were observed during the study. Members of the placebo group showed either no change or some deterioration.

A 26-week analysis of a placebo-controlled trial of a moderate dose of *Ginkgo* found that the placebo group had declines in most areas, whereas the treatment group experienced slight improvements on cognitive assessment, daily living, and social behavior.[72] As an example of the degree of positive change noted from the *Ginkgo,* 26% of the *Ginkgo* group and 17% of the placebo group showed a 4-point improvement in the measure of cognitive function.

In a 24-week prospective, randomized, double-blind study, Alzheimer's dementia and multiinfarct dementia outpatients received *G. biloba* or a placebo.[61] The *G. biloba* was found to be highly effective with few side effects. The adverse effects, which were reported by a small percentage of subjects, included headache, allergic skin reactions, and gastrointestinal complaints.

In a 1996 review of 44 randomized, placebo-controlled, double-blind studies of *Ginkgo biloba* special extract (GBSE) and the drugs nimodipine and tacrine in the treatment of Alzheimer-type dementia, vascular dementia, and a combination of the two, the three types of treatments were compared. *G. biloba* was included in 25 of the 44 studies.[74] The review confirmed the clinical efficacy of all three substances as valuable for improving behavior, psychometrics, and psychopathology. A significantly higher percentage of patients receiving the drugs nimodipine and tacrine experienced adverse side effects. A 2000 review of all the controlled trials of *Ginkgo* extracts found clinically significant improvement in memory loss, concentration, fatigue, anxiety, and depressed mood.[11] Problems were noted with the research because of small sample sizes and in particular the use of nonstandard measures.

A recent study offers some caution in the recommendation of *Ginkgo* for the problems associated with memory loss and dementia. This multicenter randomized, placebo-controlled 24-week study found no significant results between a group of people taking *Ginkgo* and those not taking it. This research evaluated both low and high doses of *Ginkgo,* and the *Ginkgo* group was again randomized into either a group continuing to receive *Ginkgo* or a placebo group at the end of the first 12 weeks of the study.[116]

Vitamin E

Vitamin E has been studied as a treatment designed to inhibit the progression of AD because of its utility as a free radical scavenger.[12] Some researchers theorize that free radicals play a role in the damaging effects of AD.[70] It is unclear whether this is because of the body's inability to repair free radical damage or because of the excessive production of free radicals.[37] Many lines of evidence suggest that oxidative stress may be important in the progression of AD. Current focus is on beta-amyloid, which acquires some of its toxicity to neuronal cell activity through the production of free radicals.[52] Vitamin E as an antioxidant may protect the body from free radical injury.

Researchers in a case-control study determined that both AD and multiinfarct dementia subjects had notably lower plasma concentrations of vitamin E and beta-carotene than the control subjects. The researchers concluded that lower levels of these antioxidants may hasten AD progression, and that further study of these substances may be beneficial in discovering their possible disease-inhibiting effects.[127] In a study comparing plasma vitamin E levels of community-dwelling early-AD patients to those of normal spouses and age-matched controls, Alzheimer's patients were reported to have lower levels of vitamin E.[91] Lower blood levels of vitamin E suggest a potential for free radical higher damage.

In a prospective study of people age 65 and older, a stratified random sample was selected from the disease-free population. At baseline, all vitamin supplements taken in the previous 2 weeks were identified, and the group was followed for the next 4.3 years. After this time, none of those taking either vitamin E or vitamin C supplements had developed AD. Interestingly, there was no relation between AD and the use of multivitamins.[85]

A Cochrane review on vitamin E and AD found only one randomized double-blind trial with sufficiently high quality that was worthy of review.[107] The 2-year RCT examined the effects of vitamin E and several other treatments on 341 patients with moderate AD. The subjects received either 2000 IU of vitamin E, 10 mg of selegiline (drug treatment for Parkinson's disease), vitamin E and selegiline, or placebo. Results showed that the vitamin E group experienced a 670-day median delay of disease progression, the selegiline group a 655-day delay, and the vitamin E/selegiline group a 585-day delay, compared with a 440-day delay for the placebo group[100] (Figure 13-1).

Music Therapy

Music therapy is a noninvasive method for treating various psychologic symptoms of AD, including depression, feelings of isolation, agitation and wandering behaviors, and loss of a sense of self.[1] Music also has potential use as a substitute for restraints for AD patients who wander.[45] Music as therapy can be effective as either a passive or an active experience. *Passive* music therapy involves the patient, alone or in a group, listening to music, whether live, prerecorded, or performed by the therapist. *Active* music therapy involves the patient and the therapist playing musical instruments, which may have added value because it helps the patient to communicate with others despite declining verbal capacity. The deterioration of communication ability may contribute to the isolation typically experienced by AD patients.

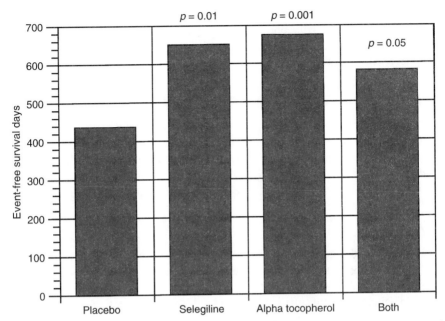

FIGURE 13–1. Median number of days of event-free survival in patients with Alzheimer's disease treated with selegiline, α-tocopherol (vitamin E), or both. Event-free survival is defined as survival until the occurrence of death, institutionalization, inability to perform activities of daily living, or severe dementia. The p values are for the differences in event-free survival between the placebo group and each of the treatment groups.

A review from 2000 found no RCTs that were of sufficient methodologic rigor to establish the efficacy of music therapy.[69] The authors noted considerable anecdotal evidence and some controlled studies with significant limitations. Overall, the review concluded that music therapy may be beneficial in treating dementia symptoms and highlighted the need for well-designed intervention studies. A different review noted that because many AD patients experience prolonged bouts of depression and other negative emotions, psychosocial interventions such as music therapy would be beneficial. Most of these conclusions come from case studies, however, and further work is needed to establish how music can benefit Alzheimer's patients.[19]

A 6-month controlled study of 60 AD patients used three groups, one of whom listened to "big band" music. The mood and ability to recall past events improved more in the music group patients than in the other two groups.[77] Another study of 20 nursing home Alzheimer's patients found that music therapy reduced their level of agitation.[23] In a study of 30 AD patients who wandered, the subjects were randomly placed in either a music or a reading group. The music group sat in or remained near the session for longer periods than the reading group.[51]

One study found that daily music therapy offered for 5 weeks decreased the levels of stress chemicals and increased the level of melatonin in AD patients.

The melatonin levels increased during the music intervention and remained higher at follow-up, whereas the epinephrine and norepinephrine levels returned to baseline when the music therapy ended. The authors hypothesized that the increase in melatonin levels may contribute to patients' increased relaxation and calm mood.[71]

CAM THERAPIES WITH SUSPECTED EFFICACY

As suggested by the research, many factors such as strokes, atherosclerosis, limited education, isolation, and oxidative damage are linked to AD. Because of the broad spectrum of links to the disease, a wide variety of treatments have provided suggestive evidence of efficacy; a few are briefly reviewed here. In each CAM area, although evidence is suggestive, it is not yet established that the treatment is effective for Alzheimer's patients.

Phytoestrogens

Lower levels of estrogen in postmenopausal women may be associated with the incidence of dementia,[13] and estrogen replacement therapy in postmenopausal women may lower the risk of AD.[57] Some studies indicate that estrogen protects against beta-amyloid damage and thus may be useful in inhibiting or preventing AD and enhancing the memory of women with the disease.[92] A recent review indicated that HRT improves cognitive ability and can decrease the incidence of dementia.[74] In a 1998 study, however, Yaffe et al.[123] cautioned against the widespread use of estrogen because of the risks involved and the weakness of the evidence of efficacy. Because of this, *phytoestrogens,* or plant-derived estrogens found predominantly in soy products, may produce similarly favorable outcomes through similar mechanisms and have lower risk than HRT. No studies to date are available to test this hypothesis.

Bioelectromagnetics

Bioelectromagnetics is the science of how electrical systems within the body are influenced by external electromagnetic fields (EMFs) and how alterations in the body's EMFs may modify physiologic, cognitive, and psychologic states.[122] It is hypothesized that changing behavior patterns regarding electrical equipment usage may be helpful in preventing cellular disturbances in the brain.

The Reagan Research Institute has reported that specific EMFs may disturb calcium ions within the brain cells.[3] In another study, researchers noted that those exposed to frequent and concentrated amounts of EMFs in the workplace were three times more prone to dementia than those who were exposed to smaller amounts.[106] Studies that examine how EMFs can be used for healing are provocative. Placebo-controlled clinical trials point to the possibility that EMFs may be influential in healing wounds and specific bone fractures.[10] No studies link EMFs to improving the condition of AD patients.

Essential Fatty Acids

Essential fatty acids (EFAs), both alone and in combination with antioxidants, are hypothesized as possible treatments for AD. In a double-blind, placebo-controlled trial in which AD patients were treated with EFAs and antioxidants, the EFA group and placebo groups both showed improvement in mood and cognitive ability, with improvements higher in the EFA group.[27] A review that examined data from the Rotterdam Study and the Zutphen Elderly Study showed that a high level of total fat and saturated fat put people at risk for dementia, whereas a high fish consumption reduced the risk of dementia.[60]

Dehydroepiandrosterone

Some evidence suggests that diminishing reserves of dehydroepiandrosterone (DHEA) may be linked to AD, particularly with regard to the amyloid precursor protein (APP), and could also be related to other forms of dementia.[125] A Cochrane review found four studies that examined DHEA's effect on cognition in healthy people. DHEA had an effect limited to women and was effective in retaining attention only after a psychosocial stressor. The review mentions that studies are under way looking at the effect of DHEA supplementation on AD patients.[59]

St. John's Wort

St. John's wort may be a useful treatment for depression in AD patients. According to a systematic review and meta-analysis of 23 randomized trials of this natural substance, St. John's wort was useful in the treatment of depression and had fewer side effects than medication. The authors note that further studies are needed, particularly to determine dosage and relative efficacy compared with standard antidepressants.[75] In a recent double-blind, RCT with 375 patients, St. John's wort extract WS 5570 was considered safer and more efficacious when compared with placebo in managing mild to moderate depression. The dosage over six weeks was 300 mg three times a day.[73a]

Massage Therapy

Massage has been used as a form of relaxation for dementia patients. In one study of residents of an Alzheimer's unit, patients were assigned to one of three groups: hand massage, therapeutic touch (TT), and control group, whose members were simply watched by another person. Although hand massage was more relaxing than TT, both had greater efficacy than simple presence of another person.[105] A demonstration project at a nursing home showed that a 1-year massage program for dementia patients could reduce anxious and agitated behavior.[101] A study that examined the effect of massage on agitated dementia found that massage did not lessen verbal agitation but did help control the physical expressions, such as pacing, wandering, and resisting.[99]

Social Support

Social support for patients with early-stage AD can provide emotional support, offer modeling, and enhance coping ability. The effect of social support increases a sense of belonging, allows for information interchanges, and provides an outlet for the expression of grief.[124] Social support has been shown to be beneficial for patients with a variety of physical conditions, and therefore it may be a useful adjunctive treatment for both AD patients and their caregivers.[29]

ℵ Osteoarthritis

Osteoarthritis (OA), the most common form of arthritis, is a degenerative joint disease characterized by the inflammation, breakdown, and eventual loss of the cartilage in weight-bearing joints. When damaged, cartilage, the protein substance that provides the "cushion" between bones, can cause severe joint pain, stiffness, and physical disability. Joints in the hips, knees, ankles, neck, lower back, and hands are the joints most often affected. Hip pain can be especially severe, making walking difficult; however, OA of the knee results in the greatest number of disabled elderly patients.[22]

OA affects an estimated 16 million Americans, mostly elderly women, and is the second leading cause of disability in adults over age 65.[80] According to the Arthritis Foundation, OA is the cause of more than 7 million visits to physicians annually. Further, a 1996 study reported that hip and knee OA accounted for at least 70% of the more than 200,000 total hip and knee replacement surgeries performed annually in the United States.[39]

DIAGNOSIS

Diagnosis is challenging because no specific laboratory test exists for OA. Physicians must rely on the accurate history of symptoms and radiographs. However, radiographic findings do not always match patient reports of pain suffered; that is, when joint destruction is demonstrated, it does not necessarily follow that a patient will have severe pain, and conversely, a patient may have severe pain with only minor x-ray findings.

Symptoms can vary greatly from patient to patient. Some patients can be debilitated by their symptoms (pain, disfigurement), whereas others may be unaware of the disease. The process of aging causes cartilage to degenerate, making the incidence of OA partly a function of age. Other precursors to the development of OA include infections, past fractures, history of other types of arthritis (e.g., rheumatism), stress on joints due to obesity, poor posture and occupational abuse, metabolic disorders affecting joints, the influence of heredity, and hormonal disturbances.[80]

In advanced cases of OA, cartilage can be completely lost, leading to extreme pain and limits of joint mobility. Inflammation of the cartilage can also stimulate new bone outgrowths (spurs, bunions) to form around the joints, thereby further limiting mobility.

CONVENTIONAL MEDICAL MANAGEMENT

Currently, there is no known cure for OA. Treatment is aimed primarily at pain relief and the reduction of disability.[121] Common conventional treatments include the following:
- Exercise (e.g., swimming, aerobics)
- Weight control
- Joint protection (rest)

- Heat/cold therapy
- Physical/occupational therapy
- Mechanical support devices (e.g., splints, canes, walkers)
- Pain relievers (e.g., aspirin, acetaminophen)
- Medications injected into the joints (e.g., cortisone)
- Nonsteroidal antiinflammatory drugs (NSAIDs) and COX-2 inhibitors
- Topical creams (e.g., capsaisin, NSAIDs)
- Surgery (arthrocentesis, arthroscopy, osteotomy, total knee/hip replacement)

Some conventional therapies, including NSAIDs, injections, topical creams, and surgery, offer relief of symptoms at a relative cost to patients, physically, financially, or both. Other treatments may cause physical or psychologic challenges and inconvenience for patients already dealing with the difficulties of OA (weight loss, exercise, mechanical support devices).

In elderly patients the use of NSAIDs poses significant risk for gastrointestinal distress. Up to 20% to 30% of hospital admissions for and deaths from peptic ulcers in elderly patients are related to NSAIDs.[50] A British review recommended NSAID use only after careful consideration of side effects and close observation during use.[32] Further, efficacy of NSAIDS has been difficult to prove due to low adherence rates in research studies. The use of medication injected into the joints can diminish pain for periods of time, but joint flare-ups can cause discomfort, and long-term use of medications such as cortisone can be damaging to tissues and bones.[117] Topical creams such as capsaicin can provide temporary relief from joint pain, but the need for constant use (four times daily) can be difficult for patients to manage. Also, side effects such as burning and stinging have been reported.[2,103] Surgery has the potential to dramatically reduce pain and restore joint mobility, but the financial cost is high and comes with the risk of complications inherent in any surgery.

Exercise for OA patients, when performed at moderate levels, can be beneficial by promoting mobility in the joints and contributing to weight loss, minimizing strain on the joints. Although strength training, resistance training, and aerobic activity have been shown to benefit patients with OA,[36] these exercises are not always appropriate for older OA patients.[83,84,102]

CAM THERAPIES

Two recent studies suggest that CAM therapies are widely used by OA patients.[95,96] Earlier studies have reported that one fourth of arthritis respondents had employed the services of CAM providers, primarily chiropractors and acupuncturists,[49] and that up to 94% had used CAM for arthritis as far back as 1984.[56]

The Arthritis Foundation estimated in 1982 that expenditures of $1.8 billion were spent on "unproven remedies." With the population over age 65 increasing in the United States, as well as the greater availability and awareness of CAM options for therapy, projected expenditures will likely be much higher.

To determine the efficacy of CAM therapies for OA, a thorough search was conducted, including books, the Internet, literature reviews, and peer-reviewed scientific journals. Clearly, general use of CAM therapies for OA is widespread. However, use of rigorous standards to evaluate CAM approaches to OA is just beginning. Although there are many anecdotal reports of effectiveness, only those CAM therapies evaluated in controlled trials found in the scientific literature are discussed here (Table 13-1).

Diet, Supplements, and Alternative Pharmaceuticals

Making sensible dietary changes can be beneficial to a person's overall health. However, there is a lack of scientific literature substantiating the claims that special diets, such as the restriction of certain foods, can aid in the reduction of OA symptoms, although research on nutritional and herbal supplements is promising.

The use of supplements has grown rapidly in the last few years, motivating investigators to review those used for the treatment of OA. Two that show the most evidence of efficacy for the reduction of pain and stiffness in RCTs are *glucosamine sulfate* (GS) and *chondroitin sulfate* (CS). A 2000 meta-analysis included 15 of 37 RCTs found and reported moderate to significant effects in treating symptoms of knee and hip OA with both GS and CS.[81] A review of GS alone by the Cochrane Collaboration in 2001 identified 16 RCTs with evidence of efficacy and safety. Four of the studies compared GS with NSAIDs directly, with two showing GS to be superior to NSAIDs and two showing the therapies as equally effective.[111] Since the publication of these reviews, at least two additional RCTs have reported positive results when using GS for symptom reduction in patients with OA.[97,109]

TABLE 13–1. **CAM THERAPIES FOR OSTEOARTHRITIS (OA)***

Therapy	EVIDENCE OF EFFICACY		
	High: Significant Scientific Evidence	**Medium: Some Scientific Evidence**	**Low: Anecdotal Evidence Only**
Diet, supplements, and alternative pharmaceuticals	Glucosamine sulfate Chondroitin sulfate	Hormone replacement therapy (HRT)	Diet (avoiding specific foods) Supplements Cell therapy Reconstructive therapy
Alternative systems and modalities	Acupuncture	Traditional Chinese medicine (TCM) T'ai chi PEMF TENS	Acupressure Osteopathy Qi Gong (Chi Kung)
Mind-body therapies	Cognitive-behavioral therapy (CBT) Social support	Yoga	Meditation Guided imagery Aromatherapy Music therapy
Manual healing		Chiropractic Therapeutic touch (TT)	Shiatsu Reflexology Massage Rolfing Craniosacral Applied kinesiology

*These CAM therapies are suggested to benefit symptoms of OA. However, given the early state of CAM research, suggestions for further research to confirm results apply to all therapies listed.
PEMF, Pulsed electromagnetic field; *TENS*, transcutaneous electrical nerve stimulation.

Other supplements advocated for the relief of OA symptoms include vitamin B$_3$ (for pain and stiffness),[42] vitamin E (for pain), vitamin D (to slow progression of OA), avocado/soybean extract (for pain), S-adenosylmethionine (for pain and stiffness), and boron (for pain and inflammation).[76] Each of these supplements is noted on the official website of the Arthritis Foundation (www.arthritis.org/) as having some scientific evidence toward efficacy in the treatment of symptoms or the prevention of OA. Although worth mentioning, these supplements lack the credible scientific evidence found for both GS and CS.

It is suggested that alternative pharmaceuticals may benefit OA patients, but few RCTs were discovered. Investigators, in at least one study of HRT, found that women taking estrogen had almost a 40% lower risk of hip OA compared with women who had never used estrogen,[88] and their risk of developing moderate to severe OA was even lower. Other alternative pharmacologic approaches, such as chelation therapy, cell therapy, reconstructive therapy, and enzyme therapy, are suggested by guidebooks to alternative medicine. A few are reportedly used in countries outside the United States, but these therapies have not been sufficiently evaluated in peer-reviewed medical journals.

Although it is unclear how particular diets play a role in the treatment or prevention of OA, dietary supplements, especially GS and CS, show promise and will continue to be evaluated as the National Institute of Arthritis and Musculoskeletal and Skin Diseases (NIAMS) and the National Center for Complementary and Alternative Medicine (NCCAM) introduce further evaluation of these agents.[89]

Alternative Systems and Modalities

This section discusses therapeutic CAM systems and the modalities found efficacious within those systems, as well as other alternative modalities.

Traditional Chinese medicine (TCM), including the use of Chinese herbs, acupuncture, and acupressure, was investigated for use by OA patients in one study using oral administration in conjunction with steaming and washing and gentle joint manipulation.[118] Of 28 patients with OA of the knee joint, seven were reported "cured" (no remaining symptoms), 13 showed marked effect (symptoms gone and reappearing only occasionally when patient tired or cold), 6 were improved (symptoms greatly improved but not eliminated), and only 2 patients showed no effect. Although no other studies using TCM were found, individual studies of acupuncture and t'ai chi are reported next.

Acupuncture has been tested for pain reduction in multiple studies with mixed results. In 1998, results from a National Institutes of Health (NIH) consensus conference on acupuncture suggested that acupuncture may be useful only as part of a comprehensive medical management program, but not alone.[87] For the conference, a thorough literature review was conducted, including articles from 1970 through 1997. More recently, a review of RCTs or quasi-RCTs for acupuncture for the treatment of OA of the knee was published.[38] Seven trials were identified, and results indicated limited evidence that acupuncture was more effective for pain and function than usual treatment. Also, evidence indicated that real acupuncture was more effective for pain than sham acupuncture, although this did not hold true when testing for function.

Results from recent trials continue to be mixed. In 1999, one RCT found acupuncture coupled with standard care to be significantly better than standard treatment alone in reducing pain and increasing function based on the WOMAC scale.[16] In 2001, acupuncture alone was compared to advice and exercise and was found to be more effective in reducing pain and increasing function, again based on the WOMAC scale.[55]

Other studies have compared real acupuncture to sham acupuncture, where the needle entry points are not part of the TCM system. In 2001, Chinese acupuncture for OA of the hip was compared to sham acupuncture, resulting in both treatments providing significant improvement of both pain and function over baseline, with no difference between groups.[40] The results from this study corroborate the results of earlier studies comparing real acupuncture[35,110] to sham acupuncture.

To explain the value of the sham acupuncture, the placebo effect is hypothesized. Clearly, physician and patient beliefs, as well as the use of acupuncture without the indication of specific points, should spark interest as an example of how healing can occur without a clear understanding of the mechanisms involved. Results have been inconclusive, but investigators from all studies cited here have encouraged more research in this area, and all indicated that acupuncture has some value in the treatment of OA.

T'ai chi and *Qi Gong*, both gentle exercises of Chinese origin and considered part of TCM, have been practiced by elderly people outside the United States for hundreds of years. Although no research studies on Qi Gong and OA were found, one RCT using t'ai chi as a therapeutic modality reported a significant reduction in OA symptoms and improvement in arthritis self-efficacy, level of tension, and quality of life after 12 weeks of practice.[54] Given the growing popularity and safety of t'ai chi for older adults and the general recommendations for exercise as a conventional therapy for OA, further research of t'ai chi is warranted.

Osteopathy, a unique system of medicine, integrates many manipulative CAM therapies (physical manipulation, craniosacral work, relaxation, nutritional guidance) and claims to have therapeutic benefit to arthritis patients in the alternative medicine guidebooks. However, no research studies on its efficacy for OA specifically were found.

Pulsed electromagnetic fields (PEMFs) in the treatment of OA of the knee and cervical spine were explored in one RCT, with positive results for OA patients.[113] Statistical significance was found in PEMF groups compared with placebo groups on measures of pain, pain during motion, overall patient assessment, and physician assessment. These results replicate an earlier pilot study by the same investigators[114] and support the suggestion that PEMF may benefit patients with OA of the knee and cervical spine. The same investigator reviewed the PEMF research more recently and arrived at similar conclusions.[112] One other study supports the use of PEMF for OA of the knee but must be considered preliminary.[28] Investigators in the PEMF field stress the need for more research.

Transcutaneous electrical nerve stimulation (TENS), a noninvasive modality of physiotherapy, has been shown to minimize postoperative pain and provide short-term pain relief in several small controlled studies on OA of the knee.[108,126] More recently, a Cochrane review pooled data from seven controlled studies on TENS for OA of the knee and found it to be significantly more effective for pain relief and knee stiffness than placebo.[90]

Mind-Body Therapies

CAM therapies grouped under the umbrella of mind-body treatments usually contain one or both of two core components: patient education and relaxation skills training. The mind-body therapies suggested for use with OA patients include but are not limited to cognitive-behavioral therapy, social support, yoga, meditation, guided imagery, aromatherapy, and music therapy.[78] These therapies may reduce suffering, in part because they induce the relaxation response, which lowers sympathetic activation. However, very few of these therapies have been studied directly with OA patients, and therefore we cannot include them in this section.

Cognitive-behavioral therapy (CBT) has been compared to patient education, a more conventional part of OA management. Both treatment approaches show similar efficacy after 1 year.[24] Keefe et al. used CBT to treat symptoms of OA with positive patient outcomes.[62-66] Results from these RCTs suggest that CBT is effective in the reduction of pain, psychologic disability, and physical disability, as well as pain behaviors. Other studies using CBT and self-management techniques have produced similar results, although some of these studies used small samples.[21] The Arthritis Self-Management Program (ASMP), developed by Kate Lorig at Stanford University and supported by the National Arthritis Foundation, is a widely used program of education, exercise, and relaxation. A 1999 review of the efficacy of psychologic and behavioral self-management interventions for various arthritic conditions concluded that both CBT and ASMP "represent well-established treatments for pain among patients with RA and OA."[20]

Social support has been shown to be particularly helpful for elderly patients dealing with health problems.[46,115] In one study investigating depression, social support, and quality of life in older adults with OA, social support was shown to be an important variable in patient reports of pain, functional limitation, and depression.[17] In studies of telephone support for patients with OA of the knee, investigators reported significant improvement in physical disability, psychologic disability, and pain in patients receiving the telephone support.[98,119] Interestingly, these same investigators conducted another RCT evaluating the effects of increased contact of health care workers to patients with OA and showed no improvement in measures of psychologic outcomes.[120]

A different approach to eliciting social support was evaluated in a recent study and showed positive results.[68] In a follow-up analysis of the effects of spouse-assisted coping skills training in the management of OA of the knee, patients reported lower levels of pain, psychologic disability, and pain behavior and scored higher on measures of coping and self-efficacy.[67] Although results have been generally consistent in the RCTs for social support and OA, personal support systems (friends, family) may have a greater impact on patient quality of life than health care worker support (phone and clinic contact). Studies evaluating the differential effects of different types of support have not yet been conducted. However, based on the many studies showing the positive response of older patients to social support and the low cost of such an adjunctive "therapy," encouragement of patients to maintain or develop strong social support systems is clearly warranted.

Yoga, a gentle form of Eastern exercise, has been systematically evaluated for patients with OA in only one study, which reported that patients with OA of the hands improved significantly in measures of pain during activity, tenderness, and finger range of motion.[43] Other studies conducted with carpal tunnel syndrome patients produced similar results.[44] Given the enjoyment and relaxation inherent in an exercise such as yoga and the need for more appropriate gentle exercises for older adults, more research into Eastern exercises such as yoga and t'ai chi is encouraged.

Manual Healing

Chiropractic is one of the more popular manual healing modalities used by patients with arthritis and is reported as second to massage therapy in CAM usage among older adults with OA.[95] Surprisingly, no RCTs were found to determine the efficacy of chiropractic alone for OA, although a few recent reviews suggest that chiropractic should be included as part of a conservative approach to the management of OA pain.[15,48]

Therapeutic touch is another manual healing modality tested for use with OA patients. Two studies were conducted in the late 1990s. One study compared TT to progressive muscle relaxation (PMR) or usual care for patients with degenerative arthritis.[93] Pain and psychologic factors improved after both treatments compared with usual care, but PMR was better for ameliorating pain and distress. The second study, an RCT comparing TT to either mock TT or standard care in patients with OA of the knee, demonstrated decreases in pain and gains in mobility for the TT groups over the control groups.[47] More research is needed, but these studies suggest some benefit of TT for patients with OA.

Other areas of manual healing suggested for OA, such as shiatsu massage, reflexology, Swedish massage, rolfing, craniosacral manipulation, and applied kinesiology, have yet to see the widespread use of chiropractic and also lack RCTs to attest to any efficacy.

Provider-Patient Relationship

Research indicates that some CAM treatments have clear indications of efficacy for use with OA patients, including GS and CS, acupuncture, CBT, self-management programs, and social support. Where there is the suggestion of efficacy with nutritional supplements other than GS and CS, t'ai chi, PEMFs, TENS, yoga, chiropractic, and TT, further work is needed to determine treatment efficacy and any contraindications. When there is no or minimal controlled research, but case study and anecdotal reports indicate that a therapy might be appropriate for OA (e.g., reconstructive therapy, Qi Gong, music therapy), CAM providers may be well situated to serve as both critical investigator and care provider.

Recent interest has emerged for the use of self-report measures of patient satisfaction and symptom evaluation as a way to track the effectiveness of CAM treatments. In this way the care provider can involve patients in an ongoing evaluation of their care as well as investigate the general efficacy of the treatments.[94] Further, given the extensive use of CAM modalities for OA, physicians should ask patients about the use of CAM therapies and develop an understanding of the many CAM therapies available.

The prevalence, suffering produced, inadequacy of medical management, and costs of treating musculoskeletal diseases in the United States will drive funding for more research into both treatment and prevention using CAM methods. According to the Arthritis Foundation, Congress provided NIAMS with $396.7 million in support of research in 2001. It is likely that investigation of the many therapies reported in this chapter will be furthered in the coming years.

SUMMARY

Alternative treatments for arthritis and Alzheimer's disease abound and are commonly used. With the dramatic rise in the number of elderly people, in particular with the rise in the numbers of people living past the age of 85, the incidence of these diseases will increase. Current medical treatment for either condition is not adequate to control the human suffering and often is not cost-effective. Although there is some excellent research into the effectiveness of CAM therapies for these conditions, it is insufficient and rarely definitive. Because surveys reliably show that people use alternative methods to manage their health, it seems a responsible approach to systematically evaluate the care that people are already receiving and to provide a scientific basis to expand the options available to patients and their families.

Since arthritis and AD show such resistance to treatment, a helpful line of research may be in the area of *prevention*. Research is needed to evaluate the effect of comprehensive lifestyle modification programs in which proper diet, exercise, emotional self-management, and enhanced self-efficacy are modeled, taught, and supported. An ounce of prevention may be superior to a pound of cure.

REFERENCES

1. Adridge D: Alzheimer's disease: rhythm, timing and music as therapy, *Biomed Pharmacother* 48:275, 1994.
2. Altman RD et al: Capsaicin cream 0.025% as monotherapy for osteoarthritis: a double-blind study, *Semin Arthritis Rheum* 23(suppl 3):25,1994.
3. Alzheimer's Association: Alzheimer's conference success, *Greater San Francisco Bay Area Chapter Newsletter* Winter:6, 1997.
4. Alzheimer's Association: Alzheimer's disease and related disorders fact sheet: an overview of the dementias, *Alzheimer Assoc Fact Sheet*, 1990.
5. Alzheimer's Association: Facts about Cognex and Alzheimer's disease, *Alzheimer Assoc Fact Sheet*, June 1993.
6. Alzheimer's Association: Facts about donepezil hydrochloride and Alzheimer's disease, *Alzheimer Assoc Fact Sheet*, December 1996.
7. Alzheimer's Association: Research round up: advances in Alzheimer's research, *Alzheimer Assoc Fact Sheet* 7:4, 1997.
7a. Alzheimer's Disease Education and Referral Center: *Alzheimer's Disease Medications Fact Sheet*, May 2002.
8. Alzheimer's Disease Education and Referral Center: Genes and APO E, *Connections* 5:3, 1996.

9. Astin JA, Pelletier KR, Marie A, Haskell WH: Complementary and alternative medicine use among elderly persons: one year analysis of a Blue Shield Medicare supplement, *J Gerontol* 55A:M4, 2000.

10. Baker M: The force may be with you, *Stanford Med* 13:18, 1996.

11. Beaubrun G, Gray GE: A review of herbal medicines for psychiatric disorders, *Psychiatr Serv* 51:1130, 2000.

12. Behl C, Davis J, Cole GM, Schubert D: Vitamin E protects nerve cells from amyloid beta protein toxicity, *Biochem Biophys Res Commun* 186:944, 1992.

13. Behl C, Widmann M, Trapp T, Holsboer F: 17-B Estradiol protects neurons from oxidative stress induces cell death in vitro, *Biochem Biophys Res Commun* 216:473, 1995.

14. Berg L: *Advances in biomedical research, Wash U Alzheimer Dis Res Ctr* 2:1, 1996.

15. Berkson DL: Osteoarthritis, chiropractic, and nutrition: osteoarthritis considered as a natural part of a three-stage subluxation complex—its reversibility, its relevance and treatability by chiropractic and nutritional correlates, *Med Hypotheses* 36:356, 1991.

16. Berman BM et al: A randomized trial of acupuncture as an adjunctive therapy in osteoarthritis of the knee, *Rheumatology* 38:346, 1999.

17. Blixen CE, Kippes C: Depression, social support, and quality of life in older adults with osteoarthritis, *Image J Nurs Sch* 31:221, 1999.

18. Bohorquez A, Liano E, Fernandez de Araoz G, Guillen F: Non-pharmacological treatments for Alzheimer's disease, mood and cognitive disorders, *Facts Res Gerontol Suppl*, 1995, p 109.

19. Bonder BR: Psychotherapy for individuals with Alzheimer's disease, *Alzheimer Dis Assoc Disord* 8(suppl 3):75, 1994.

20. Bradley LA, Alberts KR: Psychological and behavioral approaches to pain management for patients with rheumatic disease, *Rheum Dis Clin North Am* 25:215, 1999.

21. Bradley LA et al: Psychological approaches to the management of arthritis pain, *Soc Sci Med* 19:1353, 1984.

22. Brandt KD: Nonsurgical management of osteoarthritis, with an emphasis on nonpharmacologic measures, *Arch Fam Med* 4:1057, 1995.

23. Brotons M, Pickett-Cooper PK: The effects of music therapy intervention on agitation behaviors of Alzheimer's disease patients, *J Music Ther* 33:2, 1996.

24. Calfas KJ et al: One-year evaluation of cognitive-behavioral intervention in osteoarthritis, *Arthritis Care Res* 5:202, 1992.

25. Cherniack EP, Senzel RS, Pan CX: Correlates of use of alternative medicine by the elderly in an urban population, *J Altern Complement Med* 7:277, 2001.

26. Coleman LM, Fowler LI, Williams ME: The use of unproven therapies by people with Alzheimer's disease, *J Am Geriatr Assoc* 43:747, 1995.

27. Corrigan FM, Van Rhijn AV, Horrobin DF: Essential fatty acids in Alzheimer's disease, *Ann NY Acad Sci* 640:250, 1991.

28. Danao-Camara T, Tabrah FL: The use of pulsed electromagnetic fields (PEMF) in osteoarthritis (OA) of the knee: preliminary report, *Hawaii Med J* 60:288, 2001.

29. Davies H, Robinson D: Supportive group experiences for patients with early-stage Alzheimer's disease, *J Am Geriatr Soc* 43:1068, 1995.

30. Devanand DP, Levy SR: Neuroleptic treatment of agitation and psychosis in dementia, *J Geriatr Psychiatry Neurol* 8(suppl 1):18, 1995.

31. *Diagnostic and statistical manual of mental disorders,* ed 4 (*DSM*-IV), Washington, DC, 1994, American Psychiatric Association.

32. Eccles M et al: North of England Evidence Based Guidelines Development Project: Summary guidelines for non-steroidal anti-inflammatory drugs versus basic analgesia in treating the pain of degenerative arthritis, *BMJ* 317:526, 1998.

33. Eisenberg D et al: Unconventional medicine in the United States: prevalence, costs, and patterns of use, *N Engl J Med* 328:246, 1993.

34. Eisenberg DM et al: Trends in alternative medicine use in the United States, 1990–1997, *JAMA* 280:1569, 1998.

35. Eriksson S et al: Interaction of diazepam and naloxone on acupuncture induced pain relief, *Am J Chin Med* 19:1, 1991.

36. Ettinger WH et al: A randomized trial comparing aerobic exercise and resistance exercise with a health education program in older adults with knee osteoarthritis, *JAMA* 277:25, 1997.
37. Evans DA, Morris MC: Is a randomized trial of antioxidants in the primary prevention of Alzheimer's disease warranted? *Alzheimer Dis Assoc Disord* 10(suppl 1):45, 1996.
38. Ezzo J et al: Acupuncture for osteoarthritis of the knee: a systematic review, *Arthritis Rheum* 44: 819, 2001.
39. Felson DT: Weight and osteoarthritis, *Am J Clin Nutr* 63:430S, 1996.
40. Fink MG et al: Non-specific effects of traditional Chinese acupuncture in osteoarthritis of the hip, *Complement Ther Med* 9:82, 2001.
41. Foster DF, Phillips RS, Hamel MB, Eisenberg DM: Alternative medicine use in older Americans, *J Am Geriatr Soc* 48:1560, 2000.
42. Gaby AR: Natural treatments for osteoarthritis, *Altern Med Rev* 4:330, 1999.
43. Garfinkel M, Schumacher HR Jr: Yoga, *Rheum Dis Clin North Am* 26:125, 2000.
44. Garfinkel M et al: Evaluation of a yoga based regimen for treatment of osteoarthritis of the hands, *J Rheumatol* 21:2341, 1994.
45. Gerdner LA: Effects of individualized music on confused and agitated elderly patients, *Arch Psychiatr Nurs* 7:284, 1993.
46. Gliksman M et al: Social support, marital status, and living arrangement correlates of cardiovascular disease risk factors in the elderly, *Soc Sci Med* 31:811, 1995.
47. Gordon A et al: The effects of therapeutic touch on patients with osteoarthritis of the knee, *J Fam Pract* 47:271, 1998.
48. Gottlieb MS: Conservative management of spinal osteoarthritis with glucosamine sulfate and chiropractic treatment, *J Manipulative Physiol Ther* 20:400, 1997.
49. Gray D: The treatment strategies of arthritis sufferers, *Soc Sci Med* 21:507, 1985.
50. Griffin MR et al: Non-steroidal anti-inflammatory drug use and death from peptic ulcer in elderly persons, *Ann Intern Med* 109:359, 1988.
51. Groene RW: Effectiveness of music therapy in 1-1 intervention with individuals having senile dementia of the Alzheimer's type, *J Music Ther* 30:138, 1993.
52. Grundman M: Vitamin E and Alzheimer's disease: the basis for additional clinical trials, *Am J Clin Nutr* 71:630S, 2000.
53. Gwyther LP: *Stages of progression in Alzheimer's disease, care of Alzheimer's patients: a manual for nursing home staff*, Washington, DC, 1985, American Health Care Association.
54. Hartman CA et al: Effects of t'ai chi training on function and quality of life indicators in older adults with osteoarthritis, *J Am Geriatric Soc* 48:1553, 2000.
55. Haslam R: A comparison of acupuncture with advice and exercises on the symptomatic treatment of osteoarthritis of the hip: a randomised controlled trial, *Acupunct Med* 19:19, 2001.
56. Hawley DJ: Nontraditional treatment of arthritis, *Nurs Clin North Am* 19:663, 1984.
57. Henderson VW et al: Estrogen replacement therapy in older women: comparisons between Alzheimer's disease cases and nondemented control subjects, *Arch Neurol* 51:896, 1994.
58. Hofferberth B: The effect of EGb 761 in patients with senile dementia of the Alzheimer type: a double-blind placebo-controlled study on different levels of investigation, *Hum Psychopharmacol* 9:215, 1994.
59. Huppert FA, Niekerk JK: Dehydroepiandrosterone (DHEA) supplementation for cognitive function, *Cochrane Database Syst Rev* (2):CD 000304, 2001.
60. Kalmijn S: Fatty acid intake and the risk of dementia and cognitive decline: a review of clinical and epidemiological studies, *J Nutr Health Aging* 4:202, 2000.
61. Kanowski S et al: Proof of efficacy of the *Ginkgo biloba* special extract EGb 761 in outpatients suffering from mild to moderate primary degenerative dementia of the Alzheimer type or multi-infarct dementia, *Pharmacopsychiatry* 29:47, 1996.
62. Keefe F, Caldwell D: Cognitive behavioral control of arthritis, *Adv Rheumatol* 81:277, 1997.
63. Keefe F et al: Behavioral and cognitive-behavioral approaches to chronic pain: recent advances and future directions, *J Consult Clin Psychol* 60:528, 1992.
64. Keefe F et al: Osteoarthritic knee pain: a behavioral analysis, *Pain* 28:309, 1987.
65. Keefe F et al: Pain coping skills training in the management of osteoarthritic knee pain. II. Follow-up results, *Behav Ther* 21:435, 1990.

66. Keefe F et al: Pain coping strategies in osteoarthritis patients, *J Consult Clin Psychol* 55:208, 1987.

67. Keefe FJ et al: Spouse-assisted coping skills training in the management of knee pain in osteoarthritis: long-term follow-up results, *Arthritis Care Res* 12:101, 1999.

68. Keefe FJ et al: Spouse-assisted coping skills training in the management of osteoarthritic knee pain, *Arthritis Care* 9:279, 1996.

69. Koger SM, Brotons M: Music therapy for dementia symptoms, *Cochrane Database Syst Rev* 3, 2000.

70. Kontush A: Influence of vitamin E and C supplementation on lipoprotein oxidation in patients with Alzheimer's disease, *Free Radic Biol Med* 31: 345, 2001.

71. Kumar AM et al: Music therapy increases serum melatonin levels in patients with Alzheimer's disease, *Altern Ther Health Med* 5:49, 1999.

72. Le Bars PL et al: A 26-week analysis of a double-blind placebo-controlled trial of the *Ginkgo biloba* extract Egb761 in dementia, *Dement Geriatr Cogn Disord* 11:230, 2000.

73. LeBlanc ES et al: Hormone replacement therapy and cognition: systematic review and meta-analysis, *JAMA* 285:1489, 2001.

73a. Lecrubier Y et al: Efficacy of St. John's wort extract WS 5570 in major depression: A double-blind, placebo- controlled trial, *Am J Psychiatry* 159:8, 2002.

74. Letzel H, Haan, J, Feil WB: Nootropics: efficacy and tolerability of products from three active substance classes, *J Drug Dev Clin Pract* 8:77, 1996.

75. Linde K et al: St. John's wort for depression: an overview and meta-analysis of randomized clinical trials, *BMJ* 313:253, 1996.

76. Little CV, Parsons T: Herbal therapy for treating osteoarthritis, *Cochrane Database Syst Rev* 1:CD002947, 2001.

77. Lord TR, Garner JE: Effects of music on Alzheimer's patients, *Percept Mot Skills* 76:451, 1993.

78. Luskin FM et al: A review of mind/body therapies in the treatment of musculoskeletal disease with implications for the elderly, *Altern Ther Health Med* 6:46, 2000.

79. Mace NL, Rabins PV: *The 36-hour day*, Baltimore, 1991, Johns Hopkins University Press.

80. March LM: Osteoarthritis, *Rheumatology* 166:98, 1997.

81. McAlindon TE et al: Glucosamine and chondroitin for treatment of osteoarthritis: a systematic quality assessment and meta-analysis, *JAMA* 283:483, 2000.

82. McShane R et al: Do neuroleptic drugs hasten cognitive decline in dementia? Prospective study with necropsy follow up, *BMJ* 314:266, 1997.

83. Minor M: Exercise in the management of osteoarthritis of the knee and hip, *Arthritis Care Res* 7:198, 1994.

84. Minor M, Sanford M: Physical interventions on the management of pain and arthritis, *Arthritis Care Res* 6:197, 1993.

85. Morris MC: Vitamin E and vitamin C supplement use and risk of incident Alzheimer's disease, *Alzheimer Dis Assoc Disord* 12:121, 1998.

86. National Advisory Council on Aging: *Report to Congress on the scientific opportunities for developing treatments for Alzheimer's disease,* Bethesda, Md, 1995, National Institutes of Health and National Institute on Aging.

87. National Institutes of Health (NIH) Consensus Conference: Acupuncture, *JAMA* 280:1518, 1998.

88. Nevitt MC et al: Association of estrogen replacement therapy with the risk of osteoarthritis of the hip in elderly white women: study of Osteoporotic Fractures Research Group, *Arch Intern Med* 156:2073, 1996.

89. O'Rourke M: Determining the efficacy of glucosamine and chondroitin for osteoarthritis, *Nurse Pract* 26:44, 2001.

90. Osiri M et al: Transcutaneous electrical nerve stimulation for knee osteoarthritis, *Cochrane Database Syst Rev* 4:CD002823, 2000.

91. Osmand AP: Plasma levels of antioxidant vitamins in patients with Alzheimer's disease, *Neurobiol Aging* 11(abstract 270):318, 1990.

92. Paganini-Hill A: Estrogen replacement therapy and risk of Alzheimer's disease, *Arch Intern Med* 156:2213, 1996.

93. Peck SD: The efficacy of therapeutic touch for improving functional ability in elders with degenerative arthritis, *Nurs Sci Q* 11:123, 1998.

94. Pincus T: Analyzing long-term outcomes of clinical care without randomized control clinical trials: the consecutive patient questionnaire database, *J Mind Body Health* 13:3, 1997.

95. Ramsey SD et al: Use of alternative therapies by older adults with osteoarthritis, *Arthritis Rheum* 45:222, 2001.

96. Rao JK et al: Use of complementary therapies for arthritis among patients of rheumatologists, *Ann Intern Med* 131:409, 1999.

97. Reginster JY et al: Long-term effects of glucosamine sulfate on osteoarthritis progression: a randomised, placebo-controlled clinical trial, *Lancet* 357:251, 2001.

98. Rene J et al: Reduction of joint pain in patients with knee osteoarthritis who have received monthly telephone calls from lay personnel and whose medical treatment regimens have remained stable, *Arthritis Rheum* 35:511, 1992.

99. Rowe M, Alfred D: The effectiveness of slow stroke massage in diffusing agitated behaviors in individuals with Alzheimer's disease, *J Gerontol Nurs* 25:22, 1999.

100. Sano M, Ernesto C, Thomas RG, Klauber MR: A controlled trial of selegiline, alpha tocopherol or both as treatment for Alzheimer's disease, *N Engl J Med* 336:1216, 1997.

101. Sansone P, Schmitt L: Providing tender touch massage to elderly nursing home residents: a demonstration project, *Geriatr Nurs* 21:303, 2000.

102. Schilke JM et al: Effects of muscle-strength training on the functional status of patients with osteoarthritis of the knee joint, *Nurs Res* 45:68, 1996.

103. Schnitzer T et al: Topical capsaicin for osteoarthritis pain: achieving a maintenance regimen, *Semin Arthritis Rheum* 23(suppl 3):34, 1994.

104. Snowdon DA et al: Linguistic ability in early life and cognitive function and Alzheimer's disease in late life: findings from the nun study, *JAMA* 275:528, 1996.

105. Snyder M, Egan EC, Burns KR: Efficacy of hand massage in decreasing agitation behaviors associated with care activities in persons with dementia, *Geriatr Nurs* 16:60, 1995.

106. Sobel E et al: Elevated risk of Alzheimer's disease among workers with likely electromagnetic field exposure, *Neurology* 47:1477, 1996.

107. Tabet N et al: Vitamin E for Alzheimer's disease, *Cochrane Database Syst Rev* (4):CD002854, 2000.

108. Taylor P, Hallett M, Flaherty L: Treatment of osteoarthritis of the knee with transcutaneous electrical nerve stimulation, *Pain* 11:233, 1981.

109. Thie NM et al: Evaluation of glucosamine sulfate compared to ibuprofen for the treatment of temporomandibular joint osteoarthritis: a randomized double-blind controlled 3-month trial, *J Rheumatol* 28:1347, 2001.

110. Thomas M et al: A comparative study of diazepam and acupuncture in patients with osteoarthritis pain: a placebo-controlled trial, *Am J Chin Med* 19:95, 1991.

111. Towheed TE et al: Glucosamine therapy for treating osteoarthritis, *Cochrane Database Syst Rev* 1:CD002946, 2001.

112. Trock DH: Electromagnetic fields and magnets: investigational treatment for musculoskeletal disorders, *Rheum Dis Clin North Am* 26:51, 2000.

113. Trock DH, Bollet AJ, Markoll R: The effect of pulsed electromagnetic fields in the treatment of osteoarthritis of the knee and cervical spine: report of randomized, double-blind placebo-controlled trials, *J Rheumatol* 21:1903, 1994.

114. Trock DH et al: A double-blind trial of the clinical effects of pulsed electromagnetic fields in osteoarthritris, *J Rheumatol* 20:456, 1993.

115. Uchino N et al: The relationship between social support and physiological processes: a review with an emphasis on underlying mechanisms and implications for health, *Psychol Bull* 119:488, 1996.

116. Van Dongen MC et al: The efficacy of ginkgo for elderly people with dementia and age-associated memory impairment: new results of a randomized clinical trial, *J Am Geriatr Soc* 48:1183, 2000.

117. Walker-Bone K: Medical management of osteoarthritis, *BMJ* 321:936, 2000.

118. Weiheng C et al: Treating osteoarthritis of the knee joint by traditional Chinese medicine, *J Tradit Chin Med* 14:279, 1994.

119. Weinberger M et al: Improving functional status in arthritis: the effect of social support, *Soc Sci Med* 23:899, 1986.

120. Weinberger M et al: The impact of increased contact on psychosocial outcomes in patients with osteoarthritis: a randomized, controlled trial, *J Rheumatol* 18:849, 1991.
121. What can be done about osteoarthritis? *Drug Ther Bull* 34:33, 1996.
122. Workshop on Alternative Medicine: *Alternative medicine: expanding medical horizons: a report to the National Institutes of Health on alternative medical systems and practices in the United States,* Chantilly, Va, 1992, Washington, DC, 1994, US Government Printing Office.
123. Yaffe KG et al: Estrogen therapy in postmenopausal women: effects on cognitive function and dementia, *JAMA* 279:688, 1998.
124. Yale R: Support groups for newly diagnosed Alzheimer's clients, *Clin Gerontol* 8:86, 1989.
125. Yanase T et al: Serum DHEA and DHEA sulfate in Alzheimer's disease and in cerebrovascular dementia, *Endocr J* 43:119, 1996.
126. Yurtkuran M, Kocagil T: TENS, electroacupuncture and ice massage: a comparison of treatment for osteoarthritis of the knee, *Am J Acupunct* 27:133, 1999.
127. Zaman Z et al: Plasma concentrations of vitamins A and E and carotenoids in Alzheimer's disease, *Age Aging* 21:91, 1992.

SUGGESTED READINGS

Horstman J: *The Arthritis Foundation's guide to alternative therapies,* Atlanta, 1999, Arthritis Foundation.
Kahn RL, Rowe JW: *Successful aging,* New York, 1998, Pantheon Books.
Klein WC, Bloom M: *Successful aging: strategies for healthy living,* New York, 1997, Plenum Press.
Lorig K, Fries J: *The arthritis helpbook,* Reading, Mass, 1990, Addison-Wesley.
Luskin FM, Newell KA: Mind body approaches to successful aging. In Watkins A, editor: *Mind body medicine: a clinician's guide to psychoneuroimmunology,* New York, 1997, Churchill Livingstone.
Mace NL, Rabins PV: *The 36-hour day: a family guide to caring for persons with Alzheimer's disease, related dementing illnesses, and memory loss in later life,* Baltimore, 1991, Johns Hopkins University Press.
Murray MT, Pizzorno JE: *Encyclopedia of natural medicine,* ed 2, Rocklin, Calif, 1998, Prima Publications.
Pelletier KR: *The best alternative medicine: What works? What does not?* New York, 2000, Simon & Schuster.
Progress report on Alzheimer's disease: taking the next steps, NIH Pub No 00-4859, Bethesda, Md, 2000, National Institute on Aging and National Institutes of Health.
Tappen RM: *Interventions for Alzheimer's disease: a caregiver's complete reference,* Baltimore, 1997, Health Professions Press.

PART THREE

Future Directions and Goals for Complementary and Alternative Medicine

CHAPTER 14

Legal and Ethical Issues

KATHLEEN M. BOOZANG

Consumers are enthralled with integrating complementary and alternative medicine (CAM) therapies into both their health maintenance routines and their treatment regimens. CAM users believe that they are finding relief, particularly from the irritants of chronic conditions,[13,30] not only for themselves, but for their children as well.[17] Further, managed care organizations, perceived by many as the most conservative spender of the health care dollar, have begun covering alternative modalities, suggesting that CAM must have some efficacy.[18] In almost every state legislature, as well as the U.S. Congress, bills have been introduced to expand the ability of CAM providers to offer their interventions legally to the public.[40] Significantly, the presidential-appointed White House Commission on Complementary and Alternative Medicine Policy has just issued its final report, urging significant investment in CAM research and expansion of opportunities for patients to access CAM.[63]

Most observers of the CAM phenomenon assume that the appeal of unorthodox medicine is a type of "resurrection." They suggest that CAM's revival represents a backlash against the impersonality and myriad other inadequacies of conventional medicine, particularly its failure to provide the holistic care that is the hallmark of CAM. Ironically, this phenomenon is a replay of the past. The diverse array of health professionals who proliferated in the nineteenth century, when physicians were not yet the caretakers of choice, persisted even while biomedicine became predominant.[41] In short, though arguably dormant, "unconventional" health care has never disappeared.

The most significant change in current attitude is not the renewed interest in CAM by consumers, however, but that at least some traditional physicians have begun practicing CAM. These physicians are integrating CAM into their practices, referring patients to CAM providers, or at least inquiring of their patients what complementary modes they might be using so that they can avoid contraindicated medication.[14] The White House Commission urges the establishment of integrated practices, which might be physician centered, "where CAM practitioners provide services independently but under the supervision of a primary or a specialty care physician," or where physician and CAM provider practice "side-by-side as equals, collaborating both in the diagnosis and treatment of patient conditions."[63] On the other hand, most physicians remain skeptical, studiously ignoring the CAM revolution, and avoid any discussion with their patients about unconventional remedies. Physicians in both camps face ethical challenges and legal risks.

The physicians who are embracing CAM need to do so cautiously, ensuring that they are acting to serve patients' best interests and are not subjecting them to unnecessary medical risk in trying unproven CAM modalities. Further, these physicians need to protect themselves from the legal risks attendant to the harm patients may experience from reliance on unsafe or ineffective CAM interventions. Physicians employing CAM must also be cognizant of the particular care they should take when fulfilling the duty to obtain patients' informed consent. Importantly, such physicians need to ensure that they do not stray so far from the standard of care expected of doctors that they put their licenses at risk. Additionally, some states are increasingly open to the notion that health care providers may commit the tort of consumer fraud when they misrepresent the benefits of specific health care treatments to their patients.

In the other camp, physicians who ignore CAM risk prescribing contraindicated treatments to patients already ingesting herbs or dietary supplements, misdiagnosing a patient experiencing the adverse effects of some CAM treatment, or failing to offer a patient an effective CAM modality that could alleviate pain, treat symptoms, or cure the specified condition altogether. This chapter provides a brief overview of these legal issues to aid the physician confronting the challenges raised by the public's use of CAM.

◼ Importance of Adhering to an Evolving Standard of Care

The legal standard of care for physicians is established by a number of factors, including testimony of experts in the same practice specialty and professional peer-reviewed articles. Sufficient consensus exists in the literature to establish a standard of care that compels physicians to integrate oral questioning (as opposed to written questionnaires) about their patients' CAM use into the history part of the physical examination.[9] Physicians need to be sufficiently knowledgeable about CAM to interpret the information from their patients and to recognize potential contraindications. More specifically, presurgical discussions require inquiries and warnings about patients' CAM use, particularly herbal substances that should be discontinued before anesthesia or that inhibit coagulation.[11] Because patients frequently provide inaccurate information about the herbs and supplements they are taking, physicians should require their patients to bring the substances and the packages in which they were purchased to their preoperative evaluation.[11] Patients should be prepared for potential withdrawal symptoms when they discontinue herbs they have used for long periods. Some postsurgical discharge planning discussions should include warnings against prematurely returning to certain CAM practices, such as yoga after heart surgery.[42]

Emergency department (ED) physicians need be aware of the signs of ephedrine abuse[23] and must ensure that information about other supplement use is recorded in the patients' charts for reference by providers to whom the patient may be subsequently referred. The Centers for Disease Control and Prevention[23] reported that adverse events ranged in severity from tremor and headache to death in eight ephedrine users and included reports of stroke, myocardial infarction, chest pain, seizures, insomnia, nausea and vomiting, fatigue, and dizziness. "Seven of the eight reported fatalities were attributed to myocardial infarction or cerebrovascular accident."[23] Physicians writing prescriptions for their patients need to be aware of the possibility of adverse interactions with herbs. St. John's wort is not appropriate for patients taking fluoxetine (Prozac),[10] those with major depression,[27] patients with HIV/AIDS taking protease inhibitors,[54] or patients awaiting organ transplants.[11]

Merely asking patients about their CAM use is insufficient. Physicians must attend continuing educational programs that include discussions about popular alternative modalities, or they must have access to reliable CAM peer-reviewed resources, to be able to advise patients readily about the potential benefits and risks of CAM integration with conventional medicine. Physicians should also be alert to the symptoms that may result from the ingestion of contaminated herbal or other supplements.[31]

Empiric studies reveal that patients are reluctant to reveal their CAM use to their treating physicians, fearful that it will evoke the physicians' disapprobation.[9] As such, physicians should elicit information about their patients' CAM use without conveying disapproval, thereby encouraging patients to be forthcoming about how they might be supplementing their physicians' treatments. Further, physicians should be sensitive to patients' dissatisfaction or frustration with the inadequacies of their conventional care; resorting to CAM may reveal significant anxieties[21] or a patient who needs guidance on selecting alternative care because orthodox medicine is inadequate to treating the patient's pain or other symptoms.[11]

No physician should ignore CAM, even if he or she believes most of the alternative modalities used have insufficient evidence of efficacy or show little promise in the long term. Physicians must be sufficiently knowledgeable to advise patients about CAM in order to avoid contraindications and detect the side effects of complementary therapies. Other physicians are enthusiastic about the potential of integrative care and are tentatively exploring, with their patients, the benefits of this emerging approach to patient care.

◼ Ethical Issues in Referring or Integrating CAM with Conventional Care

No studies exist to support fully the efficacy of most CAM treatments.[63] Likewise, few clinical practice guidelines exist for specific CAM modalities, and few accreditation and credentialing standards exist for CAM providers. Nonetheless, many physicians are increasingly confronted with patients demanding to integrate alternative approaches with their care, whether because they are intrigued or because their managed care plan sponsors an alternative network.

Premature integration of unproven CAM therapies has raised much ethical debate in the literature. Schneiderman,[58] for example, argues strongly for maintaining the distinction between medicine and the many factors that contribute to "the good life" that are *not* medicine but alternatives *to* medicine. The ethical principle of *beneficence* "requires subjecting claims of benefits to empirical evidence."[58] Employing concepts of justice, Schneiderman asks whether, given the unjust U.S. health care system, the diversion of resources to alternative medicine is a just action, in general and specifically to the patients whose time and money are wasted on useless or harmful treatments.

At the clinical level, physicians are compelled to decide for themselves in what circumstances they believe it is ethically appropriate to integrate CAM proactively into their practices or to accede to patient desires for a CAM therapy that the physician does not believe will benefit the patient. One analytical framework from which to examine this issue is to consider whether the CAM treatment is (1) invalidated, (2) nonvalidated (plausible but not yet proven), or (3) validated (already proven to be efficacious).[20] Physicians should not hesitate to consider the comparative cost-effectiveness of any proven treatment with their patients, whether conventional or unconventional. In fact, it may violate the doctrine of informed consent *not* to offer a viable CAM alternative to a patient.

On the other hand, if a CAM modality has been established to be unsafe, physicians should neither recommend nor accede to patient demands to integrate it into the treatment regimen, even at the risk of losing the patient. Similarly, even if reason exists to believe that an alternative is safe, but it has been proven to be ineffective, the physician should not recommend the treatment. Even if the treatment is "not unsafe," it cannot be said that it will do no harm for the patient to use it. First, because the physician is offering the treatment, the message conveyed is a belief that the therapy works, which may not be true. Second, harm could result from the patient relying on an ineffective CAM modality to the exclusion of an effective conventional treatment. Third, even if this is not the case, harm may result for those to whom the patient recommends the CAM modality, saying that "the doctor" recommended it. Unless the physician is seeking to elicit the placebo effect, no justification appears to exist to offer an ineffective therapy other than the opportunity for potential revenue.

Physicians face a greater challenge if they believe that a particular alternative is ineffective but not necessarily *unsafe* (i.e., "it won't do any harm") and the patient still insists on using it. Myriad factors might affect the analysis in this case and could influence a physician's decision, such as whether the patient is healthy and desires to use CAM for health maintenance or is terminally or chronically ill, and whether the patient suffers from unrelieved pain or merely is extremely anxious. If the patient demands a useless modality instead of an effective conventional treatment that represents the standard of care, the physician should press the patient to use the standard therapy, especially if real harm could result with refusal. On the other hand, if conventional medicine offers nothing to the patient, perhaps the CAM alternative might at least result in a placebo effect.[19] The conflict might be susceptible to compromise. The patient might agree to use the physician's recommended treatment for an agreed-on time as a test before resorting to the CAM intervention, or the patient and physician might bargain to compromise their respective preferences. However, the physician and patient may be unable to agree; the treatment might deviate so far from the standard of care or present such a risk to the patient that the physician has no choice but to refuse to cooperate with the patient, even if that means their relationship is severed. Whatever the ultimate resolution, the physician should document the advice provided to the patient and the agreed course.

◼ Legal Issues in Referring or Integrating CAM with Conventional Care

However difficult the ethical issues, the legal issues are even more complicated. The White House Commission report, as well as some managed care organizations, encourages physician cooperation with CAM providers. In a few states, complementary providers may treat patients only on referral from a physician. New Jersey, for example, precludes acupuncturists from accepting patients without a physician referral or diagnosis; the physician's preevaluation must be maintained in the acupuncturist's chart.[45] Such collaborations, whether referrals between CAM and conventional provider or partnerships in integrated practice settings, present serious challenges. Because so few data exist on many complementary interventions, physicians have no guidance on when or how such integration is appropriate. Further, even if the physician determines that referral is appropriate, states are wildly divergent in their oversight of alternative providers, establishing no easily verifiable markers for identifying properly trained and competent CAM providers. The education and training of CAM providers are similarly inconsistent. Little precedent exists for developing protocols for conventional physician–CAM provider collaboration, making it difficult to obtain sample protocols.

Physicians are best positioned with respect to protecting themselves against malpractice liability if they refer to or collaborate with licensed practitioners. States have several regulatory choices to regulate CAM providers, such as mandatory licensure, title licensure, certification, and registration.[36] Washington, for example, employs such a multilevel regulatory schema for CAM practitioners,[60] which complements its "any-willing provider" law for health insurance plans.[61] Minnesota, on the other hand, takes a much more hands-off approach, establishing an Office of Unlicensed Complementary and Alternative Health Care Practice to monitor unlicensed CAM practitioners.[43] These states are unique; the majority of states either license or do not license. Chiropractors are licensed in every state, acupuncturists in 40 states, massage therapists in 30 states, and naturopaths in 11 states.[63] Although there are professional accrediting agencies for some schools of CAM providers, the only other convenient option for physicians to assist them in validating CAM providers is if a local managed care organization has a network of alternative providers who presumably have been screened.

Physicians should take care in selecting CAM providers with whom to affiliate, or to whom to refer, just as they would with conventional providers. Physicians may be liable for referring a patient to a provider whom they know or should know is incompetent, and the patient suffers harm that can be related to such referral. Further, physicians can be at risk if state law imposes on them any supervisory responsibilities over CAM practitioners to whom they refer patients, or if they voluntarily engage in such consultation or oversight.[29] Many CAM providers do not carry professional liability insurance, thereby increasing the physician's risk of exposure if liability is found.

A physician's integration of CAM therapies into clinical practice raises a number of legal issues for consideration, such as potential for negligence, duty of informed consent, licensure, and consumer fraud.

NEGLIGENCE

Physicians can be liable for professional negligence if they deviate from the relevant standard of care applicable to their own requisite training, expertise, and knowledge base of the field of practice. The plaintiff patient must be harmed and must establish that the harm is caused by the physician's provision of substandard care, as defined by experts of the physician's same specialty, as well as peer-reviewed journal articles or textbooks recognized as reflecting the standard in the field.

Negligence law can be quite threatening to physicians offering alternative treatments to their patients. By being a practitioner of "alternative therapy," the physician almost by definition is providing treatment that deviates from the standard of care and is thus "negligent."[24] This concept is illustrated in the case of *Charell v. Gonzalez,*[5] in which a physician's treatment (special diet, six coffee enemas daily) of a patient with uterine cancer was deemed negligent. The court observed that "it would seem that no practitioner of alternative medicine could prevail on such a question as the reference to the term 'nonconventional' may well necessitate a finding that the doctor who practices such medicine deviates from 'accepted' medical standards."[4]

On the other hand, the law does not seek to quash all innovation and recognizes that physicians are constantly trying new approaches to treatment of their patients.[53] In a review of the book *Complementary and Alternative Medicine: Legal Boundaries and Regulatory Perspectives,* one reviewer said, "The best defense for these activities is rigorous biomedical research, with institutional review board approval, as indicated."[53] Courts do recognize the concept of a *minority approach,* such that a physician would not be deemed to deviate from the standard of care for subscribing to an approach that experts are willing to state constitutes a respectable minority position that is generally accepted and supported in the legitimate medical literature.[64]

Currently, it is not clear that any CAM practice would garner sufficient physician support to be designated a minority approach by a court.

INFORMED CONSENT

Independent from being sued for the type of care that is provided, physicians may also be sued for violating the doctrine of informed consent if they have not properly explained everything relevant to the patient's decision in electing to use a CAM modality. The ethical and legal conceptions that underlie the requirement that physicians obtain informed consent rest on notions of patient self-determination and autonomy, the right to determine what is to happen to one's body, and the right to protect one's dignitary interests.

Essentially, the doctrine of informed consent requires physicians to disclose the patient's diagnosis, prognosis (with and without treatment), alternative treatments, and risks and benefits of each alternative.[16] A heightened standard of disclosure probably exists if the treatment can reasonably be considered "experimental,"[20] which could feasibly encompass most of alternative medicine. In such cases the physician should advise that the patient should consider the treatment to be experimental, that little or no evidence exists to suggest what outcomes can be expected, and that the physician cannot be sure of all of the risks or side effects that may result.

It is extremely difficult for physicians to judge exactly what must be disclosed to the patient, whether in terms of alternative treatments or risks of the respective treatments. Increasingly, physicians ask whether they are obliged to disclose CAM therapies that show promise or have been proven to work. On the other hand, physicians offering complementary therapies to their patients ask how far they must go in disclosing risks and uncertainties. State laws govern these questions, employing divergent approaches. Basically, states fall into two camps in articulating the test to which physicians must adhere in deciding what they must disclose to their patients: the professional standard and the lay standard.

The *professional standard* requires physicians to disclose what other physicians of the same specialty would tell their patients[33] (see Appendix D). Expert testimony is required to establish what a physician of a particular specialty would have disclosed to a patient in a similar condition.[55,62] The *lay standard* requires physicians to disclose the information that a reasonable person in the patient's position would find to be material[12] or would need to know to make an informed decision,[35] although only a handful of states apply this subjective standard. The *standard of materiality* serves to guide the physician in determining what risks and possible alternative forms of treatment(s) should be disclosed to patients.[15] Under this standard, a physician can be liable for nondisclosure if the patient would not have consented to the procedure had additional information been made available.[34]

Under either the lay or the professional standard, at present the law does not impose much obligation on physicians to discuss CAM options with their patients. Clearly, under the professional standard, one could safely suggest that physicians have little obligation to tell their patients about CAM options, because so few of their colleagues do. Cohen[25] critiques the current doctrines of informed consent for precisely this reason. Even under the lay standard, currently it is unlikely that most patients expect their physicians, whom they know prefer and are trained to provide conventional therapies, to offer CAM.

The sparse case law available supports this conjecture. The plaintiff in *Moore v. Baker*[8] sued her physician for not advising her before surgery that chelation therapy was a potential option for carotid endarterectomy. Georgia informed consent law requires physicians to disclose practical treatment alternatives that are "generally recognized and accepted by reasonably prudent physicians."[47] The defendant physician testified that he had not been taught in medical school or graduate training that chelation therapy was an appropriate option for carotid endarterectomy. He produced statements by professional societies that chelation is not recommended and is unsupported by extant evidence and that most physicians think this therapy is dangerous to patients with carotid endarterectomy. Despite testimony from experts for the plaintiff that a minority of physicians did recommend chelation therapy, it was held that, because most physicians reject chelation therapy, the defendant physician had no obligation under the Georgia informed consent statute to discuss this alternative with his patient.

It is more difficult to determine prospectively the law's expectations in any particular case regarding disclosure of *risks* of CAM therapies. Case law seems to suggest that under both the professional and the lay standards, more disclosure is better, probably because much of CAM is considered unproven. On the other hand, so little is known about many alternative therapies that the disclosure obligation probably will focus primarily on explaining to patients that much about CAM is indeed unknown.

The informed consent process can also be employed defensively to protect a physician from malpractice liability resulting from patient harm caused by the patient's selection of an alternative therapy that is ineffective. A few cases suggest that a patient who consents to receive an alternative treatment with a clear understanding of the risks either assumes the risk of harm or is considered to have contributed to the negligent situation that created the harm. As such, these patients cannot fully recover from their physician, even if the physician was negligent. Thus, if it is clearly explained to a patient that more mainstream, or conventional, treatments exist that have a record of successfully treating the medical condition in question, and the patient nonetheless opts for the CAM alternative, which is unsuccessful, the physician may be shielded from partial or total liability.

The case of *Boyle v. Revici*[6] provides an example of this scenario. Ms. Zyjewski died approximately a year after commencing treatment for cancer at the Institute of Applied Biology with Dr. Revici. The treatments consisted of "urine monitoring, urinalyses and the ingestion of various mineral compounds that Dr. Revici claimed retard and reduce the size of cancerous tumors."[7] Revici advised Zyjewski that his cancer therapy was not FDA approved and that he could offer no guarantees. Consistent with the *Gonzalez* case, Revici did not even contest the question of his negligence because he had admittedly deviated from the standard of care for cancer treatment. He was not liable for damages, however, because it was found that the patient had declined conventional care in favor of Revici's treatments with a clear awareness of the risks she was assuming. In New York at least, assumption of the risk by the patient can be a total bar to recovery, even if the physician is negligent.

In another case involving Dr. Revici's treatment of a woman with breast cancer, the court explained the rationale for the assumption of the risk doctrine as follows: "we see no reason why a patient should not be allowed to make an informed decision to go outside currently approved medical methods in search of an unconventional treatment. While a patient should be encouraged to exercise care for his own safety, we believe that an informed decision to avoid surgery and conventional chemotherapy is within the patient's right."[57] In the case of Ms. Zyjewski, the court specifically indicated that it did not matter that the patient's consent was not in writing (presumably, there was other reliable evidence to establish that she had indeed understood the risks and consented anyway, such as the physician's chart).

Even in this scenario, however, physicians could still be liable if, in administering an alternative regimen to a patient, they are negligent. Thus the physician/homeopath who selects the wrong homeopathic remedy, thereby harming the patient, who consequently does not recover, will be liable for negligence. Similarly, the physician who punctures a patient's lung while practicing acupuncture could be found negligent. Both these examples point to the necessity of physicians being properly trained in any CAM modality they choose to integrate into their practices. Significant concern exists about the threats to patient safety presented by physicians who self-train or pursue "crash courses" in CAM modalities that, when improperly administered, can seriously harm patients. At least one state, Colorado, requires that physicians who offer alternative medicine to their patients include as part of the informed consent process, in writing, the physician's education, experience, and credentials to perform the particular CAM therapy being offered.[26]

LICENSURE

Physicians who stray too far from the standard of care by integrating unproven or dangerous CAM therapies into their practices can also incur difficulties with their licensing boards, which are vested with the state's "police power" to protect the public's health, safety, and welfare.[28] Medical boards struggle greatly with questions related to assessment of any physician engaged in "fringe practices," including CAM. Boards are governed by state statutes enumerating the standards by which they are to judge allegedly errant physicians. Statutes do not necessarily require actual or even potential harm to a patient to sanction a physician for unorthodox practices.[39] Statutes frequently refer to deviations from the standards of acceptable or prevailing medical practice[44] or the failure to employ scientific methods in making treatment decisions.[48]

Medical boards also struggle in applying these standards to physicians engaged in CAM practices that are unsupported by reliable studies. Many physicians believe that some CAM therapies, such as ozone therapy or shark cartilage for cancer, constitute quackery and should be disallowed. Others question entire alternative schools, such as homeopathy, the principles of which are unsupported by biomedicine. As such, physicians frequently take the position that these determinations are obvious to a board composed of licensed physicians and should not require consideration of expert testimony. If testimony is considered, it can be difficult to select appropriate witnesses. Is the board required to hear testimony from a nonphysician homeopath to aid in assessing whether a physician homeopath is engaged in practices inconsistent with prevailing standards? Or, may the board rely on an expert who testifies that homeopathy does not reflect the medical standard of care for a particular condition?

In 1990 the North Carolina Supreme Court upheld the decision by the Board of Medical Examiners to revoke a physician's medical license because he was practicing homeopathy that, as all the testimony suggested, was inconsistent with the prevailing standards of practice in North Carolina, where no other physician engaged in homeopathic practices. The court specifically decided that the North Carolina statute did not require the board to establish that the physician had either harmed or presented a threat of harm to any patient.[3]

Legislatures have begun to react to pressure from proponents of alternative medicine to protect physicians from licensure sanctions resulting from their integration of "unorthodox medicine" into their practices. In response to the case just described, for example, the North Carolina legislature amended its licensing statute to add the following language: "The Board shall not revoke the license of or deny a license to a person solely because of that person's practice of a therapy that is experimental, nontraditional, or that departs from acceptable and prevailing medical practices unless, by competent evidence, the Board can establish that the treatment has a safety risk greater than the prevailing treatment or that the treatment is generally not effective."[44]

Oregon and Colorado have taken similar approaches, specifically stating in their licensing laws that by itself, a physician's use of alternative medicine will not be the grounds for sanction.[26,51] New York law provides that it should not be interpreted to preclude "the physician's use of whatever medical care, conventional or nonconventional, which effectively treats human disease, pain, injury, deformity or physical condition."[46] However, the Oregon physician must have an objective basis to believe that the alternative treatment has a reasonable probability of effectiveness, even if not yet proven.[52] Licensing statutes might also be used to ensure appropriate physician oversight of CAM providers with whom physicians affiliate. In Ohio, for example, the failure to supervise an acupuncturist may be grounds for sanction.[49]

A few states have articulated a right to receive unconventional treatment from a physician under certain enumerated circumstances. Ohio authorizes physicians to provide alternative treatments as long as they have complied with the informed consent process.[50] The California legislature recently enacted a statute recognizing the interest of its citizens in integrating holistic-based alternatives with their conventional care and directed the state's various medical boards to establish policies that will maintain quality of care while still providing access to CAM.[22] Texas also recognizes such a right by statute.[1] Georgia, however, limits the right of access to unconventional treatment to patients with potentially life-threatening or chronically disabling conditions.[32] Both Georgia and Indiana require the physician to determine that the unconventional treatment will not present an "unreasonable and significant risk of danger" to the patient.[32,37] In addition, both states' statutes provide that the physician must give the patient a written and oral explanation of the treatment as well as information that the treatment is experimental or unconventional, that the drug or device is not FDA approved, and the "material risks generally recognized by a reasonably prudent physician of the medical treatment's side effects."[32,38] Texas has one of the most extensive statutes, which states that "the physician may offer the patient complementary and integrative treatment pursuant to a documented treatment plan tailored for the individual needs of the patient by which treatment progress or success can be evaluated with stated objectives such as pain relief and/or improved physical and/or psychosocial function."[2]

CONSUMER FRAUD

Finally, physicians offering patients CAM therapies must ensure that they make accurate representations regarding the attributes and expected benefits of the proposed CAM treatment, lest they expose themselves to charges of fraud pursuant to state consumer protection laws, either by patients or by the state attorney general. Consumer protection statutes vary, but most include a prohibition on a seller's misrepresentation of a product's approval, performance characteristics, uses, or benefits.[59] States have applied consumer protection statutes to health care professionals, taking care to ensure that the claims are based on unfair business practices rather than medical malpractice.[56] Consequently, physicians must ensure that they accurately represent to patients the virtues of an alternative treatment, taking care not to exaggerate the results patients might expect to receive.

SUMMARY

Undoubtedly, many CAM therapies will prove to be clinically effective, and some will become the standard of care. Until then, physicians must weigh the ethical and legal risks of integrating unproven therapies in which their patients have tremendous faith. As with most of medicine, any CAM consideration is yet another "judgment call" best made by the individual physician on a case-by-case basis.

REFERENCES

1. 22 Tex Code Ann § 200.1 (2002).
2. 22 Tex Code Ann § 200.3(E)(2)(2002).
3. 393 NE.2d 383, 837-38 (ND 1990).
4. 660 NYS.2d 232 (NY Sup 1997).
5. 660 NYS.2d 665 (NY Sup 1997).
6. 961 F.2d 1060 (2d Cir 1992).
7. 961 F.2d 1062 (2d Cir 1992).
8. 989 F.2d 1129 (11th Cir 1993).
9. Adler SR, Fosket JR: Disclosing complementary and alternative medicine use in the medical encounter: a qualitative study in women with breast cancer, *J Fam Pract* 48:453, 1999.
10. Alternative medicine: what works...maybe, *Harvard Health Lett* 26:1, 2001.
11. Ang-Lee MK, Moss J, Yuan CS: Herbal medicines and perioperative care, *JAMA* 286:208, 2001.
12. *Arato v Avedon,* 858 P.2d 598 (Cal 1992).
13. Astin J: Why patients use alternative medicine: results of a national study, *JAMA* 279:1548, 1998.
14. Astin JA et al: A review of the incorporation of complementary and alternative medicine by mainstream physicians, *Arch Intern Med* 158:2303, 1998.
15. *Backlund v Univ Wa,* 975 P.2d 950, 662 n 3 (Wash 1999).
16. Berg J et al: *Informed consent,* Oxford, 2001, Oxford University Press.
17. Boozang KM: CAM for kids, *Houston J Health Law Policy* 1:109, 2001.
18. Boozang KM: Is the alternative medicine? Managed care seems to think so, *Conn Law Rev* 32:567, 2000.
19. Boozang KM: The therapeutic placebo: the case for patient deception. Whether the placebo effect is real is a current subject of much research, *Fla Law Rev* 54:687, 2002.
20. Boozang KM: Western medicine opens the door to alternative medicine, *Am J Law Med* 24:185, 1998.
21. Burstein HJ et al: Use of alternative medicine by women with early-stage breast cancer, *N Engl J Med* 340:1733, 1999.

22. Cal Bus & Prof Code Article 23 § 2500 (2002).
23. Centers for Disease Control and Prevention: Adverse events associated with ephedrine-containing products: Texas, December 1993–September 1995, *JAMA* 276:1711, 1996.
24. Cohen MH: *Beyond complementary medicine: legal and ethical perspectives on health care and human evolution,* Ann Arbor, 2001, University of Michigan Press.
25. Cohen MH: *Complementary and alternative medicine: legal boundaries and regulatory perspectives,* Baltimore, 1998, Johns Hopkins Press.
26. Colo Rev Stat Ann § 12-36-117(3)(a) (West 2002).
27. Davidson JR: Effectiveness of *Hypericum perforatum* (St. John's wort) in major depression, *JAMA* 287:1807, 2002.
28. *Dent v West Va,* 129 US 114, 122-23 (1889).
29. Doyle A: Alternative medicine and medical malpractice: emerging issues, *J Leg Med* 22:533, 2001.
30. Eisenberg DM et al: Trends in alternative medicine use in the United States, 1990–1997: results of a follow-up national survey, *JAMA* 280:1569, 1998.
31. Fugh-Berman A: Herb-drug interactions, *Lancet* 355:134, 2000.
32. Ga Code Ann § 43-34-42.1 (2001).
33. *Gorab v Zook,* 943 P.2d 423, 427 (Colo 1997).
34. *Hales v Pittman,* 576 P.2d 493, 499-500 (Ariz 1978).
35. *Hammer v Mt. Sinai Hosp,* 596 A.2d 1318, 1325 (Conn 1991).
36. Havighurst CC, Blumstein JF, Brennan TA: *Health care law and policy: readings, notes, and questions,* New York, 1998, Foundation Press.
37. Ind Code § 25-22.5-1-2.1(a)(2) (2001).
38. Ind Code § 25-22.5-1-2.1(a)(3)(A), (B), (C) (2001).
39. *In re Guess,* 393 NE.2d 383 (ND 1990).
40. Josefek KJ: Alternative medicine's roadmap to mainstream, *Am J Law Med* 26:295, 2000.
41. Kaptchuk T, Eisenberg DM: Varieties of healing. 1. Medical pluralism in the United States, *Ann Intern Med* 135:189, 2001.
42. Lin JH: Evaluating the alternatives, *JAMA* 279:706, 1998.
43. Minn Stat Ann § 146A.05 (West 2002).
44. NC Gen Stat § 80-14(6) (2001).
45. NJ Stat Ann § 45:2C-5.a(1) (West 2002).
46. NY Educ Law 6527(4)(c) (West 2002).
47. OCGA § 31-9-6.1 (d) (Sup 1991).
48. Ohio Rev Code Ann § 4731.22(A)(2)(West 2002).
49. Ohio Rev Stat Ann § 4731.22(B)(36) (West 2002).
50. Ohio Rev Stat Ann § 4731.227 (2002).
51. OR Rev Stat § 677.190(1)(a) (2001).
52. OR Rev Stat § 677.190(1)(b)(A)(i) (2001).
53. Oz MC: Complementary and alternative medicine: legal boundaries and regulatory perspectives, *J Leg Med* 20:141, 1999 (book review).
54. Piscitelli SC et al: Indinavir concentrations and St. John's wort, *Lancet* 355:547, 2000.
55. *Potter v Wisner,* 823 P.2d 1339 (Ariz App 1991).
56. *Quimby v Fine,* 724 P.2d 403 (Wash App 1986).
57. *Schneider v Revici,* 817 F.2d 987, 995 (2d Cir 1987).
58. Schneiderman LJ: Medical ethics and alternative medicine, *Sci Rev Altern Med* 2:63, 1998.
59. Uniform Consumer Sales Practices Act 3(b)(1) (1970).
60. WA Rev Code Ann §§ 18.06.010, 18.25.002, 18.36A010, 18.108.005, 18.138.010 (West 2002).
61. WA Rev Code Ann § 48.43.045 (West 2002).
62. *Wells v Storey,* 1999 WL 1065143 (Ala).
63. *White House Commission on Complementary and Alternative Medicine Policy: Final report,* Washington, DC, 2002, US Government Printing Office. Available at: www.whccamp.hhs.gov/finalreport.html.
64. *Yates v Univ W Va,* 549 SE.2d 681, 689 (W Va 2001).

SUGGESTED READINGS

Cohen MH: *Complementary and alternative medicine: legal boundaries and regulatory perspectives,* Baltimore, 1998, Johns Hopkins Press.

Novey DW: *Clinician's complete reference to complementary and alternative medicine,* St Louis, 2000, Mosby.

CHAPTER 15

Integration of Clinical Practice and Medical Training with Complementary and Alternative and Evidence-Based Medicine

OPHER CASPI, VICTORIA MAIZES, and
IRIS R. BELL

The term *integrative medicine* (IM) is sometimes used interchangeably with complementary and alternative medicine (CAM) in that the central concept involves blending the best of conventional and nonconventional medicine tools for patient care. In reality, IM challenges at least these two assumptions: (1) all CAM has to offer is more tools beyond drugs and surgery, and (2) conventional medicine, the politically dominant, technologically oriented system, is the proper and only way to provide high-quality care for patients. Such assumptions imply that approaches deemed outside the mainstream, such as some of the many modalities and systems of CAM, will simply undergo assimilation into the current model of mainstream care after rigorous scientific studies demonstrate their safety and effectiveness.

As the Institute of Medicine has concluded, however, the current health care system is deeply flawed.[54] Health care involves humanistic concerns that extend beyond those of tools and technical options. Because of the convergence of multiple factors, including severe economic and resource constraints, technologic advances, and increasing emphasis on a reductionist model for science, modern medicine, except in such areas as hospice care, has lost sight of its humanistic roots. In addition, since the relatively recent advent of the randomized, placebo-controlled trial (RCT) for drugs, medical researchers often lose sight of the much larger repertoire of methodologies for studying health care available from scientists of various disciplines, including qualitative techniques, psychologic and behavioral assessment methods, and real-world observational outcomes and health services studies.

This chapter examines complex issues that reveal *truly* integrative medicine as a new system of systems of care that differs in important ways from both the conventional and the nonconventional approaches that contributed to IM's emergence. We draw on an "evolving" conceptual approach, used at the University of Arizona, that is throught to be more comprehensive than that captured by the term "complementary medicine." Key elements of IM include the following[40,70]:

- Healing emphasis, including prioritizing low-risk low-technology options, when feasible and rational, over high-risk cures at any cost
- Patient-centered focus, with patient and provider working in a partnership relationship to accommodate the individual's unique circumstances, needs, and preferences
- Routine assessment of spiritual and religious elements of the patient's life to provide context and support for coping with health and wellness issues
- Familiarity with and routine use of conventional preventive medicine and public health strategies for primary, secondary, and tertiary prevention
- Familiarity with and routine use of current conventional evidence of disease causation, treatment options, and outcomes
- A systems theory framework for evaluating and treating the patient as an intact, individual, living system rather than as a combination of distinct parts
- Incorporation of specific CAM therapies and lifestyle strategies into treatment plans as indicated and appropriate, including knowledge of potential positive and negative interactions between these therapies and the indicated and appropriate conventional therapies
- Outcomes that involve not only absence of disease, but also the presence of positive dimensions of health and well-being, in accord with the World Health Organization's definition of health[115]
- Outcomes that go beyond health-related functionality to include satisfaction with a wide range of spiritual and biopsychosocial domains, including sense of meaning and purpose, community involvement, positive social supports and relationships, adaptive coping style, and health-promoting diet and exercise habits
- Continuing medical education on the process of integration in optimizing health care
- Incorporation of IM principles in the physician's personal self-care program

In short, any particular element of IM borrows extensively from constructs and practices already studied and sometimes used in conventional medicine, such as family practice, preventive medicine, geriatrics and end-of-life care, psychiatry, and behavioral medicine, as well as in many systems of CAM, such as traditional Chinese medicine or Ayurveda. The uniqueness of IM is the overt focus on *synthesis*.

⬛ Clinical Application of Conventional and Integrative Medicine: Case Study

Integrative medicine can serve a wide variety of patients. Natural, less invasive methods are more likely to be useful in patients with earlier stages of a disease process, those with a desire to use more natural approaches, and those who are open to mind-body connections. IM often expands options for living with a wide range of chronic diseases. Leading conditions for which patients have sought IM consultation include a wide range of cancers, rheumatologic disorders, and nonspecific syndromes (e.g., "chronic fatigue syndrome") and similar problems. In addition, at the University of Arizona, we have found that patients with immune disorders, chronic pain, gastrointestinal disturbances, pulmonary conditions, cardiovascular disease, and mental health problems often seek integrative treatment as well.

The following case study reveals important differences between the conventional and integrative methods of evaluating and treating disease.

CASE HISTORY

Conventional Medicine

The patient, Mr. S, is a 67-year old man who had been in good health until he developed a dry cough followed by left upper chest discomfort in April 2000. A chest radiograph revealed a wedge-shaped abnormality in the left upper lobe, which was believed to be an infection and was treated with antibiotics. Three days later he experienced hemoptysis of a small amount of blood. A computed tomography (CT) scan of the chest revealed a left upper lobe mass with three smaller masses in the right lung. Bronchoscopy revealed pulmonary adenocarcinoma. Metastatic work-up included brain CT, bone scan, and liver ultrasound, all of which were normal. The patient was diagnosed with stage IV lung cancer with bilateral unresectable disease.

Integrative Medicine

This case is a classic history of present illness as taught to students for the last several decades. Compared with the conventional approach, an integrative summary of the history would begin differently: Mr. S is a vital, ruddy-complexioned, 67-year-old fighter. He spent 40 years of his life in the U.S. Marine Corps, which explains his reaction to the diagnosis of stage IV lung cancer. Mr. S says, "Having cancer is like mortal combat. Understand the situation as well as you can, be alert to changes in the situation, do your very best, and deal with the consequences." He comes to the IM clinic to do all he can to live well with his cancer. This history provides a gestalt of the man with the disease. IM practitioners would then proceed with the "regular" history.

TREATMENT AND ADDITIONAL MEDICAL/SOCIAL HISTORY

Conventional Medicine

Combination chemo/radiotherapy was initiated. Mr. S received 900 cGy with a 6 MV beam over 3 fractions to the left upper lobe using anteroposterior/posteroanterior fields, followed by 2800 cGy with an 18-MeV beam to the right lower and left upper lobes. Low doses of carboplatin and paclitaxel were used as radiosensitizers. The patient tolerated the combination therapy well, except for mild esophagitis.

Mr. S' past medical history is notable for hepatitis A. Past surgical history included cholecystectomy in 1982. The patient's family history is notable for hypertension in his mother and colon cancer in his father. The patient is married and has two grown children. He retired from a military career 2 years ago. He discontinued tobacco use approximately 12 years ago after a 25-year pack/day history.

Integrative Medicine

Additional social history is an important part of an integrative history that helps shape recommendations. For example, beyond discovering his marital status, we suggest physicians ask about the nature of his relationship with his wife and children and other support systems. Of note, Mr. S describes his wife as "the rock of Gibraltar." He feels blessed by the support of his children.

MEDICATIONS AND SUPPLEMENTS

Conventional Medicine

Medications included acetaminophen as needed, about 1 or 2 tablets a day, and multiple herbs and supplements.

Integrative Medicine

"Multiple herbs and supplements" is not an adequate history. The IM provider needs to know doses, brands, frequency, duration, reason for use, and results. Past use and reasons for discontinuation are also important. Given the increasing numbers of drug-herb interactions, it is important to ask about and consider the entire list. Typically, patients taking a long list of supplements no longer remember the reason for taking some of them.

THERAPY

Conventional Medicine

Because combination therapy had resulted in a partial response with greater than 50% shrinkage, it was followed by full-dose carboplatin (area under the curve [AUC] = 5) and paclitaxel (175 mg/m^2) treatment. As Mr. S was about to resume chemotherapy, he was advised to discontinue the use of all supplements because of their unknown interaction with chemotherapy. The patient completed four cycles every 3 weeks with mild improvement, 25% further shrinkage, and then disease stabilization.

Integrative Medicine

Stopping antioxidant vitamins during chemotherapy and radiation therapy is usually advised. Any herb or supplement that might activate the cytochrome P-450 system is avoided during chemotherapy as well. Because knowledge of herbs is limited, temporarily stopping all herbal substances is a reasonable recommendation.

On the completion of the four cycles of chemotherapy, Mr. S was referred to the Program in Integrative Medicine Clinic.

It is important to ask for the patient's goals in choosing IM. Many patients may wish that "magic herbs" or alternative therapies will offer primary treatment or prevent a recurrence. Mr. S stated he did not expect to find a cure for his cancer; rather, his goal was to discover a way to live with his cancer as long as possible.

It is valuable to explore a patient's attitude and any insights the diagnosis has given. Mr. S believed that his perspective about cancer was greatly shaped by two forces: his 40 years in the Marines and his wife's intolerance for self-pity. The Marines led him to confront his own mortality at an early age. His wife's attitude taught him to transform anger and bitterness into a determination to heal. The literature on the impact of attitude on cancer is limited. Social support systems and spirituality emerge as the most constant predictors of survival among patients with advanced malignancies.[21]

Integrative treatment strategies decided by the patient and physician included nutritional approaches (including supplements), exercise, mind-body approaches, and healing therapy ("energy work"). Further information resources were shared.

NUTRITION THERAPY. The patient was advised to choose organic food whenever feasible; to increase his consumption of fresh fruits, vegetables, and omega-3 fatty acids; and to avoid processed foods and foods containing *trans* fatty acids and polyhydrogenated fats.

Intake of fruits and vegetables has been consistently related to a reduction in cancer risk.[8,101,102,114] The most commonly held mechanism for this effect is through antioxidation. *Antioxidants* are defined as compounds in our food that help protect the body from oxidative stress by suppressing free radical formation, scavenging free oxygen species, inhibiting lipid peroxidation, and repairing oxidative damage. Antioxidant nutrients, including vitamin C, vitamin E, carotenoids, and selenium, have been shown to inhibit cancer cell growth individually[36,81,82,100,108] and in combination,[80,85,93] although some studies have shown a worsened clinical course.[76,106]

Several supplements were recommended, including a multivitamin-multimineral complex, 100 mg of Co-Q10 daily, green tea extract, and products containing medicinal mushrooms: a combination product containing iceman polypore, reishi *(Ganoderma lucidum)*, maitake *(Grifola frondosa)*, chaga, shiitake *(Lentinus edodes)*, birch polypore, Zhu Ling *(Polyporus umbellatus)*, Split-Gill *(Schizophyllum commune)*, Yun Zhi *(Trametes versicolor)*, Cordyceps capsules *(Cordyceps sinensis)*, and a mushroom tea (reishi, maitake, shiitake, Zhu Ling).

Medicinal mushrooms have immunomodulating properties and a long history of clinical use in Asian cultures. Clinical trials by Ghoneum[42,43] show increases in natural killer (NK) cell activity, reduction in tumor markers, and increased survival. Several different mechanisms have been postulated. Polysaccharides in the mushrooms have immunomodulatory and antitumor effects.[38,59] It is believed that the breakdown of these large compounds may stimulate the immune system. Another compound, arabinoxylane, is a potent inducer of tumor necrosis factor alpha (TNF-α) and augments the immunomodulatory effect of low concentrations of recombinant interleukin-2 (IL-2) on the antitumor activity of NK cells.[42] The rationale for mixtures of mushrooms is to potentiate the immune system with a complex assortment of polysaccharides that may promote a synergistic effect.[42]

EXERCISE. Regular exercise was encouraged for its health-promoting effects. Most data on the benefits of exercise in cancer come from observational and epidemiologic studies. Specific information and advice as to the ideal amount, intensity, and type are not yet known.

MIND-BODY THERAPIES. Mind-body suggestions included journaling, guided imagery, and meditation. *Guided imagery* has a long history of popular use among cancer patients.[89,98] Most studies are small, and survival benefit has not been shown. NK cell activity, however, has been shown to increase.[44,116] The strongest evidence for guided imagery relates to mitigation of anticipatory nausea related to chemotherapy.[72,111] Whether imagery can enhance survival is unknown. Mr. S saw a hypnotherapist once and then developed his own form of guided imagery in which he communicates with the operating system of his body.

Group support was recommended, but Mr. S found the groups he attended depressing. Instead, he has formed his own network via the Internet, where he regularly offers his assistance and himself as a model for those with a new diagnosis of cancer.

HEALING THERAPY. Mr. S was advised to experiment with a healing circle in which his IM physician participated. *Healing circles* are a form of energy medicine practice in which group members direct healing energy towards individuals. This practice has not been studied. Energetic practices such as Qi Gong have been shown to stimulate the phagocytic activity of human polymorphonuclear leukocytes.[39]

OTHER INTERVENTIONS. Further resources for innovative and alternative cancer treatments were shared, including the book *Choices in Healing* by Michael Lerner, the Cancer Help Program at Commonweal for their week-long residential retreats, and multiple cancer research services accessible through various websites.

RESULTS

Over the past year, Mr. S has been followed regularly with physical examination and laboratory studies, including carcinoembryonic antigen (CEA) levels. He has continued without physical limitations due to his disease. His CEA levels have increased by approximately 20%, without significant change clinically or radiographically. Radiographic evaluations included CT and positron emission tomography (AET) scans. A PET scan was essentially normal when evaluated 20 months after his initial diagnosis.

Mr. S has had a better-than-expected course given the diagnosis of stage IV lung cancer. In addition to his allopathic therapy, this patient used a variety of other therapies and used a holistic approach to his cancer. His tumor may have been particularly susceptible to the radiation therapy or chemotherapeutic agents. Guided imagery, medicinal mushrooms, and antioxidants may be responsible in part for his current state of well-being. The factor most responsible may be impossible to elucidate, and the multiple therapies may have created an emergent, synergistic combination.

Mr. S was highly motivated and willing to do all he could to enhance his survival. Physician and patient partnered easily to select strategies supported by evidence and meeting the patient's preferences. The patient accepted conventional treatment and used adjuncts carefully to maximize his sense of health, well-being, and control.

CONCLUSIONS

It is important for medicine to study successful patients.[61] Exploring what makes these long-lived patients different, whether it is a function of who they are (personality, attitude) or what they do (conventional or unconventional therapies), is a worthwhile pursuit because it could lead to reproducible improved outcomes. Although it is methodologically challenging to examine a whole package of care, the groundwork for this type of research has been laid.[5] Ultimately, it will enhance our understanding of how to stimulate and support the body's natural healing system and lead us to interventions worthwhile to test in controlled trials. This approach also may lead to more cancer patients experiencing this patient's goal: "I'd like to think I will die of something else."

▧ Information and Evidence in Clinical Practice

Worldwide interest in CAM and IM is peaking.[31,109] This fascination brings with it not only renaissance for many old healing philosophies and techniques, but also some unique challenges for contemporary medicine. For example, valid concerns have been raised with respect to the best models for CAM integration into the health care delivery system,[18,22,55] the risk/benefit ratio of various CAM modalities,[2] and the competency and scope of education of integrative physicians.[112] This section focuses on yet another challenge—the information basis for the evidence-based practice of CAM and IM.

Never before in the history of medicine have information-based decisions, better known as *evidence-based medicine* (EBM), been more valued than today.[25,41,45] An ever-growing number of health care providers,[4,46,51] end consumers,[47] third-party insurers,[78] and policymakers[74] now depend on the availability of readily accessible and accurate information that will support such informed decisions in both CAM/IM and allopathy. Yet retrieving high-quality information in CAM/IM is not an easy task.[35] For example, assessments of MEDLINE sensitivity (the proportion of RCTs identified by a MEDLINE search relative to a "gold standard" of the known number of RCTs) have demonstrated that on average, MEDLINE searches yield only half of all known trials on a given topic, with CAM/IM topics usually scoring below average (e.g., 17% for homeopathy, 31% for *Ginkgo biloba,* 58% for acupuncture).[24] Furthermore, despite that more than 330 meta-analyses and systematic reviews have been published to date in CAM, the quality of many of those reviews is poor,[75] to an extent that often precludes any meaningful statistical analysis.[65] The result is often a *lack of evidence of effectiveness* rather than "evidence of lack of effectiveness," and the task of making an informed decision remains largely a matter of opinion rather than evidence.

Medicine and health care have always shown tension between the hard science of the profession and the art of healing. Traditionally, issues of clinical and public health decision making have had three main sets of influences: authority and convention, theory, and empiric assessment.[29] The predominant influence, until recently, has been that of authority and convention, the viewpoint of accumulated experience and consensus, which is based on a complex and at times a questionably rational system of appraisal of evidence. To this end, the medical community is now moving, under the umbrella of EBM, from the reliance on traditional and largely qualitative reviews of the literature (opinions) to much more structured systematic overviews (evidence) to make health care recommendations.[60] A major catalyst of that shift is the exponential growth of clinical research and the new emphasis on cost and outcome assessment of healthcare.[34]

Frequently defined as "the conscientious, explicit and judicious use of current best evidence in making decisions about the care of individual patients,"[91] EBM represents a cluster of methods aimed at solving clinical problems.[49] In contrast to the traditional paradigm of medical practice, EBM acknowledges that intuition, unsystematic clinical experience, and various domains of rationale are insufficient grounds for clinical decision making. Rather, EBM stresses the examination of evidence from clinical research by suggesting a formal set of rules that help clinicians to effectively interpret the results of such research.[45]

As a distinctive approach to patient care, whether allopathic or CAM/IM, EBM involves two fundamental principles. First, *evidence alone is never sufficient to make a clinical decision;* in other words, EBM is not meant to replace clinical judgment.[92] That is, decision makers must always trade the benefits and risks, inconvenience, and costs associated with alternative management strategies and in doing so, consider the patient's values.[45]

Second, *EBM posits a hierarchy of evidence to guide clinical decision making.* The nature of that hierarchy, however, is not free from controversy. Different hierarchies have often been suggested as a function of the issues under consideration (e.g., therapeutics vs. diagnostics), the goals (e.g., knowledge vs. recommendations), or the different epistemologic and ontologic philosophies of the authors (Box 15-1).

BOX 15–1. Hierarchy of Strength of Evidence for Treatment Decisions

Nature of investigation of therapy
N-of-1 randomized controlled trial (RCT)
Systematic review of RCT
Single RCT
Systematic review of observational studies addressing patient-important outcomes
Single observational study addressing patient-important outcomes
Physiologic studies
Unsystematic clinical observations

Modified from Guyatt G, Rennie D: *User's guides to the medical literature,* Chicago, 2002, AMA Press.

The potential applicability of hierarchy scales to CAM/IM is a subject of an intense debate between those who refuse to accept the principles of EBM when applied to CAM[107] and those who suggest a broader viewpoint of the topic, regardless of whether its applications are for CAM/IM or allopathy (Figure 15-1).[57]

Does EBM, as just described, contradict the core philosophical underpinnings of IM? Contrary to the common belief that EBM (which focuses on the need for rational, empirically proven health care decision making) is at odds with the humanistic, narrative approach to understanding an illness experience (which attends to the needs of patients), we consider the two complementary to one another. One of the best ways to integrate traditional CAM therapies with advanced contemporary therapies is to consider the "compassionate use of individual patients' predicaments, rights, and preferences in making clinical decisions about their care."[91] This is exactly what good medicine should be about—the patient and not just the procedure.

Evidence is an important part but not the only part of effective decision making. The use of evidence is most successful when patient and societal factors such as choice, efficiency, and equity are factored into the decision-making process, whether at the clinical, system, or policy level. Global evidence still needs localized decision making.[95] As the late John Eisenberg stated, "Worldwide access to evidence-based clinical decision-making must coexist with respect for individual decision making shaped by local culture and circumstances. This is the balance between globalizing the evidence and localizing the decisions that will improve delivery of health care worldwide."[28]

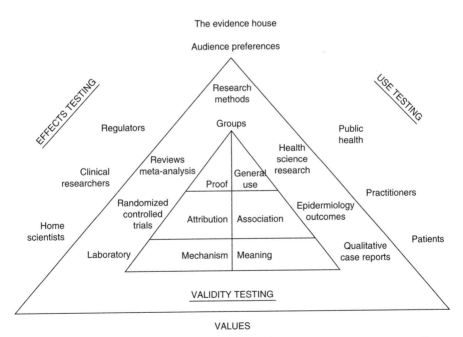

FIGURE 15–1. The "evidence house" affords greater accessibility to important information on evidence-based medicine (EBM) as a guide to CAM decision making. (*From Jonas WB: West J Med 175:79, 2001.*)

FROM EVIDENCE TO ACTION: BRIDGING THE GAP

Although the rise of EBM represents a major intellectual advance in clinical decision making and patient care, it remains largely untested.[41] Current estimates are that only 15% to 40% of allopathic medical treatments have been properly tested.[53,99] Estimates for CAM are lacking, although it has been suggested that CAM, as a popular consumer-based movement, is still almost entirely opinion based. Ernst et al.[32] recently evaluated the recommendations of seven leading CAM textbooks for specific medical conditions. They found that (1) the consistency in the recommendations of these sources was very poor; (2) treatments were recommended that, according to evidence from reliable RCT, are ineffective and in some cases even contraindicated; and (3) treatments of proven effectiveness were not recommended by some of the authors.

Even when evidence does exist, medicine is still seldom practiced in a manner consistent with the evidence.[25,66] Four major difficulties span the gap between evidence and action for the physician[97]: (1) retrieving evidence that is relevant to the clinical action, (2) critically appraising this evidence, (3) applying the evidence within a specific decision context at the point of care, and (4) assessing the change in patient outcome that can be attributed to the application of the evidence. Add to this gap, between knowledge and practice, the integration of values and preferences of both the providers and consumers,[73] which is the focus of IM, and a system of care results in which evidence may be poorly translatable to practice.

Evidence indicates that physicians do want to know about CAM to enhance communication with their patients, but the mission of acquiring the necessary knowledge base of such a diverse group of methods may seem impossible. CAM, as a categorical term, encompasses more than 100 therapeutic modalities that generally have little in common.[86] In this sense, CAM is no more than a label.[16]

If this is indeed the case, why bother? Why not let some physicians excel in CAM while others become excellent allopathic providers? The answer is quite simple: in the daily interactions with patients and their families, health care providers will be asked CAM-related questions for which they are expected to provide informed answers. Competent physicians are now expected to have a knowledge base that extends well beyond the specific diseases and disorders pertaining to their medical fields. Furthermore, patients use CAM, often without informing their providers.[27] Rather than looking for "super physicians" who are equally competent in both the allopathic and the CAM worlds, patients are looking for open-minded practitioners who listen, understand, guide, and comfort.

Thus the goal need not be to become an "all-in-one" physician. Rather, the goal is to develop a health care system that facilitates the practice of good medicine, whether its origins are conventional or complementary, based in good science that is both inquiry driven and open to new paradigms. Only in this way can the philosophies of the past become the basis for evidence in the future.[19]

DEVELOPING A KNOWLEDGE BASE

In general, there are four major domains of inquiry with respect to CAM/IM for which information is often sought and evidence is much needed, as follows.

1. *Spectrum of CAM therapeutic and diagnostic options available for a specific medical condition.* This domain includes the most common type of questions a physician typically encounters (e.g., "What else can I do to improve my diabetes?" "Do you recommend taking St. John's wort instead of or together with my conventional antidepressant?"). Allopathic practitioners probably will be asked occasionally about treatments for which they are uninformed, in which case it is advisable to consult with trustworthy CAM providers. Practitioners must say, "I don't know," when the situation warrants.

2. *Quality of data existing to support any of the therapeutic and diagnostic claims made by various CAM practices.* As already emphasized, information related to quality of data in CAM is especially problematic, often due to poor methodology and lack of validity.[35] It is advisable to consult an open-minded, "local champion" of EBM. In general, the cumulative knowledge on any one topic accounts for more than any single study. Providers must always look for a "web" of evidence, not just for anecdotes.

3. *Mechanism of action and other related methodologic issues associated with the plausibility and science of CAM.* This basic type of knowledge is best represented in textbooks and review articles. Attending workshops and conferences is an effective way to become familiar with contemporary theory. Science is not about knowledge but rather *methods* to gain knowledge. Again, it is advisable to consult trustworthy, open-minded CAM providers who have good understanding of scientific methods.

4. *Various aspects associated with the practicality of having an integrative health care system.* Such information would be available through both informal (word of mouth, the media) and formal resources (publications, communications). In the search for further information on cost, availability of services, and other areas, the retrieval of quality information and the ability to appraise it critically would be dramatically improved by collaborating with an informatics specialist. Establishing working relationships with various knowledgeable CAM providers in the community is invaluable. They can answer many questions for which data are difficult to find using conventional databases. Furthermore, even the most systematic modalities within CAM, such as homeopathy and traditional Chinese medicine, have different schools of thoughts and ways of practice. By consulting various practitioners who master a discipline, the provider is most likely to hear different opinions.

In recent years, several papers dealing with advising patients on issues related to CAM have been published.[9,17,26,103] Three main conclusions emerge from these and other papers, as follows.

1. **Never make assumptions.** CAM should never be treated as one entity. Treat each modality as appropriate. What may be alternative for one individual may be mainstream and logical for another. For many patients, routine use of mind-body practices (e.g., meditation, massage) on a monthly basis to support health and well-being and following a healthy diet supplemented with vitamins are not "alternative" at all. If the medical practitioner does not consider the patient's viewpoint, not only may the therapeutic relationship be compromised, but the result of treatment could be failure.[11]

2. **Practice open, respectful, and nonjudgmental communication with patients.**
Although the vast majority of patients use CAM along with allopathy, in many
cases the "don't ask, don't tell" approach is applied to CAM, and too often
patients feel uncomfortable disclosing their use of CAM to their physicians.[26]
Consequently, physicians might miss an important opportunity to educate their
patients about the benefits and risks of CAM. Remember that these are alternative
therapies, not "alternative patients." All patients deserve the best treatment possible
without being judged by their physicians. Talk to patients in an open and respectful
way, and try to explore their health-related practices and beliefs. Advise them
accordingly.

3. **Promote healing.** Every medical encounter is an opportunity to empower patients.
Often the reasons for which patients seek CAM point to other important underlying processes that can then be targeted to facilitate healing.[3] Rather than seeking to
expand the therapeutic options a patient might have, always ask which of the available options best facilitates healing and promotes well-being. In particular, try to
trigger the placebo effect, because this often reflects an innate healing capacity that
can dramatically shift the illness experience.[13]

INTEGRATING TRADITIONAL CAM WITH CONTEMPORARY THERAPIES

The complexity of the integration of allopathy and CAM is self-evident.[5,15] Two different lines of argument, both valid, seem to dominate the discourse about the nature of
this integration.

The first argument, the *add-on approach,* driven greatly by the evidence-based
movement, asserts that once modalities, whether alternative or allopathic, have been
proven to be effective, they should become legitimate parts of the medical armamentarium.[22] The problem with this "xenografting" approach is that modalities are all too
often assimilated without their philosophical underpinnings. This in turn results in
"combination medicine," rather than in the creation of a new emergent property.[14]

The second line of argument, the *integrative approach,* driven by the care-
rather-than-cure approach to medicine, asserts that without a true shift of the medical
paradigm from one of disease to one of humanism, no real integration will be feasible.
According to this approach, CAM integration creates a real opportunity for expanding
the horizons of medicine beyond the domain of therapeutics. Thus, for many, the crucial question is not how many CAM modalities will be integrated into the current
health care delivery system, but rather, will future physicians, whether specialists or
generalists, practice healing-oriented medicine. The problem with this holistic
approach to CAM integration is that, as yet, no substantial empiric data support many
of its claims.

Thus these two approaches represent not only mere disagreement about methods of synthesis, but also a true values battle over the future of medicine.[23]

To illustrate how we access evidence in IM and incorporate it into practice at the
point of care, we will use the case of Mr. S, the 67-year-old ex-Marine with stage IV
pulmonary adenocarcinoma. While receiving chemo/radiotherapy, the patient was

advised to discontinue the use of all supplements, including antioxidants and herbs, due to their unknown interaction with the antitumor regimen. Was that recommendation justified? To answer, we propose using a sequential five-step strategy.[1] Other useful strategies and tips are provided elsewhere.[58]

Step 1: Identify the Question

The search for evidence always starts with the construction of a well-built clinical question that focuses on specifics, for example, an individual patient with a specific health problem, a range of intervention options, or an outcome. In the case of Mr. S, a number of interesting questions can be constructed. For example, should a patient with stage IV pulmonary adenocarcinoma who undergoes chemo/radiotherapy discontinue the use of all supplements, including antioxidants and herbs? If so, should they be discontinued only during the therapy, or also when the patient is not receiving chemo/radiotherapy? For illustrative purposes, we restrict this discussion to only antioxidants (ignoring other supplements and herbs) and chemotherapy (ignoring radiotherapy). Specifically, we attempt to identify and assess the evidence for the potential interaction of antioxidants with various chemotherapeutic agents, particularly carboplatin and paclitaxel.

Step 2: Narrow the Question

Because medical decisions are typically made within the specific context and particularities of the patient for whom evidence is being sought, all the important parameters must always be defined. In this example there are two crucial variables: the patient's condition (stage IV pulmonary adenocarcinoma) and the possible agent of harm (antioxidants interacting with chemo/radiotherapy). The "intervention" or "cause" of the possible outcome is the antioxidants. However, we can further specify the questions by replacing the general constructs of chemo/radiotherapy with the exact regimen (carboplatin and paclitaxel) and by defining the exact antioxidants under consideration.

Step 3: Retrieve the Information

To retrieve the information, one must retrieve the existing body of knowledge that pertains to the question under consideration. To maximize yield, it is important to prioritize the search so that only those sources that could provide an answer are consulted. At times, textbooks are sufficient (e.g., information on the natural history of a disease or its differential diagnosis). However, for the current state of therapeutics, it is advisable to search for meta-analyses, systematic reviews, RCTs, and observational or prospective outcome data now available in various electronic databases.[33] When using electronic databases, such as MEDLINE, one should use MeSH (Medical Subject Heading) terms as key words and cross-reference those with key publication parameters, such as type of publication (review, editorial, or original), study design (e.g., RCT), and population (e.g., men, neonates). In this case we are interested in both the specific question (potential interaction between antioxidants and carboplatin and paclitaxel) and the more general question (potential interaction between antioxidants and chemotherapy).

An electronic search using MEDLINE, *Cochrane Database of Systematic Reviews* (CDSR), ACP Journal Club, *Database of Abstracts of Reviews of Effectiveness* (DARE), *Cochrane Controlled Trials Register* (CCTR), and *Allied Complementary Medicine* (AMED) found studies that indeed verify the theoretic concern that at least some antioxidants may counteract the antitumor activity of paclitaxel. For example, Marone et al.[71] found that "the isoflavonoid quercetin, a known general kinase inhibitor and an antioxidant, was able to prevent the onset of Taxol-induced cellular detachment and to protect from cell death." This should not be surprising because quercetin inhibits topoisomerase II activity, which is necessary for the formation of 6α-hydroxypaclitaxel in vitro.[77] Likewise, selenium can also interfere with the antitumor activity of cisplatin. Selenium, with chemical properties similar to those of sulfur, can bind with platinum and inactivate the antineoplastic platinum coordination complexes. Thus, caution should be used when administering selenium during chemotherapy with cisplatin and carboplatin.[20]

However, the search failed to identify any definitive human clinical trials that have studied the long-term effects of combining chemotherapeutic agents and oral antioxidants. Likewise, we found no systematic reviews or meta-analyses that synthesized results from RCTs or other prospective clinical trials in humans directly comparing the outcome of non–small-cell lung cancer patients who received chemotherapy simultaneously with or without antioxidants. Only a few small-scale nonrandomized trials have been found. For example, Jaakkola et al.[56] reported their experience with 18 nonrandomized patients with small-cell lung cancer who received, in addition to conservative chemotherapy, antioxidant treatment with vitamins, trace elements, and fatty acids. The antioxidant treatment, in combination with chemotherapy and irradiation, prolonged the survival time of patients with small cell lung cancer compared with combination treatment regimens alone, and the patients receiving antioxidants were able to tolerate chemotherapy and radiation treatment well.

In the absence of "better" evidence, a reasonable compromise is to search for comprehensive review articles that focus on one or more aspects of the issue under consideration. Critical appraisal of these articles in our case demonstrates vividly why only a small fraction of clinical care is addressed by research evidence.

Step 4: Make a Critical Appraisal of the Information

The practice of EBM, whether allopathic or CAM, depends primarily on physicians' ability to assess critically the validity and applicability of research evidence and successfully incorporate the evidence into patient care.[41,105] Decisions based on critical evaluation of evidence rely on how effectively the physician interprets research findings.[67] Critical appraisal comprises the ability to assess the validity and applicability of clinical, paraclinical, and published evidence and to incorporate the results of this assessment into patient management.[6]

Critical appraisal of the review literature that focuses on the potential benefit or harm associated with the simultaneous use of chemotherapy and antioxidants reveals contradictory findings and opposing opinions. Prasad et al.[83] reviewed the literature on high doses of multiple antioxidant vitamins and concluded, based on extensive in vitro studies and limited in vivo studies, that "multiple antioxidant vitamin supplements together with diet and lifestyle modifications may improve the efficacy of standard and experimental chemotherapy." Labriola and Livingston,[64] on the other hand, identified six factors that predict interactions between chemotherapeutic agents and antioxidant compounds: fraction of drug effectiveness that depends on reactive oxygen species, nature of the reactive species generated by the chemotherapeutic agent, dosage and concentration of reactive oxygen species, nature of the antioxidant, and concentration of the antioxidant. Based on this predictive model, it is almost certain that carboplatin (which acts through DNA cross-linking) and paclitaxel (which binds to DNA microtubules) actions will be hampered by antioxidants (Table 15-1).

After a comprehensive review of the literature, Conklin[20] concluded it is unlikely that dietary supplementation with antioxidants interferes with the mechanism whereby antineoplastic agents are cytotoxic to cancer cells, since reactive oxygen species are not involved in the mechanism of action of most anticancer drugs in current use, except bleomycin. Also, "numerous studies have also demonstrated that antioxidants do not inhibit, but actually enhance, the cytotoxic effect of antineoplastic drugs on cancer cells."[33]

Step 5: Apply the Evidence Within the Point of Care

What evidence-based recommendation should the provider then make to the patient? Should Mr. S take antioxidants during his chemotherapy treatment, or should he avoid them? Contrary to Prasad et al.,[83] who developed a specific antioxidant protocol for cancer patients who undergo active treatment, the World Cancer Research Fund and the American Institute of Cancer Research panel support the

---

TABLE 15–1. **VULNERABILITY OF CHEMOTHERAPEUTIC AGENTS TO INTERACTIONS WITH ANTIOXIDANTS**

Drug Class/Drugs	Comment
AGENTS WITH ACTIONS DEPENDENT ON REACTIVE OXYGEN SPECIES	
Classic alkylating agents	Vulnerable to interaction with antioxidants; avoid
Anthracyclines (doxorubicin, daunorubicin, epirubicin)	concurrent administration.
Mitomycin	
Bleomycin	
Podophyllum agents (e.g., etoposide, teniposide)	
AGENT WITHOUT ESTABLISHED MOLECULAR PHARMACOLOGY	
Plicamycin	Treat as though interaction is possible.
AGENTS WITH ACTIONS NOT HIGHLY DEPENDENT ON REACTIVE OXYGEN SPECIES	
Hormones	Probably not vulnerable to interactions; avoid
Biologic agents	high levels of antioxidants until long-term
Antimetabolites	studies are done.
Vinca alkaloids	
Taxanes	

role of increased fruit and vegetable consumption, but not antioxidant supplementation, even in the prevention of cancer.[114] Labriola and Livingston[64] concluded after analyzing the literature that "cancer patients who use nutritional supplements with antioxidant activity risk interfering with actions of chemotherapeutic agents that utilize reactive oxygen species as a mechanism for cytotoxicity. Ironically, these patients may improve their short-term tolerance to treatment while increasing their vulnerability to later recurrence as a result of having decreased the effectiveness of the drug." Commenting on this analysis, Ratain[87] admitted that "the dilemma for the practicing oncologist may be complex. In my own practice, I emphasize to patients that alternative therapies are drugs and, as such, complicate the administration of highly toxic therapies. I also stress that the administration of any drug, even a "natural" compound, has the potential to increase the side effects of cancer chemotherapy. In my experience, this warning usually results in patients avoiding alternative therapies, especially during the critical perichemotherapy period."

Provider-Patient Communication

Integrative medicine advocates a different form of communication with patients, one that is based on open discussion and understanding, rather than on frightening. Since our search for evidence failed to generate an unequivocal recommendation whether antioxidants should be discontinued in all patients undergoing chemotherapy, in the case of Mr. S, this seems to be a reasonable recommendation due to the type of chemotherapeutic agents he received.

CONCLUSIONS

Commenting on the extent to which practitioners know about "what works," and if researchers and policymakers are truly committed to developing and using the best evidence, Macintyre et al. said, ". . . we were struck by the lack of empirical evidence available for a government to base policies or decide on priorities, despite the large amount of research undertaken and published on the subject. . . . We were also struck by the readiness of researchers to recommend policies the effectiveness of which they knew little about in contrast to their caution in interpreting the results of epidemiological or clinical evidence."[68] The field of CAM/IM deserves more than mere opinions. We believe that for medicine to reach new horizons, a paradigm shift in medical education must occur.

N Integrative Medical Education

Conventional medical education espouses the biomedical paradigm, which is rarely acknowledged during medical training. When this paradigm is addressed, Western medicine is usually described as modern, scientific, and the preferred way of knowing about health and humans. IM training asks physicians to set aside this dogma. It acknowledges the value of Western medicine and simultaneously acknowledges that there are other ways of knowing and seeing. Thus, IM espouses a broader, more encompassing paradigm.

Studying alternative systems helps us recognize that the biomedical model is one of a number of ways of viewing health and disease. For example, the Chinese medical system's use of moxibustion to turn a "breech baby" does not fit within the Western paradigm.[12] Although the methods have been disputed,[94] the possibility of distance healing, shown to be significant in double-blind RCTs, is especially challenging.[10,48,96]

IM education asks physicians to be open-minded skeptics who explore with curiosity the great diversity of healing traditions. In addition to critical content, the training emphasizes a shift in skills and attitudes and experiential learning. IM training is a nonlinear process; content and experiences are woven together, and physicians are asked to experience alternative treatments personally to expand their understanding.

INTEGRATIVE MEDICINE PROGRAM

The University of Arizona Program in Integrative Medicine (PIM) has developed a comprehensive curriculum in IM. PIM is offered in both residential and distributed learning formats (http://integrativemedicine.arizona.edu/) by synthesizing the work of many fields, both conventional and alternative. PIM addresses deficiencies in the current medical education system while modeling a different learning culture. It remains to be determined which aspects of the curriculum fit best into undergraduate, graduate, postgraduate, and ongoing professional education. The Arizona model is not the only approach for training the full diversity of providers involved in health care. Rather, PIM represents one way to begin and to evolve a new form of medical education, subject to modifications from the characteristics, needs, and missions of local educational settings to which it may be adapted, as well as to the emergence of new evidence.

Many physicians who study and then practice IM experience a rejuvenated call to service. Their relationships with patients deepen and become more satisfying. Patients experience the humanistic, broad-minded medical care they are seeking. This synergism of the best conventional and alternative therapies has the potential to create a medicine of which we can all be proud.

CURRICULUM

The IM curriculum is divided into three didactic and four process sections. *Didactic* sections include philosophical foundations, lifestyle practices, and therapeutic systems and modalities. *Process* sections include clinical integration, personal development and reflection, research education, and leadership.

FOUNDATIONS

Integrative medicine training begins with philosophical foundations. Physicians explore the epistemology of allopathic medicine. Kuhn's theory of paradigm shift[63] and Popper's falsifiability theory[79] expose physicians to the assumptions that underlie medical science. These theories help providers to understand the nature of evidence and how to incorporate new knowledge and information into medicine.

The shift from a disease focus to a healing approach requires a shift in orientation and "way of being." Physicians examine their own beliefs about medicine and the role of the physician. The art of medicine prepares physicians for new roles as partner, coach, teacher, motivator, and healer. Medicine and culture heighten awareness of the different cultural healing systems and explore the beliefs about health and illness that underlie health behaviors among cultural groups.

Most alternative systems are holistic in their orientation; thus they create models for physicians to take a holistic approach. This approach is an essential principle of IM. The antithesis of reductionism is the value that each patient is unique. Most conventional training is *reductionist;* physicians are taught the pulmonary system or the cardiovascular system, creating disease categories into which they lump groups of patients. Whereas most alternative systems have a coherent philosophy of *health,* Western medicine focuses on disease.

LIFESTYLE PRACTICES

The lifestyle practices curricula prepare physicians for the increased focus on prevention and health promotion. Extensive training is offered in nutrition, mind-body medicine, spirituality and medicine, and physical activity. Nutritional influences on health address the central role of nutrition in healing. This educational emphasis provides a scientific basis for the integration of nutrition in medicine in order to practice preventive and therapeutic nutrition and to make appropriate referrals to nutritionists. Mind-body medicine explores the breadth and mechanics of mind-body interactions, teaches an appreciation of a broad range of applied interventions, and teaches the use of mind-body interventions in clinical care. Physicians examine the role of spirituality in themselves and their patients. They learn to assess their patients' spiritual beliefs and consider how these beliefs help (or hinder) the healing process. The physical activity curriculum teaches the benefits of physical activity, how to prescribe exercise, and how to enhance self-practice.

ALTERNATIVE SYSTEMS

Physicians are instructed in Chinese medicine, energy medicine, homeopathy, allopathic medicine, manual medicine, and Western herbalism. Common to all systems and modalities teachings is an introduction to the history, philosophy, and scientific basis of the system. Other goals are to identify different schools and styles, understand issues relating to safety and efficacy, discuss credentialing and licensing issues, effectively explain the various systems to patients, and make appropriate referrals. A central challenge is to identify methods to integrate these systems with allopathic knowledge, values, and skills. Comprehensive training in an alternative medical system is pursued by some IM physicians.

REFLECTION

Integrative medicine education emphasizes personal experience and self-care. Physicians are encouraged to experience the modalities they recommend to their patients. Time is allotted for regular exercise, and healthy nutrition is taught in an experiential manner that places value on incorporating the concepts into the lives of the physician and their families as well as their patients. Therapeutic movement is woven into the curriculum and alternates among yoga, t'ai chi, and Qi Gong.

Building on support groups in medical training programs,[30,90] a reflection process that fosters self-awareness is vital to IM education. In facilitated sessions, physicians examine their humanity, including the identity they have left behind and the physician-healer they are seeking to become. These meetings include group work, listening to music, hiking, reading plays and poetry, and participating in Sufi dancing and sweat lodge ceremonies.

During their training, physicians may mirror the healing process that patients undergo. They become more comfortable living with uncertainty. They are more willing to partner with patients with the understanding that healing originates within the patient. There may be a disassembling of identity before a new identity emerges. *Family physician, internist,* and *emergency doctor* become less accurate descriptive names, but *integrative physician* is not as clearly defined as *specialists.*

CLINICAL INTEGRATION IN PRACTICE

Clinical care offers the opportunity to put theory into practice. The life experiences and knowledge of both participants in the encounter are acknowledged and respected.[88] Listening skills, interaction skills, and motivational skills are taught and highly valued. This style, modeled in part on family practice and psychiatry,[84,104] is intended to develop a highly therapeutic physician-patient relationship. Behavioral medicine and health psychology tools that focus on improving self-care and self-efficacy are used. The boundaries of the professional relationship are examined, and a closer and perhaps more effective relationship may emerge.[37]

The initial patient visit lasts 60 to 90 minutes. Physicians begin the interview with a statement such as, "My goal is to get a sense of who you are as a person, to understand the important relationships and events in your life, in addition to the medical condition that brings you in today." As physicians and patients, we seek to understand the origins of an illness with the hope of finding ways to change that course.[69] We listen carefully to what is said and what is left unsaid. We seek to discern the origins of the disease—genetic, physical, emotional, psychological, or spiritual. Most important, we seek to promote a healing response.

PATIENT CONFERENCE

After the consultation, physicians perform a literature search and present their patients at a multidisciplinary patient care conference. This meeting is precepted by practitioners of traditional Chinese medicine (TCM), naturopathy, osteopathy, homeopathy, and energy medicine; a mind-body psychologist; a spiritual counselor; a nutritionist; and a pharmacist, in addition to physicians trained in family medicine, general practice, internal medicine, psychiatry, environmental medicine, and geriatrics.

Patients are presented in a holistic fashion. The typical "this is a 49-year-old woman with a 2-year history of diabetes mellitus" does not capture the essence of the human being in a manner that allows a spiritual provider, homeopath, or TCM practitioner to give input. Instead, the provider might begin "Debra Smith is a 50-year-old woman who says she wants her body to catch up with her mind. This is how she describes her lifelong struggle with her weight. Debra is energetic, funny, a loving wife, a good friend, and mother of four young children. She admits that she is a perfectionist in everything she does. She comes to IM to explore a new approach to managing her diabetes." Thus the physician attempts to capture the nature of the patient for the group. The presentation proceeds with a thorough medical and psychosocial history.

Patient conference is a critical part of the clinical training. The dialogues lead to a deeper understanding of the worldviews of various practitioners. A broader set of questions is developed and practiced as a result of input from the various practitioners. Over time, clarity sharpens as to which system works best for a particular patient or condition. Physicians discover situations in which symptoms cannot fit together from a Western perspective but, for example, neatly fit into a TCM diagnosis. Active dialogue and questioning are encouraged. Input from preceptors is tailored into a treatment plan. In partnership, physician and patient determine the course of action. Integration ultimately rests with the patient. Follow-up visits tailor the course of care.

Physicians are encouraged to refine their practice of IM continually and to learn from every encounter. Healing often takes very different routes.[50] This fact is affirmed by research that reveals that the strongest predictor of mortality is neither laboratory tests nor physician assessment but rather the patient's self-rated health status.[52]

RESEARCH EDUCATION

Critical to all physicians, but especially to those incorporating alternative medicine, are skills to evaluate the medical literature. Physicians participate in journal clubs and study research methodology and statistics. They write review articles, book chapters, and case studies for scholarly publications. For those pursuing academic research tracks, advanced degrees (e.g., MPH, PhD), additional practical training in senior investigators' laboratories, and didactic coursework in clinical research, CAM/IM research methodology, biostatistics and epidemiology, and research ethics are offered.

LEADERSHIP

The fellowship at the Program in Integrative Medicine is designed to develop leadership skills; our intention is for graduates to educate, inspire others, and serve as agents of change. Effective communication skills are developed to build and maintain relationships and advance IM. Leadership skills in the political, administrative, advocacy, and personal commitment arenas are taught. Opportunities are provided for practitioners to act as advocates for IM.

CHALLENGES

Acknowledging the existence of multiple paradigms does not reduce the challenge in effectively integrating them in patient care. Bridging different perspectives of health and illness is a significant challenge. Although many clinical practices now provide CAM and conventional care alongside one another, we promote the value of integration. CAM practitioners and academic faculty often have different perspectives; our goal is to create a setting in which they can work comfortably together.

Academic institutions across the United States are responding to their patients' demand for CAM by providing lectures in holistic medicine and CAM.[7,113] The content of these lectures varies. In general they are elective, survey courses describing alternative therapies and systems. Increasingly, schools are providing experiential components. Postgraduate CAM conferences and continuing medical education (CME) are broadening in availability. However, the American Academy of Family Physicians (AAFP) and more recently the American Medical Association (AMA) will not provide CME credits to learn how to "do" any form of CAM.

Guidelines for including CAM in residency curricula have been suggested by the Society of Teachers of Family Medicine Group on Alternative Medicine.[62] The Association of American Medical Colleges has formed a special-interest group in CAM. For the past 2 years, the National Institutes of Health (NIH) has offered institutions 5-year grants to develop curricula in CAM. The Education Subcommittee of the Consortium of Academic Health Centers for Integrative Medicine is developing objectives and goals for undergraduate medical education. A next step for the consortium will be to develop competency measures.

Adding to the curriculum of undergraduate or graduate medical education is a formidable challenge. Even when agreement exists on the need for education, barriers include limited resources (e.g., time, money, faculty), student and faculty resistance, and a lack of continuity among courses.[110] Completely learning an alternative system of medicine takes years of study and commitment.

SUMMARY

Integrative medicine is an emerging model for medical education and practice. To advance the field of IM, providers need to move into interdisciplinary research approaches as much as into interdisciplinary practice. That is, if IM is a system of systems of care, studying the various components in isolation can only answer reductionistic questions about the efficacy of a specific intervention. Integratively oriented research requires the capacity to study a multicomponent treatment program as a whole and to evaluate multidimensional features of the same persons. Cost-effectiveness, well-done observational research, and health services research studies become as important as the single-drug model of a double-blind RCT for building an evidence base in IM. Just as IM medical education and practice expand to include more than technical knowledge, IM research must incorporate methodologies and multivariate statistical approaches that borrow from already well-established academic fields such as anthropology, sociology, psychology, and epidemiology.

Many leaders in the field of medicine, both proponents and skeptics of CAM, have written about the concept of one medicine. That is, in the end, the ideal goal should be a fully integrated system of care in which patients receive state-of-the-art and state-of-the-science care that addresses their individualized circumstances in the most effective and safest manner possible. From an IM perspective, the process of care itself should nurture not only patients but also providers. Although still in its earliest stages, IM offers a direction for addressing the Institute of Medicine–identified flaws in medicine today and promises to enrich the quality of health care for the future.

REFERENCES

1. [Access online]: A methodology for finding "evidence" in the biomedical literature, 2002, *http://www. ahsl.arizona.edu/guides/topics/methods.html.*
2. Angell M, Kassirer JP: Alternative medicine: the risks of untested and unregulated remedies, *N Engl J Med* 339:839, 1998.
3. Astin JA: Why patients use alternative medicine: results of a national study, *JAMA* 279:1548, 1998.
4. Astin JA et al: A review of the incorporation of complementary and alternative medicine by mainstream physicians, *Arch Intern Med* 158:2303, 1998.
5. Bell IR et al: Integrative medicine and systematic outcomes research: issues in the emergence of a new model for primary health care, *Arch Intern Med* 162:133, 2002.
6. Bennett KJ et al: A controlled trial of teaching critical appraisal of the clinical literature to medical students, *JAMA* 257:2451, 1987.
7. Bhattacharya B: M.D. programs in the United States with complementary and alternative medicine education opportunities: an ongoing listing, *J Altern Complement Med* 6:77, 2000.
8. Block G, Patterson B, Subar A: Fruit, vegetables, and cancer prevention: a review of the epidemiological evidence, *Nutr Cancer* 18:1, 1992.
9. Burstein HJ: Discussing complementary therapies with cancer patients: what should we be talking about? *J Clin Oncol* 18:2501, 2000.
10. Byrd RC: Positive therapeutic effects of intercessory prayer in a coronary care unit population, *South Med J* 81:826, 1988.
11. Campbell SM, Roland MO, Buetow SA: Defining quality of care, *Soc Sci Med* 51:1611, 2000.
12. Cardini F, Weixin H: Moxibustion for correction of breech presentation: a randomized controlled trial, *JAMA* 280:1580, 1998.
13. Caspi O: Activating the healing response. In Rakel D, editor: *Integrative medicine: complementary therapy in medical practice,* Philadelphia, 2002, Saunders.
14. Caspi O: Integrated medicine: orthodox meets alternative: bringing complementary and alternative medicine (CAM) into mainstream is not integration, *BMJ* 322:168, 2001.
15. Caspi O et al: The tower of Babel: communication and medicine: an essay on medical education and complementary-alternative medicine, *Arch Intern Med* 160:3193, 2000.
16. Caspi O et al: On the definition of complementary, alternative, and integrative medicine: societal mega-stereotypes vs. the patients' perspectives, 2002 (in press).
17. Chez R, Jonas WB, Eisenberg D: The physician and complementary and alternative medicine. In Jonas WB, Levin JS, editors: *Essentials of complementary and alternative medicine,* Philadelphia, 1999, Lippincott, Williams & Wilkins.
18. Coates JR, Jobst KA: Integrated healthcare: a way forward for the next five years? A discussion document from the Prince of Wales's Initiative on Integrated Medicine, *J Altern Complement Med* 4:209, 1998.
19. Comfort A: Quantum physics and the philosophy of medicine, *J R Soc Med* 77:631, 1984.
20. Conklin KA: Dietary antioxidants during cancer chemotherapy: impact on chemotherapeutic effectiveness and development of side effects, *Nutr Cancer* 37:1, 2000.
21. Creagan ET: Attitude and disposition: do they make a difference in cancer survival? *Mayo Clin Proc* 72:160, 1997.

22. Dalen JE: "Conventional" and "unconventional" medicine: can they be integrated? *Arch Intern Med* 158:2179, 1998.

23. Dalen JE: Is integrative medicine the medicine of the future? A debate between Arnold S. Relman, MD and Andrew Weil, MD, *Arch Intern Med* 159:2122, 1999.

24. Dickersin K, Scherer L, Lefevbre C: Identifying relevant studies for systematic reviews. In Chalmers I, Altman D, editors: *Systematic reviews*, London, 1999, BMJ Press.

25. Eddy DM: Clinical decision-making: from theory to practice—three battles to watch in the 1990s, *JAMA* 270:520, 1993.

26. Eisenberg DM: Advising patients who seek alternative medical therapies, *Ann Intern Med* 127:61, 1997.

27. Eisenberg DM et al: Trends in alternative medicine use in the United States, 1990–1997: results of a follow-up national survey, *JAMA* 280:1569, 1998.

28. Eisenberg JM: Globalize the evidence, localize the decision: evidence-based medicine and the international diversity, *Health Aff* 21:166, 2002.

29. Elwood M: *Critical appraisal of epidemiological studies and clinical trials,* ed 2, New York, 1998, Oxford University Press.

30. Epstein RM et al: Perspectives on patient-doctor communication, *J Fam Pract* 37:377, 1993.

31. Ernst E: Prevalence of use of complementary/alternative medicine: a systematic review, *Bull WHO* 78:252, 2000.

32. Ernst E et al: *The desktop guide to complementary and alternative medicine: an evidence-based approach,* St Louis, 2001, Mosby.

33. Evidence-based health care, 2002, http://www.ahsl.arizona.edu/.

34. Evidence-Based Medicine Working Group: Evidence-based medicine: a new approach to teaching the practice of medicine, *JAMA* 268:2420, 1992.

35. Ezzo J, Berman BM, Vickers AJ, Linde K: Complementary medicine and the Cochrane Collaboration, *JAMA* 280:1628, 1998.

36. Fariss MW et al: The selective antiproliferative effects of alpha-tocopheryl hemisuccinate and cholesteryl hemisuccinate on murine leukemia cells result from the action of the intact compounds, *Cancer Res* 54:3346, 1994.

37. Frank E, Breyan J, Elon L: Physician disclosure of healthy personal behaviors improves credibility and ability to motivate, *Arch Fam Med* 9:287, 2000.

38. Franz G: Polysaccharides in pharmacy: current applications and future concepts, *Planta Med* 55:493, 1989.

39. Fukushima M, Kataoka T, Hamada C, Matsumoto M: Evidence of Qi-gong energy and its biological effect on the enhancement of the phagocytic activity of human polymorphonuclear leukocytes, *Am J Chin Med* 29:1, 2001.

40. Gaudet TW: Integrative medicine: the evolution of a new approach to medicine and medical education, *Integr Med* 1:67, 1998.

41. Geyman JP, Deyo RA, Ramsey SD: *Evidence-based clinical practice: concepts and approaches,* Boston, 1999, Butterworth-Heinemann.

42. Ghoneum M: Enhancement of human killer cell activity by modified arabinoxlane from rice bran (MGM-3), *Int J Immunother* XIV:89, 1998.

43. Ghoneum M: Immunomodulatory and anti-cancer properties of (MGN-3), a modified xylose from rice bran, in 5 patients with breast cancer. Presented American Association for Cancer Research (AACR) special conference: The Interference between Basic and Applied Research, Baltimore, 1995 (abstract).

44. Gruber BL et al: Immunological responses of breast cancer patients to behavioral interventions, *Biofeedback Self Regul* 18:1, 1993.

45. Guyatt G, Rennie D: *User's guides to the medical literature,* Chicago, 2002, AMA Press.

46. Halliday J, Taylor M, Jenkins A, Reilly D: Medical students and complementary medicine, *Complement Ther Med* 1(suppl):32, 1993.

47. Harris P, Rees R: The prevalence of complementary and alternative medicine use among the general population: a systematic review of the literature, *Complement Ther Med* 8:88, 2000.

48. Harris WS et al: A randomized, controlled trial of the effects of remote, intercessory prayer on outcomes in patients admitted to the coronary care unit, *Arch Intern Med* 159:2273, 1999; erratum, 160:1878, 2000.

49. Haynes RB et al: Transferring evidence from research into practice. 1. The role of clinical care research evidence in clinical decisions, *ACP J Club* 125:A14, 1996.

50. Hirshberg C, Barasch MI: *Remarkable recovery: what extraordinary healings tell us about getting well and staying well,* New York, 1995, Putnam.

51. Hopper I, Cohen M: Complementary therapies and the medical profession: a study of medical students' attitudes, *Altern Ther Health Med* 4:68, 1998.

52. Idler E: Self-assessed health and mortality: a review of studies, *Int Rev Health Psychol* 1:33, 1992.

53. Imrie R, Ramey DW: The evidence for evidence-based medicine, *Complement Ther Med* 8:123, 2000.

54. Institute of Medicine: *Crossing the quality chasm: a new health system for the 21st century,* Washington, DC, 2001, National Academy Press.

55. Integration of complementary and alternative medicine: a health services research perspective, 2002, http://grants2.nih.gov/grants/guide/rfa-files/RFA-AT-01-001.html.

56. Jaakkola K et al: Treatment with antioxidant and other nutrients in combination with chemotherapy and irradiation in patients with small-cell lung cancer, *Anticancer Res* 12:599, 1992.

57. Jonas WB: The evidence house: how to build an inclusive base for complementary medicine, *West J Med* 175:79, 2001.

58. Jonas WB, Linde K, Walach H: How to practice evidence-based complementary and alternative medicine. In Jonas WB, Levin JS, editors: *Essentials of complementary and alternative medicine,* Philadelphia, 1999, Lippincott, Williams & Willkins.

59. Jong SC, Birmingham JM, Pai SH: Immunomodulatory substances of fungal origin, *J Immunol Immunopharmacol* 11:115, 1991.

60. Khan KS, Daya S, Jadad A: The importance of quality of primary studies in producing unbiased systematic reviews, *Arch Intern Med* 156:661, 1996.

61. Klem ML et al: A descriptive study of individuals successful at long-term maintenance of substantial weight loss, *Am J Clin Nutr* 66:239, 1997.

62. Kligler B, Gordon A, Stuart M, Sierpina V: Suggested curriculum guidelines on complementary and alternative medicine: recommendations of the Society of Teachers of Family Medicine Group on Alternative Medicine, *Fam Med* 32:30, 2000.

63. Kuhn TS: *The structure of scientific revolutions,* ed 3, Chicago, 1996, University of Chicago Press.

64. Labriola D, Livingston R: Possible interactions between dietary antioxidants and chemotherapy, *Oncology (Huntingt)* 13:1003, 1999.

65. Linde K, Jobst KA: Homeopathy for chronic asthma, *Cochrane Database Syst Rev* 2:CD000353, 2000.

66. Lomas J et al: Do practice guidelines guide practice? The effect of a consensus statement on the practice of physicians, *N Engl J Med* 321:1306, 1989.

67. MacAuley D: Critical appraisal of medical literature: an aid to rational decision making, *Fam Pract* 12:98, 1995.

68. Macintyre S, Chalmers I, Horton R, Smith R: Using evidence to inform health policy: case study, *BMJ* 322:222, 2001.

69. Maizes V, Koffler K, Fleishman S: The health history revisited: an integrative medicine approach, *Integr Med,* 2001.

70. Maizes V, Schneider C, Bell I, Weil A: Integrative medical education: development and implementation of a comprehensive curriculum at the University of Arizona, *Acad Med* 77:851, 2002.

71. Marone M et al: Quercetin abrogates taxol-mediated signaling by inhibiting multiple kinases, *Exp Cell Res* 270:1, 2001.

72. Mastenbroek I, McGovern L: The effectiveness of relaxation techniques in controlling chemotherapy induced nausea: a literature review, *Aust Occup Ther J* 38:137, 1991.

73. Napodano RJ: *Values in medical practice: a statement of philosophy for physicians and a model for teaching a healing science,* New York, 1986, Human Sciences Press.

74. National Center for Complementary and Alternative Medicine: Expanding horizons of healthcare: five-year strategic plan, 2001-2005, May 2002, http://nccam.nih.gov/about/plans/fiveyear/index.htm.

75. Norton C, Hosker G, Brazzelli M: Biofeedback and/or sphincter exercises for the treatment of faecal incontinence in adults, *Cochrane Database Syst Rev* 2:CD002111, 2000.

76. Omenn GS et al: Effects of a combination of beta carotene and vitamin A on lung cancer and cardiovascular disease, *N Engl J Med* 334:1150, 1996.

77. Paclitaxel. In *Mosby's drug consult,* ed 12, St Louis, 2002, Mosby.
78. Pelletier KR, Astin JA, Haskell WL: Current tends in the integration and reimbursement of complementary and alternative medicine by managed care organizations (MCOs) and insurance providers: 1998 update and cohort analysis, *Am J Health Promot* 14:125, 1999.
79. Popper KR: *The logic of scientific discovery,* revised edition, London, 1968, Hutchinson.
80. Prasad KC: Induction of differentiated phenotypes in melanoma cells by a combination of an adenosine 3′,5′-cyclic monophosphate stimulating agent and D-alpha tocopheryl succinate, *Cancer Lett* 44:17, 1989.
81. Prasad KN, Edwards-Prasad J: Effects of tocopherol (vitamin E) acid succinate on morphological alterations and growth inhibition in melanoma cells in culture, *Cancer Res* 42:550, 1982.
82. Prasad KN, Edwards-Prasad J, Ramanujam S, Sakamoto A: Vitamin E increases the growth inhibitory and differentiating effects of tumor therapeutic agents on neuroblastoma and glioma cells in culture, *Proc Soc Exp Biol Med* 164:158, 1980.
83. Prasad KN, Kumar A, Kochupillai V, Cole WC: High doses of multiple antioxidant vitamins: essential ingredients in improving the efficacy of standard cancer therapy, *J Am Coll Nutr* 18:13, 1999.
84. Rakel RE: Compassion and the art of family medicine: from Osler to Oprah, *J Am Board Fam Pract* 13:440, 2000.
85. Rama BN, Prasad KN: Effect of hyperthermia in combination with vitamin E and cyclic AMP on neuroblastoma cells in culture, *Life Sci* 34:2089, 1984.
86. Ramos-Remus C, Gutierrez-Urena S, Davis P: Epidemiology of complementary and alternative practices in rheumatology, *Rheum Dis Clin North Am* 25:789, 1999.
87. Ratain MJ: Comments on Labriola D, Livingston R: Possible interactions between dietary antioxidants and chemotherapy, *Oncology* 13:1012, 1999.
88. Risdon C, Edey L: Human doctoring: bringing authenticity to our care, *Acad Med* 74:896, 1999.
89. Rossman ML: *Healing yourself: a step-by-step program for better health through imagery,* ed 4, New York, 1987, Walker.
90. Saba GW: What do family physicians believe and value in their work? *J Am Board Fam Pract* 12:206, 1999.
91. Sackett DL et al: Evidence-based medicine: what it is and what it isn't, *BMJ* 312:71, 1996.
92. Sackett DL et al: *Evidence-based medicine: how to practice and teach EBM,* ed 2, New York, 2000, Churchill Livingstone.
93. Sahu SN, Prasad KN: Combined effect of adenosine 3′,5′-cyclic monophosphate stimulating agents, vitamin E succinate, and heat on the survival of murine B-16 melanoma cells in culture, *Cancer* 62:949, 1988.
94. Sandweiss DA: P value out of control, *Arch Intern Med* 160:1872, 2000.
95. Schneider EC, Eisenberg JM: Strategies and methods for aligning current and best medical practices: the role of information technologies, *West J Med* 168:311, 1998.
96. Sicher F, Targ E, Moore D 2nd, Smith HS: A randomized double-blind study of the effect of distant healing in a population with advanced AIDS: report of a small scale study, *West J Med* 169:356, 1998.
97. Sim I, Sanders GD, McDonald KM: Evidence-based practice for mere mortals: the role of informatics and health services research, *J Gen Intern Med* 17:302, 2002.
98. Simonton OC, Matthews-Simonton S, Creighton JL: *Getting well again,* New York, 1992, Bantam.
99. Smith R: Where is the wisdom...? *BMJ* 303:798, 1991.
100. Sporn MB, Roberts AB: Role of retinoids in differentiation and carcinogenesis, *Cancer Res* 43:3034, 1983.
101. Steinmetz KA, Potter JD: Vegetables, fruit, and cancer prevention: a review, *J Am Diet Assoc* 96:1027, 1996.
102. Steinmetz KA, Potter JD: Vegetables, fruit, and cancer. II. Mechanisms, *Cancer Causes Control* 2:427, 1991.
103. Stubbs J, Rangan A: Discussing alternative therapies with your patients, *Aust Fam Physician* 28:877, 1999.
104. Tasman A: The doctor-patient relationship in the new century, *Isr J Psychiatry Relat Sci* 37:159, 2000.
105. Taylor R et al: A systematic review of the effectiveness of critical appraisal skills training for clinicians, *Med Educ* 34:120, 2000.

106. α-Tocopherol, β-Carotene Cancer Prevention Study Group: The effect of vitamin E and beta carotene on the incidence of lung cancer and other cancers in male smokers, *N Engl J Med* 330:1029, 1994.
107. Tonelli MR, Callahan TC: Why alternative medicine cannot be evidence-based, *Acad Med* 76:1213, 2001.
108. Turley JM et al: Vitamin E succinate inhibits proliferation of BT-20 human breast cancer cells: increased binding of cyclin A negatively regulates E2F transactivation activity, *Cancer Res* 57:2668, 1997.
109. Vickers A: Recent advances: complementary medicine, *BMJ* 321:683, 2000.
110. Waldstein SR, Neumann SA, Drossman DA, Novack DH: Teaching psychosomatic (biopsychosocial) medicine in United States medical schools: survey findings, *Psychosom Med* 63:335, 2001.
111. Watson M, Marvell C: Anticipatory nausea and vomiting among cancer patients: a review, *Psychol Health* 6:97, 1992.
112. Weeks J: What makes a physician an expert in CAM? *Med Econ* 77:109, 2000.
113. Wetzel MS, Eisenberg DM, Kaptchuk TJ: Courses involving complementary and alternative medicine at U.S. medical schools, *JAMA* 280:784, 1998.
114. World Cancer Research Fund, American Institute for Cancer Research: *Food, nutrition, and the prevention of cancer: a global perspective*, Washington, DC, 1997, American Institute for Cancer Research.
115. World Health Organization: About WHO: definition of health, http://www.who.int/about/definition/en.
116. Yan L et al: [The effect of psycho-behavioral intervention on the emotional reaction and immune function in breast cancer patients undergoing radiotherapy], *Acta Psychol Sinica* 33:437, 2001.

SUGGESTED READINGS

See also especially references 5, 7, 26, 27, 40, 57, 62, and 70.

Maizes V, Caspi O: The principles and challenges of integrative medicine: more than a combination of conventional and alternative medicine, *West J Med* 171:148, 1999.

CHAPTER 16

Complementary and Alternative Medicine in the Twenty-First Century: Future Trends and Key Focuses

JOSEPH J. JACOBS, PHUONG THI KIM PHAM,
and JOHN W. SPENCER

This chapter examines four important groups that must be kept in "focus" and that are critical to the survival of complementary and alternative medicine (CAM): (1) those who use CAM, (2) those who sell these therapies, (3) those who regulate CAM, and (4) those who attempt to integrate CAM with conventional medicine. If CAM is to remain a viable subject and part of a larger health care plan through debate, it cannot lose its focus or its contributions to any of these groups. They all contribute to a continuing formation of policies and goals for the next decade and beyond. The use of and potential implementation of *evidence-based medicine* (EBM), both as a guide or vehicle and as part of all these groups, will help to shape and validate CAM's journey into the twenty-first century.

The Consumer and CAM

The emergence of CAM as a social phenomenon has been viewed as a paradigm shift in medicine in the United States. CAM is one of several indicators of a changing health care market. One of the changes is occurring in the physician-patient relationship. The traditionally held views of provider-patient relationships are changing from a willing, passive, dependent patient to an activist health consumer who demands and seeks out timely and accurate health information. The new patient, who is also a health care consumer, is prepared to seek, lobby for, and be critical of health information and medical care practice in general. These patients no longer accept with blind faith their physicians' pronouncements or recommendations. Consumers are the primary reason that managed care organizations now offer CAM coverage.

CONSUMERS' PERCEIVED NEEDS OR EXPECTATIONS FOR CAM DELIVERY

Most health care consumers state that they want quality and access to all venues of medicine, but they also are now asking for "objective measures of evidence-based care" so that they can make a more complete evaluation of *all* the needed health information. Health consumers, armed with unprecedented access to information from numerous venues—self-help books, the Internet, seminars, and word of mouth—are becoming more "empowered" to take control of their health care destinies.

The lack of information about CAM and physicians' attempts to explain CAM as a "placebo response" or therapy with minimal scientific merit become a barrier. From the consumer's perspective, CAM is plausible, especially since it is derived from seemingly age-old principles. Patients come away from the transactional relationship with their physician feeling relatively powerless over their health care future. Turning to a CAM practitioner is a predictable and overt expression of empowerment: the patient's ability to *choose* his or her own healing paradigm regardless of the physician's recommendations.

A survey evaluating CAM usage reported that most individuals use CAM because of a "congruence with their own values, beliefs and philosophical orientations toward health and life."[3] Variables relevant to predicting CAM usage taken from a sample of 1035 patients (mail survey with a 69% return rate) were higher education, poorer health status, a more holistic orientation toward health, and a transformational change in health that influenced personal views. Approximately 40% of the respondents reported they had used some form of CAM during the past year for health conditions that included chronic pain (37%), anxiety and other health problems (31%), sprains/muscle strains (26%), addictive problems (25%), and arthritis (25%). The most common therapies were chiropractic, lifestyle, diet, exercise/movement, and relaxation. Most of these individuals used CAM not because they felt dissatisfied with conventional medicine but rather because CAM was closer to their own beliefs about health. Only a small percentage (4.4%) relied solely on CAM for treatment.

Empowerment shifts the burden of health care decision making to the patient. The patient becomes responsible for gaining access to and participating in the health care system, which includes diagnosis and treatment planning. The Dietary Supplement Health and Education Act of 1994 states that "consumers should be empowered to make informed choices about preventive health care programs based on scientific studies relating to dietary supplements."

Access is one component of empowerment. An underlying principle of the free-market system is that all its participants have equal access to all information. The health care marketplace must meet the imperative to supply information that helps health consumers make informed, rational choices about their health care.

Recently, Holmes-Rovner et al.[16] suggested that evidence-based medicine (EBM) outcomes might be linked to a technology that can be easily accessed by consumers. Direct summaries of outcomes of relevant clinical information could be delivered through electronic means (e.g., Internet), focusing on advantages and disadvantages of particular CAM therapies, including safety, for health outcomes. This information might be incorporated into an "understandable" literature meta-analysis or systematic review. The critical component, however, is that some form of "patient template" be developed for treatment options that features *focused* questions, such as options for treatments based on various measured outcomes.

With the consumer then armed with varied clinical information, *sharing information* between health care provider/physician and patient might become easier. For example, Eisenberg[10] has suggested a step-by-step approach to shared decision making between provider and patient. After a conventional medical evaluation and discussion of conventional therapeutic options with or without consultation (depending on the patient's choice), the following points are addressed before a CAM consultation:

- Ensure that the patient recognizes and understands his or her symptoms.
- Maintain a record of all symptoms, including the patient's own opinions and assumptions.
- Review any potential for harmful interactions, with possible risks and benefits.
- Plan for follow-up to review CAM effectiveness of treatment.

This approach helps to keep communication channels open between patient and practitioner so that the patient receives the most effective and safest treatment for his or her condition(s).

From the conventional physician's perspective, it is important to be knowledgeable about the various types of CAM therapies to ensure a level of trust with the patient. Patients have a stronger sense of confidence when their providers give advice from a position of knowledge. Part of the information-gathering process for the clinician is to periodically survey patient attitudes and preferences for CAM therapies. The choices made by the patients may lead to the healing of their condition as they focus more on improving their quality of life and less on a cure.

A second component of empowerment and what consumers need is the formation of *self-help groups,* a consumer-driven operation. Self-help groups assist patients who want to work in a socially supportive environment. Patients need to talk about their fears and anxieties associated with their condition and their treatment options, including CAM, in a nonhostile, open, and accepting group setting. One such group, SHARE, offers support groups in English and Spanish, a hotline in several languages, and a broad spectrum of educational programs dealing with conventional and CAM treatments. SHARE's overall goals are to enlighten, empower, educate, be an advocate for, and support patients who have breast or ovarian cancer. SHARE does not offer medical advice and only attempts to promote harmonious relationships between medical caregivers and patients. More self-help groups that at least promote discussions about CAM need to continue to grow and especially to be patient advocates.

COMMONALITY BETWEEN RESEARCH AGENDA AND CONSUMER/RESEARCHER NEEDS

Patient advocation by specialized groups suggests a potential problem between EBM and its outreach to the consumer. Tallon, Chard, and Dieppe[35] recently demonstrated that the focus of published research (e.g., evaluation of osteoarthritis of knee joint) did not agree with research preferences of consumers. Most research focus was on pharmaceuticals and surgery, whereas consumers wanted more targeting of broad-based areas, such as CAM, education, and physical therapy. The research agenda may be skewed because of factors such as commercial funding, vested researcher interests, professional dominance of research (i.e., medical and surgical professions directing research funding), publication bias, and lack of consumer involvement in research. Clearly, it will be important in the future for more detailed and complete information to be developed and presented to consumers. The focus (with consumer participation) should be not only on developing current rationales for new federal funding opportunities, but also on encouraging professional and private organizations to be more responsive to public health needs and priorities. The White House report on CAM is a good example of involvement by the federal government to listen and respond to the public concerning both clinical and research issues of CAM.

Consumers will play a large role in keeping CAM's visibility in focus and in the forefront of health care. Because their health and lives are involved, consumers now, unlike in the past, will ask questions and challenge conventional medical practices.

◼ The Market and CAM

RETAIL PRODUCTS

The use of CAM by both providers and consumers has been directed at acute and chronic diseases, health promotion, and disease prevention. The two classes of retail products that have figured most prominently are nutritional supplements and herbal therapies. The *nutraceutical* industry promotes vitamins and herbs to enhance feelings of well-being and provide therapeutic benefit. In addition, many products enhance or facilitate ambulation or performance of tasks that enable a more normal daily life. For example, "hardware" products that are not nutritional may be purchased in health food stores or pharmacies. A new chain of stores called ALIVE offers products that go beyond nutritional supplements. Included are tapes for relaxation, devices for personal massage, various "natural" skin and beauty products, and services that assess posture and provide chiropractic-designed devices to enhance posture (e.g., devices that electronically scan the foot soles to provide customized shoe insoles).

New Paradigm Ventures, a market research company, conducted a survey of consumer spending on health-related retail products.[26] In 1994, U.S. consumers spent more than $100 billion on various products not ordinarily considered part of the medical mainstream, including CAM pills, nutraceutical products, and other wellness products (Tables 16-1 to 16-3). Table 16-4 lists the number of products marketed in 1994 to address specific medical conditions. Consumer spending and usage of these products clearly reflect a strong belief in health care products outside the conventional medical mainstream.

The health consumer is caught in the natural tension between a market promoting CAM and medical directors monitoring the attitudes of the conventional medical community. More integrated networks between alternative and conventional markets are expected to occur with or without clear research findings. As the market-driven health care economy evolves, a complementary care expenditure greater than $100 billion can be expected.

An entirely different "product"—a data bibliographic and archive system (see Chapter 1)—once completely developed, will have ramifications across the field of CAM. This system includes data sets from research studies, questionnaires, and protocols used in the data sets and software programmed to answer specific questions about CAM. Potential customers include health researchers, social scientists, educators,

TABLE 16–1. **EXPENDITURES ON CAM PILLS: UNITED STATES, 1994**

Alternative Pills	Amount Spent (Billions)
Vitamins	$3.745
Herbal remedies	$0.874
Homeopathy	$0.15
TOTAL	$4.8

From New Paradigm Ventures: *Complementary medicine research project*, South Norwalk, Conn, 1996.

TABLE 16–2. **EXPENDITURES ON NUTRACEUTICAL PRODUCTS: UNITED STATES, 1994**

Nutraceutical Products	Amount Spent (Billions)
Diet, lactose, fiber aids	$0.51
Vitamins, minerals, herbal products	$5.7
Sports, herbal, and fortified beverages	$20.9
Meals, snacks, meal replacements	$37.3
TOTAL	$64.4

From New Paradigm Ventures: *Complementary medicine research project*, South Norwalk, Conn, 1996.

TABLE 16–3. **EXPENDITURES ON WELLNESS PRODUCTS: UNITED STATES, 1994**

Wellness Products	Amount Spent (Billions)
Miscellaneous home products	$2.5
Supplements	$3.5
Health and beauty aids	$14.0
Specialty foods and diets	$22.0
Fitness products	$24.5
Smoking cessation products, water and air filtration systems	$0.5
TOTAL	$67.0

From New Paradigm Ventures: *Complementary medicine research project*, South Norwalk, Conn, 1996.

TABLE 16–4. **NUMBER OF MEDICAL PRODUCTS AVAILABLE IN UNITED STATES, 1994**

Medical Category	Number of Products
Arthritis	82
Asthma and allergies	16
Backache and headache	60
Cancer	11
Diabetes	42
Diet and exercise	18
Eye care	30
New mothers	31
Osteoporosis	31
Sports medicine	38
TOTAL	359

From New Paradigm Ventures: *Complementary medicine research project*, South Norwalk, Conn, 1996

students, and policymakers. The greatest number of potential customers may be the direct-response buyers, who will use CAM information products to explore and answer questions on specific CAM treatments and their potential efficacy. This type of either primary or secondary analysis extends and defines the original work. If offered on the Internet and then downloaded in multimedia formats such as CD-ROMs, the availability of this information can be maximized.

INTEGRATION WITH MANAGED CARE

The increase in consumer usage of CAM has led both medical insurers and hospitals to reexamine their own practices and policies. Pelletier,[28] in an ongoing survey begun in 1997–1998, recently recorded information on CAM insurance coverage with six new managed care organizations. When collated with earlier results, he was able to report that the majority of insurers offered coverage for acupuncture, biofeedback, chiropractic, counseling, nutrition, osteopathy, psychotherapy, preventive medicine, and physical therapy. The primary factors driving coverage included potential cost-effectiveness, consumer interest, and usefulness of the CAM therapy. Not surprisingly, the greatest hindrance appeared to be lack of scientific support.

Hospitals have started to integrate CAM therapies such as acupuncture, massage, and meditation. The major reported obstacle for insurance companies and hospitals to include CAM was the lack of information concerning its usefulness. Evaluation of cost-effectiveness and longer-term benefits of CAM is important for further study.

As research continues to reveal the prevalence of CAM, health care providers are repositioning themselves to succeed in this health-driven economy. They are actively learning more about the managed care industry and how to participate in it. Research shows that many people still rely on indigenous healing systems for spiritual, emotional, and physical health needs. Thus many managed care organizations are grappling with ways to integrate indigenous care financially as part of their benefits package because they want to retain this unique marketing opportunity to increase their market share. Before any strategy of integration occurs, however, changes must occur in conventional health care providers' perception of CAM therapies and providers, and vice versa.

Changes can be seen in hospitals that have begun to apply conventional technologies in a "holistic" manner. For example, the Griffin Hospital in Derby, Connecticut, a 160-bed, Yale-affiliated hospital, has instituted a patient-oriented approach to the delivery of hospital care based on the Plane Tree philosophy. It has implemented community-oriented programs to address health care issues and concerns, including the use of CAM therapies. As Griffin Health Services Corporation, which includes a health maintenance organization (HMO), and other managed care organizations reposition themselves in this new health care environment, how might CAM fit into their strategic plans? A unique opportunity exists for the development of a system of care, rather than CAM and conventional medicine merely competing in a crowded market. A vertically integrated provider/payer system may easily integrate CAM practitioners into a complementary system of care.

To be competitive in a market-driven health care economy, managed care providers are focusing on the following objectives: (1) to increase market share, (2) to decrease costs, and (3) to maintain quality.

Increase Market Share

To increase market share, managed care organizations must offer a broad range of health care products and services that add clinical value to attract potential subscribers. Therapies such as acupuncture, massage therapy, and chiropractic manipulation may be considered to have "clinical value adaptivity" to conventional care. *Clinical value* may be seen in a situation in which acupuncture is an integral part of a low back pain management program and provides a less expensive, more cost-effective treatment for pain management in some patients. Clinical value may also been seen in the development of wellness centers to meet the needs of clients wanting to use different strategies to prevent the onset of diabetes, heart disease, and cancer. This strategy helps to develop a chain of wellness centers that would feature a major role for CAM. This approach may result in enhanced patient referrals and simultaneously provide a source of revenue for managed care organizations.

Interest from health insurance providers, including American Western Life Insurance Company, Oxford Health Plans, Pacific Health & Life, and to some extent Mutual of Omaha, has focused primarily on financial reimbursement through the development of policy riders to cover usage of CAM. A significant gap remains in determining how CAM clinical practices may be included under an umbrella of a more comprehensive, integrated health care system. Managed care organizations should play a major role in providing information on safe and effective medications and treatments. The large number of original prescription drugs now sold over the counter, not to mention the increase in usage of CAM, has shifted the burden of health care decision making to the consumers of these products. Managed care organizations must declare themselves to be patient advocates to attract potential clients to their programs.

Decrease Costs

Managed care organizations must provide a comparative analysis of different treatment approaches to specific conditions. Cost-effective treatment options will result in attracting new clients. How, then, is cost reduction achieved? Part of the answer lies in offering affordable products that are attractive to potential policyholders. Cost-benefit programs must compare CAM with conventional medical interventions (e.g., surgery), not only to provide patients with an overview of treatment options along with cost, but also to identify the most cost-effective treatment option.

For example, for several years a program developed by Dr. Dean Ornish[27] to reverse the progression of cardiac disease was evaluated by the Mutual of Omaha insurance company. The evaluation was relatively risk free because physicians have been advising their cardiac patients to decrease their fat intake, exercise more, decrease stress in their lives, and obtain mutual support to help them through the process. The clinical methodology used was not outside medical mainstream opinion. Mutual of Omaha was able to accomplish its rather straightforward objectives with minimal controversy. The evaluation of other CAM therapies, such as determining the benefits of prayer or magnetic therapy, presents more challenging obstacles.

Although more than 40% of the patients in Eisenberg's latest survey (see Chapter 1) were using some form of CAM, close to 60% were not. People who pay premiums for health care want assurance that their premium dollars are being expended in a cost-effective way. Most people do not want to abandon conventional care, which supports the importance of a team approach. Collaboration between conventional medicine and CAM must occur in a clinical setting and through the process of clinical evaluation for efficacy. Recently Wolsko[44] reported that patients who saw a CAM provider also likely were to have previously visited a conventional provider (a significant number of times) in the last year, were female, and used the CAM therapy for "treating diabetes, cancer or back problems." Importantly, the "extent of insurage coverage for CAM providers and use for wellness" were both strong correlates of usage by patients.

Maintain Quality

Consumers want a managed care organization to maintain quality, especially if CAM medical practices are offered. Managed care organizations need to provide a high-quality network of CAM providers. Conventional practitioners must have confidence in the CAM providers for referral purposes. To help facilitate this approach, when patients visit a CAM provider, they should attempt to elicit answers to the following questions:
- Is the CAM provider's belief in the therapy's effectiveness based on other patients' experiences with the same treatment, and are these patients available to speak with?
- What does the therapy consist of?
- How frequently is the therapy given?
- How are decisions reached (and by whom) regarding whether the treatment is beneficial?

- Are there side effects to the therapy? If so, what are those side effects?
- How much time is required to implement the therapy?
- Is insurance reimbursement available?
- Will the CAM practitioner provide findings, plans, and follow-up information to the patient?

With quality control in place, managed care organizations can shift their energy to the development of compensated services provided by CAM providers. Much of this development is rooted in basic business decisions in the marketplace. It represents changes in attitudes not only by conventional providers but also by employers and worker groups. States now provide mandates for change within individual markets, which led to the state of Washington's recent mandate for CAM reimbursement. The tax court of Canada recently allowed for a woman to claim "vitamin supplements, rehabilitative therapies including massage and therapeutic touch" as "legitimate medical expenses" on her "taxable expenses."[7]

Managed care organizations must "catch up" on their knowledge of CAM. To what extent this may hasten CAM integration with conventional medicine more universally can only be conjecture at present. It is likely that CAM will remain as part of the health care industry and that integration with conventional medicine will need to be more completely addressed in the twenty-first century.

▐ Federal Regulation of CAM: Food and Drug Administration

The move by CAM into the next decade must be followed closely by an active role of regulation at the federal level. The importance of safety remains *the* principal component of any evidence-based analysis.

The regulation of CAM at the state level ensures a close and more complete focus within the area of individual, professional, and training disciplines, including reimbursement.

Internationally, with the number of requests increasing each year regarding standards, technical guidance, and informational support on CAM, the World Health Organization (WHO) has published *Legal Status of Traditional Medicine and Complementary/Alternative Medicine: A Worldwide Review.* This resource includes information on the regulation and registration of CAM as well as policies adopted by different countries. National recognition and regulation of CAM vary considerably among different countries, and policies seem to change constantly. As part of its Traditional Medicine Program, WHO has extensively evaluated common herbal medicines since 1995, publishing results in its monographs. Through technical review panels, information on quality, safety, and clinical usefulness of various herbs is disseminated.

SCOPE AND HISTORY

The major charge of the U.S. Food and Drug Administration (FDA) is provided through the Food, Drug and Cosmetic Act (FDCA) of 1938. This oversight role involves regulation of the labeling of medicines and devices, including those relevant to CAM, such as acupuncture needles, equipment, and homeopathic medicines.

The FDA uses an evidenced-based scientific mandate to oversee most food products (other than meat and poultry), human and animal drugs, therapeutic agents of biologic origin, medical devices, radiation-emitting products (consumer, medical, occupational), cosmetics, and animal feed. The FDA has grown from a single chemist in the U.S. Department of Agriculture in 1862 to approximately 9100 employees, ranging from chemists, pharmacologists, pharmacists, physicians, and microbiologists to veterinarians and lawyers. In 2001 the FDA's budget was more than $1.2 billion. The FDA reviews applications for new human drugs and biologics, complex medical devices, food and color additives, infant formulas, and animal drugs. It also regulates the manufacture, import, transport, storage, and sales of about $1 trillion of products annually.

ROLE IN CLINICAL EVALUATION

Approval of many of pharmaceuticals, both current and proposed, including potential devices relevant to CAM, rests on the procedures and processes described below. When a new molecule of drug shows positive pharmacologic activity and minimal acute toxicity potential in animals, the sponsor, usually the manufacturer or potential marketer, will want to test its diagnostic or therapeutic potential in humans. The sponsor submits an Investigational New Drug (IND) application to the FDA. The three types of IND are as follows:

1. *Investigator IND* allows the physician who initiates and conducts an investigation, under whose immediate direction the investigational drug is administered or dispensed, to submit a research IND. Examples might include the study of a new unapproved drug or an approved product for a new indication or for use in a new patient population.
2. *Emergency use IND* allows the FDA to authorize the use of an experimental drug in an emergency situation that does not allow time for submission of an investigator IND. The emergency IND is also used for patients who do not meet the criteria of an existing study protocol or if an approved study protocol does not exist.
3. *Treatment IND* allows experimental drugs showing promise in clinical testing to be used for serious or immediately life-threatening conditions while the final clinical work is conducted and the FDA review takes place.

The IND application must contain information in three areas: animal pharmacology and toxicology studies, manufacturing information, and clinical protocols and investigator information. After the IND is submitted, the sponsor must wait 30 calendar days before initiating any clinical trials so that the FDA has an opportunity to review the IND for safety. This step ensures that research will not be subjected to unreasonable risk. The three phases of clinical trials for human testing of a new drug have been reviewed previously (see chapter 2).

The FDA can impose a clinical hold if a study is unsafe or if the protocol is deficient in design in meeting its stated objectives. This is an important consideration for CAM as it develops its own protocols.

REGULATION OF CAM PROCEDURES

Acupuncture

In 1996 the FDA reclassified acupuncture needles for general use from *class III*, a category in which clinical studies are required to establish safety and effectiveness, to *class II*, a category only requiring good manufacturing and proper labeling. However, manufacturers are required to label the needles for "single use only," and use is restricted to qualified practitioners, as determined by state laws. The manufacturer must also provide information about the device's material, biocompatibility, and sterility.

According to the National Institutes of Health (NIH) Consensus Development Conference in 1997, acupuncture shows promising results for postoperative and postchemotherapy nausea and vomiting in adults and for postoperative dental pain. For other conditions, such as addiction, stroke rehabilitation, headache, menstrual cramps, tennis elbow, fibromyalgia, myofascial pain, osteoarthritis, low back pain, carpal tunnel syndrome, and asthma, acupuncture may be effective as an adjunct treatment. It is anticipated that current and future studies funded by the National Center for Complementary and Alternative Medicine (NCCAM) will clarify both safety and efficacy concerns.

Although generally considered safe, acupuncture may cause fainting, local internal bleeding, convulsions, hepatitis B, dermatitis, nerve damage, and insertion site infection from contaminated needles when performed improperly (Table 16-5). WHO publishes several guidelines on acupuncture, including research, training, safety, and nomenclature.*

Botanical and Dietary Supplementation

In 1973 the FDA issued regulations for special dietary foods, including vitamins and minerals. The public and industry response to these regulations led The U.S. Congress to prohibit the FDA from controlling the potency of dietary supplements in 1976. Congress passed the Nutrition Labeling and Education Act (NLEA) in 1990, which included a section on the regulation of labeling as to nutrient and health claims that could be made by manufacturers of dietary supplements. Subsequently the Dietary Supplement Health and Education Act (DSHEA) was passed in 1994, classifying vitamins, amino acids, and mineral, herbal, or botanical products as "foods" and thus exempting them from regulation as drugs or food additives. Manufacturers of these "dietary supplements" do not need to prove efficacy or safety, and these substances are not regulated by the FDA. DSHEA permitted supplements to carry substantiated statements about their role in health, provided the manufacturer issued a disclaimer that the FDA had not evaluated the statements and that the product was not intended to diagnose, treat, cure, or prevent any disease. In addition, the FDA must be notified when "structure and function" claims are made, generally within 30 days after the product is marketed.

---

*At http://www.who.int/medicines/library/trm/acupuncture/acupdocs.html.

TABLE 16–5. **SAFETY OF SELECT CAM PROCEDURES: REVIEWS, 1999–2002**

Review	Study Design	Results	Comments
ACUPUNCTURE			
Yamashita et al.[38]	Case study review of 85 therapists; 65,482 treatments	<1% adverse effects	Selective sample Underreporting
Lytle et al.[21]	Evaluation of 3 electroacupuncture devices	Frequencies > 30 pulses/sec = unbalanced direct current	Importance of device regulation Potential danger to patients
Ernst, White[13]	Review of adverse effects from separate studies	Needle pain most common; bleeding second; fainting, syncope rare; 85% report relaxation	Wide variation of results Serious events rare
Brolinson et al.[5]	Survey of 515 nurses' perception of safety; 91% female	15% report herbal and macrobiodiet unsafe; 50% report acupuncture definitely safe but not among recommended therapies	Focused sampling Need other professions sampled
White et al.[37]	Survey of 78 acupuncture practitioners; 31,822 treatments	43 significant events reported; 2135 minimal, mainly bleeding and pain; 70% improvement in 1 week	Follow-up data important Underreporting possible
MacPherson[22]	Postal audit of 574 practitioners; 34,407 treatments; 4-week study period	No serious adverse effects, 43 minor (nausea, fainting); 12% report feeling relaxed; mild transient reactions in 15%; bruising, pain, bleeding <2%	Importance of follow-up and linking/communicating with provider All studies need better descriptors of training and experience of providers as covariable
BOTANICALS			
Heck et al.[15]	Evaluation of herb interactions with warfarin	Documents reports of warfarin interaction with coenzyme Q10, danshen, devil's claw, dong quai, ginseng, green tea, papain, vitamin E	Importance of systematic reporting Use of MedWatch Greater need to obtain more data
Little et al.[19]	Cochrane review of 5 studies on use of herbs for osteoarthritis	Avocado/soybean unsaponifiables found to have no serious side effects Prescription authorization	More data required
McIntyre[23]	Review of articles on safety of St. John's wort	Side effects with tyramine foods: hypertension, mental status change, tremors, headaches, restlessness Ingredients unclear 1963–1999 29 adverse drug reports filed	Training and licensing variables important Potential negative interaction between St. John's wort and conventional medicines in cancer treatment[360]

Stickel et al.[33]	Evaluation of herbal toxicity literature	Mushrooms (Jin Bulhuran, Ma-Huang, sho-saiko-to), germander, chaparral, and alkaloid-containing plants have potential for hepatotoxicity	Confusing picture; need for more accurate incidence reporting Dose-response evaluations not included
Aggarwal, Ades[2]	Interactions of herbs with cardiovascular medications	Garlic: myocardial infarction Ginseng: hypertension (blood pressure medications) Ginkgo: PAF inhibitor Ephedra: myocardial infarction, hypertension, coronary vasospasms St. John's wort: digoxin plasma concentration reduced	Unclear about number of adverse events in total population studied Systematic reporting still needed
Boniel, Dannon[4]	Use of herbs in psychiatric practice; review of 23 randomized, controlled trials	Hypericum: possible mania; some efficacy Valerian: toxicity, headaches, chest tightness, mydriasis, abdominal pain, tremors of hands and feet Ginseng: vaginal bleeding, mental status change Ginkgo: bleeding time, spontaneous bleeding; cautious use with aspirin	Importance of systematic reporting Better communication about drug usage
Liu et al.[20]	Genus Phyllanthus for chronic hepatitis; review of 22 randomized controlled trials; 1947 patients; methodology quality high in 5 double-blind studies; low in 17 others	No serious adverse event recorded	Improvement in studies Evaluation for longer-term effects
CHIROPRACTIC			
Proctor et al.[30]	Spinal manipulation for dysmenorrhea; review of 5 randomized, controlled trials; outcome measures of pain intensity (visual analog scales)	Minimal benefit; no adverse effects	Descriptive data No strong conclusions
Ernst[12]	Safety of spinal manipulation 238 patients 95 patients 625 patients, 1856 treatments 1058 patients, 4712 treatments	No adverse event lasted more than 3 days Neck pain (1) Discomfort (34%), very noticeable discomfort (10%), reduced ability to work (14%) Discomfort, at least one episode (44%) "Unpleasant feelings" (14%); no severe injuries	Longer-term follow-up needed Underreporting

Continued

TABLE 16–5. **SAFETY OF SELECT CAM PROCEDURES: REVIEWS, 1999–2002—cont'd**

Review	Study Design	Results	Comments
HOMEOPATHY			
Adler[1]	*Lobaria pulmonaria, Luffa operculata,* and potassium dichromate for 2-week treatment of acute sinusitis; open-label practice base, 119 patients	No adverse drug effect reported	Longer duration of treatment requires study
Dantas, Rampes[9]	Evaluation of published safety data through systematic review of homeopathic medicine	Mean incidence of adverse effects greater in treatment than placebo group in controlled trials (9.4:6.1); most minor effects and many anecdotal reports of effects not well documented; some current symptoms aggravated	Conclusions difficult to draw; poor study quality
Stam et al.[32]	Low back pain treated by Spiroflor SRL gel vs CCC; 19 practices; 161 patients; 1-week treatment; pain scored on 100-mm visual analog scale	Adverse effects: 11% in SRL group; 26% in CCC group Withdrawal: 0 in SRL group; 8 in CCC group Adverse drug reactions: 4% in SRL group; 24% in CCC group	Longer duration of treatment requires study, with multiple follow-ups

PAF, Platelet-activating factor; *SRL, Symphytum officinale, Rhus toxicodendron,* and *Ledum palustre; CCC,* Cremor Capsici Compositus.

DSHEA requires the manufacturer to ensure that its dietary supplements are safe before being marketed but does not require the usual tests to prove their safety and efficacy as drugs. Accordingly, the FDA has the burden of proving that a dietary supplement is misbranded or adulterated before the agency can restrict the product's use or remove it from the market. Therefore dietary supplements such as herbs are under no requirements for quality control standards, batch-to-batch consistency, or identification of the constituent products.

Although DSHEA grants the FDA authority to establish standards of good manufacturing processes for supplements, these regulations are still in preparation. Furthermore, the standards of quality for individual ingredients are lacking. For example, contamination of herbal preparations may occur with heavy metals during the manufacturing process or with microorganisms during storage.[16] Neither consumers nor researchers can be assured that the label actually reflects the product content. Repeated studies yield different results, and it is almost impossible to make a general recommendation about herbal medicines. Also, the lack of formal education or mandated licensing of herbalists or individuals selling herbal products may lead to incorrect information or partial misinformation given to consumers, as is the case when evaluating health information on the Internet.

More rigorous research is needed to establish suitable procedures for analyzing and determining the concentration of *all* active components in herbs and to ensure that *all* ingredients are present at recommended amounts with adequate dosage descriptions. Because of the lack of patentability of herbs and thus lack of market exclusivity, companies are not willing to make the same costly investment required for new synthetic drugs to prove efficacy.

The *United States Pharmacopeia*[36] (USP) sets standards for drugs as well as botanical and nonbotanical dietary supplements. A product that carries the USP symbol must fulfill the USP standards for identity, strength, quality, purity, packaging, and labeling. A product that has been used extensively with no documented adverse safety risks may carry the *National Formulary* (NF) symbol, even if it does not have FDA approval or a USP-accepted use. The American Herbal Products Association supports voluntary standardization and a guarantee of potency. Some companies use these standards as a stamp of approval to market their product quality.[14]

Homeopathy

Homeopathy is part of the *Homeopathic Pharmacopeia of the United States* and was included in the 1938 FDCA. In 1951, with the passage of the Durham-Humphrey Amendment, all homeopathic drugs became prescription drugs. Because homeopathic drugs had not been reviewed or approved by the FDA from 1938 to 1962, they did not conform to the Drug Efficacy Study Implementation standards. In 1972 the FDA once again excluded reviewing homeopathic drugs, citing the Over-the-Counter Review Act. Although the FDA established new guidelines for homeopathy in 1988, political pressure from the American Institute of Homeopathy led to the Compliance Policy Guide (CPG). CPG allows some homeopathic products to bear the prescription drug legend, whereas others were allowed to be marketed as over-the-counter (OTC) products. In 1994, 42 scientists, physicians, and consumer advocates requested that the FDA hold homeopathic drugs to the same safety and efficacy standards as other drugs; as of 2002, this had not occurred.

REPORTING OF ADVERSE EFFECTS: SAFETY ISSUES

About 2600 adverse events and 100 deaths have been associated with dietary supplements alone between 1993 and 1998.[29] Still, no central mechanism for mandatory reporting exists, possibly leading to underreporting. Therefore the amount of information required to remove a product from the market is severely limited. The FDA is forced to be reactive rather than proactive in the regulation of potentially toxic dietary supplements. Although it is required that adverse events be reported for approved drugs, no requirement is imposed on foods, including dietary supplements. A MedWatch program has been established to give health care professionals and consumers the opportunity to report serious problems that they suspect are associated with the drugs and medical devices that they prescribe, dispense, or use, including botanicals.

In the mid-1990s, investigators reviewed both direct and indirect adverse effects of certain CAM therapies.[11,17] The reviewed therapies included (1) cervical manipulation, for which the most common complications were vascular accidents; (2) acupuncture, with associated risks of infection (e.g., hepatitis C, osteomyelitis, endocarditis) through nonsterilized needles in skin or blood vessels, tissue trauma, pneumothorax, and hemothorax; (3) herbal medicine, with reactions ranging from dermatitis to anaphylactic shock, renal fibrosis, and renal failure; and (4) homeopathy, in which adverse reactions were rare, perhaps less than 3%, although toxic concentrations of arsenic and cadmium could be found in certain preparations. Systematic evaluation of reported adverse effects of CAM found that even when research methodology was strong (e.g., randomized, controlled trials with blinding procedures), herbal treatments were most often cited.[17]

Use of the botanical dietary supplement *chaparral*, which has antioxidant properties, reportedly carries important associated risks.[31] Varying degrees of hepatotoxicity were noted in 13 of 18 patients examined. Symptoms included jaundice and an increase in serum liver chemistry values. Symptoms resolved 1 to 17 weeks after discontinuation of chaparral.

Because many herbal products contain heavy metal contaminants, long-term adverse effects must be more thoroughly described. When given with orthodox medications, herbal preparations' effect on minimizing or preventing treatment effects needs further study and clarification. It is reassuring that the Office of Dietary Supplements at NIH has called for guidelines on publishing articles that evaluate botanical dietary supplements. A critical need exists to provide "accurate and complete descriptions of the botanical test material regardless of whether it is a finished product, commercial ingredient, extract or single chemical constituent."[34]

Table 16-5 reviews selected studies that recently evaluated safety issues and CAM (see also previous chapters and the Cochrane Library reviews of CAM, Appendix C). Safety information about CAM is admittedly sparse and at times allegedly controversial because of "misuse of references, misleading statements, errors in citation, and selective use of research reporting."[25] Most of the severe adverse events in CAM procedures are rare, but because of underreporting or no reporting and poor research methodology, an incomplete picture of CAM safety currently exists. Table 16-5 shows that herbal preparations remain the most problematic in terms of safety. As of 2002, NCCAM has put on hold studies evaluating the herb kava because of reports from Germany and Switzerland, as well as from the U.S. health care community, of liver failure as a result of toxicity, including hepatitis and cirrhosis. Much more information is needed. For example, a recent article[14] reviewed all systematic reviews and meta-analyses completed on efficacy/effectiveness and safety of CAM procedures between 1966 and 2000 using either Medline or the Cochrane Library. Slightly more than 25% of all studies reported safety information. Only 3% to 5% of the systematic reviews evaluated safety as a primary focus.

With the risk of malpractice liability, it is crucial that physicians are aware of the scientific evidence for CAM modalities before referring patients. Physicians need to learn about safety of CAM and the CAM modalities used by their patients so that possible adverse reactions as well as undesirable interactions with conventional treatments are avoided.

Integration of CAM with Conventional Medicine

The integration of CAM with conventional medical practices should not be considered a new endeavor. The Lifestyle Heart program developed by Ornish[27] used meditation, muscle relaxation, and yoga in addition to diet and exercise. Integrative medicine encourages the patient to "jump-start" the healing process, a process that occurs from within and is directed at defining or reintegrating thoughts and feelings with health.

The close working relationship and potential integration of CAM with conventional medicine raise important issues of medical boundaries, especially in the area of *consultation*. Each practitioner must be aware of and comfortable with the other's philosophy, approach, and respective role. Communication cannot be overemphasized. A recent study evaluated the nature and quality of communication between general practitioners in medicine and chiropractors.[6] Through survey analysis, referral to chiropractors was based primarily on whether the general practitioner had a good knowledge of chiropractic procedures and if the previous experience had been useful in terms of clear information that was free of jargon and confusing terminology. Further, although complete agreement may not exist in all cases that integrated outcomes will always be clinically favorable, well-done studies with replicable information about product and therapy safety issues will facilitate and make the process of collaboration and integration more complete.

EBM *possibly* can provide an important venue for CAM and its subsequent integration with conventional medicine. EBM forms a basis for decision making and patient care that extends to a scientifically quantifiable and replicable research base. However, EBM is also at odds with many general premises of CAM, including the importance of the individual patient. Acceptance of both the strengths and the weaknesses of the two approaches must occur with collaborative sharing.

EBM should not be seen as a threat to physicians' clinical experience and intuition. When CAM has an evidence base, as in the evolving areas of psychologic therapies (biofeedback, cognitive-behavioral, relaxation, hypnosis) and musculoskeletal approaches (massage, chiropractic) or acupuncture all for the treatment of pain, the provider should feel confident to begin discussions on integrating these palliative approaches with conventional medicine. The situation becomes more problematic, however, when a conventional therapy (radiation, chemotherapy) has not been tried or completed and a decision is made to add an alternative therapy, either to replace or to complement the cancer therapy, and subsequent side effects and efficacy are not known. The clinician's ability to educate, review safety options, use guidance from previous experience, and practice information gathering and sharing with other colleagues becomes critical. At this point EBM may not have much to offer because of the paucity of CAM research. Also, each patient brings to the clinical setting a much varied but valued individual response to illness and stress that must be factored into any treatment equation.

No set or easy answer exists to establishing a complete "cookbook" approach to integrating or using CAM with or without EBM with every patient. Experience is still the most important factor.

EXAMPLES OF CAM INTEGRATION

Chapter 14 provides one example of the integration of CAM, as conceptualized by the University of Arizona group, within the clinical hospital setting, including a teaching and training focus. Other areas in which CAM will be "tested" through "integration" might include the workplace, nursing homes, and as mentioned throughout other chapters in this text, health promotion programs. The key is learning *collaboration* skills. In the past, conventional medicine and CAM occupied separate and distinct roles, but Vickers[42] notes in his review article that now 40% of general practices in the United Kingdom offer some form of access to CAM. Popular areas include relaxation classes for promoting well-being and massage for reducing anxiety and inducing sleep. Acupuncture is provided in rheumatology clinics. Similar examples can be found at many of the funded NIH CAM centers in the United States.

In a systematic study of clinical integration, Byass[8] evaluated implementation of CAM over 2 years in a medical health palliative unit, using a clinical audit of the integration of daily massage as the measurement tool. More than 90% of the patients thought that the massage could be considered a complementary therapy to conventional medicine. Daily massage had some effect to a definite effect in decreasing anxiety, depression, and pain and promoting relaxation. Most importantly, patients said massage should be part of a standard of care.

BARRIERS TO CAM IMPLEMENTATION

With the potential integration of CAM into conventional medicine, several steps need to be taken to reassure a doubting and distrustful medical community. Strong and replicable research on CAM's usefulness and safety needs to be made available. Admittedly, however, when reviewed and evaluated, this research base has not always been incorporated into practice. NIH has held technology conferences on acupuncture for treatment of nausea and on behavioral-relaxation approaches for pain, but even favorable efficacy findings have not always led to their incorporation into standard clinical practice.

NCCAM has recently provided grant money, to evaluate the potential for integration of CAM with conventional medicine. Obstacles that need to be overcome include provider competition, fear of change and concern with debating/negotiating health decisions with patients, liability issues, lack of practice and license standards, and understanding the necessary motivation needed for change of provider bias. Again, the way the message of integration is framed seems to be important, especially as it impacts utilization issues, medical importance, and patient satisfaction. In Germany, for example, Kruse et al.[18] report that in a children's hospital, homeopathy was successfully integrated with conventional medicine. Almost 70% of the surveyed physicians agreed with and recognized a role for homeopathy, even though little research suggested its usefulness.

We argue that research on integration needs to be done not only to help form a complete picture of health care issues, but also to expand and enhance legal issues and medical boundaries (see Chapter 14). The willingness of policymakers to include CAM in an open and flexible medical system is described in the next section.

N Importance of a National CAM Policy

At the national policy level, evaluation of the entire CAM process and its potential integration across many sectors of health care have been the subjects of a White House Commission established in March 2000. The findings were subsequently released in March 2002.[37a] Four major topics were initially explored: (1) coordinated research to better understand CAM practices and products, (2) ways to produce and distribute information about CAM to the public, (3) access and delivery of CAM, and (4) education and training of CAM practitioners. The commission heard testimony from a broad range of individuals, including the general public. The more than 80 initial recommendations indicated the need for a much stronger role and more oversight by the federal government, the states, and private organizations. Recommendations and actions include the following:

1. NCCAM should take a leadership role in disseminating information about current clinical efficacy of CAM therapies, including safety.
2. Using the 10 leading health indicators, a strategy should be developed to integrate, where appropriate, CAM procedures in terms of usage and practice. This usage should have some practical significance by incorporating data collected from national surveys, such as the National Health Survey (e.g., *Healthy People 2010* [see suggested readings]).
3. More research should be devoted to understanding complex issues of CAM, such as determining the role of multicompound mixtures, effects of multiple treat-

ments, and patient-provider interactions, and incorporating a strategy for evaluating ways to customize therapies for individual patients.

4. Linkages should be formed between EBM and training of practitioners, possibly through the formation of expert panels composed of CAM and conventional providers and educators and through focused courses in CAM curricula taught in medical schools.

5. The Agency for Health Care Research and NCCAM should work collaboratively toward disseminating evidence-based information, such as practice guidelines review criteria and systematic reviews (meta-analyses), to the public and to researchers.

6. Information about CAM in any form, including that on the Internet, should be evaluated for its accuracy. Consumers should be educated in ways to evaluate health care information, including safety, risks, and cost-benefit ratios, especially in the area of dietary supplements and herbal medicine. The FDA should be a major collaborator in this endeavor.

7. Any practitioner who provides CAM services as well as marketing should be regulated in a way that ensures accountability to the public.

Other groups have also reported on similar summary reports. *The House of Lords Report*[24] reviewed both oral and written evidence that suggested that in the United Kingdom, CAM is becoming increasingly popular and is thought to be useful. As might be expected, the report argues for stricter regulation, especially of herbal medicine; more valid, complete ways for training and accreditation; strong, replicable research; and accountability of acupuncture, herbal medicine, and nonmedical homeopathy according to statutory regulations.

SUMMARY

Conventional medicine is undergoing change and reexamination of its scope and practice due in part to the issues discussed in this chapter. The extent to which CAM may be part of this change and focus in the future will depend on CAM's ability to achieve a professional, valid, deserving status while maintaining its own identity. This is especially true with consumer and clinical practice issues. The attempts described should lead to a strong and continued focus on CAM integration into health care for the next decade. However, it should also be recognized that policies become useless if there is not a sincere attempt to track progress and hold individual and corporate institutions accountable. An ongoing and continuous review by the entire medical community, making changes as necessary in both policies and procedures, will produce the best outcome for the consumer—good health.

REFERENCES

1. Adler M: Efficacy and safety of a fixed-combination homeopathic therapy for sinusitis, *Adv Ther* 16(2):103, 1999.
2. Aggarwal A, Ades PA: Interactions of herbal remedies with prescription cardiovascular medication, *Coron Artery Dis* 12(7):581, 2001.
3. Astin JA: Why patients use alternative medicine: results of a national study, *JAMA* 279(19):1548, 1998.

4. Boniel T, Dannon P: The safety of herbal medicines in the psychiatric practice, *Harefuah* 140(8):780, 2001.

5. Brolinson PG et al: Nurses' perceptions of complementary and alternative medical therapies, *J Community Health* 26(3):175, 2001.

6. Brussee WJ, Assendelft WJ, Breen AC: Communication between general practitioners and chiropractors, *J Manipulative Physiol Ther* 24(1):12, 2001.

7. Bugg G: Woman wins claim for tax deductibility of complementary/alternative medical expenses, *Can HIV/AIDS Policy Law Rev* 6(1/2):14, 2001.

8. Byass R: Auditing complementary therapies in palliative care: the experience of the day-care massage service at Mount Edgcumbe Hospice, *Complement Ther Nurs Midwifery* 5(20):51, 1999.

9. Dantas F, Rampes H: Do homeopathic medicines provoke adverse effects? A systematic review, *Br Homeopath J* 89(suppl 1):35, 2000.

10. Eisenberg DM: Advising patients who seek alternative medical therapies, *Ann Intern Med* 127:61, 1997.

11. Ernst E: Direct risks associated with complementary therapies. In Ernst E, editor: *Complementary medicine: an objective appraisal,* Oxford, 1996, Butterworth-Heinemann.

12. Ernst E: Prospective investigations into the safety of spinal manipulation, *J Pain Symptom Manage* 21(3):238, 2001.

13. Ernst E, White AR: Prospective studies of the safety of acupuncture: a systematic review, *Am J Med* 110(6):481, 2001.

14. Fisher J: The (un)regulation of dietary supplements, *SD J Med* 52(2):53, 1999.

15. Heck AM, DeWitt BA, Lukes AL: Potential interactions between alternative therapies and warfarin, *Am J Health Syst Pharm* 57(13):1221, 2000.

16. Holmes-Rovner M et al: Patient choice modules for summaries of clinical effectiveness: a proposal, *BMJ* 322:664, 2001.

17. Jonas W: Safety in complementary medicine. In Ernst E, editor: *Complementary medicine: an objective appraisal,* Oxford, 1996, Butterworth-Heinemann.

18. Kruse R et al: Can homeopathy be integrated in a university hospital? *Forsch Komplementarmed Klass Naturheilkd* 8(4):213, 2001.

19. Little CV, Parsons T, Logan S: Herbal therapy for treating osteoarthritis, *Cochrane Library* 1, 2002 (online: Update software).

20. Liu J, Lin H, McIntosh H: Genus *Phyllanthus* for chronic hepatitis B virus infection: a systematic review, *J Viral Hepat* 8(5):358, 2001.

21. Lytle CD et al: Electrostimulators for acupuncture: safety issues, *J Altern Complement Med* 6(1):37, 2000.

22. MacPherson H: The York acupuncture safety study: prospective survey of 34,000 treatments by traditional acupuncturists, *BMJ* 323:486, 2001.

23. McIntyre M: A review of the benefits, adverse events, drug interactions and safety of St. John's wort *(Hypericum perforatum)*: the implications with regard to the regulation of herbal medicines, *J Altern Complement Med* 6(2):115, 2000.

24. Mills S: The House of Lords report on complementary medicine: a summary, *Comp Ther Med* 9(1):34, 2001.

25. Morley J, Rosner AL, Redwood D: A case study of misrepresentation of the scientific literature: recent reviews of chiropractic, *J Altern Complement Med* 7(1):65, 2001.

26. New Paradigm Ventures: *Complementary medicine research project,* South Norwalk, Conn, 1996 (internal publication).

27. Ornish D et al: Can lifestyle changes reverse coronary artery disease? *Lancet* 336:129, 1990.

28. Pelletier KR, Astin JA: Integration and reimbursement of complementary and alternative medicine by managed care and insurance providers: 2000 update and cohort analysis, *Altern Ther Health Med* 8(1):38, 2002.

29. Penson RT et al: Complementary, alternative, integrative or unconventional medicine? *Oncologist* 6:463, 2001.

30. Proctor ML et al: Spinal manipulation for primary and secondary dysmenorrhoea, *Cochrane Library* 1, 2002 (online: *Update Software*).

31. Sheikh N, Philen RM, Lover LA: Chaparral associated hepatotoxicity, *Arch Intern Med* 157:913, 1997.

32. Stam C, Bonnet MS, van Haselen RA: The efficacy and safety of a homeopathic gel in the treatment of acute low back pain: a multi-centre, randomised double-blind comparative clinical trial, *Br Homeopath J* 90(1):21, 2001.

33. Stickel F, Egerer G, Seitz HK: Hepatotoxicity of botanicals, *Public Health Nutr* 3(2):113, 2000.

34. Swanson CA: Suggested guidelines for articles about botanical dietary supplements, *Am J Clin Nutr* 75(1):8, 2002.

35. Tallon D, Chard J, Dieppe P: Relation between agendas of the research community and the research consumer, *Lancet* 355:2037, 2000.

36. *United States Pharmacopeia*, http://www.usp.org/

36a. Weiger WA et al: Advising patients who seek complementary and alternative medical therapies for cancer, *Ann Intern Med* 137(11): 889, 2002.

37. White A et al: Adverse events following acupuncture: prospective survey of 32,000 consultations with doctors and physiotherapists, *BMJ* 323:485, 2001.

37a. *White House Commission on Complementary and Alternative Medicine Policy*, http://whccamp.hhs.gov.

38. Yamashita H et al: Adverse events in acupuncture and moxibustion treatment: a six-year survey at a national clinic in Japan, *J Altern Complement Med* 5(3):229, 1999.

SUGGESTED READINGS

Clark C: *Integrating complementary health procedures into practice*, New York, 2000, Springer.

US Congress House Committee on Government Reform and Oversight: *Patient access to alternative treatments beyond the FDA*, Hearings before Committee on Government Reform and Oversight, House of Representatives, 150th Congress, second session, Washington, DC, 1998, US Government Printing Office.

US Department of Health and Human Services: *Healthy People 2010*, vol 1 and 2, Washington, DC, 2000, US Government Printing Office.

CHAPTER 17

Final Summary: Goals for Complementary and Alternative Medicine

JOHN W. SPENCER and JOSEPH J. JACOBS

The preceding chapters have reviewed the available evidence on the more common and well-known complementary and alternative medicine (CAM) therapies and their proposed degree of treatment efficacy. Historically, many CAM procedures have been used in health care for centuries; however, almost half the books written about CAM have been published in the last 8 years. Many journals devoted exclusively to CAM were started during the last decade.

Definitional quality of CAM, including its description and classification, remains a continuing goal. CAM therapies and systems, including acupuncture, herbal, homeopathy, manual, and psychologic, are still widely used at the beginning of the twenty-first century. Reviewed demographic studies show an increase in CAM usage in the United States, indicating that consumers are either unaware of the intense debate over CAM treatment efficacy or simply do not care about the controversy. Interestingly, a 2001 methodologic evaluation reported that clinical trials, taken from systematic reviews of homeopathy, herbal therapy, and acupuncture, revealed various weaknesses in design, making efficacy interpretations difficult.[2] The range of positions taken by clinicians, researchers, and consumers regarding CAM efficacy comprises the following:

- A sufficient number of studies show that most, if not all, CAM therapies have no efficacy.
- Studies show that CAM therapies have some efficacy (certain therapies, certain conditions).
- Studies show that CAM therapies have broad efficacy (certain therapies, certain conditions).
- It is impossible to determine which CAM therapies are useful, partly because the research has not allowed for any definitive statements due to poor design

attributable to small samples, lack of hypothesis testing, and likelihood of subject, experimenter, or journal review bias.

With the advent of increased federal funding and focus, the evaluation may become more clear. Importantly, national research priorities should help to define the order of focus, especially in chronic and many acute medical conditions that have less complex and interacting biologic mechanisms.

Legal and ethical issues shaping the debate over CAM must focus on the importance of allopathic therapists' understanding and judgment regarding patient referral, including issues of malpractice and court testimony. Also, the increased usage of CAM requires a better understanding of integration models with allopathic medicine, as well as potential implementation of CAM therapies and a more integral role in medical education.

The reasons that CAM remains popular must be more fully understood as related to consumer beliefs and attitudes and social networking. One proposed explanation is the high cost and potential side effects of conventional medications. In addition, however, a more health-focused consumer demand exists for other, varied treatments that improve quality of life and offer prevention. This is especially true for diseases such as cancer and acquired immunodeficiency syndrome (AIDS), for which no treatment may exist to stop or slow down the disease course, but palliative issues, notably pain and nausea, remain important and researchable.

Much of the debate between conventional science and medicine and CAM has focused on improved provider-patient communication so that each can understand the other's intentions and motivations better in future interactions. Healing encompasses many parameters, including the process of patients confronting their anxiety about their illness. In addition to education, it is important for health care providers to facilitate the process by being *empathetic* and demonstrating caring and understanding. Empathy can be taught, learned, and developed. For example, in a clinical skills class, counseling students, especially women, were able to increase a self-rated composite empathy score after completing a 1-year training sequence.[3] Interestingly, self-reflection on their personal distress decreased by the end of the course. Empathy is only one of many variables, however, and future health providers should also have full knowledge about CAM, including safety and research data.

◼ Research Evaluation Goals

Based on our evaluation of the field of CAM at the beginning of the twenty-first century, in this chapter we present *emerging CAM therapies* that are accumulating favorable efficacy data but as a seminal goal need a more focused, complete, and continuing analysis (Table 17-1). Also, whereas most Western research focuses on comparable randomized groups, their relevance to much larger population distributions must be part of the evidence base, along with individual protocols and case-control studies. Health maintenance and disease prevention endeavors that include diet, nutrition, exercise, and vitamins, as well as more "borderline" conventional therapies that include chiropractic, osteopathy, and behavioral therapies, are prime areas of analysis, especially in cardiovascular treatment and pain control.

Procedures such as biofeedback and cognitive-behavioral therapy (CBT), although less "unconventional" and more "conventional," are nonpharmacologic approaches and are included here. Because of safety concerns, kava *(Kava kava)* becomes problematic for the treatment of anxiety; more research data, especially pre-clinical studies, are needed. With all studies, both *replication* and *longer-term follow-up* are important and relevant. Other important factors to study and report are *costs* associated with CAM therapies, *adverse effects* (events), and more complete "intention to treat" analysis accurately describing *population distribution*. All clinical trials need to be registered to provide future investigators with a basis for their own hypotheses and clinical trial design.

IMPROVEMENT

Research methodology continues to improve as researchers learn about the many intricacies in CAM studies. Researchers must be accurate in producing meta-analyses and should consider the use of guidelines.[4] Although systematic reviews help provide a beginning evidence base for research and health care, they can be incomplete. Many reviews simply conclude that studies have demonstrated either "no effect" or "insufficient evidence"; however, when others (besides the author of the review) evaluate the results there can be disagreements concerning conclusions reached.[1] That is, interrater reliability can be low. Is it possible that interpretations of data can become too subjective? This disparity must be examined, better understood, and improved on. While randomization is one important aspect of clinical research, full coverage should also include blocking for components in subjects' decision to undergo treatment, and in outcome analysis, comparisons should be made between more than one CAM treatment versus placebo.

EVIDENCE-BASED MEDICINE

The strength of the methodology of CAM studies will ultimately lead to providing physicians with the information necessary to make more knowledgeable referrals to CAM providers and to warn patients against unsafe procedures. Pro and con debate will continue, but evidence-based medicine (EBM) will be the accepted format used by a large percentage of researchers and health providers in the future. As such, EBM should continue to be improved and made more user friendly, as with the use of portable databases that are constantly updated.

SCOPE AND PRIORITY

The National Center for Complementary and Alternative Medicine (NCCAM) at the National Institutes of Health (NIH) should be at the forefront of prioritizing targeted areas. Centers with ongoing research must help shape the agenda, but individual grants are also needed to evaluate CAM areas that show promise. Select

TABLE 17–1. **EMERGING CAM THERAPIES REQUIRING FURTHER ANALYSIS**

Condition	CAM Therapy	Study Findings	Safety	Documentation Comment
Allergy (e.g., rhinitis)	Homeopathy Galphimia glauca Other?	9 studies; more than 1500 patients; varying effects, 0%-78% improvement	Small numbers of AEs documented	CISCO database, 1971–1998 Pub Med systematic reviews Wiesenauer, 1983, '85, '90, '95; Reilly, 1985, See Chapter 3.
Anxiety	Herbal therapy (kava, valerian)	Individual studies, systematic reviews, meta-analyses; significant improvement in anxiety scores; more than 200 patients, including complementing with benzodiazepines and then subsequently tapering off	Currently, AEs a significant concern; need more preclinical dose-response analyses	Phytother Res, Sept 200 Psychopharmacology, Sept 2001; J Clin Psychopharmacol, Feb 2000 (systematic review/meta-analysis) See Chapter 8.
Closed-head injury	Flexyx Neurotherapy System	Significant improvement in cognitive social functioning Few data directly relating brain electrical dysfunction and behavior with retraining	No AEs recorded	J Head Trauma Rehab 2001 See Chapters 7 and 8.
Depression	Herbal therapy Hypericum (St. John's wort)	More than 80% articles use RCTs with placebo and report significant effects; in mild to moderate depression	Some AEs reported; closer monitoring needed	Duke University multicenter study, 2001 did not find significant effects with placebo comparison See Chapter 7.
Fibromyalgia	Acupuncture Biofeedback Hypnosis Magnet therapy Manipulation	Well done studies with controls; adequate samples in certain studies	Few AEs reported	See Chapter 10.

Headache pain	Biofeedback Cognitive-behavioral Manipulation Hypnotherapy	Some RCTs with adequate samples but more needed	Manipulation: some AEs, but small samples	NIH Technology Assessment Conference 1995 See Chapter 10.
Low back pain (musculoskeletal)	Acupuncture Biofeedback Massage Spinal manipulation	Biofeedback and massage: numerous well-done RCTs Manipulation: meta-analysis, individual studies (150); more than 1550 patients; 55%–60% of studies report significant positive effect; 45% no effect; positive effect range: 17%–100%	Biofeedback and massage: few AEs Manipulation: sparse AE reports (vertebrobasilar, cauda equina syndrome); underreporting bias a problem	Biofeedback and massage NIH Technology Assessment Conference 1995 Manipulation: CISCO database, 1981–1998 See Chapter 10.
Nausea and vomiting (pregnancy, breast cancer treatment)	Acupuncture	Meta-analysis; reviews of 2503 patients found greater than 80% with 30%–50% improvement Recent review[5] similarly found acupuncture reasonably recommended for palliation and cancer Mind-body techniques appeared only CAM therapy recommended without reservation for stress reduction and cancer	One study reported no AEs	CISCO database, 1995–1998 Database developed by Rosenthal Center Cochrane reviews have reported fewer positive outcomes

AEs, Adverse events; RCTs, randomized, controlled trials; NIH, National Institutes of Health.

populations, especially women, children, and elderly persons, are important in research. Strategies that more completely describe CAM and ethnicity also need to be implemented.

Education

MEDICAL STUDENTS

Medical students have much to learn in their 4 years of education. CAM therapies, both theoretic and evidence-based components and including safety information, should be standardized as a course across all medical schools. A performance base should then be developed, using a section of the final clinical examination for evaluation. Questions about CAM should be on all state board licensing examinations. Also, a survey should be taken to determine the uniformity in teaching communication and clinical skills regarding CAM in medical curricula.

CONSUMERS

Because consumers are the users of CAM, the best available information about their needs, biases, and knowledge of CAM needs to be formatted for sharing among health providers to establish meaningful dialogue and communication. Providing CAM information through better indexing in the public library system needs further exploration, as well as ensuring the most accurate information on the Internet.

Clinical Integration: Holistic Approaches

Clinical integration will occur as more information is shared about CAM therapies and their applicability for use with conventional medicine, as either stand-alone or adjunctive therapies. Creative ways to share CAM procedures and integrate them in acute, chronic, and especially palliative conditions are needed. Although holistic approaches may not be feasible for all health conditions, further studies are needed to develop models such as naturopathy or Vedic medicine. Patient satisfaction measures should be included in these studies, as well as more quantifiable outcome measures.

Finally, we believe that conventional medicine will ultimately accept the integration of certain CAM therapies, based on research findings and marketplace demand through continued consumer pressure. In the last few years, there has been much more clinical and research cooperation between NIH and NCCAM, including more focused oversight and collaboration with the U.S. Food and Drug Administration (FDA). This spirit of cooperation and trust between conventional medicine and CAM, although slowly evolving, will benefit the consumer as well as effect positive changes in clinical practice and test research assumptions, with the ultimate outcome goal of a better-educated and healthier society.

REFERENCES

1. Ezzo J et al: Reviewing the reviews. How strong is the evidence? How clear are the conclusions? *Int J Technol Assess Health Care* 17(4):457, 2001.
2. Linde K et al: The methodological quality of randomized controlled trials of homeopathy, herbal medicines and acupuncture, *Int J Epidemiol* 30:526, 2001.
3. Maciak A, Spencer J: Changes in empathy in Christian counseling students during clinical skills training. Presented at National Conference of the Christian Association for Psychological Studies, Richmond, Va, 2001.
4. Moher D et al: Improving the quality of reports of meta-analyses of randomised controlled trials: the QUOROM statement—quality of reporting of meta-analyses, *Lancet* 354:1896, 1999.
5. Weiger WA et al: Advising patients who seek complementary and alternative medical therapies for cancer, *Ann Intern Med* 137(11): 889, 2002.

Definitions of Complementary and Alternative Therapies Described in the Text

⊠ Acupuncture

Thin needles are inserted superficially on the skin at locations throughout the body. These points are located along "channels" of energy. Heat can be applied by burning *(moxibustion)*, electric current *(electroacupuncture)*, or pressure *(acupressure)*. Healing is proposed by the restoration of a balance of energy flow called "Qi." Another explanation suggests that stimulation may activate endorphin receptors.

⊠ Alexander Technique

Bodywork technique in which rebalancing of "postural sets" (i.e., physical alignment) is taught by mentally focusing on the way correct alignments should look and feel and through verbal and tactile guidance by the practitioner.

⊠ Antineoplastons

Naturally occurring peptides, amino acid derivatives, and carboxylic acids are proposed to control neoplastic cell growth using the patient's own "biochemical defense system," which works jointly with the immune system (see Chapter 4).

⊠ Applied Kinesiology

Form of treatment that uses nutrition, physical manipulation, vitamins, diets, and exercise for the purpose of restoring and energizing the body. Weak muscles are proposed to be a source of dysfunctional health.

⊠ Aromatherapy

Form of herbal medicine that uses various oils from plants. Route of administration can be through absorption in the skin or inhalation. The action of antiviral and antibacterial agents is proposed to aid in healing. The aromatic biochemical structures of certain herbs are thought to act in areas of the brain related to past experiences and emotions (e.g., limbic system).

⊠ Ayurveda

Major health system that emphasizes a preventive approach to health by focusing on an inner state of harmony and spiritual realization for self-healing. Includes special types of diets, herbs, and mineral parts and changes based on a system of constitutional categories in lifestyle. The use of enemas and purgation is for the purpose of cleansing the body of excess toxins.

⊠ Biofeedback

Mind-body therapy procedure in which sensors are placed on the body to measure muscle, heart rate, and sweat responses or neural activity. Information is provided by visual, auditory, or body-muscle cell activation to increase or decrease physiologic activity, which when reconstituted, is proposed to improve health problems (e.g., pain, anxiety, high blood pressure). In some cases, relaxation exercises complement this procedure.

⊠ Brachytherapy

Ionizing radiation therapy with the source applied to the surface of the body or located a short distance from the treated area.

⊠ Bristol Cancer Help Center (BCHC) Diet

Stringent diet of raw and partly cooked vegetables with proteins from soy; claimed to enhance the quality of life and attitude toward illness in cancer patients.

⊠ Cell Therapy

Healthy cellular material from fetuses, embryos, or organs of animals is directly injected into human patients to stimulate healing in dysfunctional organs. May also include blood transfusions or bone marrow transplantations.

▨ Chelation Therapy

Involves the removal—through intravenous infusion of a chelating agent (synthetic amino acid ethylenediaminetetraacetic acid [EDTA])—of metal, toxins, lead, mercury, nickel, copper, cadmium, and plaque to treat certain diseases (e.g., cardiovascular). Ancillary treatments include the use of vitamins, changes in diet, and exercise.

▨ Cognitive Therapy

Psychologic therapy in which the major focus is on altering and changing irrational beliefs through a type of "socratic" dialogue and self-evaluation of certain illogical thoughts. Conditioning and learning are important components of this therapy.

▨ Craniosacral Therapy

Form of gentle manual manipulation used for diagnosis and for making corrections in a system made up of cerebrospinal fluid, cranial and dural membranes, cranial bones, and sacrum. This system is proposed to be dynamic with its own physiologic frequency. Through touch and pressure, tension is proposed to be reduced and cranial rhythms normalized, leading to improvement in health and disease.

▨ Dance Therapy

Movement-based therapy that aids in promoting feeling and awareness. The goal is to integrate body, mind, and self-esteem. It uses different parts of the body such as fingers, wrists, and arms to respond to music.

▨ Diathermy

Use of high-frequency electrical currents as a form of physical therapy and in surgical procedures. The term, derived from the Greek words *dia* and *therma,* literally means "heating through." The three forms of diathermy employed by physical therapists are short-wave, ultrasound, and microwave.

▨ Dimethylaminoethanol (DMAE)

Pharmacologic therapy that uses a natural substance found in certain foods and the human brain. DMAE is a precursor to the transmitter acetylcholine. It is proposed to have a stimulant effect on the central nervous system if used as a supplement.

N Electrochemical Treatment (ECT)

Method using direct current to treat cancer. It involves inserting platinum electrodes into tumors and applying a constant voltage of less than 10 V to produce a 40-mA to 80-mA current between the anodes and cathodes for 30 minutes to several hours.

N Electroencephalographic Normalization

Frequencies of electroencephalogram (EEG) are changed through self-induced or external stimulation entrainment to a more uniform pattern of response. Potentially, certain health conditions such as depression and anxiety are improved.

N Environmental Medicine

Practice of medicine in which the major focus in on cause-and-effect relationships in health. Evaluations are made of such factors as eating and living habits and types of air breathed. Testing in the patient's own environment is performed to determine what precipitators are present that may be related to disease or other health problems. A treatment protocol is developed from this information.

N Eye Movement Desensitization and Reprocessing (EMDR)

Technique that proposes to remove painful memories by behavioral techniques. Rhythmic, multisaccadic eye movements are produced by allowing the patient to track and follow a moving object while imaging a stressful memory or event. By using deconditioning, including verbal interaction with the therapist, the painful memory is extinguished and health improved.

N Feldenkrais Method

Bodywork technique in which its founder used the integration of physics, judo, and yoga. The practitioner directs sequences of movement using verbal or hands-on techniques or teaches a system of self-directed exercise to treat physical impairments through the learning of new movement patterns.

N Flexyx Neurotherapy System

A type of neural conditioning technique in which brain-specific EEG frequencies are reset through sequenced low-intensity external stimulation (i.e., light).

◪ Hallucinogen Therapy (for substance abuse)

The controversial use of lysergic acid diethylamide (LSD) to reduce anticraving and promote tolerance of and decrease dependence on certain illicit drugs such as cocaine.

◪ Hatha Yoga

Branch of yoga practice that involves physical exercise, breathing practices, and movement. These exercises are designed to have a salutary effect on posture, flexibility, and strength for the ultimate purpose of preparing the body to remain still for long periods of meditation.

◪ Hellerwork

Bodywork technique that treats and improves proper body alignment through the development of a more complete awareness of the physical body. The goal is to realign fascia for improvement in standing, sitting, and breathing using " body energy," verbal feedback, and changing emotions and attitudes.

◪ Herbal Medicine

The use of herbs to treat various health conditions. Herbal medicine is a major form of treatment for more than 70% of the world's population.

◪ Homeopathy

Form of treatment in which substances (minerals, plant extracts, chemicals, or disease-producing germs), which in sufficient doses would produce a set of illness symptoms in healthy individuals, are given in microdoses to produce a "cure" of those same symptoms. The symptom is not thought to be part of the illness but part of a curative process.

◪ Hydergine

Phytotherapeutic method that combines extracts from the ergot fungus. Originally proposed to be used as an antihypertensive agent.

Hydrazine Sulfate

Pharmacologic treatment proposed to treat certain cancers (see Chapter 4).

Hyperbaric Oxygen

Therapy in which 100% oxygen is given at or above atmospheric pressure. An increase in oxygen in the tissue is proposed to increase blood circulation and improve healing and health and influence the course of disease.

Hyperthermia

Use of various heating methods (e.g., electromagnetic therapy) to produce temperature elevations of a few degrees in cells and tissues, leading to a proposed antitumor effect. This is often used in conjunction with radiotherapy or chemotherapy for cancer treatment.

Immunoaugmentative Therapy

Cancer treatment that proposes cancer cells can be arrested by the use of four different blood proteins; this approach is also proposed to restore the immune system. Can be used as an adjunctive therapy.

Jin Shin Jyutsu

Bodywork technique that uses specific "healing points" at the body surface, which are proposed to overlie energy flowing (Qi). The therapist's fingers are used to "redirect, balance, and provide a more efficient energy flow" to and throughout the body.

Laetrile

Pharmacologic treatment using apricot pits that has been proposed to treat certain cancers (see Chapter 4).

Light Therapy

Natural light or light of specified wavelengths is used to treat disease. This may include ultraviolet light, colored light, or low-intensity laser light. The eye generally is the initial entry point for the light because of its direct connection to the brain.

N Magnetic Therapy

Magnets are placed directly on the skin, stimulating living cells and increasing blood flow by ionic currents that are created from polarities on the magnets. Both acute and chronic health conditions are suggested to be treatable by this procedure.

N Manual Manipulation

Group of therapies with different assumptions and, in part, different areas of treatment. The major focus includes both stimulation and body manipulation, which are proposed to improve health or arrest disease, or both. Includes soft tissue manipulation through stroking, kneading, friction, and vibration. Types include massage, adjustment of the spinal column *(chiropractic),* and tissue and musculoskeletal *(osteopathic)* manipulation.

N Mediterranean Diet

Diet that is thought to provide optimal distribution of daily caloric intake of different nutrients and includes 50% to 60% carbohydrates, 30% fats, and 10% proteins. The diet is derived from the eating habits of people in the Mediterranean area, who were shown to have reduced rates of cardiovascular disease.

N Mind-Body Therapies

Group of therapies that emphasize using the mind or brain in conjunction with the body to assist the healing process. Mind-body therapies can involve varying degrees of levels of consciousness: (a) *hypnosis,* in which selective attention is used to induce a specific altered state (trance) for memory retrieval, relaxation, or suggestion; (b) *visual imagery,* in which the focus is on a target visual stimulus; (c) *yoga,* which involves integration of posture and controlled breathing, relaxation, and meditation; (d) *relaxation,* which includes lighter levels of altered states of consciousness through indirect or direct focus; and (e) *meditation,* in which there is an intentional use of posture, concentration, contemplation, and visualization.

N Muscle Energy Technique

Manual therapy with components of both passive mobilization and muscle reeducation. Diagnosis of somatic dysfunction is performed by the practitioner, after which the patient is guided to provide corrective muscle contraction. This is followed by further testing and correction.

▟ Music Therapy

Use of music in an active or a passive mode. Proposed to help allow for the expression of feelings, which helps to reduce stress. Other types of "vibratory" sounds can be used, mainly to reduce stress, anxiety, and pain.

▟ Native American Therapies

Therapies used by many Native American Indian tribes, including their own healing herbs and ceremonies that use a focused spiritual emphasis.

▟ Naturopathy

Major health system that includes practices emphasizing diet, nutrition, homeopathy, acupuncture, herbal medicine, manipulation, and various mind-body therapies. Focal points include self-healing and treatment through changes in lifestyle and emphasis on health prevention.

▟ Neuroelectric Therapy

Transcranial or cranial neuroelectrical stimulation (*transcutaneous electrical nerve stimulation*, TENS), once called "electrosleep"; originally used in the 1950s for the treatment of insomnia. In a typical TENS session, surface electrodes are placed in the mastoid region (behind the ear) and, similar to electroacupuncture, stimulated using a low-amperage, low-frequency alternating current. It has been suggested that TENS stimulates endogenous neurotransmitters such as endorphins that produce symptomatic relief.

▟ Newcastle Disease Virus (NDV)

NDV is a paramyxovirus that causes Newcastle disease in a variety of birds but only minor illness in humans. There are two strains of NDV, lytic and nonlytic. *Lytic* NDV is used for its ability to kill cancer cells directly, but both strains have been used to make vaccines to stimulate the immune system to fight cancer.

N   Ornish Diet

Life choice program based on eating a vegetarian diet containing less than 10% fat. The diet is high in complex carbohydrates and fiber. Animal products and oils are avoided.

N   Orthomolecular therapy

Therapeutic approach that uses naturally occurring substances within the body, such as proteins, fat, and water, which promote restoration or balance (or both) by using vitamins, minerals, or other forms of nutrition to subsequently treat disease or promote healing, or both.

N   Oslo Diet

Eating plan that emphasizes increased intake of fish and reduced total fat intake. Diet is combined with regular endurance exercise.

N   Pilates

Educational and exercise approach using the proper body mechanics, movements, truncal and pelvic stabilization, coordinated breathing, and muscle contractions to promote strengthening. Attention is paid to the entire musculoskeletal system.

N   Piracetam

Pharmacologic treatment proposed to be useful in the treatment of dementia. Uses a cyclic relative of the transmitter gamma-aminobutyric acid (GABA).

N   Prayer

Offering of prayers to some higher being or authority for the purpose of healing and arresting disease. May be practiced by the individual patient, by groups, or by others with or without the patient's knowledge (*intercessory prayer*).

◼ Pritikin Diet

Weight management plan that is based on a vegetarian framework. Meals are low in fat, high in fiber, and high in complex carbohydrates.

◼ Qi Gong

Form of Chinese exercise-stimulation therapy that proposes to improve health by redirecting mental focus, breathing, coordination, and relaxation. The goal is to "rebalance" the body's own healing capacities by activating proposed electrical or energetic currents that flow along meridians located throughout the body. These meridians, however, do not follow conventional nerve or muscle pathways. In Chinese medical training and practice, this therapy includes "external Qi," which is energy transmitted from one person to another for the purpose of healing.

◼ Raja Yoga

Yoga practice that includes all the other forms of yoga practice. The practitioner is instructed to follow moral directives, physical exercises, breathing exercises, meditation, devotion, and service to others to facilitate religious awakening.

◼ Reconstructive Therapy

Nonsurgical therapy for arthritis that involves the injection of nutritional substances into the supporting tissues around an injured joint. The intent is to cause the dilation of blood vessels, which will allow fibroblasts to form around the injury and begin the healing process.

◼ Reflexology

Bodywork technique that uses reflex points on the hands and feet. Pressure is applied at points that correspond to various body parts with the intention of eliminating blockages thought to produce pain or disease. The goal is to bring the body into balance.

◼ Reiki

From the Japanese word meaning "universal life force energy." The practitioner serves as a conduit for healing energy directed into the body or energy field of the recipient without physical contact with the body.

▲ Restricted Environmental Stimulation Therapy (REST)

Procedure that uses a completely sensory-deprived environment for the purpose of increasing physical or mental healing through a nonreactive state.

▲ Rolfing

Bodywork technique that involves the myofascia. The body is realigned by using the hands to apply a deep pressure and friction that allow more sufficient posture, movement, and the "release" of emotions from the body.

▲ Shark Cartilage

Cancer therapy that proposes shark cartilage can interrupt blood supply to a tumor(s) and subsequently "starve" it of any nutrients by using the antiangiogenic properties and other substances contained in the cartilage (see Chapter 4).

▲ Shiatsu

A Japanese form of acupressure in which a bodywork technique involving finger pressure at specific points on the body is used mainly for the purpose of balancing "energy" in the body. The major focus is on prevention by keeping the body healthy. The therapy uses more than 600 points on the skin that are proposed to be connected to pathways through which energy flows.

▲ T'ai chi

A technique that uses slow, purposeful motor-physical movements of the body for the purpose of control and achieving a more balanced physiologic and psychologic state.

▲ Therapeutic Riding

Form of animal-assisted therapy in which either passive or active movements are produced to aid in approximating the human gait. In certain cases, physiotherapeutic exercises are performed.

Therapeutic Touch (TT)

Body energy field technique in which hands are passed over the body without actually touching to recreate and change proposed "energy imbalances" for restoring innate healing forces. Verbal interaction between patient and therapist helps to maximize effects.

Traditional Chinese Medicine (TCM)

Ancient form of medicine that focuses on prevention and secondarily treats disease, with an emphasis on maintaining balance through the body by stimulating a constant, smooth-flowing Qi energy. Herbs, acupuncture, massage, diet, and exercise are also used.

Trager Psychophysical Integration

Bodywork technique in which the practitioner enters a meditative state and guides the client through gentle, light, rhythmic, nonintrusive movements. "Mentastics" exercises using self-healing movements are taught to the clients.

Transcranial Electrostimulation

Pulsed electrical stimulation of 50 mA or less is applied between two electrodes attached to the ear. The stimulation is proposed to activate endogenous opioid activity, which may assist in the treatment of certain health problems, such as substance abuse and physical pain.

Twelve-Step Program

Program such as Alcoholics Anonymous that is based on a series of 12 steps, or tasks, which participants are asked to complete. As members progress through the 12 steps, they are expected to gain courage to attempt personal change and develop a greater acceptance of themselves. Programs emphasize the group process through the sharing of stories and experiences and through social interactions with other group members. Most 12-step programs incorporate a spiritual component and ask members to turn their lives over to a higher power.

APPENDIX B

Selected Resources for Complementary and Alternative Medicine

American Academy of Medical Acupuncture
4929 Wilshire Blvd.
Suite 428
Los Angeles, CA 90010
(323) 937-5514
www.medicalacupuncture.org/

American Association of Naturopathic Physicians
8201 Greensboro Dr., Suite 300
McLean, VA 22102
(877) 969-2267
(703) 610-9037
(703) 610-9005 fax
mbianchi@naturopathic.org
www.naturopathic.org/

American Association of Oriental Medicine
433 Front St.
Catasauqua, PA 18032
(888) 500-7999
(610) 266-1433
(610) 264-2768 fax
aaom1@aol.com
www.aaom.org

American Association of Professional Hypnotherapists
4149-A El Camino Way
Palo Alto, CA 94306
(650) 323-3224
www.aaph.org

American Botanical Council
PO Box 144345
Austin, TX 78714-4345
(512) 926-4900
(512) 926-2345 fax
www.herbalgram.org

American Chiropractic Association
1701 Clarendon Blvd.
Arlington, VA 22209
(800) 986-4636
(703) 243-2593 fax
www.amerchiro.org/

American Dietetic Association
216 W. Jackson Blvd.
Chicago, IL 60606-6995
(312) 899-0040
www.eatright.org

American Holistic Nurses Association
PO Box 2130
Flagstaff, AZ 86003-2130
(800) 278-2462
www.ahna.org

American Massage Therapy Association
820 Davis St., Suite 100
Evanston, IL 60201-4444
(847) 864-0123
(847) 864-1178 fax
www.amtamassage.org

American Osteopathic Association
142 East Ontario St.
Chicago, IL 60611
(800) 621-1773
www.aoa-net.org

American Society of Alternative Therapists
PO Box 703
Rockport, MA 01966
(978) 281-4400
asat@asat.org
www.asat.org

Biofeedback Certification Institute of America
10200 W. 44th Ave., #310
Wheat Ridge CO 80033
(303) 420-2902
(303) 422-8894 fax
bcia@resourcenter.com
www.bcia.org

Research Council for Complementary Medicine (RCCM)
Suite 5, 1 Harley St.
London W1G 9QD
Info@rccm.org.uk
www.rccm.org.uk

◾ Other Resources

Alternative Health Benefit Services
www.alternativeinsurance.com

Alternative Medicine Alert
www.ahcpub.com/ahc_root_html/products/newsletters/ama.html

Health Information, National Institutes of Health
Numerous data relevant to consumer information about health, various institute research-clinical consensus statements, as well as health alerts.
www.nih.gov/health/

Integrative Medicine Service at Sloan-Kettering Cancer Center, New York
www.mskcc.org/mskcc/html/44.cfm

National Center for Complementary and Alternative Medicine Clearinghouse
PO Box 7923
Gaithersburg, MD 20898
Info@nccam.nih.gov

National Center for Homeopathy in the United States
801 N. Fairfax St.
Suite 306
Alexandria, VA 22314
(703) 548-7790
(703) 548-7792 fax
www.homeopathic.org/

NIH Consensus Program Information Center
PO Box 2577
Kensington, MD 20891
Includes consensus statement on acupuncture, November 1997.

Oncolink-Complementary Medicine
www.oncolink.upenn.edu/specialty/complementary/

Quackwatch
www.quackwatch.com

Therapeutic Touch
www.phact.org/e/tt/

Townsend Letter for Doctors and Patients
tldp.com
Provides reviews of health journal articles and books.

UK Chiropractic
www.chiropractic.org.uk/

US Society for Clinical and Experimental Hypnosis
www.sunsite.utk.edu/IJCEH/scehframe.htm

◣ Publications

Acupuncture Electrotherapy Research
Elmsford, NY, Oxford University Press

Advances in Mind-Body Medicine
Inno Vision Communications
169 Saxony Rd., Suite 104
Encinitas, CA 92024
(760) 633-3910
(760) 633-3918 fax
www.fetzer.org/resources/resources_mindbody.htm

Alternative Health News Online
www.altmedicine.com/

Alternative Therapies in Health and Medicine
Inno Vision Communications
169 Saxony Rd., Suite 104
Encinitas, CA 92024
(760) 633-3910
(760) 633-3918 fax
www.alternative-therapies.com

Alternative Medicine Review
Sandpoint, Idaho
Thorne Research
www.thorne.com/altmedrev/index.html

American Journal of Acupuncture
Felton, CA, Acupuncture Research

The American Journal of Chinese Medicine
Garden City, NY, Institute for Advanced Research in Asian Science and Medicine

Biofeedback and Self-Regulation
New York, Plenum Press

BMC Complementary Alternative Medicine
London, Biomed Central
www.biomedcentral.com

BMJ (British Medical Journal) Collected Resources in Complementary Medicine
http://www.bmj.com/cgi/collection/complementary_medicine

Chinese Medical Journal
Beijing Chinese Medical Association
Pergamon Press

Complementary Therapies in Medicine
London, Churchill Livingstone, Elsevier

Complementary Therapies in Nursing and Midwifery
London, Churchill Livingstone, Elsevier

The Directory of Complementary and Alternative Medicine
Opus Communication
Marblehead, MA 01945
2000 (Greeley, Banas, editors)
Listings of CAM therapies with education and training requirements, licensing, certi-fication, and professional associations, including international listings.

European Journal of Oriental Medicine
London NW1 6DX
www.ejom.co.uk

Homeopathy
London, Churchill Livingstone

International Journal for Vitamin and Nutrition Research
Bern, Switzerland, Hans Harber

Journal of Alternative and Complementary Medicine: Research on paradigm, Practice and Policy
May Ann Liebert, Inc.
2 Madison Ave.
Larchmont, NY 10538

Journal of Ethnopharmacology
Limerick, Elsevier Sequoia

Journal of Manipulative and Physiological Therapeutics
PO Box 4109
Huntington Beach, CA 92605-4109
(714) 230-3150
www.chiroweb.com

Journal of Music Therapy
National Association for Music Therapy
Washington, D.C.

Journal of Natural Products
Cincinnati, Ohio
American Society of Pharmacognosy

Journal of Palliative Medicine
Mary Ann Liebert, Inc.
2 Madison Ave.
Larchmont, NY 10538

Nutrition and Cancer
Hilldale, NJ
Lawrence Erlbaum Associates

Phytomedicine
New York, Verlag

Scientific Review of Alternative Medicine
Amherst, NY, Prometheus Books
www.hcrc.org/sram/

Centers for the Study of Complementary and Alternative Medicine (Currently, 2001, federally funded by National Institutes of Health)

U.S. National Guideline Clearinghouse
www.guideline.gov

Addictions

Minnesota Medical Research Foundation
Program Evaluation Resource Center
914 South 8th St., Suite D9
Minneapolis, MN 55404
Thomas J. Kiresuk, Principal Investigator

Aging/Women's Health

Center for Complementary/Alternative Medicine
Columbia University College of Physicians and Surgeons
630 W. 168th St., Box 75
New York, NY 10032
Fredi Kronenberg, Principal Investigator

Arthritis

Department of Complementary Medicine Program
University of Maryland School of Medicine
Kernan Mansion, Kernan Hospital
2200 Kernan Dr.
Baltimore, MD 21207
Brian Berman, Principal Investigator

◣ Botanicals

Department of Foods & Nutrition (Age-related diseases)
Purdue University
1264 Stone Hall
West Lafayette, IN 47907
Connie Weaver, Principal Investigator

Department of Medicine
University of California at Los Angeles
900 Veteran Ave., Room 12-217
Los Angeles, CA 90095
David Heber, Principal Investigator

Department of Pharmacology/Toxicology
University of Arizona
PO Box 210207
Tucson, AZ 85721
Barbara Timmermann, Principal Investigator

Program for Collaborative Research (Women's Health)
University of Illinois at Chicago
833 South Wood St., MC 877
Chicago, IL 60612
Norman Farnsworth, Principal Investigator

◣ Cancer

Cancer Institute of New Jersey
Robert Wood Johnson Medical School
195 Little Albany St., Room 2002B
New Brunswick, NJ 08901
William Hait, Principal Investigator

Comprehensive Cancer Center
Wake Forest University
Bowman Gray School of Medicine
Medical Center Boulevard
Winston-Salem, NC 27157-1082
Frank Torti, Principal Investigator

Johns Hopkins Oncology Center
North Wolfe St., Room 157
Baltimore, MD 21287-8943
Martin Abeloff, Principal Investigator

UCSF Cancer Center & Cancer Research Institute
Univ. California at San Francisco
2340 Sutter St., Box 0128
San Francisco, CA 94115-0128
Frank McCormick, Principal Investigator

◼ Cardiovascular

Center for Natural Medicine
Maharishi University of Management
Fairfield, IA 52557
Robert Schneider, Principal Investigator

Section of Thoracic Surgery
University of Michigan School of Medicine
1500 E. Medical Center Drive
2120D TC, Box 0344
Ann Arbor, MI 48109-0344
Steven Bolling, Principal Investigator

◼ Chiropractic

Consortorial Center for Chiropractic Research
741 Brady St.
Davenport, IA 52803
William Meeker, Principal Investigator

◼ Craniofacial

Center for Health Research
Kaiser Foundation Hospitals
3800 N. Interstate Ave.
Portland, OR 97227-1110
B. White, Principal Investigator

N Hyperbaric Oxygen and Cancer

Department of Medicine
Institute for Environmental Medicine
University of Pennsylvania School of Medicine
1 John Morgan Bldg/3620 Hamilton
Philadelphia, PA 19104-6068
Stephen Thom, Principal Investigator

N Neurodegenerative Diseases

Department of Neurology
Emory University
1639 Pierce Dr., Suite 6000
Atlanta, GA 30322
Mahlon Delong, Principal Investigator

N Neurological

Department of Neurology
Oregon Health Sciences University
3181 SW Sam Jackson Park Rd., CR 120
Portland, OR 97201-3098
Barry Oken, Principal Investigator

N Pain

University of Virginia Center for the study of CAM
School of Medicine & Nursing
McLeod Hall
15th and Lane Sts.
Charlottesville, VA 22903-3395
Ann Gill Taylor, Principal Investigator

N Pediatrics

Department of Pediatrics
University of Arizona Health Sciences Center
1501 N Campbell Ave.
PO Box 245073

Tucson, AZ 85724-5073
Fayez Ghishan, Principal Investigator

◼ Useful Websites

www.cfsan.fda.gov/%7Edms/ds-warn.html
US Food & Drug administration Center for Food Safety & Applied Nutrition, Dietary Supplements

www.consumerlab.com/index.asp
Conducts independent tests on products.

www.ncahf.org/
The National Council Against Health Fraud

www.who.org
World Health Organization

APPENDIX C

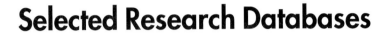

Selected Research Databases

BC Cancer Agency: *Unconventional cancer therapies,* ed 3
On-line manual written "to provide objective information for patients and their families, relating to alternative and complementary therapies." Includes descriptions of 46 unconventional therapies. Each therapy is summarized and includes quotations from peer-reviewed book and journal literature about the benefits, risks, and costs of the therapy.
http://www.bccancer.bc.ca/uct/

Center for Complementary Medicine at the University of Maryland
Cochrane Collaboration in complementary medicine (field) to help "establish and promote and facilitate the production of systematic reviews."
www.compmed.umm.edu

Combined Health Information Database (CHID)
Online database developed by several health-related agencies of the U.S. Federal Government. Provides for titles, abstracts, and availability information, including Chinese medicine
http://chid.nih.gov

Herb Research Foundation
Has private library of papers covering botanic issues. A fee for searching is charged.
www.herbs.org

International Bibliographic Information on Dietary Supplements
National Institutes of Health (NIH) database that provides research information on dietary supplements.
http://odp.od.nih.gov/ods/databases/ibids.html

Medlineplus—Alternative Medicine
National Library of Medicine's Medlineplus includes a section on alternative medicine. The section is composed of links to other websites divided into

subcategories, including "Children," "Clinical Trials," and "Specific Conditions/ Aspects."
http://www.nlm.nih.gov/medlineplus/alternativemedicine.html

National Cancer Institute (NCI) *Cancer Facts*
Collection of fact sheets that address a variety of cancer topics. Fact sheets are frequently updated and revised based on the latest cancer research. This page links to specific CAM topics, including overviews, results of human/clinical studies, adverse effects, and references.
http://cis.nci.nih.gov/fact/index.htm

National Center for Complementary and Alternative Medicine at NIH
Section entitled "CAM on PubMed," which can be used to access articles specific to alternative and complementary medicine. Can also access "Clinical Trials" on the web, which includes information concerning ongoing clinical research at NIH and throughout the United States.
www.nccam.nih.gov

PDQ (Physician Data Query)
NCI database that contains the latest information about cancer treatment, screening, prevention, genetics, and supportive care, plus clinical trials.
http://www.cancer.gov/cancer_information/pdq/

PSYCHINFO and psychology articles
Abstract or full-text database of peer-reviewed psychologic literature, 1887–present. Abstracts are free; there is a charge for full-text articles.
www.apa.org

Quackwatch
Quackwatch, Inc., a member of Consumer Federation of America, is a nonprofit corporation whose purpose is to combat health-related frauds, myths, fads, and fallacies. It examines claims about paranormal phenomena and fringe science from a skeptical point of view.
http://www.quackwatch.com

Research Council for Complementary Medicine
Clinical, research, and educational database that includes abstracts from the CISCO reviews. Includes 30,000 holdings and is thought to be one of the most thorough databases of CAM in the world. Fees for search are assessed.
http://www.homeopathyhome.com/reference/rmmc/rmmc.shtml

Richard and Hinda Rosenthal Center for Complementary and Alternative Medicine
Center at Columbia University has a listing of major biomedical bibliographic databases, main databases specific to alternative medicine and medical-pharmaceutical-traditional therapy, and researcher-listed databases.
http://cpmcnet.columbia.edu/dept/rosenthal/Databases.html

University of Texas–M.D. Anderson Cancer Center
Contains evidence-based reviews of complementary or alternative cancer therapies as well as links to other authoritative resources. Detailed scientific reviews are provided to assist health care professionals in guiding patients who would like to integrate these therapies with conventional treatments.
http://www.mdanderson.org/departments/cimer/

Informed Consent Process Checklist for Physicians Integrating Complementary and Alternative Medicine

KATHLEEN M. BOOZANG

A physician's education and discussions with his or her patient about the CAM modality comprise the informed consent process. A consent form represents the evidence that the physician has provided the information appropriate to, and has obtained the patient's consent to (or rejection of), the proposed treatment. Documentation in the patient's chart also satisfies the recommendation that physicians record having obtained the patient's consent to treatment. Whatever documentation method the physician uses, the following represents a nonexclusive list of considerations for inclusion in the informed consent process for CAM therapies:

- The known benefits of the CAM modality
  - If no reliable data regarding therapeutic benefits exist, the physician should so advise the patient. The physician may describe anecdotal experience, emphasizing that it is indeed anecdotal, or describe what proponents of the treatment suggest it accomplishes, without endorsing those representations.
  - If data establish that there are no benefits, the physician should so advise the patient, and without strong reasons to do so, should decline to provide the requested CAM intervention.
  - If the physician considers the CAM modality to be experimental, he or she should so advise the patient.
- The potential risks and side effects of the proposed CAM modality
  - This discussion should include difficulty in dosaging common with many herbs and supplements and the potential for contamination or adulteration of certain CAM products.

- In addition to discussing contraindications generally, the physician should advise the patient of contraindications for combining certain herbal and dietary supplements with other herbs and supplements, as well as certain prescription medications.
- In appropriate circumstances, the physician should discourage the patient from relying on a CAM therapy to the exclusion of a proven conventional treatment.
- The physician should inform the patient of his or her training and experience in providing the proposed CAM therapy (e.g., acupuncture).
  - The physician should ensure that the patient understands the alternatives to the CAM intervention under consideration, as well as the attendant risks and benefits of those alternatives.
  - If the physician is selling the recommended herbal or dietary supplement, the price should not reflect a profit to the physician, or if it does, the physician should so advise the patient.

Glossary

Acquired immunodeficiency syndrome (AIDS) Condition associated with infection by the human immunodeficiency virus (HIV).

American Diabetes Association guidelines Clinical practice recommendations dealing with prevention, screening, and diagnosis of diabetes. In addition, standards of medical care for patients with diabetes mellitus are established and published.

Anecdotal health reports Impressionistic information that may or may not be collaborated by other sources regarding whether a health intervention was useful.

Angiogenesis Formation of new blood vessels.

Antioxidant Chemical that inhibits oxidation, a process that causes deterioration of DNA in cells. Oxidation of low-density cholesterol particles in the artery wall appears to be a key process in the development of atherosclerosis, and some evidence indicates that selected antioxidants reduce the rate of initiation or progression of atherosclerosis.

Autoimmune process Antibodies that attack specific cells and cell functions are produced within the body. In the case of diabetes, beta cells of the pancreas are attacked by antibodies and are eventually destroyed.

Bacille Calmette-Guérin (BCG) Product of the treatment of tuberculosis organisms that is used as a vaccine against this disease, causing an increase in immune reactivity.

Barthel index Standardized instrument for the assessment of functional outcomes such as independence in self-care and mobility. This reliable, well-validated index is widely used in U.S. medical rehabilitation settings.

Beck Anxiety and Depression Scales Beck Anxiety Inventory (BAI) has 21 items, each representing an anxiety symptom rated on a four-point scale (0 to 3) ranging from "Not at all" to "Severely, I could barely stand it." The Beck Depression Inventory (BDI) is designed to assess the severity of depression in adolescents and adults and also uses a 21-item inventory assessing an individual's complaints, symptoms, and concerns related to his or her current level of depression.

Boston Motor Inventory Developed for use in studies of patients with hemiplegia or paralysis; measures isolated, active range of motion for four leg movements and three arm movements.

Brief Psychiatric Rating Scale Multisymptom category rating tool originally designed for use by clinical observers of inpatient psychiatric populations in pharmacologic outcome studies. The items are rated on a seven-point severity scale (1 to 7) and assess psychotic symptoms such as hallucinations, unusual thought content, conceptual disorganization, bizarre behavior, self-neglect, and suicidality. Administration is by a trained interviewer. Symptoms can be readily graphed over time, so baseline changes can be detected and interventions mounted.

Brief Social Phobia Scale Observer-rated scale designed to assess the characteristic symptoms of social phobia using three subscales: fear, avoidance, and physiologic arousal. Results are then combined for a total score.

CAM Complementary and alternative medicine.

Carcinogenesis Formation of cancer.

Cervical dysplasia Appearance of abnormal cells on the cervix, possibly a precursor to cervical cancer, usually associated with the human papillomavirus (HPV), which causes genital warts.

Clinical practice guidelines Statements and official guidelines for patient health care and treatment.

Clusters In epidemiologic research, groupings of people or tendencies within a population.

Coenzyme Q10 Naturally occurring, fat-soluble antioxidant that is used for energy production in body cells. Coenzyme Q10 occurs in the lipid core of inner mitochondrial membranes. It functions in the electron transport chain that produces adenosine triphosphate (ATP), the basic cellular energy-producing molecule. Coenzyme Q10 is also known as *ubiquinone*. It has been promoted for a variety of cardiovascular disorders.

Conductivity Refers to electrical conductivity; in the body, the higher the water content, the higher the conductivity.

Contract-relax-antagonist-contract technique Proprioceptive neural facilitation (PNF) technique used to facilitate muscle relaxation and lengthening in the agonist muscle (see Chapter 7).

Cytochrome P-450 enzymes Oxygenating catalysts for a wide variety of reactions responsible for detoxification of many drugs.

Derailment Moving in random fashion from one topic, thought, or behavior to another. A psychotic state descriptive term used in a mental status examination.

Dong quai (Angelica sinensis) Root used in traditional Chinese medicine (TCM) formulas for menopausal symptoms and other conditions in patients who meet specific criteria in TCM diagnosis. Currently it is being sold as a single-ingredient product in U.S. health food stores and is used by women for menopausal symptoms. Also spelled *dang gui, tang kuei.*

Double-blind study Experimental clinical research technique in which neither the patient nor the researcher is aware of whether treatment given is active (medicinal) or inactive (nonmedicinal).

Drug court Special court given the responsibility of handling cases involving less serious drug-related offenses. Offenders are given the opportunity to complete a treatment program under intensive supervision instead of harsher penalties such as incarceration. The judge wipes clean all record of arrest if the offender graduates from the program; otherwise the client may have to serve his or her sentence in full. The design and structure of drug court programs are - developed at the local level, to reflect the unique strengths and needs of each community.

DSM IV, TR, 2000 *Diagnostic and Statistical Manual of Mental Disorders,* ed 4, American Psychiatric Association Press, 1994; standardized classification of mental disorders.

Dysplasia Abnormal size, shape, and organization of adult cells.

Echinacea Narrow-leafed perennial member of the daisy family native to the central United States. Originally used by Native Americans, its rhizome and roots seem to exert an immune-stimulating effect.

Eicosanoids Biologically active substances derived from arachidonic acid.

Electrolysis Process in which electrical energy causes a chemical change in a conducting medium, usually a solution or a molten substance. Electrodes, usually pieces of metal, induce the flow of electric energy through the medium. Electrons enter the solution through the cathode and leave the solution through the anode. Negatively charged ions, or *anions,* are attracted to the anode; positively charged ions, or *cations,* are attracted to the cathode.

Electroosmosis Movement of fluids through diaphragms as a result of the application of an electric current.

Electrophoresis Migration of the electrically charged solute particles present in a colloidal solution toward the electrode with an opposite charge when two electrodes are placed. This technique is widely employed in biochemical analysis, for example, in the separation and study of plasma protein.

Endorphins Any of a group of proteins with potent analgesic (pain-killing) properties that occur naturally in the brain.

Enkephalins Pentapeptides are molecular chains of amino acids containing five amino acid residues; the enkephalins have a marked affinity for opioid receptors and thus have opiate and analgesic activity. They occur naturally in the brain and spinal cord.

Epidemiology The study and reporting of the presence, spread, and cause of disease within a population.

Epstein-Barr virus (EBV) Member of the herpesvirus family. Causes mononucleosis and may be involved in some forms of chronic fatigue syndrome.

Eysenck Personality Inventory (EPI) Self-report questionnaire used to measure the personality dimension of neuroticism-stability *(N)* and extraversion-introversion *(E)*, including a lie scale *(L)*. The EPI consists of two parallel forms, thus making possible retesting after experimental treatment without interference from memory factors.

Flexner Report Report written in the early twentieth century concerning strengths and weaknesses of medical education in the United States.

Fluoxetine, sertraline, and ritanserin Fluoxetine (Prozac) and sertraline (Zoloft) are orally administered antidepressants. The drugs are presumed to inhibit the central nervous system (CNS) neuronal uptake of serotonin. Ritanserin (Ondansetron) is a 5HT-3 antagonist. It is used clinically as an antiemetic (to treat nausea and vomiting).

Genotype The genetic constituents of the organism.

Hamilton Anxiety and Depression Scale Rating scales that have been used for decades in the assessment of anxiety and depression. They are completed by clinician interviewers and use a semistructured interview format with the patient. Hamilton scales are thought to be more systematic in evaluating neurovegetative symptoms than cognitive symptoms, a strength of Beck rating scales.

Heating pattern Distribution of rate of temperature rise in a human body or model. The unit of measure is degrees Celsius per minute per watt.

Human immunodeficiency virus (HIV) Retrovirus contributing to acquired immunodeficiency syndrome (AIDS).

Hypnotic induction profile test Evaluates hypnotic capacity—the degree to which an individual can control dissociation, become absorbed, and accept suggestion.

Immunoglobulin A (IgA) Immunoglobulin found in body fluids. IgA protects the body's mucosal surfaces from infection.

Immunoglobulin G (IgG) Prominent type of immunoglobulin existing in the blood. Also called *gamma globulin.*

Intermittent claudication Complex of symptoms characterized by an absence of pain or discomfort in a limb when at rest and the commencement of pain, tension, or weakness after the limb is put to use, attributable to reduced blood flow through narrowed arteries. The symptoms can intensify to become disabling but subside again after a period of rest.

In vitro In an artificial environment outside the organism.

In vivo In the organism itself.

Iridology Study of the iris of the eye to define the disease entity in the body.

Isocyanates Compounds with a functionality group $(N = C = O)$. Such compounds have been found to elicit an asthmatic response in some individuals and to help reduce the asthmatic response in others.

Isoflavones, lignans, and coumestans Three main classes of phytoestrogens, which are plant compounds with estrogen-like biologic activity.

Jenkins Activity Survey Self-report, multiple-choice inventory designed to assess the coronary-prone behavior pattern known as type A behavior. *Type A behavior* has been implicated as an independent risk factor in the etiology of coronary heart disease, including both myocardial infarction and coronary atherosclerosis.

Kampo formulations Combinations of herbal components used in Japan that have free-radical scavenging activity with efficacy that shows concentration-dependent properties. Kampo has been evaluated with regard to cerebral ischemia and brain damage.

Leukotrienes Biologically active compounds consisting of 20-carbon carboxylic acids formed from arachidonic acid, which function as regulators of allergic and inflammatory reactions.

Likert Self-Report Self-reporting method for measuring attitudes; the scale provides options on a continuum of various numbers (1, strongly disagree, to 7, strongly agree). It is suitable for measuring the strength and dimensionality of attitudes.

Locus of control Concept that describes how patients attribute responsibility for disease management. Patients with diabetes may believe that control of their illness depends on themselves (internal) or powerful others (external) or is governed by chance.

Low-density lipoprotein cholesterol Cholesterol is produced in the liver and is needed to form cell membranes, nerve coating, and certain hormones. When a lipoprotein contains more fat than protein, it is called a *low-density lipoprotein* (LDL) and increases the risk of atherosclerosis because it contributes to a fatty buildup in the arteries.

Mesh terms Individual words or terms used to access, through database and computer searches, research information related to particular health issues. For example, in CAM such terms might include "acupuncture," "homeopathy," or "alternative medicine."

Meta-analysis Technique in which scientific data from several unrelated clinical trials are reviewed by interpreting treatment effects as to consistency and magnitude of effect.

Metaplasia Change in type of adult cells.

National Acupuncture Detoxification Association (NADA) Formed in 1985 as a membership and training organization. At present, NADA trainers have taught more than 4000 acupuncturists, counselors, nurses, and physicians how to perform acupuncture for substance abuse in the United States and almost that many in Europe.

National Health and Nutrition Examination Survey (HANES) Ongoing survey conducted by the National Center for Health Statistics. NHANES-III was conducted from 1988 to 1994 and contains data on 33,994 persons 2 months of age and older. Five domains of data are monitored: household adult, household youth, medical examination, laboratory, and dietary recall data.

Nei Guan point Acupuncture point (also called point *P6* or "inner gate") above the inner wrist that is used in treating nausea and vomiting. In traditional Chinese medicine practice it is used in conjunction with other points.

N-of-1 design Type of an evaluation in which goals, diagnosis, treatment, and outcomes are directed and assessed for one specific patient under study.

Nottingham Health Profile Brief self-assessment of physical, emotional, and social health, with emphasis on evaluating patients' subjective perception of their health status.

Nurses Observation Scale for Inpatient Evaluation Psychometric tool that assesses the ward behavior of psychiatric inpatients. Nursing personnel use a 30-item paper-and-pencil observational inventory to evaluate patient status and change. The six factors measured are social competence, social interest, personal neatness, irritability, manifest psychosis, and psychomotor retardation.

Pelvic inflammatory disease Condition usually brought on by untreated gonorrhea and chlamydial infection. Symptoms include severe pelvic pain and high fever.

Perceived Guilt Index (PGI) Self-report measure of guilt experienced by an individual based in part on his or her own interpretation of emotions such as anxiety, guilt, or obsessions and their intensity in everyday life.

Persimmon tannin Condensed derivative isolated from persimmon. These condensed tannins exhibit concentration-dependent free-radical scavenging activity.

Placebo A substance or intervention that contains no active medicinal ingredient.

Poultice Soft, moist mass, about the consistency of cooked cereal, spread between layers of muslin, linen, gauze, or towels and applied hot to a given area to create moist local heat and to cause absorption of bioactive compounds from the mass into the skin and surrounding areas.

Power analysis Statistical technique used to determine the number of patients required to accurately reject the hypothesis that no differences exist between experimental or control groups.

Preclinical studies Experiments to determine the value of treatments. They include basic studies, which study the effects and mechanisms, and clinical trials, which consist of Phases I to III trials.

Pritikin Longevity Center Teaches the principles of the Pritikin diet, as well as exercise and stress management, in 1- to 4-week residential programs.

Profile of mood state Tool that assesses dimensions of affect or mood in individuals 18 years of age and older. It is used to measure outpatients' response to various therapeutic approaches, including drug evaluation studies. The 65-item paper-and-pencil test measures the following dimensions of mood: tension-anxiety, depression-dejection, anger-hostility, vigor-activity, fatigue-inertia, and confusion-bewilderment.

Prooxidant Agent that causes oxidation in the cell, a process often harmful to DNA.

Proprioceptive neural facilitation System of evaluation and treatment of neuromusculoskeletal dysfunction based on neurophysiologic principles. The practitioner uses sensory stimulation from manual contacts and verbal and visual cues to elicit efficient and functional movement.

Prostaglandins Compounds derived from arachidonic acid via the cyclooxygenase pathway that regulate a diverse group of physiologic processes.

Provider practice acts Descriptions of scope of practice and licensing/certification requirements for health providers, generally enacted through individual state legislatures.

Psychoneuroimmunology Field of medical research that explores linkages between behavior, the nervous system, and the immune system.

Purpose in Life test Test that measures the degree to which an individual has found meaning in life. It is useful with addicted, retired, handicapped, and philosophically confused individuals for purposes of clinical assessment, student counseling, vocational guidance, and rehabilitation. Subjects rate 20 statements, complete 13 sentence stems, and write an original paragraph describing their ambitions in life. The test is based on Victor Frankl's *Will to Meaning* and embraces his logotherapeutic orientation.

Randomization Experimental procedure in which subjects are assigned to either a treatment or a nontreatment group purely on chance.

Resorcylic acid lactones Phytoestrogens produced by molds that often contaminate cereal crops.

Retinoids Compounds similar to vitamin A.

Scarification Production in the skin of many small, superficial scratches or punctures, as for introduction of a vaccine.

Sishencong points Group of four acupuncture points located on the highest point of the head. According to ancient Chinese belief, these points function to "tranquilize" the mind and regulate the CNS to promote sleep.

State-Trait Anxiety Inventory Short (40-item) measurement tool that provides information about a person's level of both state and trait anxiety. Anxiety has been viewed as having two distinct forms. The *state* form of anxiety is the transitory feeling of fear or worry that most of us experience from time to time. The *trait* form of anxiety is the relatively stable tendency of an individual to respond anxiously to a stressful situation. Thus the level of trait anxiety reflects the proneness to exhibit state anxiety.

State-Trait Anxiety Inventory for Children Short (40-item) self-report measurement tool that provides information about a child's level of both state and trait anxiety.

Structural equations Comprehensive statistical approach that deals with complex, multidimensional relationships between research variables.

Succussion Procedure in which shaking of a dilute solution reduces its medicinal and biochemical concentration. Used quite often in the practice of homeopathy.

Sulfonylurea drugs Type of medication, taken orally, that stimulates the pancreas to produce and secrete more insulin. These drugs are used to lower blood glucose in type 2 diabetes mellitus. The first- and second-generation sulfonylureas are similar in lowering blood glucose by decreasing insulin resistance and increasing insulin secretion. The second-generation drugs are more potent and more effective but have an increased risk of hypoglycemia.

Symptom Checklist 90R A 90-item self-report inventory designed to assess the psychologic symptoms of psychiatric and medical patients. The inventory measures somatization, obsessive-compulsive symptoms, interpersonal sensitivity, depression, anxiety, phobic anxiety, psychoticism, paranoid ideation, hostility, and global indices of psychopathologic conditions.

Syncytial virus Virus in the multinucleated mass of protoplasm produced by the merging of cells.

Thermogram Photographic record of the amount of heat radiated from the surface of the body, obtained by an infrared sensing device, revealing a "hot spot" of potential tumors or other disorders. This technique has been used in conjunction with "phantoms" to study heating patterns inside the human body.

Thromboxane One of two compounds that are potent inducers of platelet aggregation.

Type 1 (insulin-dependent) diabetes mellitus Autoimmune disorder of metabolism. Antibodies are produced that damage the insulin-producing beta cells of the pancreas. Insulin becomes deficient, and the cells cannot use glucose efficiently. Blood glucose levels are elevated, and injected insulin is necessary to control blood glucose.

Type 2 (non-insulin-dependent) diabetes mellitus Disorder of metabolism characterized by tissue resistance to insulin and hyperglycemia. The beta cells of the pancreas become unable to secrete enough insulin to counteract decreased sensitivity (resistance) of the tissues to insulin. Oral medications and diet may be sufficient to normalize blood glucose, but a significant percentage of patients eventually need insulin for adequate control.

U.S. National Health Interview Survey (NHIS) A 1991 survey conducted by the National Center for Health Statistics containing more than 900,000 records, including five core areas (condition, doctor visit, hospital, household, person) and six supplemental areas (AIDS knowledge and attitudes, cancer control, cancer epidemiology, health insurance, immunization, youth risk behavior).

Venesection Phlebotomy; incision of a vein.

"Word salad" Symptom of a psychotic state exemplified by complete incoherence of speech, with a mixture of words lacking meaning and logical coherence.

Yale Brown Obsessive-Compulsive scale Ten-question scale with severity options ranging from 0 to 4; useful for quantifying the level of obsessive-compulsive disorder symptoms.

Index